Fourth Edition

Handbook of

Psychiatric
Emergencies

Fourth Edition

Handbook of
Psychiatric
Emergencies

Andrew E. Slaby, MD, PhD, MPH
Clinical Professor of Psychiatry
New York University

Adjunct Clinical Professor of Psychiatry
New York Medical College

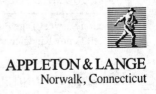

APPLETON & LANGE
Norwalk, Connecticut

Notice: The author and the publisher of this volume have taken care to make certain that the doses of drugs and schedules of treatment are correct and compatible with the standards generally accepted at the time of publication. Nevertheless, as new information becomes available, changes in treatment and in the use of drugs become necessary. The reader is advised to carefully consult the instruction and information material included in the package insert of each drug or therapeutic agent before administration. This advice is especially important when using new or infrequently used drugs. The publisher disclaims any liability, loss, injury, or damage incurred as a consequence, directly or indirectly, of the use and application of any of the contents of this volume.

ISBN   0-8385-3624-7

9 780838 536247   90000

Production Service: Tage Publishing Service
Designer: Penny Kindzierski

PRINTED IN THE UNITED STATES OF AMERICA

Contents

Preface

A psychiatric emergency is defined by an individual, or by an individual's family or community, as a psychiatric or psychosocial problem that requires immediate attention. A belligerent intoxicated person is brought to the emergency room by the police; a depressed man undergoing a divorce rings up his therapist at three o'clock in the morning thinking he wants to kill himself; a young law student is brought to a university health service by her roommate, psychotic after smoking marijuana that was contaminated with phencyclidine—all these instances are events that call for prompt and decisive intervention. They are times of crisis when the attending clinicians must summon all of their professional skills to obviate a catastrophic or even fatal outcome for patients or someone close to them. Emergency clinicians must have knowledge not only of psychodynamics, diagnostic psychiatry, psychopharmacotherapy, brief psychotherapy, and interviewing skills, but also general medical and administrative know-how in order to provide effective management at the time of human crisis. In emergency situations they must use common sense, reasoning skills, empathy, and intuitive resources in such a way as to resonate best with each unique clinical situation. The ability to tolerate anxiety and ambiguity and to blend flexibility and firmness, as well as a readiness to tactfully contend with fear and anger, are needed to stand the clinician in good stead.

Emergency psychiatry requires careful listening and observation as well as an element of risk taking and pragmatism. A diplomatic cautiousness tempered with courage is required to handle the threats to personal safety and self-esteem that sometimes occur. Emergency clinicians must constantly guard against being too provocative or too permissive. Much can be gained by consistently maintaining a professional demeanor and a necessary degree of authoritarianism. Clinicians who divest themselves of their dignity or invite a patient to do this to them court trouble both for themselves and their patients.

It is ironic that while emergency psychiatry is the one area wherein the possibility to do good or harm is greatest and most immediate, less emphasis is placed on training and supervision in this area than in the more traditional, long-term psychotherapies. Clinicians who choose or who are assigned to work in emergency facilities often feel demoralized and emotionally and physically drained. Burn out is a recurrent problem and staff turnover is frequently high. Emergency psychiatry is extremely taxing and time consuming. The drain on psychological resources that occurs in the practice of emergency psychiatry explains to some degree why it is so difficult "to shift gears" to this approach when necessary. It is more convenient and less emotionally taxing for a therapist practicing in the community to tell a patient in distress to go to the emergency room of a nearby hospital or CMHC than to attend to the emergency personally. In order to be fully effective at a time of crisis, it is sometimes necessary to move from a more highly stylized mode of therapy to more active intervention.

The fourth edition of *Handbook of Psychiatric Emergencies* is divided into two principle sections. The first consists of four chapters discussing basic principles of emergency care. These chapters have been expanded to include a discussion of how one may use the information provided in Chapter 5 on over 250 specific psychiatric emergencies to develop patient care monitors and protocols that allow the development of treatment plans *specific* to each patient's unique needs. The problem-oriented approach used in this book allows not only for the provision of the highest possible quality of care, but also allows that care to be provided in the most efficient, cost-effective way. The quality may later be reviewed retrospectively to serve a heuristic role of assuring ever improved quality of care in the future.

Chapter 5 is a review of common psychiatric emergencies with reference to the most recent literature pertaining to their clinical presentation, historical background, differential diagnosis, diagnostic-specific treatment, anticipated side-effects of treatment, and management of these side-effects. A unique and new feature of the fourth edition is discussion where appropriate of quality assurance monitors and ethical–legal concerns. The material presented can be used to develop protocols to evaluate care on a continuous basis and to improve both quality and efficiency in delivery. Chapters 6 and 7 respectively address burn out and disaster planning.

Psychiatric emergencies that may be encountered both in community and general medical hospital settings are discussed. Emphasis is placed on essential historical and clinical data that lead to appropriate diagnosis and management. An outline format has been used to provide clinicians with direct and concise information that is practical in the emergency setting, with over 2,000 relevant references at the end of the book. Doses and routes of administration of standard medications have been included, and wherever possible, alternative approaches to particular emergencies have been discussed.

Although the majority of emergency psychiatric care is rendered in the emergency room of general medical hospitals, or on crisis units of CMHCs, the material presented here is equally applicable to clinicians working in health maintenance organizations, university health centers, outpatient clinics, inpatient treatment facilities, private offices, and as part of home visit teams. The emphasis is pragmatic, with theory introduced only to the degree that it will help clinicians function in the environment where they must and should provide care. It is our hope that by reading this volume clinicians will not only be able to enrich their skills in handling psychiatric emergencies, but will also acquire a renewed awe of the complexity of human response to internal and external stresses.

Andrew E. Slaby, MD, PhD, MPH

Introduction

Nowhere in the spectrum of mental health care is as much psychiatric expertise and clinical acumen immediately demanded as in the evaluation and management of patients presenting with psychiatric emergencies. It is in the emergency psychiatric setting that we observe in bold relief how biologic, psychologic, social, and existential factors converge to create the person in sickness, and in health, and how an understanding of the interaction of these forces is necessary for effective management of a psychiatric emergency.

The goal of emergency psychiatry and crisis intervention is not merely technical resolution of a disturbance of mood, thought, and behavior. In most instances, that feat is relatively simple in the hands of a properly trained clinician who understands the natural course of a psychiatric illness untreated and treated, differential diagnosis, diagnostic-specific interventions, general principles of psychiatric management, and treatment of anticipated side effects of treatment. In addition to state-of-the-art psychiatric care, the most difficult task is for the patient and his or her family to grow through resolution of an unanticipated crisis that results in loss of control of how they feel, think, or act.

Crises are frightening. However, misfortune also provides an opportunity for an individual to grow in a way that may not have otherwise been. An ancient Chinese proverb advises: "Welcome crises." In fact, the Chinese character representing crisis is a combination of the characters for danger and opportunity. The challenge to the emergency clinician is not merely to mollify anxiety or ameliorate depression. It lies in the ability to uncover hidden strengths to buffer future stresses so that further life crises or exacerbations of a chronic psychiatric illness do not create a similar need for acute care.

Psychiatric care has radically changed since the publication of the first edition of this book a decade and a half ago. At the time of the book's first printing, emergency psychiatry was seen by some as a necessary but compromised form of psychiatric care. Resources were available for diagnostic purposes and extended inpatient or outpatient care. Diagnostic-specific treatments were in the nascent phase. The concept of differential diagnosis, which has been a consistent feature throughout the various editions of this book, was initially seen by some as highly "innovative." Those who were more psychodynamically oriented viewed the emphasis on diagnostic psychiatry and epidemiology as reductionistic. Those opposed to the differential diagnosis approach contended that it was "too medical" and that it drew clinicians away from more "critical psychosocial issues." While I never intended the approach to be only concerned with biological psychiatry, it was misperceived to be so. The approach to both diagnosis and treatment in this edition of this book, and all previous editions, is biopsychosocial. Essentially, the underlying philosophy has been that the onset of illness and its resolution involves an understanding of the complex interaction of biologic, psychologic, social, and existential forces.

Today, the concept of the evaluation of alterations in mood, thought, and behavior in such a way as to enumerate a preliminary differential diagnosis, establish a diagnosis, and provide diagnostic-specific treatment treatment is the cornerstone of state-of-the-art, quality psychiatric care. Reduction in resources for both outpatient and inpatient care has led to a continuing review of what is most cost-efficient and effective in all areas of medicine. This concept is also having its impact in psychiatry and has introduced major challenges to meet social-economic needs and yet provide quality care.

Psychiatric illnesses are no different from other medical illness. The term "mental" illness should be abandoned. It suggests that the changes in behavior that we treat are not physical illnesses. This could not be further form the truth. Anxiety disorders, affective illnesses, schizophrenia, substance-abuse disorders, and other serious psychiatric illnesses involve specific neuropharmacologic changes that induce the symptoms that emergency psychiatric interventions are directed to correct. The quality of care provided and the impact of a therapeutic intervention can be monitored in exactly the same manner one monitors care provided to patients with endocrinopathies, hypertensive disease, migraine headaches, seizures, and Parkinson's disease.

The fourth edition of *Handbook of Psychiatric Emergencies* differs from previous editions in an even greater emphasis on differential diagnosis and diagnostic-specific treatment. Advances in understanding how various illnesses, as well as both recreational drugs and prescription medications, impact behavior have improved our diagnostic capabilities and have allowed more specific psychopharmacological interventions. The approach presented here therefore is not only critical for providing acute psychiatric care but also has fundamental application for providing care in the full range of psychiatric settings, be it in a health maintenance organization, a community mental health center, a consultation–liaison service in a general hospital, or in a private office. The techniques discussed in this book represent the highest quality of care that can be provided and are presented with consideration of the same issues of cost-effectiveness, efficacy, and quality that have already taken hold in other clinical specialties, such as medicine and surgery.

The chapters on psychopharmacology, legal issues, and psychiatric ethics that appeared in the three earlier editions have been deleted. A general discussion of these subjects seems less relevant to the practicing clinician today than more formal examination of these issues where appropriate in the discussion of a specific emergency. Therefore we now include sections within specific emergencies, where indicated, on how one may monitor the quality of care provided and handle relevant legal and ethical concerns. For instance, what are the biological causes of depression that should be considered in evaluation of a mood disorder? What are the critical psychiatric questions when evaluating suicidal and homicidal behavior? What therapeutic options are available to present to patients and their families? What specific information may be obtained from family history to corroborate a diagnosis? What parameters (e.g., white cell count with carbamazepine and valproic acid) should be monitored during the course of treatment to minimize adverse outcome? How does one monitor for the neuroleptic malignant syndrome?

Comparably, what are critical legal and ethical questions? How should one obtain requisite studies on HIV reactivity in a patient presenting as psychiatric who has had a transfusion, is an intravenous drug user, or has been potentially sexually exposed to infection? What are legal concerns in managing someone who is self- or other-destructive? These issues along with information in quality assurance will be discussed under the sections on specific emergencies.

The material presented in this fourth edition allows a clinician to readily assess specific information regarding diagnosis and treatment as well as provides a basis for discussion with a clinician who may have referred a patient for consultation and with a patient's family. All illnesses are family illnesses. When one close to us hurts, we are all affected. Understanding does not reverse a course of history. A crisis has occurred and a family, like a patient, feels out of control. All of us, however, can better tolerate that which we cannot control by controlling that which we can. The information provided here provides a basis for quality care and in so doing affords the patient, the family, and the clinician awareness of what state-of-art psychiatry may offer to make the best of an adverse circumstance. In administering the highest quality of care, a clinician provides hope to a patient and his or her family . . . and we all need hope.

Andrew E. Slaby, M.D, Ph.D., M.P.H.

Basic Principles of Emergency Psychiatric Care | 1

When clinicians begin to work on a psychiatric crisis or emergency service, they find themselves anxious and suffer a pervasive sense of uncertainty as to what the future may bring. At this time psychiatric clinicians may entertain thoughts of dropping out of a training program or of limiting their professional work to office practice. They may develop distressing somatic or psychological symptoms. In one instance, a psychiatric resident had recurrent diarrhea throughout the course of his rotation on an emergency service. Another, worried over her decision not to hospitalize patients who had suicidal ideation, found herself reading obituary columns of local newspapers.

PATIENT POPULATION

Emergency psychiatric clinicians frequently have catastrophic fantasies about the types of patients that they are going to confront. Bizarre patients do at times present, but the usual lot is much more mundane. One can generally expect to see many schizophrenics, alcoholics, depressives, and individuals in acute situational crises.

Information gathered from a number of studies over the past several decades indicate clear trends in the composition of patient populations. Awareness of what a clinician may expect to have to evaluate and manage allows the development of options for treatment (Cohn, 1989). Knowledge is power and serves to reduce anxiety. If you have developed a number of approaches to treat the patients you may see, worry over lack of diagnostic acumen or treatment skill is reduced. This book has been developed to provide options for management of anticipated emergencies and to reduce care giver anxiety.

TRENDS

1. The most commonly encountered diagnoses are affective disorders, substance abuse disorders, and antisocial personality disorders (Robins E et al, 1977).
2. Increasing numbers of younger patients are being seen (Bristol et al, 1981).
3. Users of emergency services are more frequently single, divorced, or widowed.
4. Users are more frequently nonwhite.
5. Use rates are inversely proportional to socioeconomic status.
6. Use rates are inversely proportionate to distance from the hospital.

7. Outpatient management is increasingly being used in preference to hospitalization.

8. Variables reported, in order of importance, in hospitalization of adolescents include suicidal tendencies, physical abuse, primary diagnosis of schizophrenia, age, and number of suicide attempts (Hillard et al, 1987). Adolescents are less likely to receive the diagnosis of personality disorder and psychosis and are more likely to receive a diagnosis of conduct and adjustment disorders, with as high as 40% presenting with self-destructive ideation or behavior (Hillard et al, 1987).

9. Variables predicting hospitalization of adults include delusions, aggressive behavior, suicidal tendencies, and a primary diagnosis of schizophrenia or affective illness (Hillard et al, 1988).

10. Social isolation and poverty are linked both to having multiple episodes and a disposition to a public facility (Slaby and Perry, 1979; Bassuk et al, 1983a).

11. In some states, the emergency psychiatric service has become a screening center for admissions to other community mental health facilities, allowing cost containment through focal deployment of limited resources (Ellison and Wharff, 1985; Cohn, 1989).

12. Children who are hospitalized have more symptoms not tolerated by persons in the child's normal environment such as fire setting, frequent fighting, dangerousness to self and others, and stealing and tend to have histories of a previous psychiatric evaluation and history of evaluation at a younger age (Kashani and Cantwell, 1983).

13. Older emergency psychiatric patients, like younger patients, tend to have weak social supports; but unlike younger patients, older patients tend to present more with somatic complaints (Bassuk et al, 1983a).

14. For many chronic psychiatrically ill patients living in the community, the psychiatric emergency service is the sole source of treatment (Gerson and Bassuk, 1980).

15. The patients seen in many emergency psychiatric settings are first seen elsewhere in the emergency setting or by a primary care clinician. *It is incorrect to assume that such patients have been appropriately evaluated by nonpsychiatric physicians and to assume that any medical or surgical cause of the alteration in mood, behavior, or thought has been accurately ruled out.*

16. Primary care physicians, regardless of the level of training and experience, vary remarkably in their ability to make accurate assessments of patients' psychiatric symptoms. Those who are outgoing, self-confident physicians with high academic ability are most likely to identify patients with psychiatric problems (Goldberg D et al, 1982).

17. Even when internists feel they have sufficient data to make accurate predictions, their perceptions have been found erroneous, even in areas of critical importance for patient care such as the evaluation of substance use and suicidal ideation.

18. In a study of 100 state hospital psychiatric admissions to a research ward, 46% were found to have a medical illness that either exacerbated or caused their psychiatric illness and 80% had a physical illness requiring treatment. Of these, 4%

had precancerous conditions or illness (Hall RCW et al, 1980; 1981). Physical and psychiatric examination coupled with SMA-24, urinalysis, ECG, and sleep-deprived EEG was sufficient to identify 90% of the medical illnesses in the population.

20. Data from the National Institute of Mental Health Epidemiologic Attachment Area studies indicate that the mean age of onset for major depressive illness is 24 years; for anxiety disorders, 15 years; for drug abuse disorders, 19 years; and for alcohol abuse, 21 years (Christie et al, 1988).

21. Young adults (ages 25 to 44 years) have the highest rates for most psychiatric disorders, with depressive episodes and phobias predominating in women and antisocial personality and alcohol abuse and dependence most common in men (Robbins LN et al, 1984).

22. The best predictors of the number of outpatient visits by lower income groups are diagnosis, source of referral, previous use of services, and presenting complaint (Figueredo and Boerstler, 1988). Psychiatric history and scores on the Global Assessment Scale predict who is referred by nonpsychiatric physicians for psychiatric evaluation in an emergency room (Fenichel and Murphy, 1985). Other factors associated with treatment and disposition are psychotropic medications on entry to emergency room, age, "rudeness," and diffuseness of medical complaints (Murphy JG et al, 1984).

23. Appropriate referrals for consultation of patients with affective disorder and anxiety disorder by primary care physicians are directly related to the experience of those physicians (Andersen and Horthorn, 1990). In one study of a group of patients followed by primary care clinicians (Kessler LG et al, 1985) it was found that despite the fact that 35% of patients exhibited at least one Research Diagnostic Criteria disorder and two-thirds of those had significant changes on SADS-L data, only 10% were correctly diagnosed by their primary care givers.

24. In community studies, chronic medical conditions are associated with increased lifetime prevalence of substance use disorders and recent anxiety and affective disorders. Cancer, arthritis, lung disease, neurologic disorder, physical handicaps, and heart disease are more associated with psychiatric disorders than are diabetes or hypertension (Wells KB et al, 1988).

25. Patients seen in an emergency setting and who require immediate attention tend to be male, 20 to 39 years or above 80 years, and present with abusive or suicidal behavior or an organic mental disorder (Fulop and Strain, 1986).

The deinstitutionalization movement, with its decreased emphasis on inpatient care, has resulted in emergency rooms becoming the sites of ongoing medical and psychiatric care of the chronically mentally ill (Voineskos, 1983). These patients demand multifold interventions that minimize impairment and enhance compliance with treatment, requiring continuing re-evaluation of the roles of emergency psychiatric clinicians and, in some instances, major changes in what and how services are provided.

DIFFICULTIES FACING EMERGENCY PSYCHIATRIC CARE CLINICIANS

Violence

Some patients, particularly those who are acutely intoxicated substance-abusing males or actively psychotic paranoid schizophrenics, present a great potential for violence. However, the actual risk of physical harm coming to clinicians is usually exaggerated. In many instances, violent patients who have already perpetrated an assaultive act are brought to the emergency room by police officers or friends who usually serve to reduce the patient's immediate potential for violence. In other instances, there are certain precautions that clinicians can take to protect themselves against harm. These include the following:

1. Meeting patients outside the office to determine whether it is prudent to see them alone in the confines of an office.
2. Interviewing patients with a member of the hospital security force present.
3. Leaving the door open during the interview.
4. Allowing patients access to the door so that they do not feel "trapped." (In such instances, if there is a real concern for violence, security officers should be made aware of the fact that the patient may attempt to escape and should station themselves outside the door waiting inconspicuously for such a possibility).
5. Medicating the patient appropriately and by the proper route.

Suicide

Psychiatric clinicians often fear that they may fail to recognize a suicidal patient who, if not hospitalized, will successfully complete the self-destructive act. Fortunately, there are clinical, epidemiologic, and sociologic correlates of suicidal behavior that help identify people who represent major suicidal risks (requiring hospitalization) from those who manipulatively threaten suicide. However, no criteria are infallible. As surgeons are taught early in their careers, "Man proposes, but God disposes." Suicide is particularly difficult to predict in some groups, especially schizophrenics, and in that subpopulation variously referred to as "borderline personality" disorders and narcissistic character disorders. It usually is easy to recognize the antecedents of an act after it has been executed. It is less easy to identify with precision those same features in individuals before they attempt to take their life. A thorough assessment using the format outlined in this book serves to facilitate identification of those individuals who constitute high suicide risk and who should be hospitalized.

Difficult Dispositions

Dispositions are a problem in the emergency room setting. It frequently is difficult or impossible to find a setting that offers a treatment program that is consistent with what we feel best suits the patient's needs. Lack of funds or inadequate insurance may necessitate that patients be hospitalized far from their home setting. Knowledge of available facilities in the immediate area and of possible sources of payment facilitates disposition of the patient to the best possible treatment setting given the realistic limitations of any health care setting.

Commitment

Psychiatric clinicians may be concerned by the occasional need to hospitalize patients against their will through the use of a physician's certificate. The clinician's concern is usually highest when beginning work on a crisis unit, but no one ever becomes entirely inured to a patient's protestations. The realization, however, that failure to hospitalize suicidal patients may result in their untimely death leaves the evaluating clinician with no other ethical choice but to "commit." Patients' motivations to take their own or other lives often result from factors that are part of their illnesses, factors that we hope will be positively impacted by treatment (e.g., antipsychotic agents in the treatment of paranoid patients). Obviously not all destructive behavior is a consequence of psychosis; and, if a person brought to an emergency service following a violent act but is not found to be psychotic, he or she may need to be assigned to the appropriate legal authorities. This action protects both the innocent patients and the hospital psychiatric staff from the violence of such people. It also serves to reduce the inaccurate belief held by some that, in its therapeutic armamentarium, psychiatry harbors answers for all forms of violence. We do not have, and cannot afford to pretend to have, such answers.

Too Many Patients to Evaluate

The number of patients who present to an emergency room varies from setting to setting and, in any given setting, from day to day. Nothing can guarantee that a psychiatric clinician will not be inundated. If a number of patients arrive in rapid succession, it may be necessary for clinicians to triage the patients personally. The most disturbed patients, those who are potentially self- or other destructive or exhibit behavioral manifestations of acute medical and surgical problems, should be seen first. It is possible to be concurrently involved with the management of more than one patient. A clinician should be pragmatic (e.g., enlist the help of other emergency room personnel in tasks such as arranging transportation, hospitalization, or administering medication). An emergency room psychiatric team consisting of a psychiatrist, psychiatric social worker, a psychiatric nurse, and mental health workers serves to reduce the pressure brought to bear on any one clinician when an unexpected number of patients arrive. Frequently patients are inappropriately triaged into psychiatry. For instance, a patient who presents with shortness of breath and anxiety may be triaged to psychiatry by an emergency room nurse. However, these symptoms should alert the psychiatric clinician to seek alternative explanations for the behavior. One such patient, with a history of four hospitalizations for schizophrenia, was sent to psychiatry only to be found to have a pulmonary embolus as the cause of her anxiety and hours later her death.

Uncertainty as to Who Will Present

Uncertainty as to what the next patient will present with is a constant source of anxiety to emergency clinicians. Only experience provides sufficient repertoire of psychotherapeutic, sociotherapeutic, and pharmacotherapeutic techniques that can be generalized to most of the patients the clinician sees. Predominantly, substance abusing and depressed patients present in the emergency setting, with only a small percentage of patients presenting with neuroses, character disorders, and transient situational crises. Patients with organic mental disorders other than those that are substance abuse-related present infrequently to the psychiatric clinician. Therefore, the psychiatric clinician should maintain a high level of suspicion for fear of missing the occasional patient with AIDS, lupus, a subdural hematoma, or hypoglycemia.

Demand for Rapid Decision Making

Emergency room psychiatry is unique in the demand for rapid decision making it places upon psychiatric clinicians regarding the diagnoses of the causes of altered behavior, thought, or mood and their immediate management. There is no easy way to learn this other than by working in an emergency room setting for a period of time under adequate supervision and by supplementing the experience with directed reading in the areas of pharmacotherapy, crisis intervention, brief psychotherapy, and diagnostic psychiatry. Recently, as the emergency room has evolved into the only treatment site of many chronically mentally ill patients, emergency clinicians have been required to count management of deinstitutionalized and other patients with chronic psychiatric illnesses among their necessary skills (Marson et al, 1988).

Responsibility for Patients

Other than in instances where no treatment is required or where a patient is hospitalized, the psychiatric clinician assumes the responsibility of maintaining a supportive and guiding contact with the patient, and at times with the patient's family, until the crisis has approached or achieved resolution. When a clinician helps a patient follow through with treatment recommendations, there is a greater incidence of successful linkage to treatment than when a patient is simply provided the name of a treatment center or another psychiatric clinician. For effective crisis intervention, clinicians must have a strong sense of personal responsibility to their patients in order to provide the best care possible—given the obvious social or environmental limitations—at the time of crisis. This responsibility is sensed by patients, their families, and other members of the patient care teams and facilitates patient involvement in continuing care.

Sleep Deprivation

Some of the clinicians' anxiety, while working on an emergency room service, results from real loss of sleep experienced during hours on duty. Emergency room psychiatry is extremely taxing. If psychiatric clinicians are working 24-hour shifts, they find themselves to be exhausted, tense, and irritable by the time they see their twentieth patient. It is unreasonable to assume that any individual can perform at peak efficiency throughout a 24-hour shift, especially a psychiatric clinician who is very dependent upon subtle cues while working with patients. Therefore, wherever possible, arrangements should be made, either by the psychiatric clinician or by the administration, to limit emergency room work to 8- to 12-hour shifts.

Financing Treatment

As lamentable as it may be, a critical factor in determining disposition is the patient's ability to pay for treatment. Clinician concern is often greatly reduced if a city, state, or federally funded community mental health center is available for referral. In such circumstances, clinicians who are concerned that patients be treated within their communities rather than sent to remote state hospitals are able to provide patients with what they believe is the most viable treatment program. Nonetheless, the number of beds available in such hospitals is often limited. It may become necessary, therefore, to hospitalize patients elsewhere. If there is no medical coverage available through Medicare, Medicaid, insurance, or from private resources, it may be necessary to send patients to a remote and poorly staffed state hospital. In such circumstances, clinicians are placed in the unfortunate situation of having to rationalize this state of affairs to themselves as well as to patients and their families. Guilty explanations at 4 AM do not improve self-esteem or disposition. Comparably, the clinician's exhilaration experienced after obtaining a bed on a favored unit is frequently followed by the helpless realization that another clinician has just filled that unit and any further patients requiring hospitalization will have to be sent to a less desirable location.

Receiving Staffs' Reaction to the Emergency Clinician's Presumptive Diagnosis and Treatment Plan

Clinicians must do what is best for each patient and use their full store of diagnostic and treatment acumen in arriving at each clinical decision. Often, however, a need to hospitalize is equivocal due to inadequate information. In addition, patients with a variety of presenting symptoms recover dramatically within a day or two following hospitalization. Clinicians must be prepared to tolerate a certain amount of criticism from receiving clinicians concerning admission, but should not allow this to interfere with the resolve to hospitalize patients when it is felt that there are clear indications to do so.

PATIENT CONCERNS

Medical Problems Superimposed on Psychiatric Problems

Psychiatric patients may be hypochondriacal, have somatic delusions, or present with conversion symptoms. In addition, real somatic illnesses such as migraine headaches, bronchial asthma, and ulcerative colitis may exacerbate at times of stress. Of great significance in an emergency room setting are the myriads of medical complications consequent to long-term ingestion of alcohol or drugs. Patients with localized or systemic organic disease will also present at times to psychiatry with symptoms of concurrent psychiatric disorders or with psychiatric symptoms resulting from the underlying organic disease. Careful history taking, including a medical, surgical, and obstetrical history; clinical observation of the patient; and a physical examination serve as guideposts toward a correct diagnosis. One should never hesitate to use specialty consultations (e.g., neurology, internal medicine) where questions of diagnosis arise. In a study of 83,175 person-years (Zilber et al, 1989), excess mortality was found in patients of all diagnostic groups, with the highest mortality due to infectious and respiratory diseases within all of the groups (but especially among alcohol and other substance abusing patients). Excess mortality from cancer was only found among patients under 40.

Resistance to Treatment Recommendations

Consequent to the primary task of arriving at accurate diagnosis and appropriate disposition is the major challenge—at times—of dealing with patients' or families' resistance to acceptance of a treatment plan. As in psychotherapy, such resistance must be diagnosed in its psychohistorical and current social context. Strong resistance may indicate that a treatment plan is doomed to failure. Clinicians should be willing to discuss with patients how a decision was arrived at based on the information the patient or others provided about the various personality traits; psychopathology; social, cultural and economic factors; personal values; and extant myths and taboos (Lieb and Slaby, 1975a). Concern over being labelled "mentally ill" is often pre-eminent in importance in diverting a patient from considering either outpatient treatment or hospitalization. Additional uninformed notions about psychiatric hospitals frequently induce a rejection of psychiatric hospitalization in patients or family. Great patience, endurance, and a tolerance for anger are often required before it is possible to reach a point at which the patient and the family can accept a recommendation of treatment. At times a firm, somewhat authoritarian approach will succeed where other approaches have failed. However, a clinician may not be able to reason with an acutely psychotic schizophrenic or a patient with an organic psychosis. In such instances, commitment may become necessary.

Patient compliance with the recommendation to enter outpatient therapy varies. In one study (Wilder et al, 1977), older Puerto Rican and white women carrying the diagnosis of depression were most likely to follow through on an emergency psychiatric clinician's recommendation to enter outpatient therapy. Blacks and patients diagnosed as schizophrenic were least likely to follow through.

Difficult Families

At times of stress, we all tend to be curt, defensive, anxious, and short of temper. Family members of patients often have a greater amount of diagnosed and undiagnosed psychopathology, which may make it difficult to work rationally with them to form a therapeutic alliance. Even if a family seems relatively healthy, guilt may militate against a smooth working relationship when time and resources are limited. Clinicians should present the results of their evaluation and their management recommendations to the family in as nonthreatening and clear a manner as possible, with the awareness that the development of mental illness in a family member represents just as much of a crisis to a family as does a sudden loss or other misfortune. In a study comparing perceptions of 60 families from self-help psychoeducational groups with 26 hospital-based emergency mental health service providers (Morgan, 1989), families reported that obtaining emergency care involved contacts with numerous agencies over months. Both families and emergency clinicians expressed considerable dissatisfaction with the emergency care system. Clinicians were less likely than patients' families to construe the family's belief of the patient's need for care to be credible. The need for coordinated care sensitive to the patient's and family's unique needs at a very stressful time requires that skills in crisis intervention and management of social systems be enhanced by flexible use of strategic principles (Perlmutter and Jones, 1985).

Concern That Patients Get the Care Needed

In some cases, it is painfully obvious that a single emergency room visit will have little or no effect on the trajectory of a patient's illness. A person who has been an alcoholic for several years with recurrent emergency room visits when intoxicated is unlikely to follow through on treatment recommendations. This situation frustrates clinicians and engenders anger in them at the realization that they are helpless in the face of the obvious need to provide treatment. In other instances, despite the knowledge that hospitalization and proper medication provides symptom reduction, it is impossible to guarantee that patients will continue on medication and in treatment once released from the hospital. A graphic example is that of the recurrently hospitalized paranoid schizophrenic who refuses to take medication once released from the hospital and who will not consent to intramuscular injections of a long-acting fluphenazine or haloperidol. It is helpful if clinicians recognize their own limitations in effecting a perfect disposition and treatment plan in all cases.

Knowledge of Available Dispositions for Patients

The entry of patients into treatment programs depends on the clinician having good working relationships with individuals responsible for admissions to treatment systems. Clinicians should, in addition to acquiring a knowledge of public and private hospitals in the area, social agencies, church and school-related treatment programs, community based crisis centers, and private therapists, strive to develop personal working relationships with individuals from these resources at the first possible opportunity. Clinicians who have had long experience in the emergency room learn how an interested and appreciative attitude towards ambulance drivers can make a quantifiable temporal difference in how rapidly patients are picked up and brought to an inpatient unit. Clergy and community workers may know of treatment resources for psychiatric and substance-abusing patients or partial hospital programs or halfway houses that clinicians, less involved in the local communities, are unaware of.

Legal Backup

Legal consultation should be available for both patients and clinicians. When questions arise as to whether a patient can be hospitalized involuntarily when the patient's family opposes such a decision, forensic psychiatrists provide information that facilitates the best care consistent with the civil rights of the individual. Other questions that frequently arise result in appropriate disposition and treatment for individuals who are under arrest for homicidal and other criminal acts (Mills, 1988). Patients retained in the hospital (whether or not they are new to a system or have a history of multiple hospitalizations) rate higher on indicators of dangerousness to others or self, are more symptomatic, are more frequently given major diagnoses (Segal et al, 1988a) (especially of psychosis and mania), and are more likely to meet statutory criteria for grave disability (Hoge et al, 1988). In a study of 251 evaluations in five California public psychiatric emergency rooms, Segal and his coworkers (1988b) found that the combination of mental disorder and dangerousness predicted disposition of 88% of recidivist patients and 93% of new patients. The most influential factor of the mental disorder determining action was impulsivity. Unfortunately, this emphasis on dangerousness can direct emergency care providers to hospitalize less seriously ill patients who are impulsively violent (but less likely to "improve" with treatment) rather than the nonviolent but more seriously ill (and more likely to improve with hospitalization). A return to "need for treatment" criteria would serve to improve access to care of the more seriously ill (Segal et al, 1988a). Ironically, there is little support from research of the ability of clinical workers to accurately predict which patients will become violent, and the usual circumstances of an emergency room sadly enhances the likelihood of impulsive outbursts; these include small cramped examining rooms, few male staff members, high emotional intensity, unstructured social organization, and the expectation of violence (Moldin, 1985).

EMERGENCY ROOM REQUIREMENTS

Appropriate Examining Area and Equipment

Effective evaluation and management of individuals presenting with psychiatric emergencies is best achieved in a setting that meets the following standards:

1. There should be an interviewing room that is sufficiently soundproof so that the patient and his or her family and friends may talk confidentially with the evaluating clinician. It should also be secure so that violent or potentially self-destructive patients do not harm themselves or others. The room should be of sufficient size to allow potentially violent patients to have their "territory."
2. There should be no large, glassed areas, medication stores, or sharp objects (e.g., surgical blades) in the area where patients are evaluated.
3. Security guards should be readily available and alerted by an alarm button that is readily accessible to the clinician if attacked.
4. The door to the interviewing room should be unable to be locked from either the inside or the outside.
5. The interviewing room should be so located that other staff can easily get to it if needed; ideally the room should have two doors to assure rapid entry and exit if needed.
6. Parenteral and oral psychotropic medications should be available if required for use.
7. A pharmacy should be available to provide patients with the amount of medication they may need to take between the visit to the emergency room and the time

that patients, friends, or relatives can reasonably have a prescription filled by and/or have a follow-up visit.

8. The ambiance and furniture should be sufficient to allow a patient and significant others (who may include attending police officers, spouse, lover, children, or friends) to be seen at the same time if deemed necessary by the clinician.

9. Humane restraints should be available if management of the patient requires their use.

10. Blood pressure cuff, ophthalmoscope, and other instruments required for physical examination should be available.

11. A nurse or female attendant should be available if required for the examination of a female patient.

Ideally, community mental health centers, general medical hospitals, health maintenance organizations, and other institutions providing emergency psychiatric services should have holding beds so that a patient's treatment response may be evaluated over the course of 1 to 3 days. Some acutely psychotic patients and individuals with the potential to harm themselves or others recompensate quickly with a combination of crisis-oriented psychotherapeutic techniques and appropriate doses of psychotropic medication. Having holding beds available for use at the discretion of the emergency psychiatric clinician allows brief treatment and medication stabilization, so that the need for further hospitalization in an inpatient setting is minimized. In a study (Gillig et al, 1989) comparing the rates of hospitalization between an emergency room with an extended evaluation unit or holding area (used for up to 24 hours of evaluation) and a similar one without the holding beds, it was found that the rate of hospitalization for the service with holding bed capacity was 36% compared to a rate of 52% for the unit without holding beds.

A recent advance in facilitating patient flow has been the introduction of computerized technology into assessment and treatment planning in acute care units. In addition to the fact that automated modes of evaluation and treatment plans facilitate generation of legible prompt reports for referring clinicians, consultants, and clinicians receiving the patient, they allow for the creation of records that make it easier to review the progress of chronic patients using the emergency service as the primary care giver and to interpret computer-generated laboratory and clinical diagnostic data and consultant reports. Quality assurance is more easily monitored, and use and review data is more immediately available, saving clinicians much valued time. In emergency services that are part of a continuum of care, an initial treatment plan with goals and objectives can be generated (indicating the need for hospitalization) to accompany the reports of the psychiatric exam and physical examination performed to the unit.

Clinical Laboratory

Twenty-four-hour availability of a laboratory that can perform basic blood and urine screening tests as well as for toxic substances is a requisite for a quality emergency psychiatric evaluation service. In addition, access to a radiologic department for x-rays and CT scans, if needed, is required.

Methadone

Attitudes toward the liberal distribution of methadone to addicts vary from clinician to clinician, but federal regulations governing methadone distribution are strict and are regularly monitored. Individuals who are in registered treatment programs may receive methadone. Methadone-maintained programs often have working relationships with emergency room services to provide partial doses to those who have been recorded as having missed a dose on a given day. Methadone programs should make available a list of their medical backups for ready consultation if needed. In general, giving half the usual dose or less will be sufficient to prevent withdrawal symptoms when patients miss one of their daily doses. Methadone-maintained patients, particularly those who are female, have long histories of addiction, have been addicted for a larger percent of their life spans, are older, and have long histories of drug-free urinalyses, have fear of methadone maintenance detoxification (Milby et al, 1986). However, studies indicate that inpatient treatment with subsequent abstinence is associated with more significant, meaningful, and positive changes that are internally consistent than the changes found if a patient spends an equivalent amount of time in an outpatient methadone maintenance program (Craig RJ et al, 1990). Patients maintained on methadone tend to evince increased dependency needs.

Emergency Psychiatric Clinician Accessibility

There are periods when the immediate presence of psychiatric clinicians is needed in the emergency room. If they are unavailable, patients unduly suffer and staff morale is reduced by the awareness that a compromised standard of medical care is being provided. The use of a paging system or portable "beepers" facilitates the easy location of a psychiatric clinician, but should this fail, it is a recommended practice to provide the charge nurse with a telephone number where the psychiatric clinician may be contacted.

Pediatric Social Services

In instances when a single parent has to be hospitalized, the emergency room pediatric social workers should be contacted for help in temporary placement of the children. Additionally, should it become apparent that there is a history of child abuse, pediatric social workers will facilitate proper reporting and evaluation of the suspected occurrence.

Index Cards on Emergency Room Repeaters

Some patients appear in the emergency room so frequently that an index card file or computer bank with data and diagnoses, current medication, available friends and relatives to call, and the therapist's phone number becomes the only way to guarantee continuity of care. Such a filing system allows information to be fed into the emergency room by community workers, clergy, physicians, and psychotherapists. The 7 to 18% of total patients who are repeaters (as reported in various studies) account for up to a third of all emergency room visits (Ellison et al, 1986). The repeater population tends to be made up of chronic patients without social supports but who were often in psychiatric treatment at some time, indicating need to call the therapist of record to provide continuity of care.

Security

Hospital security officers may be needed to watch a suicidal patient who is being reluctantly hospitalized or to minimize the abusive and assaultive behavior of substance-abusing and psychotic patients receiving treatment or awaiting disposition. The more security officers are made to feel that they are part of a medical treatment team, that their interventions are valued, and that clinicians are willing to explain those interventions to them, the more they are willing to act in a prompt and humane way to protect patients and clinicians.

Medical and Surgical Consultation

Medical and surgical consultation should be available when needed but particularly in instances where there is

1. A history of previous neurologic disease, which could explain the patient's present symptoms and signs
2. A physical examination suggestive of neurologic dysfunction
3. A history of or recent onset of seizures
4. A history suggestive of amnesia, head injury, unconsciousness, or progressive deterioration of motor, sensory, or cognitive functioning
5. A mental status examination suggesting an organic mental disorder

Medical consultation should be obtained for all patients with a history of recent alcohol abuse. These individuals are at high risk for occult medical disease such as pneumonia, subdural hematomas, and gastrointestinal bleeding. Liver disease or alterations of central nervous system functioning may be responsible for the behavioral disturbance. Patients suspected of endocrine disturbances, cardiovascular disease, or pulmonary problems are examples of individuals requiring medical consultation. Any suspicion of a problem requiring medical or surgical intervention requires emergency room consultation before the patient is referred to a psychiatric hospital, unless the referring psychiatric clinician feels totally confident that the hospital to which they are sending the patient has adequate medical consultative services.

Emergency Psychiatric Evaluation Forms

Forms used to direct the taking of a psychiatric history, the performance of a mental status examination, and the development of treatment plans vary. Apart from obvious teaching and research significance, these forms are helpful in assuring quality in evaluation and in providing a vehicle by which clinicians on a team can easily work together and exchange information. The same form used on the emergency service can be used on all other services of the hospital (i.e., inpatient, outpatient, and consultation), reducing the need for duplication of data gathering. Clinicians working on an inpatient unit or in an outpatient clinic can supplement the social worker. In the ideal situation the data base, including physical examination, case formulation, differential diagnosis, diagnosis, and initial treatment plan, are all generated in the emergency room. Automation of this procedure facilitates both communication (due to increased legibility of documents) and the rapid transfer of information, which in turn helps to provide continuity of care.

Quality Assurance Monitors

The differential impact and power of acute psychiatric intervention has evolved to such a level of sophistication that it is not only possible but necessary to monitor the quality of care provided. This monitoring includes periodic review, not only the elements of evaluation of suicidal and homicidal potential and of a differential diagnosis, diagnosis, and diagnostic-specific treatment, but of charts to ascertain that the information obtained was legible, treatments performed were state-of-the-art, appropriate follow-up was arranged, patients and their families and lovers were provided information critical to understanding the nature of their problem and treatment, appropriate components of the physical exam were performed, and indicated diagnostic tests were obtained. In a sentence, the objective of quality assurance monitors is to ensure that the psychiatric care provided is consistent with standards of acceptable medical practice (Fauman, 1989). Information for review is usually obtained from progress notes and monitored at regular cycles, depending upon the severity of need for the monitor and the number of patients involved.

Examples of monitors of both suicidal risk and of use of seclusion and restraints are provided in Tables 1–1 and 1–2, respectively. The format provided for these two critical elements of emergency care may be modified for use in various settings. Other indicants of quality assurance are suggested at the end of the sections on specific emergencies.

Table 1–1. Quality Assurance Monitors of Suicidal Risk Assessment and Management.

Suicide attempts in the hospital

Suicide in the hospital

Patients discharged within 48 hours of discontinuation of suicide precautions

Determination of current suicidal risk and need for suicide precautions for patients admitted with identified suicide attempt or gestures toward suicide within the last 60 days (current or by history)

When current suicidal risk is identified, suicide precautions are ordered and initiated

Discontinuation of suicide precautions is preceded by an assessment that the patient is no longer considered to be a suicidal risk

Suicidal risk is assessed prior to therapeutic leaves (passes)

Suicidal risk is assessed prior to discharge

All clinical staff have been inserviced annually on clinically validated signs of suicidal risk

The least restrictive mode of restraint is used, given the patient's current and evolving clinical status

Table 1–2. Quality Assurance Monitors of Use of Seclusion and Restraints.

Seclusion/restraint is initiated after ascertainment that patient is dangerous to self or others

The time when seclusion/restraint was initiated is provided, a time limit clearly stated, and the justification provided

Methods other than seclusion/restraint were deployed without success prior to use of seclusion/restraint

Patients discharged within 48 hours of use of seclusion/restraint are reviewed

Patients restrained more than 12 hours are reviewed

Patient/staff injuries during seclusion/restraint reviewed

Physicians' orders for seclusion/restraint indicate clinical justification, specifics of type of seclusion/restraint to be used, time limitations, and specific behavioral criteria for discontinuation

EMERGENCY PSYCHIATRY TRAINING AND CONTINUING EDUCATION

There is no other setting in the psychiatric care system where as much information critical to diagnosis and treatment and the understanding of the cause of psychiatric illness may be mastered as in the emergency setting (McPherson, 1984). Unfortunately, the activity of many of the illnesses seen and the level of skill required to manage the population—coupled with limited resources—places some constraints on the use of a crisis care unit as a teaching site. If, however, there is proper training prior to experience on site, appropriate supervision, and a clear delineation of tasks and accountability, much can occur that is to the benefit of patients, their families, attending emergency clinicians, and the student of emergency psychiatry. Proper training in history taking and in the use of standardized forms facilitates accuracy of information, which in turn allows the senior attending physician to develop a differential diagnosis, diagnosis, and diagnostic-specific treatment. Many families, lovers, and friends need an opportunity to ventilate their feelings, which is frustrated by staff and time limitations. Trainees offer an expression of the opportunity for significant others to react and to provide supplementary information. Although there exists no consensus as to when in the training experience an emergency psychiatry rotation should occur (Hoffman and Forssmann-Falck, 1984), the skills acquired are critical to successful management of patients at all other points along the trajectory of psychiatric care. Mastering the essentials of differential diagnosis and of the evaluation and management of the suicidal and violent patient serves to reduce clinician stress and facilitate both good care and the deployment of psychosocial aspects of crisis intervention. In addition to clinical skills in differential diagnosis, diagnosis, management of violence, suicide, and crisis intervention, training in emergency psychiatry should include enhancing knowledge of legal and ethical issues, psychopharmacotherapy, management of drug and alcohol problems, required staffing patterns, referral patterns, inter-agency and agency cooperation, institutional contracts, and funding (McPherson, 1984).

ETHICAL ISSUES

The ever-evolving legal constraints on providing care when indicated to the most seriously psychiatrically ill and limited resources for disposition of these patients inevitably create ethical dilemmas for both the novice and seasoned emergency clinician. Clinical acumen and a stable sense of moral direction can facilitate coping with ethical problems as they arise (Sider, 1986). Legal and ethical problems specific to particular psychiatric emergencies (e.g., management of children and adolescents, suicide, other-directed violence, sexual abuse, AIDS) are addressed in the specific sections on each subject.

OUTCOME STUDIES

Outcome studies of the hospitalization of severely ill psychiatric patients (e.g., those with chronic schizophrenia and severe character disorders) provide conflicting results, but on the whole tend to suggest that briefer hospitalizations with emphasis on family therapy and community placement are associated with better outcome. Edicott et al (1979) found that, in general, standard treatment was inferior to brief hospitalization with or without day care. Herz et al (1979) found little differential effect between brief and standard hospitalization on families. When a difference did occur, however, it tended to favor brief hospitalization. Sylph and Kedward (1977) found that hospitals play a major role in the lives of chronic patients regardless of the hospital facilities available. Lamb (1979) found that the use of community social rehabilitation programs was directly related to provision and use of transportation. Board and care homes appeared to offer asylum for life's pressures, a degree of structure, and some treatment (usually in terms of medication supervision). Blouin and coworkers (1985) found several patient and therapeutic factors predicted the outcome of a crisis intervention program. Middle-aged, higher socioeconomic patients with a single mild to moderate life stressor did best. Techniques that were positive, forward-looking, and supportive were predictive of improvement. Techniques emphasizing the past and negative thoughts, or focusing on maladaptive responses, were counterproductive.

Mortality rates are particularly high among psychiatric patients, probably due to a combination of the risk of suicide and other self-destructive behavior, such as accident proneness and substance abuse; increased vulnerability to physical illness in a stressed, psychiatrically ill population; impaired judgement resulting in unsafe sex practices leading to AIDS and other sexually transmitted disease; poor nutritional status; and failure of the clinician to evaluate and diagnose physical and surgical illness in a polysymptomatic and sometimes delusional population with impairment of the ability to identify correctly and communicate their physical distress. A study of 500 randomly selected psychiatric outpatients followed for a mean of 7 years using age-, sex-, and race-adjusted methods (Martin RL et al, 1985a, 1985b) produced a mortality rate that was twice that expected from a reference population. Excess mortality predominated in younger (but not older) patients, black and white men, white women, and homosexuals. Black women did not show increased rates of mortality. Schizophrenia, drug and alcohol addiction, organic brain diseases, and antisocial personalities were the diagnoses with greatest recorded increase in mortality. Affective illness unattended by any other illness (e.g., alcoholism) was not associated with increased mortality. In a 6 to 12 year followup of 500 patients (Martin RL et al, 1985b) death from unnatural causes (e.g., suicide and homicide) was 3.5 times normal with death from natural causes (e.g., myocardial infarction) 1.5 times normal. Affective illness was associated with excess mortality when another illness associated with excess death antedated the onset of a mood change, drug and alcohol abuse disorders, or antisocial personality. In this study, homosexuals, younger patients, and all racial groups except black women showed increased rates of mortality.

Emergency Psychopharmacotherapy | 2

The ability to properly diagnose psychiatric disorders, knowledge of diagnostic-specific pharmacologic intervention, and recognition and management of side effects are essential to appropriate psychopharmacotherapy. Failure to diagnose affective disorders (and/or an ideological unwillingness to treat them with lithium or antidepressants) raises both legal and ethical questions. Prompt initiation of lithium or antidepressants where appropriate can literally be lifesaving. While a complete response to medication may take as long as 3 weeks to 3 months, the response that occurs within the first few days of therapy may be significant and provide hope for a cure.

GENERAL INFORMATION

1. Drugs are metabolized at different rates by different individuals. The effective serum level of two patients on the same oral dose of an antidepressant may be remarkably different.
2. Barbiturates induce liver microsomal enzymes, increasing the rate at which other drugs are degraded.
3. The degradation of alcohol, barbiturates, and narcotics is inhibited by monoamine oxidase inhibitors (MAOIs).
4. A syndrome similar to atropine poisoning characterized by delirium, convulsions, and excitation may occur when tricyclic antidepressants are taken with an MAOI.
5. Neuroleptics may enhance the hypotensive effectiveness of the antihypertensive agents.
6. The atropine-like side effects of anticholinergics, antihistamines, antiparkinsonian drugs, and phenothiazines are enhanced by the tricyclic antidepressants.
7. Both the thioxanthenes and phenothiazines lower the convulsive threshold in susceptible individuals, necessitating in some patients an increase the amount of anticonvulsant medication taken.
8. Physostigmine may be effective in the treatment of an atropine psychosis but has side effects of its own that limit use.
9. Low doses of neuroleptics (e.g., 5 mg fluphenazine decanoate every 2 weeks) once thought to be homeopathic have been shown to be as effective in the management of chronic, recurrently hospitalized patients as are higher doses (e.g., 25 mg every 2 weeks) (Van Patten and Marder, 1986).
10. Although patients improve at a slower rate with low-dose neuroleptics, they re-

18

port less dysphoria and fewer side effects, particularly akathisia (Van Du Hen and Marder, 1986; Dubin et al, 1986).

EMERGENCY PSYCHIATRY PHARMACOPOEIA

Routine psychiatric medications (e.g., hypnotics, neuroleptics, benzodiazepines, lithium carbonate, thymoleptics, and antiparkinson agents) should be available for patients whose prescriptions have expired at a time when all pharmacies are closed; a variety of liquid and parenteral medications should be readily available for use in emergencies. These include thioridazine concentrate and liquid forms of chlorpromazine, fluphenazine, haloperidol, perphenazine, thiothixene, and trifluoperazine. Parenteral lorazepam alone or coupled with a parenteral neuroleptic such as thiothixene or haloperidol is the treatment of choice for most agitated psychotic states seen. In rare instances, parenteral droperidol may be used. Parenteral Cogentin and Benadryl are needed to manage acute dystonic reactions. Dalmane, Benadryl, Restoril, Halcion, and chloral hydrate are helpful for patients presenting with sleeping difficulties. A supply of the various antidepressants should be kept in stock to tide over patients presenting with sleeping difficulties and, together with lithium carbonate, kept in stock to tide over patients whose supplies run out. It is not a recommended policy to commence antidepressant or lithium therapy in the emergency room setting unless the evaluating clinician will personally follow the patient.

Side Effects

Identification and management of side effects play a significant role in emergency psychopharmacotherapy. Misidentification of side effects may have deleterious consequences. For instance, akinesia secondary to neuroleptic drugs may be diagnosed as depression and treated with an antidepressant rather than with an antiparkinsonian drug. Abdominal pain caused by a tricyclic antidepressant may result in an unnecessary consultation with a gastroenterologist if it is not recognized as a side effect.

There are a number of references that can and should be used for investigating established or potential side effects. These resources include the *Physician's Desk Reference,* the *Monthly Index of Medical Specialties, The Medical Letter,* and the *Adverse Drug Effect Bulletin.* Many hospitals now have drug information centers to assist clinicians in drug selection, dosage, side effect recognition, and management. Clinical pharmacists are an added resource in the management and prevention of side effects and of drug/drug interactions.

Psychosocial Issues

Inquiry should always be made as to which persons in the patient's social circle are on medications that the patient may have access to and use to overdose. Two or more members of the same household may be taking psychoactive medication. Children may accidentally take their mother's or father's medication. The outcome could be fatal if a child is taking dextroamphetamine for hyperkinesia and his or her mother or father is taking an MOAI for depression.

The pharmacist is an important figure for influencing patient and family. He or she can constructively enhance compliance and provide useful additional information. However, pharmacists, by omission or commission, occasionally undermine a physician's treatment plan.

Compliance

Each patient is primed by his or her previous experiences with medicines. Positive previous response to medication enhances compliance. Patients who must control, however, will often not comply. Poor compliers usually remain poor compliers unless the physician undertakes active intervention to bring about change.

Patients often become alarmed on learning of the dosage of medicine that they are to take. Patients accustomed to low milligram doses of a phenothiazine or antianxiety drug may become alarmed to learn that lithium carbonate is generally prescribed in a daily dosage range of 600 to 1800 mg. Patients frequently know of someone else who received the same medication, and lament that they have to take such a "big dose" when a friend "only had to take three of these capsules a day." Conversely, patients may complain about what they consider to be low doses (e.g., "My cousin used to take ten of them a day. Do you really think I'm going to get well on just two?").

Many patients have an inherent bias against taking medicines, often expressed in terms of feeling a loss of autonomy or an implied weakness or failure. While some patients insist that their illnesses have nothing to do with developmental experiences and are happy to take medicines, others insist that they became ill because of earlier experiences and fear that medication prevents emotional resolution of traumatic childhood events.

Personal attributes determine response to side effects. Patients who are highly concerned about appearance may stop phenothiazines, antidepressants, or lithium after weight gain has occurred, whereas underweight patients may welcome the weight gain. Patients requiring constant accurate vision (e.g., students) may not tolerate blurry vision, just as a lawyer objects to dry mouth. Thioridazine may bring a welcome inhibition of premature ejaculation for one patient, while worsening potency problems for another.

Cost of treatment, including cost of medicine, may be a significant factor in compliance. Compliance improves when patients are informed of the estimated cost of the medicine. In the United States, outpatient prescriptions have a built-in dispensing fee. It is generally less expensive to have one prescription for 100 tablets or capsules filled than two prescriptions for 50 each. Weighed against this is the hazard of dispensing a large number of tablets or capsules to a patient at risk for suicide.

Although the topic of compliance has been widely discussed in the literature in recent years, the predominant (and generally ignored) issue is of the effectiveness of the treatment. Noncompliance is much less likely to occur when the drug regimen is effective and when side effects are minimal and the physician's instructions to the pharmacist are conveyed in the form of a written prescription to confirm a verbal (usually telephone) order.

It is important that patients understand and follow the directions for use. Preferably, patients know exactly what it is that they are taking, the dose, and the dosage schedule. The physician must be assured that patients clearly understand the instructions. If there is insufficient space on the prescription blank for clear instructions, a separate note can be sent to the pharmacist. The physician may also compile a detailed list of instructions to review with a patient and his or her family until the physician is satisfied that the patient understands the instructions and can follow them.

Legal constraints on provision of medication to the most critically psychiatrically ill who refuse medication vary. The *Rogers* decision maintained that antipsychotic medication cannot be given to a consenting hospitalized patient unless the patient is competent to provide consent. A psychiatrist can make an assessment as to whether a patient is competent to refuse or accept medication but only a judge can declare a patient legally competent (Beck and Staffin, 1986). Medication can only be given involuntarily in an emergency and where there is danger of irreversible, substantial immediate harm (Beck and Staffin, 1986).

A patient's right to refuse treatment when committed at times places well meaning staff in a compromised position regarding delivery of quality care in a timely manner to reduce pain and embarrassment to the patient and family (Appelbaum, 1988). The basic issues germane to legislation regarding the right to refuse treatment include due process, patient competency, risks versus benefits, patient advocacy, and possibility of physician threat (Prehn, 1989).

Crisis Intervention | 3

Individuals present in crises with medical, psychiatric, and social problems. Clinicians should have at their command the necessary expertise to recognize the crisis situation and deal with it appropriately. Specific crises call for specific remedies. Thorough familiarity with medical and social resources both within and outside of the emergency setting is a must. It is essential to attempt to assess the exact nature of a crisis. This requires both a cross-sectional and a longitudinal assessment of the patient in order to effect more permanent changes than those possible by crisis intervention alone. For instance, individuals with bipolar disorder or relapsing schizophrenia often decompensate under environmental circumstances, which for them have untoward real or symbolic connotations. A patient's presenting symptoms may include flight of ideas, elation, and infectious gaiety, with the most likely diagnosis being manic psychosis. On interviewing a family member, clinicians may learn that the patient has had similar episodes in the past but has responded well to phenothiazines and never required hospitalization. Clinicians may also learn that no one has ever taken the trouble to discuss maintenance lithium carbonate with the patient and his or her family. A family member may further inform a clinician that the patient has always responded poorly to anniversaries and that his or her fortieth birthday is upcoming. All this data provides a clinician with the groundwork for an immediate plan: a neuroleptic and/or benzodiazepine to reduce acute symptoms; referral to an outpatient clinic for lithium carbonate therapy; and supportive psychotherapy around the upcoming birthday is probably all that is immediately needed.

GENERAL PRINCIPLES

Pragmatism and Innovation

Successful resolution of crises requires pragmatism with a knowledge of and willingness to employ a variety of therapeutic techniques. These may involve supportive psychotherapy, with or without the use of antianxiety or antipsychotic agents in the emergency situation, coupled with a few follow-up visits. At other times, it may be necessary to bring in other family members, friends, or a heterosexual or homosexual lover. Brief hospitalization for 1 to a few days may be required for chronically ill psychiatric patients for a diagnostic reassessment or reinstitution or adjustment of medication. In other instances, an intensive inpatient or outpatient workup may be needed to differentiate medical or neurologic problems from the more purely psychiatric causes of behavioral disturbances.

Confidentiality

Effective crisis intervention sometimes requires a broadening of the definition of confidentiality to include, with the patient's permission, their families, spouses, friends, or lovers so that a clearer picture of what is troubling them may be obtained and sufficient social support provided. A quick resolution of a crisis may at times then be facilitated by sociotherapeutic manipulations (when indicated). Obviously, if a patient is obtunded, psychotic, comatose, suicidal, or homicidal, the psychiatric clinician must decide who should be contacted to best effect expeditious and accurate diagnostic assessment so that definitive therapeutic interventions may be initiated without undue delay. When possible, written consent should be obtained before others are contacted.

Ready Availability of the Clinician

What appear to be insurmountable crises or therapeutic impasses are often resolvable to a considerable degree if patients and their families feel that the clinician seeing them in the emergency room setting is available for consultation and an extra visit, if indicated. One often finds that when a patient or family feels that a clinician is available, seemingly urgent matters seem less pressing.

Awareness of What Was Effective in a Previous Crisis

It has been said that one who fails to know the past is doomed to repeat it. Awareness of what has contributed in the past to successful resolution of the patient's crises often reduces the need to attempt therapeutic manipulations that are doomed to failure. One might, for instance, call a patient's therapist or a family member in order to learn what may have been used effectively in the past to resolve a crisis. Calling the patient's therapist, in addition to being an obvious courtesy, is part of ideal emergency psychiatric care. It allows therapists to be aware of the patient's crises and provides for continuity of care by allowing the emergency room clinician to obtain more information (e.g., the doses of medication a patient is on). The involvement of a patient's own therapist and the establishment of a follow-up appointment often reduces the need for hospitalization and other more disrupting therapeutic interventions.

Reduction of Patient Drop-Out Rate

Repeated users of the emergency room often are individuals who, if they were seen in a long-term therapy arrangement, would not use the emergency room service. If a clinician arranges a follow-up visit to see if the patient is in treatment, or in some cases just calls a week later, the referral drop-out rate can be reduced.

Psychiatric History and Mental Status Examination

By necessity, an evaluation of a disturbance of mood, thought, or behavior undertaken in the emergency room cannot be as comprehensive as an extended evaluation in a private therapist's office, an outpatient clinic, or an inpatient hospital setting. However, there are certain basic questions that should be asked in every emergency evaluation. If a patient is unable to provide the answers to these questions, a perusal of old charts or an interview with a relative or a friend may yield the required information. This information is needed to provide the best assessment of a patient's problem from a medical, social, and psychological perspective. Should hospital records or a psychiatrist's private files be subpoenaed for legal reasons or be called upon for utilization review, a written record of a comprehensive emergency psychiatric consultation demonstrates that the evaluation was complete, how a diagnosis was arrived at, and for what reasons certain therapeutic interventions, including hospitalization with or without medical certification, were performed.

Ability of the Clinicians to Handle Their Own Anxiety

Crisis intervention involves many quick decisions. For instance, what is the diagnosis? What type of treatment should be given? Does the patient need to be on long-term medication? Who should be called in to participate in the treatment process? Is hospitalization necessary?

Arriving at a decision is always somewhat anxiety provoking; however, it is even more so when the data base and time are limited. Psychiatric clinicians who are adept at techniques of crisis intervention often take a quick hold of an electric situation. They readjust a family's equilibrium and overcome interpersonal impasses. They do not hesitate to employ medication to relieve intrapsychic pain. Given the time frame, they solicit information from as many sources as possible, with care for accuracy. They use the information, obtained discriminatively, avoiding the common pitfall of being forced into a position they do not want to take.

Use of Multiple Sources of Data in Evaluation

Psychiatric patients in the emergency room are not always as able to provide as complete and coherent a history as are candidates for psychoanalysis. They may, in fact, be unable to provide a history at all because of an acute schizophrenic psychosis, a drug-induced state, or dementia. In such instances, the clinician should not hesitate to contact other possible sources for historical information. These include:

1. Family members
2. Friends
3. Lovers
4. Employer or fellow employees
5. Clergy
6. Police officers who may have brought them in
7. Primary physician
8. Therapist

Charts may show that patients have long standing medical or psychiatric conditions that explain part or all of their present clinical picture. In addition, a former therapist or an old chart may provide baseline data to which the current clinical status can be compared.

Research studies indicate that defensiveness (a tendency not to report unfavorable information about oneself) is inversely correlated with lifetime prevalence of any psychiatric disorder and with self-reported symptoms (Lane et al, 1990). Test/retest reliability for most questions tends to be high with the exception of alcohol-related questions and anxiety disorders (Wittchen et al, 1989). When eliciting a family history, information based on direct interview of as many family members as possible is superior to information obtained indirectly from a patient or family member (Andreasen et al, 1986; Zimmerman M et al, 1988a).

MEETING THE PATIENT

Patients presenting in an emergency room are usually quite upset and see their problem as requiring immediate attention. Although this may prove not to be the case when a patient is interviewed, it is good practice for clinicians to introduce themselves to a new arrival shortly after they have registered, even if this means that clinicians have to excuse themselves for a few minutes from a patient they are already interviewing. This tactic serves several functions:

1. Patients require evaluation as to their relative need for immediate attention. A patient with an acute organic brain disorder secondary to a medical condition (e.g., transient cardiac arrhythmia) or a patient with an uncontrolled schizophrenic psychosis may require immediate attention.
2. Prompt introduction reduces the anxiety of more integrated patients who then know a clinician is aware of their presence, despite the fact that they cannot be seen immediately.
3. Nurses and other emergency room staff respect clinicians who are aware of the fact that "psych" cases are not a homogenous group. Some patients need more immediate care than others. Prompt treatment of disruptive psychotic behavior reduces staff tension in the emergency room.
4. The presence of a psychotic patient in the waiting room frightens other patients who are waiting to be seen for medical or surgical problems. A grief-stricken woman awaiting news as to whether her husband is still alive after being rushed to the hospital with chest pain is not comforted by a paranoid patient's delusions. Also, a schizophrenic patient may respond in an exaggerated and bizarre manner to the sight of blood or mutilation.

Emergency room psychiatric residents and team leaders should devise mechanisms whereby they can be alerted intermittently to the number of patients waiting to see them and their ostensible complaints. Close liaison with admission personnel and emergency room nursing staff and orderlies can be of great help in this regard. A few minutes spent with such personnel prior to on-call duty can be of inestimable advantage. They should be requested to inform the clinician if a patient seems to be in great distress. A few minutes spent with such patients shortly after they have registered can help them to organize their fantasies and get their anxieties under control.

Initial Observations

A patient's response to a simple introduction can provide a wealth of data that may prove useful in the evaluation. How does the patient comport themselves? How do they walk? Are they guarded or do their eyes gaze about furtively as they talk? How do they dress and speak? Do they seem to be responding to voices or visual phenomena that don't exist? Psychiatric clinicians can create a sense of competence as they carefully and conscientiously watch patients approach their office. Seasoned clinicians often find that they tend to develop preliminary ideas as to diagnosis in the first few minutes of an interview, and that data obtained by the interview serves to corroborate the initial diagnostic impression.

Chief Complaint

The chief complaint should be stated in the patient's own words; for example, "I feel my head is exploding." If the patient is unable to provide a chief complaint, the reasons why they were brought to the emergency room should be stated; for example, "The patient was brought in because he was walking naked down Main Street."

PATIENT HISTORIES

History of Present Illness

1. When did the patient's symptoms begin? Have they been constant? Increased? Decreased? Fluctuated in intensity?
2. How does the patient describe the symptoms (e.g., the patient states he feels "worthless," "sinful," and "dirty")?
3. Has there been any change in somatic functioning? Sleep disturbance? Weight changes? Appetite change? Change in sexual interest or performance? Constipation and other gastrointestinal difficulty? Headache or other pain? Palpitations and other cardiovascular symptoms? Respiratory, excretory, or neurologic changes?
4. What were the circumstances when the symptoms began? Recent death or loss? Job loss or advancement? Divorce or separation? Impending jail sentence? Menopause or loss of potency? Injury? Diagnosis of severe illness or impending surgery? First or difficult sexual experience? Pregnancy? Change of residence or job? Impending retirement? Financial reversal? Beginning or ending of school? Marital reconciliation? Mortgage due? Loss of friend through death or separation? Other difficulty at home, work, or play? Does the problem that precipitated the difficulty persist? Reporting of life events is always limited (greatest recall is for the most recent 6 months) casting doubt on the validity of some retrospective studies of the relationship of life events to onset of illness (Neugebauer, 1983).
5. During the evaluation of the illness, has there been a change in the patient's mental status? Have they had auditory, visual, gustatory, olfactory, or tactile hallucinations? Ideas of reference? Paranoid ideation? Delusions of grandeur, persecution? Racing thoughts? Feelings that his or her head is going to explode?

Obsessions? Compulsions? Ritualistic behavior? Hypochondriasis? Somatic delusions? Overwhelming anxiety? Free-floating anxiety? Depression? Feelings of elevated mood? Intense anger or fear? Derealization? Depersonalization? Identity or sexual confusion? Homicidal or suicidal ideation or attempts? Phobias?

6. What is the patient's past psychiatric history? If they have been hospitalized, for how long and where? Have they been or are they currently on any medication? What and how much? Has the patient been taking it? Have they ever had electroconvulsive therapy? Who is or was his or her therapist? How frequently and for how long were they seen? Have they had any difficulty with the law? Has the patient ever been incarcerated? If yes, where, for what, and for how long? Does the patient know what his or her diagnosis was?

7. If the patient is suicidal or homicidal, do they have a plan of action, a weapon, or other lethal means of ending their own or another's life? Have they attempted before? If so, how many times? With what and where? Did they leave a note or tell someone, or would they have died if not found? Does the patient have religious or other reasons not to commit suicide? Does the patient see people looking at them as dead? Have they given away any possessions, especially prized ones? Do they have command hallucinations (i.e., voices telling the patient to kill themselves or others)? Is the patient dissociated? Do they talk about themselves in the third person?

Past Psychiatric Treatment

1. Has the patient ever seen a psychotherapist or counselor before? For what and for how long? Do they know the diagnosis? Were they given medication or ECT? Who was or were the patient's therapists? When is the last time they sought psychiatric help? Did treatment help?

2. Has the patient ever been hospitalized for psychiatric reasons? How many times? Where? For how long? What modes of therapy were used? Did the patient feel that the treatment helped?

Medical and Surgical History

1. What medical illnesses and operations has the patient had? Do they have a chronic illness? Could this illness explain his or her present symptoms? Are they presently in treatment? Are his or her symptoms worse now? Have they ever been hospitalized for any serious illness? How long?

2. Has the patient ever had a serious accident? Are they accident prone? Are the number of accidents increasing?

3. Does the patient presently have any medical or neurologic symptoms? (These may give clues to an organic illness that may be the basis of the presenting symptom(s).)

Drug History

1. What medications are the patient presently on and at what dosage? Have they

ever been on any medications previously for a long period of time? Could these explain the present symptoms?

2. Has the patient ever smoked marijuana? Taken LSD? DMT? STP? PCP? MDA? Amphetamines? Mescaline? Psilocybin? Other hallucinogens? Cocaine? Crack? How many times and for how long? Have the drugs ever caused the patient difficulty? Are they currently using drugs? Could this explain the symptoms? What is the route of drugs taken?

3. Does the patient drink alcohol? How much? How many days a week? Alone? In the morning? Is it needed to perform a task (e.g., go to work)? Have they ever had delirium tremens? When and how was it treated? Do they belong to Alcoholics Anonymous? Have they ever been hospitalized for alcoholism? Where and for how long? Has it interfered with his or her performance at work, home, or school?

4. Does the patient regularly take any sedatives (e.g., barbiturates) or tranquilizers? If so, how much? Has this increased? Is the patient dependent on them? Do they get withdrawal symptoms?

5. Has the patient ever been or are they presently addicted to heroin? How much? For how long? Have they ever been in a treatment program? Where? Did they get off the drug at the time? Are they withdrawn? When was their last dose? Do they use other drugs in addition to heroin?

6. Is there any history of use of glues, gases, or solvents?

7. Is the patient allergic to any medication? If so, which medication and what was the response?

Family History

1. Is there any history of comparable problems among members of the patient's family? If so, what? At what ages were they treated? What drugs did they receive? Were they hospitalized? For how long? What are their relationships to the family? Did treatment work?

2. Is there a family history of suicide? Dementia? Depression? Alcoholism? Mania? Bankruptcy (as an indicant of mania)? Schizophrenia? Epilepsy? Drug abuse? Jail sentences? Panic disorder? Any nervous or mental disease? Are there any particularly strange or bizarre relatives? Are there any long, unexplained hospitalizations in the family?

Comparison of diagnoses based on direct interviews of affected relatives and diagnoses based on family history indicate that the specificity for the family history method is high but the sensitivity is low. Accuracy is better for alcoholism and affective illness than for less severe disorders. Offspring and spouses provide more accurate information than siblings or parents. Sensitivity is somewhat increased by the use of multiple informants (Thompson et al, 1982).

Past Personal History

1. Where was the patient born? Was there any difficulty around their birth? What was their birth order? How many brothers and sisters does the patient have? Are the siblings alive? What are their ages? Where do they live? What do they do?

Are they married? Are the patient's parents alive? When has the patient last seen them? If they are dead, when and of what did they die? How old were the parents, or any sibling or spouse, when they died? How old was the patient when the parents died?

2. Where did the patient go to school? How many years did they complete? What were their grades like? Was there any change in their academic performance? Were there any discipline problems at school? What was their major?

3. What role does sex play in the patient's life? How did a woman respond to her menarche and/or menopause? When was her last period? How does she feel about her menses? Did the patient engage in sexual play as a child? Do they masturbate for release? Has the frequency changed recently, and how does he or she feel about masturbating? What is the theme of sexual fantasies? How old was the patient when they first began to neck? Pet? Have intercourse? If unmarried, how frequently do they date? Have they had any homosexual experiences? How frequently, and how does the patient feel about them? Do they have a lover? Do they reach orgasm? How many people have they had intercourse with? How old were they when they became engaged? Married? How old is their spouse or lover? How is the sexual relationship between the patient and partner (i.e., mutual satisfaction)? Frequency? Orgasm? How many children does the patient have? Any adopted? Was the patient's spouse at the time of the birth of the patient's children the coparent? If the patient is female, have there been induced or spontaneous abortions? Miscarriages? How did she respond to the birth of her children? Any post-partum depression? How does the patient and his or her spouse get on? Any physical violence? Extramarital affairs (heterosexual and homosexual)? Talk of divorce? If divorced, what were the grounds? Does the patient still see his or her ex-spouse? How many subsequent marriages were there? If subsequent divorce, what were the grounds? Does the patient live with anyone? Any plans for marriage? Feelings about lack of commitment? Birth control? Desire for or not to have children? If sexually active with multiple partners, do patients know their HIV status?

Social History

1. Where and with whom does the patient live? What are the living conditions (e.g., crowded, rats, no heat, dangerous neighborhood)?

2. How much does the patient earn? Do they earn enough for food, housing, etc.? How many meals a day do they eat and what do they eat? Do they get along with the person(s) with whom they live?

3. Did the patient have any close friends growing up? How many? Have they withdrawn from people? When? How many close friends do they have now? How frequently do they see them? Do they offer support? Are the relationships characterized by mutual satisfaction and warmth?

4. Does the patient belong to any clubs or organizations? Are they religious? Do they belong to any men's or women's groups? Is this supportive? What other social activities does the patient engage in?

Occupational and School History

1. Where does the patient work? How long have they been at the job? How do they get on with their employer and fellow employees? Does the patient enjoy the work? The working conditions? The hours? The other employees? The employer?
2. How many jobs has the patient held in their life? For how long? Why did they quit? Are jobs being held for shorter periods of time? Is their performance at work decreasing? Are they holding jobs below their level of competence or professional training?
3. What is the patient's current salary? Is it sufficient to meet their expenses? What are their expenses? Do they have any outstanding debts?

EXAMINATIONS

Physical Examination

A complete physical examination is usually not part of the routine psychiatric emergency consultation. This relates in part to the fact that a psychiatrist's expertise lies in the performance and evaluation of parts of the physical examination that relate to alterations of mood, thought, and behavior, much as a cardiologist's expertise lies in the examination of the heart. However, if either history or presentation suggests that there is some underlying disease requiring more careful medical, surgical, or neurologic attention, then a physical examination should be performed either by the psychiatrist or an appropriate specialist. In all instances, vital signs should be taken (i.e., blood pressure, pulse, temperature, and respiratory rate) and if organicity is suggested, a neurologic exam should be performed. Level of consciousness should be assessed as part of a determination of whether or not an organic etiology may be responsible for the change in behavior. Any suggestion of a chronic or acute mental disorder requires that the psychiatrist further evaluate the patient. One should be particularly alert to stigmata of endocrine disorders such as moon-shaped face, buffalo hump, prognathism, and large hands. Changes in mental status may accompany a variety of alterations of cardiac rate or rhythm (e.g., bradycardia, tachycardia, or heart block) as well as radical changes in blood pressure.

Use of narcotics may be suggested by pupillary changes and needle marks on the arm. Withdrawal may be indicated by goose flesh, rhinorrhea, and lacrimation. Inspection of the skin and conjunctiva may reveal evidence of liver disease through the presence of jaundice. Scars on the head, especially fresh ones, should make one think of a subdural hematoma. The pupillary size, symmetry of pupils, and their reaction to light and accommodation are important. Pupillary inequality suggests the possibility of a subdural hematoma, which may present with a history of seizures or alcoholism. Cyanosis, dyspnea, and pyrexia are also indicators of an organic process. A cachectic individual presenting with dementia may have an occult neoplasm, as yet undiagnosed, that has metastasized to the brain or have mental changes as the result of "distal effects" of a tumor without direct invasion of the brain. Examination of the breasts or a chest x-ray may reveal a mammary carcinoma or pulmonary tumor that may have metastasized and caused the changes. Smelling an obtunded individual's breath may suggest alcoholism, diabetes (acetone breath) or hepatic or renal disease (fetid breath).

Elevated temperature coupled with an alteration in mental status suggests an infection of the central nervous system, especially in patients who may be immunologically compromised such as a patient with diabetes, AIDS, and cancer and those on steroids and immunosuppressant drugs. The probability that behavioral changes are due to an underlying organic cause increases with the number of medical problems a patient has (Goldberg VJ et al, 1989).

Mental Status Examination

1. Do patients have racing thoughts? Feel their head is exploding? Do they feel people are after them? Talking about them as they walk down the street (ideas of reference)? Do they have auditory, visual, olfactory, gustatory, or tactile hallucinations? Do they feel unreal (derealization)? Feel apart from themselves, like actors on the stage (depersonalization)? Are their associations loose? Are they tangential? Circumstantial? Do they have clang associations? Deja vu? Deja entendu? Deja lu? Jamais vu? Verbigeration? Word salad? Do they have nihilistic, somatic, or other delusions? Are they markedly ambivalent? Do they have obsessive thoughts or phobias? Do they respond slowly or not at all?

2. Is the patient depressed? Euphoric? Manic? Anxious? Fearful? Do they feel worthless? Guilty? Dirty? Bad? Is their affect flat? Inappropriate? Do they have emotional incontinence?

3. Are they autistic? Negativistic? Catatonic (waxy flexibility or excited)? What is their appearance like? Facial expression, dress, and behavior? Are they affected? Angry? Pompous? Retarded or agitated? Engaging? Warm? Affable? Fearful? Seductive? Do they have compulsions? Tics? Unusual mannerisms? Tremors? Unusual posturing? Are they relaxed or tense? Do they pace the floor?

4. Do patients know who they are? Who the examiner is? Where they are? What the date is? What does their level of intelligence appear to be? What is their fund of knowledge like? Can they name the past five presidents beginning with the most recent? Do they know something current in the news? What is their recent and past memory like? (Clues to this come when taking the history.) Can they remember three objects after 10 minutes? What is their arithmetic ability like? Can they subtract 7 from 100 and continually go down by 7's (e.g., 100, 93, 86, 79, 72, etc.)? How many numbers can they repeat backward and forward? (Most can do 7 forward and 5 backward.) Can they perform simple mathematics (e.g., 70 − 30, 50 × 3, 10 − 2)? Are they concrete or abstract? Can they interpret proverbs correctly (e.g., People who live in glass houses shouldn't throw stones; A stitch in time saves nine.)? Can they tell how an apple and a pear are alike? Is their judgement good? What would they do if they were in a movie theater and smelled smoke? Can they identify a simple object (e.g., a pen) and its purpose? Is there evidence of a catastrophic reaction during the interview? Confabulation? Occupational delirium?

Examination and interpretation of mental status is often difficult, particularly in cases of children with temperament problems (Mazeade et al, 1990) casting doubt on validity (Rosenthal MJ, 1989). Results must be interpreted in a cultural, educational, and clinical perspective.

Clinical Studies

Every alcoholic who presents with an altered mental status should have a serum alcohol and drug screen drawn to document whether the changes may be explained by intoxication. A toxicology screen will help to identify what a patient might have overdosed on. Urine and blood sugar analysis help to identify patients presenting with mood, thought, or behavioral disturbances secondary to hyperglycemia or hypoglycemia. Serology, HIV, and thyroid function tests may be indicated and the results reviewed prior to a patient's return for a follow-up visit. A CBC and differential should be drawn if an infection or anemia is suspected. An electrocardiogram should be performed in the emergency room if cardiac dysfunction is suggested by history or alteration of pulse.

DIAGNOSES

Differential Diagnosis

Crisis intervention involves the establishment of a differential diagnosis of the behavior changes and tentative diagnosis to direct diagnostic-specific treatment. For instance, a 45-year-old woman without a previous psychiatric history is brought into the emergency room by her family because of an altercation with a neighbor, and is found to be suspicious, distrustful, and have ideas of reference. The differential diagnosis includes the following:

1. Paranoid schizophrenia
2. Delusional depression
3. Delusional disorder
4. Paranoid personality
5. Amphetamine, cocaine, and other sympathomimetic psychoses
6. Other organic states (chronic and acute) such as dementia

Simple verbal intervention with the family is seldom sufficient to manage such a patient in crisis.

Diagnostic Formulation

Following the evaluation, clinicians should integrate their data and write down a presumptive diagnosis and a reasonable differential diagnosis. The *DSM-III-R (Diagnostic and Statistical Manual III, Revised)* of the American Psychiatric Association serves as a guide to this task.

Diagnosis using the *DSM-III-R* is made on five axes. Axis I is concerned with the clinical psychiatric syndrome. Axis II is concerned with personality and specific developmental disorders and Axis III is concerned with physical disorders. The severity of psychosocial stress and the highest level of adaptive functioning during the past year are rated on Axes IV and V. For instance, if an obsessive-compulsive lawyer (who is a senior partner in a large international law firm) without any medical or surgical illness presents acutely intoxicated after she is told that her husband and three children had just burned to death in the family home, her diagnosis using the five axes of the *DSM-III-R* would be as follows:

Axis I	303.00 Alcohol intoxication
Axis II	301.40 Compulsive personality disorder
Axis III	None
Axis IV	Loss of wife and three children unexpectedly in a fire; loss of house and all personal property; severity: 6 catastrophic
Axis V	Highest level of adaptive functioning in the last year: GAF = 85; Current GAF = 60.

In this volume we have complied, wherever possible, with the guidelines of the nosological schema outlined in the *DSM-III- R.*

Diagnostic reliability for broad diagnostic categories such as depression, alcoholism, and psychoses tends to be accurate in the emergency room. Specific diagnosis of psychiatric subtypes such as schizophrenia and bipolar disorder is somewhat less reliable, and there is a tendency to overlook nonalcoholic substance abuse disorders (Lieberman and Baker, 1985).

TREATMENT

Treatment Plan

Sometimes, definitive treatment may be given in the emergency room and the initial treatment plan formulated. For instance, a drug-induced psychosis secondary to LSD (lysergic acid diethylamide) or PCP (phencyclidine) ingestion may be adequately treated with oral or intramuscular benzodiazepines or neuroleptics in the emergency room. Even in such a case, however, a follow-up visit is usually indicated to determine how patient is doing 1 or 2 weeks later and to ascertain if a patient's substance abuse is comorbid with another illness. Comparably, a chronic schizophrenic patient who has an acute exacerbation of symptoms may be treated in the emergency room and not have to enter a hospital.

Use of Restraints

Acutely agitated patients and those who are at imminent risk of harm to themselves or others may need to be restrained in an emergency situation. In every instance, the least restrictive and most humane option—given the circumstances—should be chosen. Chemical restraints (e.g., lorazepam, chlorpromazine, haloperidol, and thiothixene) are preferable to the use of physical restraints. They are both more humane and less restrictive than physical modes of retention. Careful titration of the minimum dose of medication necessary to control the patient's violent or agitated behavior allows the patient to participate more fully in the development of a treatment plan as well as to allow them some freedom to return to more usual activities such as eating, toilet care, and dressing.

Chemical restraints may be contraindicated or insufficient to calm a patient with considerable self- or other-destructive potential in a number of instances. These include when:

1. Violent behavior is part of an underlying organic process that is undiagnosed. Medication may confuse the clinical picture. For instance, phenothiazines, thioxanthenes, and butyrophenones cause generalized slowing on the electroencephalogram. If a cause of a patient's agitation is inflammation of the brain or its meninges, the examining clinician may discount the significance of the generalized slowing of the electroencephalogram as being due to medication if a patient has been given one of the major tranquilizers.
2. Use of significant amounts of medication may be contraindicated. A person who is acutely agitated or self-destructive following a closed head injury in an automobile crash may be vomiting. Patients regurgitating in a sedated state may aspirate and die or develop aspiration pneumonia.
3. Medication takes time to act. Staff may be unable to manage the patient in the interim or may be insufficient in number given the size of a patient or the magnitude of the disturbance.
4. The medication chosen or the amount that can be safely used may be insufficient to calm the patient. Side effects or the medical state of the patient may dictate that physical rather than chemical restraints be used. An older person may have a cardiac condition. Many of the drugs used for acutely agitated patients have strong anticholinergic side effects such as hypotension or increased cardiac irritability. Haloperidol (Haldol) and thiothixene (Navane) are remarkable for their relative safety at high dose levels. Lorazepam has few side effects.

In all of the above mentioned instances, physical rather than chemical restraints may be indicated.

When physical restraints are necessary, the following guidelines should be adhered to:

1. Leather restraints are considered the safest, most effective, and preferred mode of control.
2. If leather restraints are unavailable, heavy webbing may be used with precaution. If a jacket-binder is used, leather restraints should be used in addition to prevent a patient from becoming entangled in the restraint.
3. Rope, wire, chain, elasticized bandages, gauze, and cloth should not be used. These are either inhumane (e.g., chains, rope, and wire) or entail a risk of strangulation of an extremity, which may lead to ischemia of a limb.

4. Staff members should be educated in the indications and use of physical restraints.
5. Regular patient checks should be made to assure that a patient is not unduly restrained, to re-evaluate the possibility of a substitution of chemical for physical restraints, to assure that a patient is not being injured by the restraints, and to maintain the restraining devices.
6. Seclusion rooms, where present, should be considered. If used with good clinical judgment, these are more humane than physical restraints. Patients who have concomitant medical or surgical problems are seldom appropriate for management in a seclusion room (e.g., an acutely suicidal patient who has sustained several fractures when jumping from a building).
7. Patients who are restrained should be placed so as to allow frequent observation by staff.
8. Records should be kept of the rationale for restraint and a notation made indicating why physical restraints rather than other modes of restraint have been used. All such cases should be reviewed.
9. The responsible physician should always be kept alert to changes in a patient's status so that restraints may be removed as soon as possible.
10. Ward structure should minimize the need of both chemical and physical restraints. A staff ratio of at least 1:4 (staff to patient) is preferred but not always possible. The use of staff name tags and regular patient–staff meetings are factors that facilitate management of patients with minimum use of restraints.
11. If there exists an undue number of instances of use of physical restraints, attempts should be made to examine what is happening on the ward. Severely ill psychiatric patients are particularly sensitive to tensions among staff members or between patients or staff and act out more at times of conflict.
12. Frequency of patient behavior leading to restraint and seclusion appears, in part, directly related to stimulation caused by the presence of many other patients and staff members (Phillips and Nasr, 1983).
13. Cold, wet sheet packs are seldom used today but provide a safe alternative to restraint in selected cases when used by experienced individuals (Ross DR et al, 1988).

Patients who are most likely to require restraints are young and of involuntary legal status (Way and Banks, 1990).

Refusal of Medication

The basis of lack of compliance with a consulting psychiatrist's recommendation for medication varies from patient to patient. Common reasons include the following:

1. The patient's lack of understanding of what the etiology of their illness is thought to be and the role of medication in the management of it.
2. The patient's, relatives', and friends' fears of medication and its side effects (e.g., fear of becoming a "zombie").

3. The patient's fear that medication is being used to "control" them (which, of course is true).
4. A lack of rapport between the patient and the psychiatrist medicating the patient.
5. A feeling that medication is being provided in lieu of, rather than as an adjunct to, psychotherapy and sociotherapy.
6. A fear of becoming dependent on medication.
7. A previous bad experience with medication (e.g., the patient had a severe extrapyramidal reaction such as an oculogyric crisis).

A patient's struggle with the clinician over medication may be a re-enactment in a regressed state of the patient's struggles with parents centering around feeding or toilet training.

Management

1. Attempt to develop a relationship with the patient and his or her family and friends. No one likes to be dealt with impersonally. A few moments with a patient and his or her significant others is time well spent and may obviate problems over taking medication in the emergency situation as well as regarding hospitalization and follow-through on outpatient therapy.
2. Explain to the patient the assumed etiology of his or her difficulty and the role and probable mechanism of action of medication in the management of symptoms.
3. Be direct, frank, and authoritative in a discussion of the cost–benefit ratio of the use of medication in a given situation. Every drug has potential side effects. Some are relatively minor but a few are potentially harmful. Comparably severe psychiatric illness has some minor and several major consequences such as job loss, loss of relationships, and self- and other-destructive behavior. A patient and family must weigh options.
4. Avoid complicated schedules of drug administration for ambivalent patients and use the route of intake that is most acceptable. Some patients will refuse oral but accept intramuscular medication. The psychodynamic interpretation at that moment is less important than the need for the patient to have the medication. If it is possible to give all the medication as a single pill, capsule, liquid, or injection without serious side effects, do so.
5. If a patient requiring antipsychotics (such as a paranoid schizophrenic) is recurrently reluctant to take oral medication, use long-acting fluphenazine or haloperidol decanoate or enanthate. If given an appropriate schedule, this will usually hold a patient's symptoms in check.
6. Minimize unnecessary medication.
7. Use psychotropic drugs with minimum side effects. Patients who are ambivalent about taking medication to start with may use side effects as an excuse to discontinue the drug.
8. If a patient is particularly sensitive to a particular side effect of a drug, choose another member of the same class of drugs with the least risk of that effect.
9. Elicit the help of the individuals who have the best relationships with the patient

to encourage the patient to take the medication. These may be family members, friends, clergy, the primary care clinician, or therapist.

State laws vary concerning administration of medication to involuntary or incompetent patients. The general rule of thumb is that, if required in an emergency situation, medication may be given against a patient's will. Incompetent patients usually may be treated if the next of kin or guardian of the patient provides written consent until such a time that the patient may provide it. Certification of commitment alone in some states is not sufficient license for the physician to provide chemotherapy without the consent of the patient (Malmquist, 1979).

Decision to Enter Therapy

In some instances, intervention in a crisis results in the identification by individuals or their families of chronic problems that have been overlooked and that have contributed to bringing about the crisis. During a crisis, clinicians may provide clarification and articulation of problems felt by all and guide a patient into a long-term therapy arrangement. This may prevent further crises and reduce the patient's progression to a psychological state where hospitalization cannot be avoided. If a patient shows evidence of a major depressive disorder, referral to a psychiatrist for antidepressant medication may prevent the development of a psychotic depressive state, especially if a patient has a history of previous psychotic depressive episodes or has a family history of affective illness. Likewise, involvement in couples therapy or family therapy after a patient presents with a drinking problem and depression of a few weeks or months may serve to turn the tide of a potential alcoholic career. Both of these are examples of secondary prevention (i.e., prevention of progression of an illness early in its course with restoration to normal functioning).

Outpatient Care

Outpatient care varies according to a patient's needs and desires. One patient may only wish immediate reduction of anxiety. Another may seek long-term treatment, with the hope that future exacerbations of anxiety or depression can be avoided. Schizophrenics, bipolar patients, and patients addicted to alcohol or drugs may require long-term programs because of the nature of the treatment of these problems. In many instances, exacerbations of illness in this last group occur without apparent cause.

Hospitalization

It is good policy to maintain a readily accessible list of hospitals and the types of services they provide, the specialty inpatient services available in the area, and the types of financial or insurance coverage required in the emergency room. This list allows clinicians to present to patients and their families a number of treatment alternatives when hospitalization is necessary.

Inpatient psychiatric treatment may be required if there is an absence of adequate or responsible social support. In some cases, regardless of the nature of the patient's social matrices and the degree of responsibility of their relatives and friends, hospitalization is required. Such cases would include the following:

1. Markedly suicidal patients
2. Markedly homicidal patients
3. Patients with psychosis without rapid remission
4. Demented patients who can no longer be cared for at home
5. Manic patients
6. Stuporous, depressed patients
7. Patients in catatonic stupor or excitement
8. Schizophrenic patients with command hallucinations

Disposition is governed by adequacy of social support. A moderately suicidal patient with supportive family and friends may not require inpatient care, whereas a mildly suicidal patient who is middle-aged, divorced, male, friendless, homeless, homosexual, and alcoholic may require hospitalization.

Crisis Psychotherapy

Crisis-oriented therapy tends to be an amalgam of many types of therapy, particularly supportive psychotherapy and cognitive therapy. Supportive psychotherapy as is practiced in an emergency setting is more than a supportive relationship. The technique is characterized by a style of communication that includes elements of respect, self-disclosure, interpretation, advice, and praise (Winston et al, 1986). Cognitive therapy approaches involve active intervention with the cognitive process mediating the perception of environmental information and the consequent behavioral response (Davis and Casey, 1990).

The goal of crisis intervention is to minimize impairment, to rapidly restore an individual to asymptomatic functioning, and to facilitate individual growth. Ideally, individuals should be better for having been through a crisis that allows them (and those close to them) to become aware of what their resources and values are, what their liabilities are, and how they may be minimized. Hospitalization, particularly in a psychiatric setting (as opposed to a general medical setting), is to be avoided whenever possible. This entails a heightened awareness of what resources are available in a community and how they may be brought to bear on resolution of the crisis outside of the hospital (Stein and Test, 1980; Weisbrod et al, 1980). Social support is sought to facilitate the patient in mastering a stressful situation in the form of cognitive guidance and emotional support that compensates for the reduction in problem-solving capacity resulting from stress-induced emotional arousal (Caplan, 1981). Successful crisis therapy entails a sophisticated awareness of how each individual may uniquely rally his or her defenses to facilitate functioning at a time of stress. The use of denial, for instance, may augment or diminish risk in life-threatening physical illness crises such as that associated with coronary heart disease (Dimsdale and Hackett, 1982).

After diagnosis there arises the question of what immediate psychotherapeutic or psychopharmacologic interventions should be employed and whether the patient should be hospitalized. Not hospitalizing a patient, as many clinicians well know, often requires more effort than that which is involved in expeditious hospitalization. Many chronically psychotic and some acutely psychotic patients can be managed as outpatients if clinicians themselves have the time or if other agencies have resources to provide careful monitoring of both the patient's pharmacotherapy and the individual and/or family therapy that may be needed. Many patients in the emergency room can be managed either by crisis intervention with one or two follow-up visits or by referral to an outpatient therapist or agency. The remainder may require hospitalization for alcohol or narcotic detoxification, or because their behavior is so self- or other-destructive that they cannot be managed outside of a hospital. There is a group of patients who are hospitalized primarily because they lack the social supports of family and friends.

Alternatives to Hospitalization

Dispositions other than outpatient or inpatient care are available, and in some cases are more effective than more traditional psychiatric care. These include the following:

1. Alcoholics Anonymous
2. Methadone maintenance programs
3. Drug treatment programs
4. Church groups
5. Women's and men's centers
6. Half-way houses
7. Family services
8. Ethnic and community health clinics
9. Acute non-hospitals (Brunton and Hawthorne, 1990)
10. Crisis houses and lodges (Weisman G, 1985)
11. Board and care homes (Floisman, 1989)

Acute non-hospital programs provide an alternative to entirely inpatient treatment in some instances or for the latter component in those who are initially on a locked ward or who are involuntary patients (Weisman G, 1985; Brunton and Hawthorne, 1990). Structure is similar to a hospital without the specifics of a medical environment. Board and care homes, on the other hand, provide unlocked shelter, three meals a day, and supervision of medication for recently discharged psychiatric patients. They do not have the structure of a non-hospital unit and do not have a scheduled program of therapy and rehabilitation activities.

Self-Help Groups

Nothing helps one to understand as much as to be understood. Hearing words that you think spoken by others and emotions that you feel and have felt articulated by others is healing and gives you a sense of control as you learn that how you think, feel, and act in response to a life crisis is to be expected and has a particular course. Survivor groups help those who have survived the loss of a loved one to suicide. Compassionate friends help families who have lost a child to illness or trauma. Depression and manic-depressive groups help those who suffer affective illness and their spouses. The list of self-help groups is almost infinite: AA, NA, CA, Eating Disorder Groups, gay groups, single parent groups, Alanon, Alateen, women's groups, men's groups, post-colostomy groups, post-mastectomy groups, urinary incontinence groups, AIDS groups, relatives of AIDS patients groups, etc. Circumstances of contemporary life have eroded the natural supportive structures—the family and the church—that have long provided external support when internal crises arise following adverse or positive life events. Historically, women have provided this more for each other than have men (Goldberg MC, 1990), but today, women, especially single parents and professional women, find supportive relations lacking. The goals for seeking support from self-help groups vary and include relief of symptoms, desire for a supportive community, help in recovery from trauma, opportunity to help others, and help in coping with bereavement (Young and Williams, 1988). Self-help groups, alone or as an adjunctive intervention, are an important resource used in crisis intervention.

Transportation of Acutely Psychotic Patients

1. Patients who are to be transported to another treatment site should be appropriately medicated. There are a variety of methods available to sedate agitated patients and a number of side effects that the clinician must be alert to. If patients receive intramuscular doses of medication and are sent off without allowing some time for observation, they may arrive dystonic (especially after haloperidol, thiothixene, and fluphenazine). Therefore, some time should be allowed to lapse in order to assess the possible extent of any adverse side effects to medication.

2. Ambulance drivers should be informed of possible difficulties. If patients are potentially homicidal, they should be humanely but adequately restrained. If suicidal or homicidal, they should be searched after commitment for concealed weapons (e.g., a loaded gun or knife) or concealed drugs (e.g., a supply of barbiturates or cocaine).

3. Unless there is evidence that patients are currently overtly violent, they should be given an opportunity to cooperate before they are labeled dangerous. Patience, understanding, and calm reassurance are valuable tools in managing potentially dangerous patients. If there is concern on the part of the clinician, or concern voiced by patients that they may erupt, oral medication should be given to calm the patient. When a patient has recognized a need for more medication and has volitionally taken more oral medication, they feel they have some control over what is happening to them.

4. Patients who are not committed cannot be forced against their will to be taken to or from a hospital. Unless a patient has been committed, they must be assumed to be within their legal rights to protest hospitalization and transportation to or from a hospital. To do so against their will could constitute liability for a suit for kidnapping.

5. Patients should never be deceived about their destination. Families may have told patients that they were going to see a nonpsychiatric physician. The psychi-

atrist should not collude with this deception as it undermines further faith in the physician's word.

6. An ambulance service may require that all patients, even those with no potential for violence, be restrained. If patients are to be restrained, they should be told they will be, or that it is ambulance policy. If they are violent and it is necessary to restrain them for both their own protection and that of the ambulance crew, it should not be undertaken until adequate personnel are available to help. Family members and patients' friends may be of great value in calming them. Once in restraints, many patients feel more comfortable and secure, resting assured that they are controlled and their violent behavior in check.

7. A woman should always accompany a female patient in the ambulance. A delusional patient may fantasize that she was sexually abused. The presence of a female attendant as witness assures protection for both patient and crew.

8. It is seldom that psychiatric patients require speedy arrival at a hospital, particularly if properly restrained and medicated by an evaluating physician. Rapidly blinking lights and a loud siren may aggravate a patient's already decompensated condition. Driving at the usual speed with calm, mature attendants is usually the best transportation that can be provided for a disturbed patient.

9. If there is any question of a serious nonpsychiatric medical problem, the patient should be medically and surgically cleared before being transported over a great distance to a receiving psychiatric hospital from an emergency room. Neither ambulance personnel nor the staff of a large psychiatric hospital, public or private, are equipped to handle medical emergencies as well as a staffed general hospital emergency room. Sometimes nonpsychiatric medical staff are unaware of the limitations of psychiatric hospitals in managing medical and surgical problems. If they are reluctant to examine a psychiatric patient or if they perform only a cursory exam, they should be tactfully reminded that just as they are not experts in the evaluation and treatment of psychiatric patients, neither are psychiatrists expert surgeons and internists.

10. It is not possible to overemphasize the importance of maintaining good rapport with nonmedical members of the community who work with acutely disturbed patients. Included in this group are ambulance drivers, clergy, police officers, and firemen. High-quality care at a time of crisis requires smooth communications among a number of concerned care givers. One way to achieve this is by the participation of emergency room staff in educational programs for the community. Seminars provide excellent opportunities for the exchange of information about frequently encountered problems, and as a forum to develop ways inwhich all members of caregiving teams can better work together at times of crisis.

Special Techniques | 4

SERUM PSYCHOTROPIC DRUG LEVELS

1. Failure to respond to antidepressants may relate to inadequate plasma drug concentration.
2. Most dose–response curves are such that the greater the dosage, the more likely the response.
3. Nortriptyline is unique in that plasma a concentration of 50 to 150 ng/ml defines a therapeutic range. This is referred to as a "therapeutic window." Concentrations both below and above are inadequate to treat depression (Sorensen et al, 1978).
4. While it is valuable in some cases to monitor serum antidepressant levels in specific instances, routine monitoring is not usually required (Hollister et al, 1980).
5. Individuals receiving customary doses of tricyclic antidepressants have been found to have serum levels in the toxic range (Hollister, 1979). In addition, individuals vary in both clinical and toxic response to serum levels of a drug within so-called normal ranges.
6. The variability in rates of tricyclic and tetracyclic metabolism is so great that some individuals will develop significant and sometimes fatal alterations in cardiac contractibility and conductivity upon receiving doses that are safe for other patients.
7. High tricyclic and tetracyclic serum levels may lead a clinician to mistakenly assume a patient has overdosed (Coryell and Sherman, 1982).
8. Tricyclic antidepressants have a quinidine-like effect (Kantor et al, 1978). Quinidine-like drugs and tricyclic antidepressants, when given together, will act additively.
9. Phenothiazines, when administered alone or in combination drugs such as Triavil (perphenazine and amitriptyline), increase steady state levels of tricyclic antidepressants (Gram and Overo, 1972).
10. Electrocardiographic indication of a widened QRS interval arouses suspicion that antidepressant dosage is inappropriate. Dosage should be lowered in such instances to prevent further alterations in conduction that may lead to cardiac arrest

BARBITURATE TOLERANCE TEST

When a patient gives a history of barbiturate abuse, or denies it but physicians feel there is a strong likelihood that the patient does abuse barbiturates, they may want to conduct a barbiturate tolerance test in order to ascertain whether or not the patient must be covered for withdrawal symptoms. The test is usually performed on the morning after a patient has been admitted to an inpatient unit. The usual procedure is as follows:

1. A test dose of 200 mg of pentobarbital is given orally.
2. One hour later the patient is examined for signs of clinical toxicity.
3. If the patient is not tolerant at the end of 1 hour, they will be soundly asleep but arousable.
4. If a patient is tolerant to a dose of less than 500 mg, gross ataxia, pseudotoxicosis, nystagmus, somnolence, and Romberg's sign are present.
5. If tolerant to 500 or 600 mg, the patient will show mild ataxia, nystagmus, and perhaps dysarthria.
6. Nystagmus would be the only sign in a patient tolerant to 700 to 800 mg.
7. If the patient is tolerant to 900 mg or more of pentobarbital, they should show no signs of intoxication 1 hour after a 200 mg test dose. In such instances a test dose of 300 mg should be tried.

For a valid interpretation of the above test, it is assumed the patient is not presently withdrawing nor intoxicated. Agitation and severe anxiety may raise the tolerance. The elderly and very debilitated may require only a 100 mg dose of pentobarbital. The clinician should be certain that the patient received and took the entire test dose.

DEXAMETHASONE SUPPRESSION TEST

1. The dexamethasone suppression test (DST) is often used to access neuroendocrine dysfunction in patients suffering from depression (Carroll et al, 1981) and other types of psychiatric disorders, and to monitor the course of recovery (Rothschild and Schatzberg, 1982).
2. It is postulated that because central serotonergic activity stimulates the pituitary–adrenal axis and noradrenergic activity inhibits the axis, response to dexamethasone can be used to predict response to antidepressants (Fraser AR, 1983).
3. The usual procedure is to give the patient 1 mg of dexamethasone at 11:00 PM and to obtain blood samples at 4:00 PM and 11:00 PM the following day and determine the patient's cortisol level by fluorimetry (Carroll et al, 1981).
4. Abnormal plasma cortisol concentrations are reported to occur almost exclusively in endogenously depressed patients. Carroll et al (1981) claim a sensitivity of 67% and a specificity of 96% if the version of the DST test described above is employed. However, abnormalities are also reported to occur with a number of other conditions including degenerative dementia (Raskin et al, 1982), recent weight loss (Edelstein et al, 1983), and chronic schizophrenia (Dewan et al, 1982).
5. Nonsuppression is helpful in distinguishing individuals with primary unipolar

depression from secondary unipolar depression (i.e., depression in a person with a pre-existing nonaffective psychiatric disorder such as panic disorder, obsessive–compulsive disorder, anxiety disorders, drug dependence, schizophrenia, senile dementia, or alcoholism) (Schlesser et al, 1980; Brown and Shuey, 1980; Evans et al, 1983a; Pesslow et al, 1983; Peterson et al, 1985a).

6. Patients with unipolar affective illness who are nonsuppressors tend to have a good response to thymoleptic treatment (Brown and Shuey, 1980).

7. Patients who are nonsuppressors and psychotic tend to have mood-congruent psychoses (Schatzberg et al, 1983).

8. The DST has been found to vary in its usefulness in identifying adolescents with primary unipolar affective illness (Extein et al, 1982; Targum and Capodanno, 1983).

9. Despite prominent depressive symptoms, the majority of patients with the diagnosis of a borderline disorder have a normal DST (Soloff et al, 1982).

10. In some instances, the DST has been useful in distinguishing pseudodementia (depression associated with cognitive deficits) from delirium or dementia (McAllister et al, 1982).

11. The fact that several researchers have failed to find abnormal DSTs in patients with panic disorder and agoraphobia suggests that panic attacks and unipolar affective disorders are separate illnesses and that the antipanic properties of drugs such as phenelzine and imipramine are separate from their antidepressant actions (Curtis et al, 1982).

12. Preliminary data on children who meet Research Diagnostic Criteria and *DSM-III-R* criteria for major depressive disorders suggests that the DST is less useful in identifying severely depressed children (Geller B et al, 1983; Petty et al, 1985).

13. Bipolar depressed patients tend to be nonsuppressors more than bipolar manic patients (Evans and Nemeroff, 1983; Arana et al, 1983).

14. Outpatients with major depressive disorder are more likely to be nonsuppressors than those outpatients with other illnesses (Jaffe et al, 1983).

15. DST appears useful in screening for primary affective illness among recently abstinent alcohol abusers (Swartz and Dunner, 1982).

16. Patients with bipolar affective illness show increased variability in hormonal response using multiple neuroendocrine indices including the thyrotropin-releasing hormone test, the insulin tolerance test, the gonadotropin-releasing hormone test, and the DST (Amsterdam et al, 1983).

17. Response to the DST is used as an indicant of clinical progress in patients receiving antidepressants (Greden et al, 1983; Krishnan et al, 1983). Most non-suppressors have progressive normalization of the DST with clinical improvement. Failure to normalize is associated with poor clinical outcome. Some patients with baseline nonsuppression become nonsuppressors again upon withdrawal of antidepressants.

18. The use of the DST should be preceded by an assessment of the validity of the cortisol level determinations in the critical range (in the laboratory used), as values vary with the technique employed (Meltzer and Fang, 1983).

19. Nocturnal increase in plasma cortisol concentration occurs significantly closer to sleep onset in depressed patients (Jarrett et al, 1983).
20. One-milligram doses of dexamethasone are more effective than 2-mg doses in identifying depressed patients who are nonsuppressors (Brown WA et al, 1983).
21. An initial positive result on the DST test in major depression does not increase the likelihood of response to antidepressants nor is lack of a positive response reason for withholding antidepressants (APA Task Force on Laboratory Tests in Psychiatry, 1987).
22. While age does not correlate significantly with post-dexamethasone cortisol levels measured by competitive protein binding assay, it does when levels are measured by radioimmunoassay (Rosenbaum AH et al, 1984).
23. Information from the DST is maximized using receiver operating characteristic analyses to assess the test's overall performance and to select cortisol cutoffs (Mossman and Somoza, 1989).
24. Post-dexamethasone beta endorphin may prove to be the most specific reflection of a disorder in the negative feedback seen with dexamethasone in depression. Cortisol values and post-dexamethasone beta endorphin levels are positively correlated with nonsuppressors exhibiting higher post-dexamethasone beta endorphin levels (Maes et al, 1990).
25. Withdrawal from psychotropic medication (i.e., antidepressants, benzodiazepines, neuroleptics) is an unappreciated, confounding variable in DST studies with increased positive DST tests reported in patients recently withdrawn from psychotropic drugs (Kraus et al, 1987).

COMPUTED TOMOGRAPHY

1. Computed tomography (CT) scans have been used to identify structural abnormalities of the brain such as enlarged ventricular spaces, widened sulci, and space-occupying lesions.
2. There is some suggestion (Golden CJ et al, 1981) that there are primary structural deficits in some schizophrenic patients in and around the anterior areas of the left (dominant) hemisphere, although not all researchers find differences between the normal and schizophrenic brain subjects (Jernigan et al, 1982b).
3. Senile patients characteristically exhibit changes in the medial temporal lobe, anterior frontal lobe, and head of the caudate on CT scan (Bondareff et al, 1981).
4. Ventricular enlargement and cortical atrophy may predate the onset of psychosis in a subset of schizophrenic patients (Weinberger et al, 1982). These changes are not found in all schizophrenics (Jernigan et al, 1982b).
5. The enlargement of the ventricles reported in bipolar patients appears unrelated to age, as is the case with schizophrenia, whereas enlargement with depressed patients does relate to age, cognitive impairment, substance abuse, response to treatment, history of ECT, and other clinical variables that do not correlate with the ventricular changes in bipolar patients (Andreasen et al, 1990).
6. Review of outcomes of CT scans on groups of 45 (Battaglia and Spector, 1988)

and 4,600 patients (Beresford et al, 1986) indicates that CT scan for an initial episode of psychosis should be an option based on clinical judgment rather than routine. Findings on mental status examination are more predictive of abnormal CT scans than is focal pathology (Beresford et al, 1986).

METHYLPHENIDATE TEST

1. Mood elevation after ingestion of methylphenidate predicts positive response to imipramine or desipramine but not to nortriptyline or amitriptyline (Sabelli et al, 1983).
2. Patients who fail to improve their moods with methylphenidate often respond to nortriptyline or amitriptyline but not to desipramine.
3. Lack of response to nortriptyline of patients who respond to methylphenidate puts into question the assumption that nortriptyline blocks norepinephrine uptake.

MHPG

1. Plasma and urinary MHPG (3-methoxy-4-hydroxyphenethyleneglycol) levels are used in studying noradrenergic functioning in normal and abnormal behavioral states.
2. Depressed patients with decreased MHPG excretion do significantly better on nortriptyline than high excreters suggesting MHPG excretion may predict response to specific antidepressants (Hollister et al, 1980).
3. Drugs that act on the noradrenergic system produce more symptomatic relief for depressed patients with low MHPG than do those that impact on serotonergic systems (Rosenbaum et al, 1980). The tricyclic imipramine and the tetracyclic maprotiline exert potent effects on norepinephrine uptake (Maas, 1978; Maitre et al, 1975).
4. Patients who are at less than 80% of their ideal weight (e.g., patients with anorexia nervosa) have low 24-hour urinary MHPG levels regardless of mood (Gerner and Gwirtsman, 1981).
5. Very high positive correlation exists between urinary free cortisol and MHPG in depressed patients but *not* in control subjects (Rosenbaum et al, 1983).
6. No significant correlations are found between plasma free and conjugated MHPG or between plasma free MHPG and total urinary MHPG (Sweeney et al, 1980).

POSITRON TOMOGRAPHY

Regional cerebral glucose consumption is measured by means of a technique employing glucose labeled with fluorine with positron-emission tomography (PET scan). The technique has been applied to the study of regional abnormalities of brain metabolism in patients with a variety of neurologic and psychiatric disorders. Individuals with schizophrenia have been shown to have lower glucose use in the frontal regions than normal control subjects (Buchsbaum et al, 1982). These findings are consistent with those of cerebral blood flow that comparably has been found to be lower in the frontal regions (Ingvar, 1980).

NUCLEAR MAGNETIC RESONANCE IMAGING

1. Nuclear magnetic resonance imaging (MRI) is useful for both pathophysiologic and pathoanatomic investigation (DeMyer et al, 1985).
2. Images derive from chemical interactions within the tissues, revealing information about energy transfers within the intact brain.
3. MRI is best used after a CT scan has not been able to definitively evaluate a psychiatric symptom or presentation or in lieu of CT scan when type or location of a neuropathologic liaison is better visualized by MRI techniques (Garber et al, 1988).

BRAIN MAPPING

Brain mapping is a term used for topographic mapping and frequency analysis derived from electroencephalographic techniques such as the EEG and evoked potentials. Several color displays allow somewhat simpler interpretation than the conventional EEG (Nower, 1989). There are advantages and disadvantages to the technique, which limit its clinical usefulness. A number of features of the routine EEG may be missed and new artifacts introduced by the computer. Epileptogenic spikes may, for instance, be overlooked or deemed artifactual and transient slowing may be missed (Nower, 1989). Assessment of results entails specific reference to standards for age, state of alertness, gender, medication, and other factors (Nower, 1989). Brain mapping appears most useful as a complement to other diagnostic techniques (Garber et al, 1988) and has limited value in the emergency setting.

SODIUM AMYTAL INTERVIEW

1. Narcosynthesis is used in the emergency setting for evaluation of conversion symptoms, psychogenic amnesia, catatonia, hysterical stupor, and unexplained mutism, and for distinguishing between organic, depressive, and schizophrenic stuporous states.
2. Patients who are in psychogenic, catatonic stupor may become violent when given sodium amytal. However, the usual response is that of facilitating the patient in providing a history for the evaluating clinician.

3. Patients with organic illnesses may become symptomatically worse when given sodium amytal.
4. Sodium amytal may be used for treatment of post-traumatic stress disorder, for recovery of function in conversion hysteria, and for recovery of memory in psychogenic fugue and amnesic states.
5. Amytal interviews should not be given to patients who are paranoid, who refuse the drug, and who fear being abused or assaulted.
6. Contraindications to use include severe hepatic or renal impairment, a history of porphyria, barbiturate addiction, hypotension, and presence of upper respiratory inflammation that may obstruct the airway (Perry and Jacobs, 1982).
7. Adverse effects seldom occur in appropriately chosen patients.
8. The usual procedure is injection of a 5% solution of sodium amytal (500 mg of amytal dissolved in 10 cc of sterile water) at a rate no greater than one cc/min (50 mg/min) to prevent sleep or sudden respiratory depression, through a narrow bore scalp vein needle until drowsiness, slight slurring of speech, or sustained rapid lateral nystagmus is noted. This point is usually reached between 150 mg (3 cc) and 350 mg (7cc). At this point the patient is interviewed as in any other psychiatric situation. One-half to one cc additional amytal solution may be needed every five minutes or so to maintain the level of narcosis (Perry and Jacobs, 1982).

TSH TEST

1. Serum thyrotropin (TSH) response to thyrotropin-releasing hormone has been found to be deficit in some euthyroid-depressed patients.
2. The deficiency is believed to reflect a defect in central regulation of the pituitary–thyroid axis (Loosen and Prange, 1982).
3. It is felt that the blunted TSH response may serve as a trait marker for depression and possibly alcoholism.
4. Patients who exhibit TSH blunting have been found to have reduced TSH (but normal prolactin) levels before and after TSH administration although their thyroid hormone and cortical levels are normal (Loosen et al, 1983).

LACTATE TOLERANCE TEST

Intravenous infusion of sodium lactate has been found to produce panic attacks in some patients with panic disorder. The mechanism of production of the attacks by lactate infusion is unknown. Normal controls and patients with psychiatric disorders other than panic disorder are less sensitive to lactate (Cowley and Arana, 1990). Absence of data on the sensitivity and specifics of this test and of objective criteria for lactate-induced panic limit the clinical usefulness of the test (Cowley and Arana, 1990). Clinical history is of greater value in most instances. This test holds some promise of value in subtyping panic disorder patients. The fact that catecholamines may be elevated in some types of panic suggests that there may be other biologic parameters such as cholesterol that may vary with cause of the illness and its treatment (Lancer et al, 1990).

HYPNOSIS

Hypnosis is used in the emergency setting to facilitate abreaction as well as specifically in the treatment of conversion symptoms. In both instances its use is somewhat comparable to that of narcosynthesis. Altered states of awareness occur rapidly and spontaneously in patients who have undergone severe trauma such as rape or have survived a plane or auto crash, making hypnosis an especially important adjunctive therapy in the emergency situation (Wain and Amen, 1986).

Psychiatric Emergencies | 5

ABDOMINAL PAIN OF PSYCHOGENIC ORIGIN

Children and adults present with abdominal pain of psychogenic origin. Only 5 to 10% of children (Hodges et al, 1985) and 60% of adults in one study (Eisendrath et al, 1986) have been identified to have recurrent abdominal pain of organic origin. The other 90 to 95% of children and 40% of adults suffer psychogenic abdominal pain.

History
1. The modal patient tends to be a woman with a history of loss (Drossman, 1982).
2. Characterologic patterns of those seen vary but include patients with borderline personality disorders, histrionic personality disorders, major and minor depressive disorders, hypochondrias, and somatization disorders.
3. Psychogenic abdominal pain may accompany pain of organic origin much as pseudodementia may accompany true dementia.
4. Absence of personality disorder and short duration of pain are associated with a better prognosis (Drossman, 1982).
5. Recurrent abdominal pain is the most common complaint of children age 6 to 15 years, with only 5% having an identifiable organic etiology (Schoefer and Millman, 1979). Several studies have indicated that as great as 10% of school children are so affected that their functioning is compromised (Astrada et al, 1981).
6. Psychiatric correlates of psychogenic abdominal pain in children vary with age and sex. Anxiety disorders were found commonly among younger children while conversion disorders were found to occur more with older children and girls (Astrada et al, 1981).
7. There is some evidence to suggest that 25 to 40% of children with recurrent abdominal pain may suffer from lactose intolerance (Liebman, 1979; Barr et al, 1979).
8. Children with the disorder and their mothers and fathers report significantly more anxiety than healthy children and their parents (Hodges et al, 1985).
9. Psychogenic abdominal pain patients are characterized by the prominence of guilt, past evidence of somatization and polysymptomatic behavior and a history of physical abuse by spouse or parent (Eisendrath et al, 1986).

Management
1. Surgical and medical consultation is required to investigate nonpsychogenic causes of abdominal discomfort. As some of these causes may demand

immediate intervention (e.g., acute appendicitis, dissecting aortic aneurysm, acute porphyria, renal stone, ruptured spleen) it may be necessary to seek emergency medical or surgical consultation.

2. Psychotherapeutic and psychopharmacologic management of abdominal pain associated with a specific disorder (e.g., somatization disorder, generalized anxiety disorder, major depressive disorder) depends on diagnosis.

3. When no specific disorder is found to accompany the psychogenic pain, psychotherapy may be used. Pain rarely entirely resolves but improvement in psychosocial functioning may occur (Drakkman, 1983).

Quality Assurance Issues

1. Proper assessment of the patient is an essential element in assuring quality emergency care for abdominal pain.

2. The patient experiencing abdominal pain and crisis must be stabilized to assure proper assessment.

3. Establishing the absence of an organic basis for the patient's discomfort is critical.

4. The identification of psychosocial problems is a rate-limiting step that requires sensitizing emergency room clinicians to the range of factors that are psychosocial and their presence in a particular patient (Bingham et al, 1990).

5. The presumptive diagnosis and urgency surrounding the crisis should lead to successful referral to the next appropriate level of care, be it medical, surgical or psychiatric (Sateia et al, 1990).

Ethical/Legal Issues

1. The patient in emergency crisis is in a compromised state and may be unaware of his or her rights for proper disclosure of diagnosis and treatment options and to provide informed consent (President's Commission Report, 1982).

2. Clinicians in emergency rooms handling the patient with abdominal pain must adhere to acceptable standards of care for arriving at a differential diagnosis, set of treatment options, and appropriate referral (Tancredi, 1982).

ABUSE: PHYSICAL

Children, parents, and spouses of both sexes may report being physically or psychologically abused by a "family" member.

History

1. In some instances, clinicians identify burns, cuts, bruises, or fractures that appear to have resulted from human abuse rather than unintentional injury, despite the patient's statement to the contrary.

2. Abused patients may deny physical abuse because of fear of future physical assault, fear of abandonment financially and psychologically, and low self-esteem.

3. The "battered elder syndrome" and "battered parent syndrome" entail active

physical assault, verbal and psychological assault, misuse or theft of money or property, withholding basic life resources, financial dependence and exploitation, misuse and abuse of drugs, forced entry into a nursing home, and failure to provide care for the physically dependent (Rathbone-McCuan and Voyles, 1982).

4. Several separations from an abusing spouse may occur before the fantasy of change within a marriage ends and a firm separation occurs (Hilberman, 1980).

5. Abused spouses and parents may refuse help from a caregiver because they fear it will not be effective.

6. Abused children may fail to cooperate with a caregiver for fear of reprisal from an abusing parent.

7. Factors that limit constructive resolution of a problem of abuse include victims' depression, passivity, self-blame, and learned helplessness, and external factors such as physical disability, economic dependence on the abuser, or homicidal threats from the abuser (Hilberman, 1980).

8. In one study, it was found that the average length of abuse for a group of women was 6.7 years before seeking help. Eighty percent stated that abuse began in the first year of the relationship, and for 48% it occurred regularly at the rate of more than once a month.

Signs

1. Lacerations and abrasions on the eyes, lips, and other parts of the body.

2. Chain and rope burns from confinement, cigarette burns, and burns caused by other means such as a hot stove or boiling water.

3. Head injuries such as signs of hemorrhage beneath the scalp and absence of hair due to vigorous hair pulling.

4. Welts and bruises on the legs, shoulders, back, chest, or arms (Rathbone-McCuan and Voyles, 1982).

Management

1. The first step in appropriate management involves recognition of physical indicators, fearful behavior by the victim, and the abusing family member's disinterest or aggressive behavior (Rathbone-McCuan and Voyles, 1982).

2. Careful assessment must be made of intrapsychic and environmental factors that limit or can be mobilized to facilitate constructive resolution (Hilberman, 1980).

3. All resources available that may be used to constructively solve the problem should be rallied. These may include personal strengths, concerned family and friends, and institutional resources for economic, vocational, educational, and legal support.

4. If an abused individual has medical or psychiatric problems (e.g., fractures or depression) that need attention (e.g., orthopedic consultation, antidepressant medication), such should be provided.

5. Battered spouse groups are helpful in the process of separating from an abusing spouse or lover.

6. Shelters should be identified where a battered spouse may go during the transi-

tion from the site of abuse to an alternate living arrangement, until legal protection can be afforded to allow the spouses or lovers to recover their just property.

7. The best approach to the management of child and elderly abuse is a team approach with sufficient representation on the team to allow all resources to bear on the problem. Child abuse and elderly abuse teams are usually composed of a pediatrician or gerontologist, social worker, nurse, psychiatrist, psychologist, case worker, and legal consultant.

8. In the case of an emergency or when an abuse team is not available for referral, it may be necessary for a clinician to intervene directly with child protection and social service agencies, hospitals, and law enforcers (Hilberman, 1980). Successful intervention entails anticipating the worst and preparing for it.

9. When prescribing antidepressant medication to depressed victims of abuse who feel trapped by circumstances, clinicians should be aware of both the danger of overdose, as the victim may attempt suicide, and of the violence potential of victims. Abused individuals may seek help both when they see their own lives as threatened as well as when they feel they are losing control of their own aggressive urges toward parents, spouse, lover, or children.

10. Hospitalization is indicated when:

    a. Protection is needed for a minor until social welfare and legal resources may be mobilized to facilitate a more appropriate disposition.
    b. Physical injury is so severe that immediate medical care is indicated.
    c. A psychiatric illness is present of sufficient severity to require management in an inpatient facility.

11. Coordinated treatment of an abused child, spouse, lover, or parent entails resources for immediate protection and crisis intervention; clothing, shelter and food; psychiatric, legal and medical help; psychotherapy and counseling; and alternate living arrangements.

12. Small doses of antianxiety agents or antidepressants may be necessary for the sleep disturbance and agitation associated with leaving a relationship of great abuse.

13. Medical facilities are needed for medical and psychiatric treatment and reproductive advice in the case of battered women.

14. Legal resources are needed for court procedures, protective custody, temporary guardianship, warrants, and separation and divorce agreements.

15. Social service agencies are required for emergency shelter, clothing, housing, financial assistance and food stamps, and access to child protective agencies.

16. Criminal justice resources are needed for protection against further violence.

17. Vocational rehabilitation programs are needed for abused spouses in need of training for employment to enable them to provide for themselves.

18. The abuser should be referred for evaluation. Where it appears the abuser's behavior is the result of a treatable mental illness, he or she should be referred for appropriate psychiatric management (Goodstein and Page, 1981).

Quality Assurance Issues

1. Determine the effectiveness of the emergency room staff to recognize and

document the presence of abuse of children, parents, and spouses. The responsibility does not end with diagnosis but includes the provision of appropriate care and meeting legal reporting requirements. Determination of effectiveness can be established through intensive case review involving varying levels of severity (Caplan et al, 1991).

2. The diagnostic process, of course, includes the appropriate ruling out of alternative explanations. Given the significance of abuse both legally and socially, the proper valuation of alternative explanations is essential.

3. Quality care includes family assessment. This involves meeting with immediate family members, especially care-givers, to ascertain the nature of their relationship with the patient, and reasons for physical signs of abuse.

Ethical/Legal Issues

1. In all 50 states, the physician is obligated to report child abuse if suspected. Some states extend that obligation to other clinicians and individuals such as teachers and school administrators in the position to know if abuse is occurring. Many states include reporting of the abuse of elderly persons as mandatory. Where not required, the physician may still report to protect a patient or others. In states where reporting is required, the legislation generally includes a defense against claims of invasion of privacy or defamation of character.

2. To whatever extent possible, the law leans in the direction of maintaining the integrity of the family, perhaps with involvement of protective services (part of comprehensive state programs for child welfare) for abused or neglected children to effect changes within the family structure (Kemp and Helfer, 1972). However, where it is virtually impossible to correct a family situation, it may be necessary to resort to the legal system. Juvenile courts are empowered to review alleged cases of neglect and, where necessary, can remove children from the family.

3. State laws also provide for intervention in the care of children (and incompetent individuals) where parents and caretakers refuse a necessary treatment. Such refusals may be for religious or personal reasons rather than motivated by abuse or neglect and may well be honored where an adult decides for himself, but not when he or she decides for a child or incompetent adult. The state's power for intervention comes under *parens patriae*, the assumption that refusal of essential and particularly lifesaving treatment is a type of "neglect."

ACCIDENTS

Accidents, homicides, and suicides taken together are the leading cause of death in the age group 1 to 39 years.

History

1. While violent deaths have tended to decrease since 1900, the violent death rate is currently the highest ever recorded among 15- to 24-year-olds.

2. Accidental deaths, suicides, and homicides are not unrelated. All represent self-destructive tendencies.
3. Homicides may be victim-precipitated and represent suicides.
4. Low tension tolerance, substance abuse, paranoia, personality disorders, and immaturity are risk factors for accidents (Tsuang et al, 1985).
5. Depression with concomitant suicidal tendencies may lead to risk-taking and accident-proneness resulting in fatal or near fatal vehicular accidents.
6. The increased importance of violent deaths as a cause of mortality reflects the decrease in importance of other causes of death (such as infectious illness) among the young.
7. A small number of single-vehicle accidents have been demonstrated to be suicides.

Management

1. All accident victims should be evaluated as to the degree that self-imposed risks or self-destructiveness have contributed to an accident.
2. If an individual has a history of reported accidents or appears overly depressed, a referral for treatment should be made.
3. Some individuals' risk-taking behavior or self-destructiveness may be complicated by an alcohol or other substance abuse problem necessitating combined therapy for the substance abuse problem and underlying depression.

Quality Assurance Issues

1. Was an accident just an accident or is there a pattern of self-injury? Such a pattern might suggest a physical condition, such as failing vision and hearing or cardiac induced syncope, or an evolving neurologic disease as well as depression. Was the patient referred for neurologic or psychiatric evaluation and treatment?
2. Are the accidents a result of occult or overt alcohol or other substance abuse? Were serum alcohol and drug screens drawn? It is also necessary to evaluate any medications that the patient may be using to determine if they are being used in correct dosages or if legitimate drugs have been prescribed by one or more physicians, which in combination cause serious adverse effects.

Ethical/Legal Issues

1. If other people have been accidentally injured or killed by a patient, what obligation does the mental health care professional have for documenting information surrounding the event? It is sufficient to conduct a psychiatric examination (including interviews of those available where the patient is incompetent) and document the examination and findings?

ACUTE PSYCHOSIS

The history of an evolving psychosis provides clues to the diagnosis, which in turn directs diagnostic-specific treatment. The specifics of the natural course of the various psychoses is provided in the diagnostic-specific sections of this handbook.

History

1. If onset is extremely acute, a serious medical malady such as a drug psychosis (e.g., atropine psychosis from eye drops) or cardiovascular condition (e.g., internal bleeding, arrhythmia, pulmonary embolism, septic embolism to the brain, hypertensive encephalopathy) should be suspected.

Management

1. Treatment is dictated by diagnosis.
2. The first step is evaluation for a life-threatening medical or surgical condition with referral for treatment.
3. Immediate symptomatic management entails rapid tranquilization with benzodiazepines alone or together with neuroleptics.
4. If a patient has a psychosis due to a compromising respiratory condition, or the patient suffers chronic obstructive lung disease, a benzodiazepine such as lorazepam should not be used.
5. If the patient is toxic from a drug with strong anticholinergic effects, a neuroleptic with atropine-like side effects may enhance the intensity of the psychoses.
6. Low dose neuroleptics may be as effective as higher doses for acute psychoses (Garcia et al, 1990), with fewer side effects.
7. Anxiety may be a precipitant, consequence or part of a psychosis. Two to 8 mg per day of lorazepam may prevent hospitalization of a schizophrenic patient when a neuroleptic is reduced to minimize risk of tardive dyskinesia. The lorazepam and other benzodiazepines may mollify anxiety that seems to precipitate or exacerbate a psychosis, or they may potentiate the effects of neuroleptics on dopamine pathways via the GABA system (Garcia et al, 1990).

Quality Assurance Issues

1. Was a differential diagnosis elaborated and diagnostic-specific treatment provided?
2. Was the patient evaluated to ascertain if he or she was suicidal, homicidal, or required hospitalization to assure compliance with treatment or to provide support if malignant side effects (e.g., cardiac arrhythmia) developed?
3. If restraints were required, were adequate measures taken to assure patient comfort?

Ethical/Legal Issues

1. Was the minimum amount of neuroleptic used to prevent the development of tardive dyskinesia and neuroleptic malignant syndrome (Tancredi, 1982)? Were signs of change of the patient's condition properly monitored and handled with modification of the treatment?
2. Were seclusion and/or restraints used according to acceptable criteria and the amount of time kept to the most minimal possible (Tardiff, 1983)?

ADOLESCENTS IN CRISIS

A crisis in adolescence is indicated by a number of behavioral changes such as drug use, promiscuity, poor or declining school performance, difficulty with the law, truancy, difficulty with peer relationships, pregnancy, venereal disease, abortion, alcoholism, and running away.

General Points

1. In general, an adolescent population exhibits the same trends seen in adult populations studied, with girls scoring higher on depression scales than boys.
2. Lowest levels of adolescent depressive mood is correlated with higher levels of attachment to peers and parents. Sex difference in depressed mood is attributed to masked depression and the increased delinquency among boys as compared with girls (Kandel and Davies, 1982).
3. Approximately 20% of one population of adolescents with major depression studied were found to have bipolar affective illness (Strober and Carlson, 1982). Bipolarity was predicted by a family history of bipolar illness, a history of rapid onset with psychomotor retardation, and mood-congruent psychotic features and pharmacologically induced hypomania.
4. Fire setting, enuresis, and cruelty to animals are thought to be associated with increased delinquency, although this is not a consistent finding (Shanok et al, 1983).
5. Comparison of delinquent and nondelinquent adolescent psychiatric inpatients indicates that hallucinations, learning disabilities, being diagnosed as psychotic, evidence of neurologic impairment, and delusions do not separate the two groups (Shanok et al, 1983). Significantly more of those diagnosed as delinquent have a history of engaging in violent acts and being previously hospitalized for psychiatric reasons. The mothers of the delinquent children have a greater history of being hospitalized for psychiatric reasons.
6. Incidence of delinquency, suicide attempts, anorexia nervosa, substance abuse, suicide, and schizophrenia increases during adolescence. Rutter estimates 40% of adolescent psychiatric problems are conduct disorders, 40% emotional or movement disorders, and 20% a mix of conduct and emotional disorders (Smith and Mitchell, 1987).
7. Management of adolescents within the community in which they live allows continuity of management across the inpatient and outpatient phases of treatment (Stelzer and Elliott, 1990).
8. Adolescence and young adulthood have been found in NIMH Epidemiologic Catchment Area Program to be critical periods for development of drug and alcohol abuse, phobias, bipolar illness, and depression (Burke KC et al, 1990).
9. Depressed children and adolescents are at greater risk in adult life for affective illness, psychiatric treatment, and hospitalization, but not for other psychiatric conditions (Harrington et al, 1990).
10. Psychiatrically disturbed adolescents, like adults with psychiatric disorders, are remarkably unrecognized and untreated (Whitaker et al, 1990).

11. A 10-year follow-up study of socialized and nonsocialized delinquents revealed that socialized delinquents have less chance of being convicted of a crime or being imprisoned (Henn et al, 1980).

12. Although as high as 23% of adolescents admitted to a correctional facility meet the Research Diagnostic Criteria for major affective disorder (Chiles et al, 1980), no pattern of "acting-out" or antisocial behavior is associated with the depressed group. A family history of depression or alcoholism predicted depression in the delinquent group.

13. Stressors precipitating adjustment disorders in both adolescents and adults may be chronic rather than acute. In one study, 59% of the stressors for adolescents and 36% of those for adults have been present a year or more (Andreasen and Wasek, 1980). Adolescents tend to have many behavioral symptoms and adults many depressive symptoms.

14. Violent and/or suicidal behaviors are characteristic of psychotic hospitalized adolescents. Boys tend to be more violent than girls. In hospitalized psychotic populations, boys may be more suicidal than girls. The combination of violent and suicidal behavior is suggestive of psychosis in an adolescent population (Inamdar et al, 1982).

History

1. Children and adolescents are very sensitive barometers of the state of their parents' marriage. Careful history should be taken as to how their parents get on. Have they discussed divorce or separation? Is one or are both parent having an extramarital affair?

2. If an adolescent appears psychotic, remember that not all psychoses in adolescence are schizophrenic. Is there a family history of affective disorder?

3. Did the patient have a childhood history of phobias? Bed wetting? Fire setting? Sleep walking? Head banging?

4. Has there been any recent conflict with parents or siblings? Are the parents—one or both—drinking? Has there been any recent loss for the patient or his or her parents (e.g., job, money, death)?

5. Was there a recent newcomer to the family such as new siblings, returned divorced sibling, or grandparent?

6. Has there been a recent change in thinking, mood, or behavior? Has the patient chronically been withdrawn or behaved idiosyncratically?

7. Is there a change in school, the structure of school, or a conflict in the school hierarchy?

8. Patients with adjustment disorders with depressed mood tend to score higher in ratings on Axis IV and lower on severity of illness ratings than patients with major depression (Snyder et al, 1990).

9. Conduct disorders are frequently found in the history of adolescents with drug abuse (Roehrich and Gold, 1986–1987).

10. Historical variables most likely to predict borderline personality disorders include maternal neglect, number of father and mother surrogates, sexual abuse,

physical abuse, and a history of disrupted attachments. The families of border-line adolescents were chronically disrupted (Ludolph et al, 1990).

Management

1. Clinicians should be aware of state regulations regarding the treatment of adolescents. These regulations vary on the need to contact parents, the age at which a patient is allowed to sign themself into hospital, and the age at which a patient may have an abortion without parental consent.
2. Hospitalization may be indicated if an adolescent is psychotic, homicidal, or suicidal. Does he or she need an alternate living arrangement? Where is he or she presently living and what alternatives are available to him or her?
3. It may be necessary to call the parents in to evaluate them and the family situation. School counselors and clergymen may be other sources of further historical elaboration, as well as possibly being able to provide a viable disposition.
4. Allow the adolescent to ventilate in a supportive psychotherapeutic situation. In some instances if the problem is not serious and adequate social and family supports are available, all that may be needed is evaluation with a couple of follow-up visits.
5. Medicate the patient as indicated.
6. If the crisis appears symptomatic of a more deeply rooted disturbance, referral to long-term psychotherapy is indicated.
7. An effort should always be made to manage an adolescent outside of a hospital or other institutional setting. This serves several purposes. It avoids the labeling of the patient by peers, teachers, and others in the community as "crazy." The patient does not feel tainted or in some way inferior to those with a "better" capacity to cope. Finally, it prevents the parents from seeing the problem as solely their adolescent's adjustment difficulty. The family must work together with the therapist to reduce intrafamilial tension so that the adolescent who is open to feeling external pressures may move more freely along the path of growth and self-actualization.
8. In some instances successful management will entail a coordinated program of care with chemical abuse and psychiatric components. Parents of dually diagnosed adolescents may be resistant, enabling, or codependent, but they should be given firm recommendation that treatment include withdrawal of their child from the drugs of abuse, psychoeducation of parent and child about the disorder and its diagnostic-specific treatment, and establishment of the capability of physical abstinence and of compliance with treatment (Niven, 1986).
9. Longer-term care (greater than 6 months) may be required to impact on young chronic patients with histories of repeated failure in outpatient or brief-stay programs (Caton et al, 1990).

Quality Assurance Issues

1. Was a differential diagnosis and diagnostic-specific treatment provided?
2. If substance abuse was present, was an attempt made to see if it was comorbid with another psychiatric disorder?

3. Were parents and patients provided information on the nature of the disorder and its treatment?
4. If the decision was not to hospitalize the adolescent, was the family evaluated to determine their ability to cope with the adolescent's acute problems?
5. Were the adolescent and his or her family referred for additional evaluation and treatment?
6. Was hospitalization provided if severity of psychosis or self or other destructive intent or behavior required it?
7. If restraints or seclusion was required, was it limited in time to the period of absolute necessity and were individual humane needs attended to (e.g., food, drink, toilet privileges)?

Ethical/Legal Issues

1. Was the adolescent evaluated with respect to his competency to seek treatment? Most states have provisions allowing adolescents in their early teens (frequently age 13) to obtain treatment for substance abuse and contraceptives without parental consent. Until recently, adolescents were allowed to obtain abortions without parental consent and notification. The latter changed in 1990 when the U.S. Supreme Court held that a state had the right to require parental advance notice *(Ohio v. Akron Center for Reproductive Health)*. Although *Roe v. Wade* was not ruled out in the recent 1992 U.S. Supreme Court abortion case (Hodgson v. Minnesota), the case nonetheless provided the states with more power to regulate the conditions and circumstances of abortion.
2. Were proper precautions instituted to avert suicidal behavior and assault of others?
3. Increasingly in many jurisdictions, adolescents are accorded the same rights that adults have to refuse psychotropic medications when they are competent. This would not apply in the acute emergency situation where such drugs would be necessary to avert a crisis, such as dangerousness to self or others. Would an incompetent adolescent have the right to refuse psychotropic medications and hospitalization?

AFFECTIVE ILLNESS

The essential feature of affective illness is mood disturbance. Prolonged emotional disturbance colors all aspects of an individual's life. The alteration in mood may be episodic (i.e., last for days or months) or chronic (i.e., last for years). It may appear alone or be part of another psychological or medical disorder. The principle disturbances of mood are depression and mania.

Epidemiology

1. The point prevalence of depressive symptoms is between 9 and 20% (Boyd and Weissman, 1981).
2. The lifetime risk of bipolar illness is less than 1% (Boyd and Weissman, 1981).

3. The annual incidence of bipolar illness is 0.009 to 0.015% for men and 0.007 to 0.03% for women (Boyd and Weissman, 1981).
4. The lifetime risk of nonbipolar depression is 8 to 12% for men and 20 to 26% for women (Boyd and Weissman, 1981).
5. There is a strong association between measures of depression and demoralization and self-reported disability (Craig and Van Nattan, 1983).

History

1. In a study of a mid-sized urban community (New Haven, Connecticut) by Weissman et al (1981b), the current rate (not lifetime prevalence) of probable and definite major depression was 4.3% and the current rate of minor depression was 2.5% yielding a combined point prevalence of 6.8% for major and minor depression. In the New Haven study and another of Almeida County, California by Roberts and Vernon (1982), the number of those who sought help from a mental health professional or any other source was quite low (About 20% sought help from a mental health professional). Men sought help less than women. In New Haven, persons with depression were more likely to seek help from a non-psychiatric physician than were those with other diagnoses.
2. In a study of ambulatory medical patients (Neilsen and Williams, 1980) the prevalence of depression was 12.2% when at least mild depression was used as a criterion and 5.5 and 0.6% when "moderate depression" and "psychotic depression," respectively, were used.
3. Studies of geriatric medical patients (Okimato et al, 1982) show particularly high rates of moderate depressions.
4. In younger populations, depression may occur in relationship to substance abuse (Schuckit, 1982b).
5. Major depressive disorder is seen more frequently among children considered to have specific developmental disorders, suggesting that some children are depressed due to their inability to handle academic problems (Kashani et al, 1982).
6. Contrary to general belief, depression is a clinical entity observable in children.
7. Patients experiencing depression tend to exhibit both qualitative and quantitative alterations in how information is processed due to disruptions in arousal-activation (Weingartner et al, 1981) causing clinicians to diagnose them as having organic mental disorders.
8. Chronic minor depression may accompany major depression (a phenomenon referred to as "double depression"). This has been reported in as many as 26% of individuals with major depression (Keller et al, 1983). Chronic minor depression reduces the perceived effect of predictors of recovery and relapse of major depression.
9. Rates of affective illness are higher in relatives of depressed individuals than in normal controls (Weissman et al, 1982). Bipolar probands are found to have more bipolar relatives than unipolar probands (Baron et al, 1985). The magnitude of the differences in rates of depression between relatives of depressed probands and relatives of normal probands ranges between twofold and fivefold (Weissman et al, 1982).

10. Both men and women with affective illness appear to have a higher incidence of parental loss before age 17 (Roy, 1981a).

11. The term atypical depression is used to indicate depression accompanied by either severe anxiety or atypical vegetative symptoms (increased sleep, appetite, weight, and libido). Both types tend to be associated with early age of onset, mild intensity, outpatient status, rarity of attempted suicide, nonbipolarity, minimal psychomotor change, and nonendogenicity. Atypical depression is more common in women and tends to respond to monoamine oxidase inhibitors such as tranylcypromine (Parnate), isocarboxazid (Marplan), or phenelzine (Nardil).

12. Approximately 24% of patients with major depressive illness tend to relapse within 12 weeks at risk and 12% within 4 weeks (Keller et al, 1982). Factors associated with increased rate of relapse include an accompanying chronic minor depression ("double depression") and three or more previous affective episodes.

13. Impairment of social support is seen with major affective illness. Improvement in social relationships is seen more frequently with treatment of major depression than it is with treatment of minor depression (Blazer, 1983).

14. Factors predicting recovery from major depression include acuteness of onset of depression, severity of depression for patients without superimposed illness, and superimposition of an acute episode or chronic minor depression (Keller et al, 1982).

Management

1. Individuals with acute onset, nonpsychotic, nonbipolar depressive illness who are treated with psychotherapy in addition to thymoleptic treatment tend to do better on measures of social functioning at 1 year follow-up (Weissman et al, 1981a).

2. Efficacy studies comparing amitriptyline hydrochloride and phenelzine sulfate indicate that both have antidepressant and antianxiety effects, with similarities between the two exceeding the differences. Amitriptyline tends to be more effective in reversing weight loss and improving sleep, and phenelzine exerts a stronger antianxiety action. Frequently sedation and orthostatic hypotension occur equally with both; amitriptyline, however, causes more dry mouth (Ravaris et al, 1980).

3. Amoxapine, a dibenzoxazepine compound, has been reported to produce as much moderate and marked global improvement at a daily dose of 200 mg as 200 mg of imipramine (Rickels et al, 1981).

4. Methylphenidate has been used successfully in treatment-resistant depression as an adjunct to tricyclic antidepressant therapy. The ability to potentiate tricyclic responsiveness is related to its dopaminergic activity (Drimmer et al, 1983).

5. Methylphenidate has been used alone to treat successfully depressed geriatric patients who either had a medical illness that contradicted tricyclic therapy or had been unable to tolerate tricyclic antidepressants without adverse effects (Katon and Raskind, 1980).

6. ECT is a safe alternative for treatment-resistant patients.

Quality Assurance Issues

1. Was a differential diagnosis performed that included medical and surgical causes of mood disturbance?
2. Was diagnostic-specific treatment provided?
3. Was a history of substance abuse elicited to ascertain if a patient is self-medicating?
4. Were symptoms of anxiety present? If present, was the depression secondary to the anxiety or was the anxiety due to the depression. In some instances, an anxiety disorder such as a panic disorder will be comorbid with an affective illness.
5. Was it ascertained whether a patient was suicidal or homicidal and were appropriate precautions taken to avert harm to self or others?

Ethical/Legal Issues

1. Was a differential diagnosis and diagnostic-specific treatment provided?
2. Was a determination made of suicide and homicide risk and appropriate precautions taken?
3. In the absence of suicidal and homicidal risk which would justify medical/legal intervention such as commitment, what should be the therapist's obligation where the patient is engaging in subthreshold level behaviors which may be viewed as destructive such as expenditure of monies or promiscuous sexual conduct?
4. How should the therapist handle the communication of issues regarding the patient's behavior with other members of the family are those who have taken the patient into the emergency room?

AGORAPHOBIA

History

1. Agoraphobia is fear of open spaces.
2. It is an extremely crippling phobia because of the ramifications of the phobia on nearly all activities of those so effected (Zitrin et al, 1980).
3. Patients with agoraphobia frequently have a history of being "refractory to treatment."
4. Agoraphobic and phobic patients with spontaneous panic anxiety may appear in an emergency situation seeking immediate and longer-term management of their anxiety.
5. Agoraphobic patients appear to differ from patients with social phobias and other monosymptomatic, specific phobias by a frequent family history of affective illness in first-degree relatives (Munjack and Moss, 1981).
6. Patients with agoraphobia and social phobias more frequently report a history of alcoholism in the family than patients with other specific phobias (Munjack and Moss, 1981).
7. Depression is a common symptom associated with agoraphobia. During periods

of depression, agoraphobic patients are indistinguishable from patients with affective disorder.

8. Alcohol and sedative abuse are malignant complications of all phobic and panic disorders.

9. In a family study of panic disorder, agoraphobia, and normal controls (Harris et al, 1983), risk of all anxiety disorders was 33% among first-degree relatives of patients with panic disorder, 32% among agoraphobics, and 15% among controls. Alcoholism was also found in excess, especially in male relatives.

10. Onset of panic disorders with agoraphobia is generally in early adulthood although onset has been reported over age 65 (Luchins and Rose, 1989).

11. Agoraphobia and panic disorder have been reported in children with separation anxiety, fear and avoidance of crowds and public places, and panic (Ballenger et al, 1989). The same psychopharmacotherapy is used as in adults (alprazolam [Xanax] and imipramine [Tofranil]).

12. Agoraphobia with mitral valve prolapse may be undistinguishable form mitral valve prolapse without it (Mavissakalian et al, 1983).

Management

1. Alprazolam and clonazepam (Klonopin) are effective in the management of panic anxiety in the emergency situation.

2. The beneficial effect of imipramine on agoraphobia is dose related, generally requiring 150 mg or more per day (Mavissakalian and Perel, 1985).

3. Treatment with imipramine and psychotherapy appears to be superior to group or individual psychotherapy alone, group exposure in vivo, flooding, and imagined desensitization (implosion) for the prevention of future attacks (Zitrin et al, 1980).

4. Patients who are refractory to imipramine may respond to monoamine oxidase inhibitors or fluoxetine (Prozac). Response rate is significantly increased if depressive symptoms are present.

5. Patients who are not substance abuse prone can be maintained on alprazolam or clonazepam.

6. An evaluation of suicide risk should be obtained, as risk for attempt is increased in panic disordered patients and patients with panic not comporting to the *DSM-III-R* criteria of panic disorder.

Quality Assurance Issues

1. Were benzodiazepines avoided in patients with a personal history of substance abuse?

2. Was a differential diagnosis and diagnostic-specific treatment provided? Were depression and alcoholism properly ruled out in the patients suffering from agoraphobia? Were physical conditions such as mitrovalve prolapse considered and ruled out?

3. Was an evaluation of self-destructive risk obtained?

Ethical/Legal Issues

1. A certain number of panic prone patients using benzodiazepines become drug

dependent from the treatment for this and similar conditions. In these iatrogenic addictions, what determines if the clinician is negligent?

2. How would negligence be established in cases of iatrogenic addiction? What would be the responsibility of the clinician who provides benzodiazepines to patients who are either not warned of the side affects or ignore the warnings and engage in potentially dangerous behaviors to third parties such as driving vehicles?

AIDS
(Acquired Immunodeficiency Syndrome)

AIDS, like tuberculosis and syphilis, is a great masquerader. Its clinical manifestations are myriad, impacting both the infected and uninfected. The illness itself may present as an organic mental disorder with affective and delusional features (Nurnberg et al, 1984), schizophrenia, *Pneumocystis carinii* pneumonia and other opportunistic infections, malignancies such as Kaposi's sarcoma (Skeen, 1985), AIDS dementia complex (Dickson and Ranseen, 1990), depression, mania, substance abuse disorders, anxiety disorders, paranoid disorders, adjustment disorders, and anxiety disorders. Those not affected but concerned because they are caregivers, members of high-risk groups, relatives, friends, lovers, or those suffering depression, schizophrenia, or paranoia may present with AIDS-related delusions (but without infection), Munchausen's AIDS, phobias, and anxiety and factitious disorders (Cohen MAA, 1990). Virtually no one can assume that they have *not* been exposed unless they are sexually abstinent, are not abusing intravenous drugs, and have not been a recipient of blood or blood products. No person, regardless of how long they have been married, knows for certain how many sexual partners a spouse or lover had, who, or how recently. High-risk groups include hemophiliacs, prostitutes, homosexual and bisexual men, recipients of transfusions, infants born to high-risk mothers, male prisoners, and female sexual partners of those in high-risk groups (Skeen, 1985). AIDS victims face severe illness, economic drain, social isolation, neuropsychiatric disorders, discrimination, and death (Cohen MAA, 1990).

History
1. In patients documented to suffer the lymphadenopathy syndrome, a precipitous decline in the T-helper cell count is often a harbinger of the diagnoses of AIDS (Kaplan JE et al, 1988).
2. While widespread application of routine HIV antibody testing of blood and plasma products and removal from the pool of donors those most likely to be infected has minimized the risk of contracting AIDS through transfusion, anyone reporting a transfusion still should be deemed at risk.
3. Low-risk, depressed heterosexuals may present with obsessive concern over having AIDS (Brothman and Forstein, 1988).
4. Caregivers suffer fear and anxiety in caring for individuals who are at risk for

AIDS or who have the illness, necessitating a continuing program of education regarding the disease and its mode of transmission and providing psychological support for caregivers (Blumenfield et al, 1987).

5. AIDS is a significant risk factor for suicide with the relative rate 36 times that of men without the diagnosis and 66 times that of the general population in one study (Marzuk et al, 1988) of men age 20 to 59 with the disease.

6. The initial presentation of AIDS may be neuropsychiatric rather than infectious, hematologic, or oncological (Price and Forejt, 1986).

7. Hemophiliacs suffer from fear of sexual intimacy, health preoccupation, interference with parent–child intimacy, and fear of contagion since the advent of AIDS (Agle et al, 1987). As a result, there is increased parental anxiety, hypochondriasis, social isolation, and increased psychiatric disorders among hemophiliacs and their families and friends.

8. AIDS patients seen on consultation-liaison services require more time and are more likely to require one or more repeat consultations than non-AIDS patients (O'Dowd and McKegney, 1990).

9. Family breakup and abandonment of AIDS sufferers is not uncommon (King, 1990).

10. Heterosexual promiscuity and contact with female prostitutes is associated with heterosexual transmission of AIDS (Haverkos and Edelman, 1988).

11. Despite the fact that mood disturbances and organic mental disorders have been found to be as great as 83% and 65% respectfully in AIDS patients (Perry and Tross, 1984), these complications are underdiagnosed and undertreated.

12. Factors contributing to psychiatric morbidity in AIDS patients include guilt associated with sexual transmission, fear of contagion, disclosure of drug use or homosexuality, central nervous system involvement, threat to life, and severe physical debilitation.

13. In one study of a cohort of 1034 homosexual single men (Winkelstein et al, 1987), the only sexual practice that was identified to produce a significantly higher risk of HIV infection was receptive anogenital contact.

14. Chronically ill psychiatric patients and intoxicated, intravenous drug-using patients may not recall sexual contact or sharing needles. Both these groups may also have histories of loss of friends and contacts to AIDS, which contributes to depression and anxiety (Cohen and Weisman, 1986).

15. The majority of individuals suspected of suffering an AIDS-related psychiatric disorder will provide a history of a high-risk factor (Castro et al, 1988).

16. HIV infection is associated with a history of syphilis and serologic evidence of syphilis but not with a history of other genital infections such as that of herpes simplex virus or antibody to *Chlamydia trachomatis* (Stamm et al, 1988).

17. A study of 20 employed, educated women who were not intravenous drug abusers but HIV seropositive (Brown and Rundell, 1990) indicated heterosexual transmission was the cause, with 20% having HIV-seropositive spouses. Sixty percent of the women failed to practice safe sex despite repeated education. Twenty percent met criteria for new-onset hyperactive sexual desire disorder. All women were largely asymptomatic early in the course of the disease.

18. Impulsivity, poor judgment and hypersexuality are factors contributing to increased rates of HIV infection among psychiatric patients (Sachs et al, 1990).

Symptoms
1. Paranoia (Bundell et al, 1986).
2. Suicidal ideation.
3. Depression (Ingraham et al, 1990).
4. Panic.
5. Generalized anxiety (Chuang et al, 1989).
6. Mania (Kermani et al, 1985).
7. Drug abuse.
8. Alcohol abuse.
9. Delusions (Atkinson et al, 1988).
10. Self-imposed isolation.
11. Sadness.
12. Malaise (Beckett et al, 1987).
13. Lethargy.
14. Loss of sexual drive (Nurnberg et al, 1984).
15. Command hallucinations (Cummings MA et al, 1987).
16. Dysthymia (Dilley et al, 1985).
17. Acute psychoses (Perry and Jacobsen, 1986).
18. Thought disorder (Kermani et al, 1985).
19. Agitation (Swenson et al, 1989).
20. Impairment of long-term and short-term memory (Ingraham et al, 1990).
21. Inability to calculate.
22. Expressive aphasia.
23. Acalculia.
24. Impairment in concept formation.
25. Diminished motor speed.
26. Dysattention.
27. Ataxia (Navia et al, 1986).
28. Tremor.
29. Leg weakness.
30. Blindness.
31. Loss of fine motor coordination.
32. Weight loss (Ginzburg and MacDonald, 1986).
33. Incontinence.
34. Mutism.
35. Paraplegia.
36. Myoclonus.
37. Peripheral neuropathy (Snider et al, 1983).
38. Diarrhea.
39. Chronic, unexplained fever.
40. Oral candidiasis (thrush).
41. Generalized lymphadenopathy (Wolcott et al, 1985).

42. Rashes.
43. Cough.
44. Troubled sleep (Ostrow et al, 1989).
45. Idiopathic thrombocytopenic purpura (Wolcott et al, 1990).
46. Psychomotor retardation.
47. Hyperreflexia.
48. Spastic–ataxic gait.
49. Hemiparesis (Beckett et al, 1987).
50. Kaposi's sarcoma.

Clinical Studies

1. T-helper cell count below 400 cells/mm.
2. Thrombocytopenia (Ginzburg and MacDonald, 1986).
3. Lower T-helper/T-suppressor cell ratio (Wolcott et al, 1985).
4. Positive HIV serology.
5. Human immunodeficiency virus on CSF culture (Beckett et al, 1987).
6. Diffuse slowing on EEG (Perry, 1990).
7. Mild cerebral atrophy CT scan (Perry, 1990).
8. Nonspecific hyperdensities on brain MRI (Perry, 1990).

Course

1. The course is usually steadily progressive although at times there may be periods of abrupt acceleration (Navia et al, 1986).
2. Some patients may fraudulently gain admission to hospital with factitious AIDS and in some instances fit the description of Munchausen's syndrome (Bialer and Wallach, 1990; Baer, 1987).
3. At least one-third of patients with AIDS develop neurologic symptoms prior to death (Wolcott et al, 1985).
4. Approximately two-thirds of AIDS patients will have an opportunistic infection (i.e., viral, fungal, protozoal, or mycobacterial infections) (Wolcott et al, 1985).
5. About one-third of AIDS patients develop a neoplasm (Wolcott et al, 1985).
6. Substance abuse and other psychiatric illnesses may have preceded the onset of AIDS (Atkinson et al, 1988) and may not be related to the neuropathic changes.
7. Severe cognitive dysfunction occurs in over 50% of patients with AIDS (Atkinson et al, 1988).
8. In some instances the illness may progress as rapidly in weeks or months to global dementia and incontinence (Beckett et al, 1987).
9. In one autopsy study (Navia and Price, 1990), after patients with focal diseases such as toxoplasmas and metabolic encephalopathies obscuring clinical pathological correlation were excluded, it was found that two-thirds of the brains of patients with AIDS showed evidence of a premortem dementing process.
10. Depressed gay or heterosexual individuals and substance abusers may attempt to contract AIDS when they feel depressed (Flavin et al, 1986).
11. The HIV-III virus may directly infect the CNS causing psychiatric symptoms

before neurologic signs or cognitive impairment appears (Perry and Jacobsen, 1986).

12. Symptoms and signs emerging during the course of treatment may be a reaction to having a fatal and stigmatizing disease (due to infection of the CNS), a complication of the HIV infection, or due to treatment.

13. Lymphoma developing during the course of the illness, as in the instance of a focal infection, would be heralded by the emergence of focal signs and symptoms (Loewenstein and Sharfstein, 1984).

Management

1. AIDS is a family illness. In some instances the awareness that a member has AIDS comes contemporaneously with the knowledge that a spouse, parent, lover, or child is a substance abuser, promiscuous, or homosexual. Other stresses include the fear of contagion and of imminent death. Family, couples, or group therapy or counseling together with the provision of accurate information, peer support, grief counseling, and a nonjudgmental approach helps counter the sense of helplessness, depression, and isolation experienced by the family (Frierson et al, 1987).

2. Alcohol, marijuana, and inhalants can suppress the immune system (Flavin et al, 1986). Therefore, all patients should be discouraged from using recreational drugs and alcohol.

3. Psychostimulants such as dextroamphetamine (Dexedrine) and methylphenidate (Ritalin) have been used successfully in bringing about prompt remission of depressive and cognitive symptoms without adverse effects (Fernandez et al, 1988a). These are used in cases of primary and secondary affective disturbance as well as when depression arises from a specific organic mental disorder. Changes reported in energy, appetite, memory, affect, concentration, and attention after initial loading have been maintained on as little as 10 mg a day (Fernandez et al, 1988a,b).

4. Intravenous molindone (Moban) and haloperidol (Haldol) have been used for panic and psychosis (Levy and Fernandez, 1989).

5. Benzodiazepines such as alprazolam (Xanax), lorazepam (Loxitane), and oxazepam (Serax) have been used to alleviate anxiety (Levy and Fernandez, 1989).

6. Patients with AIDS are more prone to extrapyramidal reactions when treated with neuroleptics for psychoses or antiemetics such as prochlorperazine and metroclopropramide. Extrapyramidal reactions must be distinguished from depression, dementia, and delirium in AIDS (Swenson et al, 1989).

7. Tricyclic, tetracyclic, and the newer drugs such as fluoxetine (Prozac) have been used to treat depression with AIDS (Jenike and Pato, 1986) at the usual doses, unless organic changes are such that there is increased drug sensitivity.

8. Benzodiazepines, when used to facilitate sleep in AIDS patients, may cause a paradoxical reaction given the presence of an organic mental disorder. Chloral hydrate is preferred.

9. Zidovudine (AZT) can reverse or delay cognitive deficits (Perry, 1990).

10. High-potency neuroleptics may cause neuroleptic malignant syndrome in patients with AIDS (Perry, 1990).
11. No major exacerbations of HIV infection have been reported as a result of imipramine treatment (Rabkin and Harrison, 1990).
12. Health care professionals' attitudes toward treating AIDS patients vary reflecting the predominate subculture's biases and misinformation about the disease and its transmission (Gerbert et al, 1988). Caregivers require support and continuing education regarding the disease so that caregiver factors enhance rather than impede successful management of the patient.
13. AIDS patients are notoriously noncompliant with treatment, although patients who acquired the illness through transfusion and nonpromiscuous sexual contact would be expected to be more compliant. In one study, AIDS patients' refusal rate for a procedure or treatment was four times that of non-AIDS patients (Blumenfield et al, 1990).
14. Psychotherapeutic techniques that are particularly helpful in treating AIDS include support, clarification, and abreaction. Unique problems in therapy include irrational fears of contagion and regression associated with the sick role. Early approach may entail attention to somatic rather than psychological complaints (Perry and Markowitz, 1986). Patients who are seropositive but yet without overt illness benefit from stress inoculation, psychoeducation, and problem-solving techniques (Perry and Markowitz, 1986).
15. Work is required in communities to assure that AIDS patients receive the privileges associated with other physical illnesses, including proper insurance coverage and lack of discrimination at the worksite (Siegel K, 1986).

Neuropathologic Mechanism

The exact mode of impact of the virus on the CNS is uncertain, but it appears the virus crosses the blood–brain barrier contained within macrophages. When the virus is released in the brain, a subclinical or clinical meningoencephalitis ensues. Due to the immune suppression, the virus replicates causing a multifocal encephalopathy with relative sparing of the cortex. The major neuropathologic changes are seen in subcortical areas such as the brain stem, the thalamus, and the basal ganglia (Perry, 1990).

Quality Assurance Issues

1. Was an evaluation performed to ascertain whether symptoms were psychiatric due to a response to the illness, psychiatric and preceded the illness, due to treatment (e.g., extrapyramidal reaction to phenothiazines), or due to concurrent neuropathic changes or a concurrent nonrelated illness?
2. Was diagnostic-specific treatment provided?

Ethical/Legal Issues

1. Were patients provided education regarding precautions necessary to minimize spread of the illness (Carmen and Brady, 1990)?
2. If patients are chronic drug users, they should be alerted to sources of clean nee-

dles (if permitted by state law) to prevent spread by sharing needles (Krely, 1986).

3. In those jurisdictions where a Tarasoff type ruling exists (the duty of the therapist to warn or protect third parties) what are the legal as well as ethical obligations of the therapist to third parties? To what extent is a therapist obligated to personally warn third parties of potential dangers?

4. Pre- and post-test counseling should be provided patients who are tested for AIDS and who are HIV-positive.

5. Caregivers and other patients should be provided the measures necessary to avoid contagion on a unit (e.g., prevention of sexual abuse when a patient who is positive has poor control over his or her sexual impulses).

6. Education has proven successful in reduction of nonsafe sexual practices among homosexual male patients and university students (Klein DE et al, 1987). Programs designed to reduce spread should be tailored to the unique characteristics of specific subgroups at risk (Klein DE et al, 1987).

AKATHISIA

Akathisia, a subjective desire to move and not remain seated, is a common source of calls to therapists and visits to an emergency room when a patient is on neuroleptics or a drug with neuroleptic properties.

History

1. Patients report akathisia or appear agitated, with a history of the use of a drug that has extrapyramidal side effects.

2. Nonphysician therapists unaware of the side effects of antipsychotic medication may misconstrue the symptoms as exacerbation of the underlying illness (e.g., schizophrenia, schizoaffective disorder, Tourette's disorder).

3. In one study (Van Patten et al, 1984), 40% of a group of schizophrenics experienced akathisia within 6 hours of taking 5 mg haloperidol (Haldol). With 10 mg at bedtime, by the seventh day 75% experienced akathisia. With 5- and 10-mg doses of thiothixene (Navane), the figures were 20% and 46% respectively. Twenty percent is the average reported in most studies (Adler et al, 1985).

4. Akathisia cannot be suppressed in up to one-half of patients experiencing it. (Van Patten et al, 1984).

5. Treatment-resistant akathisia may be reported as depression or anxiety.

6. The symptoms may occur days or weeks after a dose is initiated or increased.

Management

1. Antipsychotics not causing extrapyramidal side effects or those with significantly fewer side effects (generally the high-dosage, low-potency antipsychotics with more anticholinergic properties) may be used in lieu of those more frequently causing akathisia.

2. Antipsychotics can be used at smaller dosage to control psychotic agitation if

contemporaneously provided to the patient with a benzodiazepine such as diazepam (Valium) or lorazepam (Ativan), 2 to 5 mg/day.
3. Propranolol (Inderal), 20 to 30 mg/day, is reported to be effective in reducing neuroleptic-induced akathisia (Adler et al, 1985).

Quality Assurance Issues
1. What is the obligation of the therapist to avoid akathisia in patients? The physician may confront decision-making circumstances where a higher dose of a neuroleptic may be beneficial for treating the underlying psychosis but may result in the development of akathisia. What calculus should the therapist use in determining the trade off between those two possibilities, ie, the benefit from high dosage and the potential side effects of akathisia?
2. What alternative drugs could be used to prevent the development of akathisia or to mitigate the dosage level of the neuroleptic so as to lessen the development of this condition?

Ethical/Legal Issues
1. The important ethical and legal issue addresses the role of informed consent in providing a neuroleptic to patients. How does the therapist determine the competency of the patient to understand information regarding side effects such as akathisia? In the absence of a competent patient, what are the obligations of the therapist for obtaining a legally acceptable informed consent?
2. Have the patient and family been informed that the symptoms of akathisia may look like an exacerbation of psychosis? The clinician, if unaware of this, may increase the dosage of the neuroleptic rather than decrease it. Decreasing the dosage would be the appropriate treatment for the akathisia. How would negligence be determined in such a situation?

ALCOHOL AMNESTIC SYNDROME
(Korsakoff's Syndrome)

The alcohol amnestic syndrome may develop insidiously, or follow delirium tremens.

History
1. It is most frequently seen with alcoholic polyneuritis, but also occurs with other disorders such as the polyneuritis of pregnancy.
2. Age of presentation is the same as that for alcoholic polyneuritis. Since prolonged use of alcohol is necessary to develop the disorder, it is seldom seen before age 35.
3. Men are affected more commonly than women.
4. Generally, patients have a history of several years of alcohol dependence with poor dietary intake.

5. Degree of peripheral nerve involvement may be minimal to quite severe, with occurrence of convulsions common.
6. The core feature is short-term memory disturbance due to prolonged heavy alcohol use. Immediate memory is not disturbed. The individual has a normal digit span but cannot remember the name of three objects after 20 minutes.
7. The irreversible memory defect usually follows an episode of Wernicke's encephalopathy and may be avoided if Wernicke's encephalopathy is treated in the early stages with large doses of thiamine, before the short-term memory defect becomes permanent.
8. Impairment is often severe, requiring custodial care.
9. Both Wernicke's encephalopathy and Korsakoff's syndrome are believed due to thiamine deficiency. Prolonged, heavy alcohol use leads to a malabsorbtion syndrome even if dietary intake is sufficient. However, malnutrition alone can predispose the individual to this disorder.
10. This condition is rare, and has become even rarer because of the prophylactic use of parenteral thiamine whenever individuals with a history of alcohol dependence are seen in the health care system.

Symptoms
1. Short-term but not immediate memory disturbance.
2. Confabulation in a clear sensorium.

Management
1. The patient should be given thiamine 50 mg PO tid or qid as well as high potency vitamin B complex preparation.
2. The patient should be withdrawn from alcohol.
3. If polyneuritis is present, the affected muscles should be supported and massage exercises prescribed as tenderness subsides.
4. Propranolol (Inderal) has been used to control the violence and rage in a patient with the alcohol amnestic syndrome, alcohol withdrawal, and convulsions (Yudofsky et al, 1984).

Quality Assurance Issues
1. Is the clinician aware that the patient may have had an anonymous homosexual or heterosexual relationship during the period of amnesia and therefore may have potentially contracted AIDS?
2. Is the patient and his or her family made aware that the patient may have such episodes and during these periods may drive and cause an accident?
3. What is the obligation of the clinician to inform the patient's workplace that the patient may have such episodes? What if the patient is working with a highly sensitive type of machinery where there may be injury to third parties during the amnestic period?
4. Is the clinician aware that anyone who suffers from alcoholic amnesia should be in treatment for alcoholism and that the patient's family should be made aware of this?

Ethical/Legal Issues
1. What is the responsibility of the clinician to third parties who may be injured by a patient suffering from this condition?

ALCOHOL HALLUCINOSIS

Alcohol hallucinosis is syndrome in which hallucinosis persists after an individual has recovered from the symptoms of alcohol withdrawal and is no longer drinking.

History
1. Some authors feel that it occurs in individuals with an underlying predisposition to schizophrenia.
2. Onset is 1 to 2 weeks or more after cessation of drinking.
3. Because many patients deny a history of alcohol abuse (especially upper-middle-class housewives and executives), friends or relatives of the patient may be needed to confirm the history.
4. The patient usually is a male between the ages of 30 and 50, although the disorder may occur at any age.
5. Duration of drinking, prior to the abstinence in which the hallucinosis occurs, must have been sufficient so that the individual has become dependent.
6. Course varies from several weeks to years without remission.
7. Incidence of this condition is so small that the disorder is considered very rare.

Symptoms
1. Hallucinations, usually auditory, in a clear sensorium with orientation to time, place, and person intact. The voices heard by men often accuse them of, or threaten them with, homosexual attack. Women are frequently accused of promiscuity. Auditory hallucinations may at times be of a command or imperative type.
2. Olfactory hallucinations.
3. Delusions of persecution.
4. Violent self-destructive (e.g., suicide) or other destructive (e.g., assaultive) behavior.
5. Ideas of reference.
6. Rarely visual hallucinations.
7. Apprehension.
8. Litigious behavior.
9. Panic.
10. Fear.
11. Distractibility.
12. Anger.

Differential Diagnosis
1. Alcoholic hallucinosis.
2. Hyperthyroidism.
3. Acute toxic reactions (e.g., amphetamine, cocaine psychoses, and PCP psychoses).
4. Schizophrenia.
5. Affective illness with auditory hallucinations.

Management
1. Patients should be hospitalized to protect them from harming themselves or others.
2. Sedation may be necessary. In some instances, 50–100 mg of intramuscular chlordiazepoxide (Librium) or 5–10 mg of lorazepam (Ativan) will suffice. In other instances, an antipsychotic agent such as 5–10 mg perphenazine (Trilafon) IM or haloperidol (Haldol), or 5–10 mg thiothixene (Navane) IM may be needed.
3. If violent and destructive, physical restraints may be needed to protect the patient and staff.
4. The patient should be medicated sufficiently so that he or she can sleep at night.
5. Careful attention should be given to assure that the patient's diet and vitamin intake is adequate.
6. Every attempt should be made to keep the patient oriented to reality. Procedures should be explained as they are performed, and the room should be well lit. At night, this would take the form of a night lamp.

ALCOHOL IDIOSYNCRATIC INTOXICATION
(Pathological Intoxication)

Alcohol idiosyncratic intoxication is a term used for an uncommon condition seen in a group of patients who, after drinking only a small amount of alcohol, act as if they had consumed much more.

History
1. Onset is usually sudden and dramatic with subsequent amnesia for the behavioral change.
2. Alcohol idiosyncratic intoxication can last only minutes or for as long as 24 hours or more.
3. Some authors feel it occurs in people with an epileptic predisposition and that alcohol serves as the trigger mechanism.
4. The usual behavioral change consists of aggressive or assaultive behavior that is atypical of the person when not drinking. During the episode, the individual appears out of contact with others.
5. Usual age of onset is early in life.

6. A small number of individuals with this disorder are found to have temporal lobe spikes on the electroencephalogram after receiving small amounts of alcohol.
7. The usual brain injuries associated with this disorder are encephalitis and trauma. The loss of tolerance is permanent or temporary.
8. Use of tranquilizers and sedative hypnotics that have additive effects with alcohol, fatigue, and debilitating medical illness are felt to contribute to a lower tolerance to alcohol with a tendency to respond inappropriately to small amounts.

Symptoms
1. Uninhibited behavior.
2. Illusions.
3. Assaultive, irrational, combative, and destructive behavior.
4. Transitory delusions.
5. Hallucinations.
6. Increased activity.
7. Impulsivity.
8. Anxiety.
9. Rage.
10. Depression.
11. Suicidal behavior.

Signs
1. Impairment of consciousness.
2. Confusion.
3. Disorientation.

Clinical Studies
1. Serum alcohol level helps to corroborate the diagnosis; however, the clinician should always be aware of superimposed conditions, such as temporal lobe epilepsy, that may be set off by drinking and be present in addition to acute alcohol intoxication.

Management
1. If untreated, these episodes usually terminate in a long sleep, with amnesia for the episode on wakening.
2. If violent or aggressive, the patient should be protected from injuring himself or others. This may require sedation and physical restraints.
3. Sedation can be provided by intramuscular or oral lorazepam (Ativan) or diazepam (Valium).

Quality Assurance Issues
1. Was a neurologic scan and electroencephalogram performed to identify any neurologic disease (e.g., epilepsy) as the etiology?

Ethical/Legal Issues
1. How does the clinician assess the competency of an individual suffering from this condition?
2. Where the patient engages in criminal acts, what imputation can be made about preordained knowledge and how would this affect the way the legal system would handle this patient? What would be the role of the clinician in assisting the legal system and how would this conflict with the rights of the patient to confidentiality?

ALCOHOL INTOXICATION

The acute management of alcohol intoxication entails both skill in managing someone with an acute toxic psychoses, but in addition, clinical experience with the evaluation and diagnosis of alcoholism, of dual diagnosis, and of underlying medical conditions contributing to the behavioral disturbance such as concomitant drug intoxication and withdrawal, diabetes, and subdural hematomas (Koranyi et al, 1990).

History
1. Patient or their friends will usually report that the patient drank to excess. Usually there is a history of several such previous episodes.
2. The clinical effects of alcohol are usually seen when the blood alcohol level is above 100 mg%. Above 400–500 mg%, coma usually sets in, and levels above 600–800 mg% are usually fatal. Unconsciousness usually occurs before an individual can drink enough to die.
3. Initial effects of alcohol are usually disinhibitory, but as a person continues to drink, inhibition predominates.
4. Duration of intoxification varies depending on amount of alcohol consumed; ranging from several hours to as long as 12 hours after cessation of drinking.
5. Alcohol is metabolized at the rate of 1 ounce of drinking alcohol (80 proof) per hour. Symptoms of intoxication usually appear more obvious as blood alcohol levels are rising than falling.
6. Alcohol intoxication is associated with a marked increase in automobile accidents, household accidents, industrial accidents, drownings, and airplane crashes. Obviously, an unconscious or conscious self-destructive dynamic is often operant when one drinks and has an accident, and thus, evaluation for depression is indicated (by dual diagnosis).
7 Medical complications include fractures, subdural hematomas, frostbite, and sunburn.
8. More than one-quarter of suicides occur after one has been drinking and more than one-half of murderers and victims of homicides are intoxicated at the time of the act. Incest, rape, and spouse and child abuse are also associated with alcohol intoxication.

9. Schuckit and Morrissey (1979) found that misuse of prescription drugs was more prevalent among alcoholics. Misuse is found to be greater among young alcoholics and older, middle socioeconomic status female alcoholics. The drugs most frequently abused are depressants, usually obtained from physicians by prescription.

10. Sixty percent of women above age 18 drink, with 6% of the adult female population having serious alcohol problems. Alcoholism is frequently associated with other abuse of recreational and prescription drugs and with occult psychiatric problems. Only a small proportion of women who have serious alcohol problems are in treatment (Yandow, 1989).

11. A Danish prospective study indicated more disrupted family conditions during childhood, and poor impulse control and poor verbal ability more prevalent among those most likely to become alcoholic (Schulsinger et al, 1986).

12. While prevalence of alcoholism varies among areas of North America populations, age of onset of symptoms, associated risk factors, and symptomatic presentation are similar (Helzer et al, 1990).

13. Alcoholism is a heterogeneous diagnostic entity. Some people cannot abstain once they commence drinking. Others go long periods without a drink but cannot terminate a pattern of periodic binges (Irwin et al, 1990).

14. Alcohol addiction (dependence) entails preoccupation with acquisition of alcohol, compulsive use, and recurrent or relapsing use of alcohol (Miller and Gold, 1987). Stressors may set off alcoholism in a genetically predisposed person. They do not, however, cause it in the absence of biologic susceptibility. The latter group may become intoxicated at a time of stress but not develop a pattern consistent with the diagnosis of alcohol dependence.

15. When death occurs, it is usually from respiratory paralysis or aspiration of vomitus.

Symptoms

1. Slow thinking.
2. Decreased self-control.
3. Distractibility.
4. Decreased sensory perception.
5. Decreased retention.
6. Decreased muscular control.
7. Euphoria or depression.
8. Impaired memory for recent events.
9. Labile emotion with weeping or laughter.
10. Exaggeration of underlying personality traits.
11. Rage.
12. Self- and other-directed violence.
13. Emergence of repressed and suppressed desires.
14. Irritability.
15. Loquacity.
16. Interference with social or occupational function.

17. Failure to meet responsibilities.
18. Exaggeration or muting of personality traits.
19. Amnesia for events taking place while the individual is intoxicated but fully alert (blackouts).
20. Psychiatric symptoms, past and current, does not indicate a personal or family history of schizophrenia. However, these are found more frequently in alcoholics with less early life stability, greater use of other illegal drugs, and adult antisocial behavior (Schuckit, 1982a).

Signs

1. Smell of alcohol on breath.
2. Incoordination.
3. Slurred speech.
4. Vertigo.
5. Vomiting.
6. Tremors.

Management

1. Alcoholic intoxication may be accompanied by other medical conditions that contribute to the clinical picture or it may be primarily responsible for the clinical picture. These other conditions should be treated. Physical examination and history may reveal bleeding from one of the body orifices, cardiac arrhythmias, pneumonitis, or one of the alcoholic syndromes such as Korsakoff's psychosis or Wernicke's encephalopathy.
2. If necessary, 50–100 mg of chlordiazepoxide (Librium) or 10–20 mg of diazepam (Valium) may be given orally or intramuscularly to sedate the patient.
3. Patients should be placed in a room with minimal distractions to be calmed and should be prevented from bringing harm to themselves or others. Physical restraints may be needed.
4. Some patients, both occasional drinkers and chronic alcoholics, when acutely intoxicated, may respond to coffee and support and become sober.
5. The best disposition after an acute episode of alcohol intoxication is usually home with supportive relatives or friends, who will watch the patient until he or she has entirely recovered. If this is impossible, of if for medical reasons, patients need to be observed further, they should spend the night in a bed in the emergency room or be hospitalized. Other dispositions include religious or otherwise privately supported hostels for people without a place to go for the night, the local YMCA or YWCA, the Salvation Army, and some inexpensive hotels. If the patient has physically harmed a person or property and has no acute medical problems, jail is an alternative that must be considered, especially if the patient is a repeated threat to the well-being of the community.
6. Recurrent alcohol use despite a good treatment history sometimes indicates dual diagnosis—alcoholism secondary to a primary psychiatric disorder. Primary affective illness with secondary alcoholism is associated with greater use of alcohol and illicit drugs (Schuckit, 1983a).

7. The 12 Step program is critical to the success of management of both primary alcoholism and secondary alcoholism. Even when alcohol and other drugs are used to medicate a primary psychiatric disorder, it may become such a habit that successful management of the dually diagnosed patient entails both diagnostic-specific therapy of the primary psychiatric disorder and of the alcohol abuse disorder (Zweben, 1987).

8. Suicide is always a risk among those intoxicated (as well as those who are dually diagnosed) as depression and anxiety symptoms become more predominant after cessation of alcohol. Alcohol itself decreases judgement and disinhibits, resulting in more impulsive behavior such as intravenous drug use, promiscuous sex with exposure to AIDS, and reckless driving (particularly among youth). Studies of alcoholics indicate a lifetime risk of suicide of about 3.4%. Likelihood of suicide in the conservatively diagnosed alcoholic is about 60 to 120 times that of the rest of the population. Alcoholism contributes to about 25% of suicides (Murphy and Wetzel, 1990).

9. Slow, reversible, organic mental disorders have been reported among alcoholics after prolonged abstinence (Grant I et al, 1987).

10. When alcohol is used to self-medicate a primary anxiety disorder an anxiolytic (with low potentiate for abuse and minimal ability to potentiate the effects of alcohol) such as buspirone (Buspar) should be used (Mayer, 1986).

Prevention

1. Alcoholism and affective illness appear to be independent diseases (Schuckit, 1986). If there is a family history of alcoholism, family members should be made aware that alcohol use may lead to alcohol dependence. If there is a family history of affective illness—not alcoholism—an acutely intoxicated person may be suspected of self-medication of a primary affective illness (by dual diagnosis).

Quality Assurance Issues

1. Was a patient evaluated for a concurrent medical, surgical (e.g., subdural hematomas), and primary nonalcoholic psychiatric illness?
2. Was an evaluation made of concurrent "drug" usage?
3. Was an evaluation made of a patient's suicide and homicide potential?

Ethical/Legal Issues

1. Professionals with high-risk occupations, such as physicians and airline pilots, must be placed in the care of those who are aware of the need to assure absolute compliance to treatment to avoid physical harm to others (Brewster, 1986).
2. Should a psychiatrist, knowing a patient is an abuser of alcohol, have an obligation to inform the state's motor vehicle department?
3. In many states, if an alcoholic can no longer control his drinking and is also potentially dangerous to himself and others, he may be committed for treatment (Tancredi, 1982).

ALCOHOL USE PROBLEMS

Evidence is growing that there is a biogenetic predisposition to development of alcoholism, particularly in sons of men with early onset alcoholism (Charness et al, 1989). Alcoholism alone runs in families, or it may be seen together with a family history of suicide or manic–depressive disease. In some instances, alcohol is used to self-medicate anxiety, an affective disorder, or schizophrenia.

History

1. It is difficult to obtain an accurate history of alcohol intake. The amount stated by the patient frequently represents a conservative minimum. Relatives and friends may be needed to obtain a more realistic estimate. Early in an individual's career as an alcoholic, his or her drinking is generally limited to evenings and weekends. As tolerance increases, these individuals begin to experience periods of memory loss, with loss of consciousness referred to as "blackouts." When these occur frequently with moderate amounts of alcohol intake alcohol addiction is probably near. An individual at this time begins to sneak drinks and at times has episodes of losing control. Eventually the individual imbibes to intoxication each evening and awakens the next morning with a hangover. Drinking alone may begin at this stage. Alibis are developed to excuse the individual from social events and work. Individuals begin to miss more and more work at this stage and eventually quit their jobs or are fired. Drinking begins to occur in the morning, and it may continue for periods of several days ("binges"). As individuals' tolerance increases, drinking becomes nearly constant, and they progressively deteriorate. Sudden cessation of alcohol may result in shakes, tremors, or frank delirium tremens. With passing years, the physical stigmata of chronic alcohol abuse appear. In the absence of drinking the individual notices that tremor, an indefinable fear, and difficulty performing simple motor tasks appear. Taking a drink relieves these symptoms.
2. Symptoms of abuse and dependence are generally seen within 5 years of the onset of regular drinking. A history of heavy drinking in adolescence is associated with a high incidence of alcohol-related problems in adult life.
3. Buydens-Branchey et al (1989a) found individuals with onset of alcoholism prior to age 20 had a greater incidence of paternal alcoholism and were twice as likely to have been incarcerated for crimes of violence, three times as likely to be depressed, and four times as likely to have attempted suicide than those with later onset alcoholism. Depression and aggressive tendencies in those with early onset alcoholism was found associated with low serotonin levels (Buydens-Branchey et al, 1989b). This is interesting, as low serotonin levels are known to be associated with impulsivity as manifested in suicide and homicide.
4. Alcoholism is a rising problem among career women and the elderly who live alone. Fixed budgets with rising inflation result in decreased money for food. Alcohol may be delivered to an apartment gratis, whereas, an infirm older person may have to pay someone to deliver groceries.

5. Drinking may be continuously heavy, restricted to weekends with lighter drinking during the week, or may be limited to binges (heavy daily drinking that lasts for weeks). All of these increase psychological and medical morbidity and mortality.

6. Long-term use of alcohol leads to a number of medical complications which, associated with alterations in mood, thought, and behavior, further complicate the picture. These include vitamin deficiency, neurologic diseases, and liver disease.

7. Suicide risk is greater among alcohol-dependent people and may occur in either the sober or intoxicated state.

8. Alcohol dependence occurs when there is a compelling desire to use alcohol with an inability to reduce or stop drinking. Continuous or episodic use should have occurred for at least 1 month and be associated with social complications such as decreased functioning at work, arguments with family members or friends over excessive use of alcohol, or legal difficulties such as arrests for driving while intoxicated. The individual is tolerant (i.e., requires increasing amounts of alcohol to achieve the desired level) and experiences malaise or "shakes" that are relieved by drinking.

9. Awareness of a positive family history of alcoholism is increased significantly when resource persons other than the patient are questioned in addition to the patient (Schuckit, 1983b). Men who have alcoholic relatives tend to have more severe alcohol-related pathology and earlier social problems.

10. The rate and severity of depressive symptoms is greater among subjects who relapse in an alcohol and drug abuse population than among those who do not (Hatsukami and Pickens, 1982).

11. The best data supporting the genetic influence on the development of alcoholism come from studies of individuals who have been adopted (Schuckit and Bernstein, 1981). There is a four-fold increase in the rate of alcoholism in children of alcoholics separated from their parents close to birth when compared to both children of nonalcoholics who have been adopted and to the general population (Goodwin D, 1976).

12. With alcoholic patients without primary affective illness, depressive symptoms decrease with weeks of abstinence when standard depression scales are used (e.g., Beck Depression Inventory). This is not true when patients were self-medicating a primary affective illness (Dorus et al, 1987).

13. Alcoholic men with a family history of alcoholism tend to differ from alcoholic men without a family history of alcoholism by the former group having more antisocial behavior, more severe alcoholic symptomatology, worse social and academic performance in school, more severe physical symptoms related to alcohol, less stable employment histories, and a background of families of lower socioeconomic status and more psychopathology (Frances RJ et al, 1980).

14. A relationship has been identified between childhood conduct disorder and the development of alcoholism as an adult (Cadoret et al, 1980).

15. Abstinence tends to be associated with finding substitute dependencies and new relationships such as religious or Alcoholics Anonymous involvement (Vaillant and Milofsky, 1982).

16. Postnatal environment determines the severity and frequency of expression of the most common form of genetically inherited alcoholism (Cloninger et al, 1982b).

17. There appears to be a three-fold excess of alcohol abusers among adopted daughters of alcoholic biologic mothers compared with other daughters. Fathers with extensive treatment for criminality and for alcoholism do not have an excess of alcoholic daughters while fathers with history of alcohol abuse but without criminality do (Bohman et al, 1981).

18. Patients with low psychiatric severity tend to improve from most approaches to alcohol treatment while those with high psychiatric severity tend to show virtually no improvement (McLellan et al, 1983).

19. Severe depression in alcoholics ("secondary depression") tends to be associated with greater intake of drugs in addition to alcohol (Schuckit, 1983a).

20. In a 10-year follow-up study of alcoholic native Americans, it was found that those who remained abstinent after treatment were characterized by stable marriages and/or employment, less depression, and stronger interpersonal relationships than those who relapse despite repeat treatment (Westermeyer and Peake, 1983).

Quality Assurance Issues

1. Has a complete family history been obtained with focus on affective illness, alcohol abuse, and sociopathy?

2. Has the patient's history of ability to function in employment been properly assessed?

3. Has the medical status of the abuser been thoroughly evaluated?

Ethical/Legal Issues

1. Is the alcohol abuser competent to accept treatment or to volunteer for hospitalization, if that is necessary?

2. Has the patient engaged in violent acts resulting in harm to a third person prior to coming to the hospital?

ALCOHOL WITHDRAWAL DELIRIUM
(Delirium Tremens)

The probability that alcohol withdrawal delirium will occur relates to the amount and duration of drinking before cessation of use of alcohol. Onset of symptoms usually occurs 2 to 10 days after cessation or reduction of heavy alcohol ingestion.

History

1. Duration of the delirium ranges from several days to only a period of hours. The

mortality rate due to such complications as hyperthermia or circulatory collapse is between 4% and 20%.

2. Clinical presentation and course may be complicated by a number of medical problems, including infections such as pneumonitis, profound dehydration with electrolyte imbalance, hyperthermia, vascular collapse, malnutrition, meningitis, cerebral laceration, anemia, gastritis with hematemesis, and cirrhosis.

3. Because of the alcoholic's proneness to head trauma due to falls, muggings, and seizures, the possibility of an epidural or subdural hematoma complicating the picture should be entertained, and when suspected, investigated by careful neurologic examination, skull films, lumbar puncture, and CT scan.

4. Concurrent physical illness predisposes to alcohol withdrawal delirium.

5. Only about 5% of patients being treated for alcohol withdrawal develop delirium.

Symptoms

1. Nightmares.
2. Panic attacks while attempting to fall asleep.
3. Insomnia.
4. Illusions.
5. Vivid hallucinations.
6. Agitation.
7. Delirium.
8. Increasing psychosis.
9. Disorientation.
10. Hallucinations, either of rapidly moving small animals such as snakes or Lilliputian hallucinations (auditory hallucinations are rare).
11. Suggestibility.
12. Restlessness.
13. Dizziness.

Signs

1. Coarse, persistent hand tremor.
2. Diaphoresis.
3. Tachycardia.
4. Dilated pupils.
5. Increase in temperature.
6. Seizures.
7. Restlessness.
8. Hyperactivity.
9. Ataxia.
10. Clouding of consciousness.
11. Disturbance of speech with slurring, thickness, and word distortion.
12. Elevated blood pressure.
13. Coated tongue.
14. Dry lips.

15. Stigmata of chronic alcohol abuse such as hepatomegaly and peripheral neuropathies.

Differential Diagnosis.

Differential diagnosis includes all other causes of delirium tremens such as fever and central nervous system depressant withdrawal (e.g., barbiturate, meprobamate, and benzodiazepine withdrawal).

Management

1. Patients should be placed in a well-lit room. As procedures are performed (e.g., blood drawing), they should be explained simply. If available, a family member should be present to help calm patients. Patients' location on a service should be where their delirium will cause minimal disturbance to other people.
2. Mechanical restraints may be needed—in addition to medication—to help calm patients.
3. Of extreme important in the treatment is maintenance of fluid and electrolyte intake. As much as 6 liters of fluid may be needed per day, of which $1\frac{1}{2}$ liters should be normal saline, to counter the extreme fluid loss through profuse perspiration and agitation. Serum electrolytes and BUN should be monitord to guide the treatment.
4. Sedation should be liberally used to reduce agitation, to prevent exhaustion, to make the patient more comfortable, and to produce rest and sleep. Many different methods have been tried, and currently, diazepam (Valium), chlordiazepoxide (Librium), and lorazepam (Ativan) are quite popular. The dose of chlordiazepoxide is 50–100 mg every 4 hours, up to 300–400 mg/day or more in cases of severe agitation. Paraldehyde is a frequently used agent with up to 10 mL given orally, or in an oil retention enema every 2 hours. Chloral hydrate may be given in doses of up to 1 g every 4 hours. Physicians should be aware of the danger of oversedation as it may mask symptoms of an epidural or subdural hematoma. This can be minimized if the physician reassesses the situation before each new dose of medication is ordered and then writes a new order at that time. Intramuscular administration of paraldehyde is minimized to prevent sterile abscesses and nerve damage.
5. Patients' temperatures are monitored. Physicians must be alert to the possibility of a superimposed infection, such as pneumonitis. In the absence of any infection, sponge baths, cooling blankets, and aspirin can be used to keep temperature down. Obviously, if infection is superimposed, appropriate antibiotics are employed.
6. Chronic alcoholic patients are usually vitamin deficient. Therefore 50–200 mg of thiamine is given intramuscularly followed by 100 mg of thiamine bid orally.
7. Ideally pulse, blood pressure, and temperatures are recorded at half-hour intervals at the height of the illness, in order to minimize occurrence of lethal complications and alcohol withdrawal delirium, circulatory collapse, and hyperthermia. If these occur, they are immediately treated with the appropriate measures. Whole blood transfusions, fluids, and vasopressors are used to combat shock, and ice packs and a cooling mattress are used to treat hyperthermia.

8. Prophylactic anticonvulsant medication is usually not needed for simple alcohol withdrawal. If convulsions or status epilepticus occur, these are appropriately treated.
9. If hypoglycemia accompanies the alcohol withdrawal, glucose is administered.
10. Other medical problems such as cirrhosis and gastritis are attended to. Skull and chest films are taken and a lumbar puncture is routinely performed.
11. Depression secondary to alcoholism improves during withdrawal (Bokstrom et al, 1989). If it does not, primary affective illness with self-medication with alcohol (dual diagnosis) should be suspected and treated with antidepressants.

All the drugs used in the management of alcohol withdrawal delirium have their limitations. Some authors feel the benzodiazepines (chlordiazepoxide and diazepam) are not effective in severe cases. Paraldehyde is addicting and sudden death may follow its use. Hepatotoxicity has been reported with phenothiazines and they lower the seizure threshold. Barbiturates are addicting and can produce paradoxical excitement.

Once it has been established that a patient is in alcohol withdrawal delirium, he or she is to be considered a medical emergency and must be hospitalized.

Quality Assurance Issues
1. Were a neurologic examination and diagnostic studies conducted to rule out complicating features of head trauma?

Ethical/Legal Issues
1. Given the acute emergency nature of the condition, when a patient presents with florid DTs, the emergency nature of the condition allows for the administration of treatment even if the patient is incompetent to give consent. Efforts must be made to locate the appropriate next of kin or other authority to give consent.

ALCOHOLIC JEALOUSY

Patients presenting with alcoholic jealousy usually have long histories of alcoholic use. This may be denied by the patient, requiring clinicians to obtain corroboration of the diagnosis from the patient's friends or relatives.

History
1. The premorbid history of these patients often reveals the absence of mature heterosexual relationships.
2. The paranoid delusions have been interpreted by some as a defense against unconscious homosexual desires.
3. Since delusions of jealousy can occur in both alcoholic and nonalcoholic states, alcohol may just serve as a precipitant of a delusional disorder. Alcoholic jealousy may not represent a separate diagnostic entity. It may be a delusional disorder associated with alcohol use.

Symptoms
1. Anger.
2. Suspicion.
3. Resentment.
4. Ideas of reference.
5. Delusions of jealousy.
6. Distrust.
7. Assaultive behavior with homicidal risk.
8. Self-destructive behavior with suicidal risk.
9. Accusations that spouse is having illicit sexual affairs with friends, strangers, children, or relatives.
10. Accusations that spouse has insatiable sexual desires.
11. For men, claiming to find seminal stains of other men about the house.
12. Suspecting spouse of changing underwear in preparation for an affair.
13. Accusing spouse of being colder than usual.

Differential Diagnosis
1. Alcoholic jealousy.
2. Paranoid schizophrenia.
3. Delusional disorder.
4. Paranoid personality disorder.
5. Other forms of schizophrenia with paranoia.
6. Major depressive disorder with paranoia.
7. Amphetamine psychosis.
8. Cocaine psychosis.
9. Organic mental disorders with paranoia.

Management
1. The prognosis of patients is guarded.
2. Symptoms of alcoholic jealousy are usually controllable in a hospital with appropriate psychopharmacotherapy. Unfortunately, paranoid patients are especially prone to discontinuation of medication because of their delusions of persecution. Soon after a patient stops medication, symptoms tend to return.

Quality Assurance Issues
1. Has a proper evaluation been conducted to rule out alternative biological explanations for this condition?

Ethical/Legal Issues
1. When a patient reveals serious jealous feelings and suggests harmful behavior to third parties, is the therapist obligated to "warn" the third party that he may be harmed by the patient (Tarasoff, 1977)?

ALZHEIMER'S DISEASE

Patients with Alzheimer's disease may present de novo in the emergency room with a psychiatric disorder other than Alzheimer's, confusing diagnosis for both the clinician and the patient's family, or may present as a patient known to have Alzheimer's disease with psychiatric symptoms requiring acute evaluation and treatment. In some instances, a patient may be depressed and suicidal. When Alzheimer's disease is misdiagnosed as depression, it is known as pseudodepression. When depression is misdiagnosed as dementia it is called pseudodementia. Alzheimer patients with major depressive disorder have significantly more first- and second-degree relatives with depression than do nondepressed Alzheimer patients (Pearlson et al, 1990). A study of 217 outpatients with presumed Alzheimer's disease (Mendez et al, 1990) indicated that 40% had depressive symptoms such as hopelessness, helplessness, and sad affect; 35.5% had paranoia and suspiciousness; 30.9% had fearfulness and anxiety; 30% had delusions; 24.9% had aggressive acts; and 18.4% formed visual hallucinations.

Management

Psychiatric symptoms are managed with symptom-specific treatment just as with nonorganic psychiatric disorders. Doses of antipsychotics, anxiolytics, mood stabilizers, and antidepressants necessary for therapeutic impact are smaller in older people and those with organic mental disorders, regardless of age. Primary treatment of Alzheimer's disease entails referral to a neurologist or gerontopsychiatrist.

Quality Assurance Issues

1. Was the patient evaluated to ascertain whether what appeared to be Alzheimer's disease was pseudodementia requiring antidepressant therapy?
2. Was the patient evaluated to ascertain whether antidepressants or ECT would enhance cognitive performance?

Ethical/Legal Issues

1. Patients with Alzheimers pose serious ethical issues for the clinician. The deficit of short term memory calls into question the validity of any self-determinative act. Can a patient with Alzheimers give informed consent to treatment? What about clinical experimentation? What role does memory have in an act of autonomy?

ALPRAZOLAM-INDUCED DISORDERS

Alprazolam (Xanax) is an excellent medication for the diagnostic-specific management of panic disorder. It has few notable side effects. Those reported are common to benzodiazepines (such as addiction) or seen specifically with alprazolam. Those specific to alprazolam are due to the fact that it is believed related to the fact it may have antidepressant qualities. For instance, alprazolam has been reported to produce reversible stuttering (Elliott and Thomas, 1985) and mania in patients with shortened REM latency, and nonsuppression on the dexamethasone suppression test suggestive of underlying affective illness (Peckhold and Fleury, 1986). The precipitation of these symptoms is suggestive evidence for pharmacologic effects similar to tricyclic antidepressants. Alprazolam-induced dyscontrol in patients with borderline personality disorder is consistent with the fact that it is a triazolobenzodiazepine (Gardner and Cowdry, 1985). Benzodiazepines increase behavioral outbursts such as aggressive behavior and hostile outbursts. The fact that the doses of 2–10 mg per day are generally required for efficacious therapy of panic disorder and depression increases risk of addiction.

Symptoms of Withdrawal
1. Agitation.
2. Tachypnea.
3. Palpitations.
4. Depersonalization.
5. Perceptual distortion.
6. Seizures.
7. Anxiety.

Management
1. Mania, when induced, is managed with major tranquilizers after cessation of alprazolam.
2. Stuttering and episodic dyscontrol remit with cessation of alprazolam.
3. Withdrawal symptoms can occur while the patient is on the drug but with the dosage reduced, after rapid cessation, and after gradual withdrawal to the drug-free state (Juergens and Morse, 1988; Mellman and Uhde, 1986). If symptoms persist after dosage is reduced, return to the original dosage and withdraw more gradually (e.g., 0.125- or 0.25-mg increments per week).
4. To minimize withdrawal symptoms, reduce dose by 0.25 mg weekly until patient is drug free.
5. Advise patients they may suffer some symptoms (e.g., muscular aches) in the drug-free state for a few weeks.
6. Some patients require hospitalization to successfully withdraw from the drug.

Quality Assurance Issues
1. Alprazolam should not be prescribed for a patient with known addiction to alcohol or drugs except for extraordinary reasons that are documented in the patient's chart.

Ethical/Legal Issues
1. The clinical planning to use alprazolam must balance the marginal benefit to be achieved over the alternative medications against the marginal cost in terms of addiction potential. Given that calculus, would alternatives be more desirable?

What circumstances would justify alprazolam over clonazepam (Klonopin) or buspirone (BuSpar), for example?

AMANTADINE INTOXICATION, HALLUCINOSIS, AND DELUSIONAL STATES

One of the few side effects of the antiparkinsonian agent amantadine is psychotic delirium (Hausner, 1980).

History
1. Hallucinations occur either alone or in conjunction with cognitive disturbances such as delusions and disorientation (Butzer et al, 1975).
2. While all antiparkinsonian agents may cause psychosis, that caused by amantadine is more insidious in onset and more difficult to recognize (Hausner, 1980).
3. Patients successfully managed for symptoms of schizophrenia may have an exacerbation when given amantadine.
4. Onset of amantadine-induced psychosis may be several months after commencement of the drug, leading a clinician to the conclusion that the psychosis seen is not drug-induced (Harper and Knothe, 1973).
5. Visual hallucinations alert a clinician to the fact that the psychosis is drug related.

Management
1. Symptoms disappear upon reduction or cessation of the use of amantadine.

Quality Assurance Issues
1. What factor or factors would alert you to the possibility of amantadine psychosis?

Ethical/Legal Issues
1. Would the possibility of psychosis from amantadine need to be disclosed to the patient in informed consent? How would this be done?

AMNESIA

Recovery from transient global amnesia may include periods of transient partial amnesia, confusing diagnosis for the emergency clinician. Nonverbal memory is reported to recover prior to verbal memory (Okada et al, 1987).

Management
1. Episodes tend to commence suddenly and last 2 to 12 hours with gradual clearing or disappearance with sleep (Okada et al, 1987).

Quality Assurance Issues
1. Were all causes for amnesia considered in the differential diagnosis? Was diagnostic-specific therapy used?

Ethical/Legal Issues
1. Would a consent given during amnesia be valid in informed consent? How important is memory in identifying competency?

AMOXAPINE-INDUCED DISORDERS

A number of symptoms have been reported during use of the antidepressant amoxapine (Asendin). In addition, dyskinesia has been associated with abrupt withdrawal (McMahon, 1986; Lesser, 1983; Weller and McKnelly, 1983) including orofacial dyskinesia (Gammon and Hansen, 1984). Parkinsonism and tardive dyskinesia occurring during its use indicate that its neuroleptic effects are significant (Thornton and Stahl, 1984). The disorders seen are attributed to acute or chronic blockade of striatal dopamine receptors by the amoxapine metabolite, 7-hydroxyamoxapine (Gammon and Hansen, 1984).

Management
1. Amoxapine should be administered with the same precautions afforded use of other neuroleptics.
2. The akinesia characterized by mutism, psychomotor retardation, apathy, and lack of spontaneous movement may be construed to be depression, and usually remits with cessation of the drug.
3. Reduction of dosage or concomitant treatment with anticholinergics alleviate the parkinsonism, akathisia, and acute dystonia (Weller and McKnelly, 1983).
4. Withdrawal dyskinesia, an assumed early stage of tardive dyskinesia, may disappear after weeks of cessation of use of the drug.
5. Amoxapine is a tricyclic dibenzanthracene that is the demethylated metabolite of the neuroleptic loxapine (Loxitane) and therefore can produce an irreversible tardive dyskinesia (Weller and McKnelly, 1983).

Quality Assurance Issues
1. Was the patient advised of the possibility of tardive dyskinesia with use of amoxapine?
2. Did the clinician periodically evaluate the patient for early signs of tardive dyskinesia?

Ethical/Legal Issues
1. Does the fact that effective alternatives (that do not have tardive dyskinesia as a side effect) exist for depression mean that using amoxapine is negligence?

AMPHETAMINE AND OTHER SYMPATHOMIMETIC INTOXICATION, DELIRIUM, AND DELUSIONAL STATES

Oral or intravenous use of amphetamine and similarly acting sympathomimetics lead to states of intoxication, delirium, and delusion. Cessation of use may lead to profound depression with risk of suicide. If an individual presents with the physiological, psychological, and behavioral effects of the use of such substances and evidence of delirium or delusion, the syndrome is referred to as intoxication. If signs of delirium such as fragmented thinking, dysattention, confusion, and difficulty in goal-directed behavior develop within 24 hours of taking the substance, the clinical picture is referred to as delirium.

Paranoia and other evidence of delusional thinking may follow prolonged use of moderate to high doses of sympathomimetics. This states is referred to as amphetamine or other sympathomimetic delusional disorder.

History

1. Patients who develop sympathomimetic intoxication, delirium, or delusional disorders have a history of recent use of sympathomimetic substances. These include amphetamine, dextroamphetamine, methamphetamine, and substances differing from substituted phenylethylamine that have amphetamine-like actions such as methlyphenidate (Ritalin) and a variety of diet pills.
2. Popular names for sympathomimetic substances taken for recreational use are "bennies," "dexies," "speed," "crank," "ice," "black beauties," and "crystal meth."
3. Sympathomimetic substances may be taken orally or intravenously.
4. Signs of intoxication usually begin within 1 hour of use. Delirium, when it occurs, develops within 24 hours of intake. Prolonged intake of moderate- or high-dose sympathomimetic substances are required for development of a delusional state. If the substance is taken intravenously, symptoms may begin nearly immediately. Delusions should not develop after a single dose unless preceded by prolonged use. If delusions are seen after a single dose, the clinician should think of the possibility of the presence of other underlying psychopathology such as paranoid schizophrenia.
5. Symptoms of psychoses are common in individuals who have taken more than 90–100 mg of amphetamines per day. A hallucinating panic state may occur after a single dose in a predisposed person.
6. The degree of paranoia seen vacillates in a chronic user dependent on the amount taken on any given day.
7. It is common for individuals in the drug culture, as well as for professional people with access to a number of euphorigenic and sedating substances, to mix drugs. This practice confuses the clinical picture and increases the risk of unattended withdrawal, as withdrawal from a number of "downers" can lead to delirium tremens with its risk of mortality. The use of heroin in combination with cocaine or amphetamines is known as a "speedball" or "croak." Heroin may be used alone to bring an individual down from an amphetamine binge.

8. Amphetamine, cocaine, and other sympathomimetic delusional states are sometimes virtually indistinguishable from paranoid schizophrenia. In addition, sympathomimetic substance delusional states may accompany schizophrenia or other major psychiatric disorders and complicate clinical presentation. The characteristics of cocaine intoxication are identical to that of amphetamine and other sympathomimetic psychoses with the exception that when the symptoms are due to the latter, they persist long beyond the time of substance use. Delusions and hallucinations seen with cocaine use are always transient unless there is some underlying psychopathology.

9. Symptoms of a sympathomimetic delusional state develop rapidly with paranoia being the predominant feature.

10. The clinical picture of sympathomimetic intoxication, delirium, or delusional state always represents an interaction of the patient's premorbid psychological and physical condition, the dose and duration of sympathomimetic intake, the environment in which the substance is taken, and the number and the quantity of other drugs taken. One individual may look like an emotionally labile hypomanic with paranoid features; another may look like a paranoid schizophrenic.

11. Symptoms of intoxication and delirium (when present) usually are over within 6 hours of cessation of drug intake whereas the delusional symptoms may last for as long as a year.

12. The usual course of a sympathomimetic delusional syndrome is a week or less. Delusional syndromes are seen more frequently than delirium.

13. Patients who are toxic or delusional from sympathomimetic substances usually remain oriented.

14. Corroboration of the diagnosis of amphetamine intoxication can be made by urinary or serum tests for amphetamines.

Symptoms of Sympathomimetic Intoxication
1. Euphoria.
2. Hyperarousal.
3. Grandiosity.
4. Irritability.
5. Loquacity, sometimes to the extent of pressured speech.
6. Emotional lability.
7. Hypervigilance.
8. Anorexia.
9. Aggressiveness and hostility.
10. Anxiety.
11. Panic.
12. Resistance to fatigue.
13. Restless wakefulness (insomnia).
14. Changes in body image.
15. Chronic muscular tension.
16. Severe abdominal pain, sometimes mimicking an acute abdomen.
17. Impaired judgement.

18. Interference with social and occupational functioning.
19. Chest pain.

Signs of Sympathomimetic Intoxication
1. Dilated but reactive pupils.
2. Tachycardia.
3. Elevated temperature.
4. Elevated blood pressure (both tachycardia and elevated blood pressure may be absent in chronic users).
5. Dry mouth.
6. Perspiration or chills.
7. Nausea and vomiting.
8. Psychomotor excitement.
9. Tremulousness.
10. Hyperactive reflexes.
11. Furtive glancing about the room.
12. Malnutrition (especially apparent after prolonged intravenous use of large doses).
13. Repetitious compulsive behavior.
14. Biting stereotypes may cause ulcers on the tongue and lips.
15. Teeth may be worn from bruxism.
16. Needle marks on the arm if the drug is taken intravenously.
17. Cardiac arrhythmias and subdural and subarachnoid hemorrhage are occasional complications of the elevated blood pressure and tachycardia.
18. Skin flushing.
19. Cutaneous abscesses and excoriation.

Symptoms of Sympathomimetic Delusional Disorders
In addition to the symptoms and physical signs seen with sympathomimetic intoxication, individuals with an amphetamine or similar acting sympathomimetic delusional disorder have

1. Though disorder.
2. Ideas of reference.
3. Auditory hallucinations, frequently of voices commenting, criticizing, and accusing the patient of misconduct. The voices may threaten the patient with violence or have an imperative or command quality necessitating hospitalization.
4. Paranoid ideation with delusions of persecution with a clear sensorium.
5. Visual hallucinations, sometimes with distortion of faces and disturbances of body image.
6. Formication (hallucination of bugs or vermin crawling under the skin, sometimes leading individuals to scratch themselves with resultant excoriations of the skin).

Sympathomimetic Delirium
In addition to the other symptoms and physical signs seen with sympathomi-

metic intoxication or delusional disorder, an individual with amphetamine or similarly acting sympathomimetic delirium shows the usual symptoms of delirium such as dysattention, fragmented thinking, and fluctuating levels of consciousness. Affect is labile, and both olfactory and tactile hallucinations may be seen. Individuals with a sympathomimetic delirium may become so violent that restraints may be required.

Differential Diagnosis
1. Amphetamine psychosis.
2. Cocaine psychosis.
3. Other sympathomimetic psychoses.
4. Paranoid schizophrenia.
5. Alcoholic hallucinosis.
6. Reactive psychoses.
7. Hypomania.
8. Catatonic schizophrenia (excited phase).
9. Obsessive–compulsive disorder.
10. Phencyclidine ("angel dust") psychoses.

Management
1. Symptoms of psychoses usually subside 2 to 3 days after cessation of amphetamines. Visual hallucinations usually remain 24 to 48 hours, while delusions (when present) last for 7 to 10 days. Rarely, delusions in an attenuated form may remain as long as a year.
2. Within 24 hours of the final dose, a patient may be found to be spending increasing amounts of time sleeping. In some instances, this may be as much as 18 to 20 hours a day for up to 3 days with considerable dreaming. "Crashing"—depression sometimes accompanied by suicidal ideation—may occur and increase over the weeks following discontinuation of use. Without treatment, this depression may last a considerable period of time. Characteristically such individuals show a greater amount of fatigue, apathy, and flattening of affect than in the usual depression.
3. Clinicians evaluating individuals with sympathomimetic intoxication should always be aware of the patients' potential to act out violently and should be prepared to protect themselves. It is recommended that these patients be treated on an inpatient service where appropriate sedation and restraints can be provided if necessary.
4. Patients should be placed in a quiet room, reassured, and kept as calm as possible during the acute stages of intoxication. Two to five milligrams of haloperidol (Haldol) intramuscularly followed by 2–4 mg tid is usually sufficient to handle even delusional patients. Frequently no medication is required after 1 day.
5. Amphetamine intake is discontinued immediately; gradual reduction of dosage is not necessary.
6. Phenothiazines and other antipsychotic drugs including haloperidol should not be given if it is known the patient has ingested significant amounts of antipsychotic drugs with strong anticholinergic properties in addition to the sympatho-

mimetics. Diazepam (Valium) 10–20 mg PO or IM or another similarly acting benzodiazepine is a satisfactory alternative.
7. In rare instances, life support measures may be necessary. In such instances, transfer to a medical ward may be necessary where ice packs, gastric lavage, and other needed measures may be instituted.

Quality Assurance Issues
1. Were serum or urinary screens performed to ascertain if the patient used cocaine, amphetamines, PCP, or other recreational or prescribed drugs?
2. Was a differential diagnosis developed and alternate or concurrent disorders ruled out?

Ethical/Legal Issues
1. Should the psychiatrist explore the history of proneness to violence of patients in this population? What if the psychiatrist discovers that the patient may have seriously injured a person in his or her path? What are the psychiatrist's obligations to the patient and to the putative victim?

AMPHETAMINE AND SIMILARLY ACTING SYMPATHOMIMETIC WITHDRAWAL

Symptoms and physical signs of withdrawal from amphetamines or similarly acting substances generally commence within 3 days of cessation of use and peak within 2 to 4 days.

History
1. Depression and irritability may persist for months and, in some cases, necessitate the use of antidepressants or electroshock because of the risk of suicide.

Symptoms and Physical Signs of Sympathomimetic Withdrawal
1. Depression.
2. Increased dreaming.
3. Fatigue.
4. Disturbed sleep (with increased REM activity on EEG).
5. Agitation.
6. Suicidal ideation.
7. Irritability.
8. Apathy.

Management
1. *The most critical aspect of managing patients who are withdrawing from amphetamines is a heightened sensitivity to their capacity to attempt to take their*

own lives. Suicide precautions and hospitalization may be required with profound depression.

2. Individuals presenting intoxicated on amphetamine or another sympathomimetic substance should be given haloperidol (Haldol) or thiothixene (Navane) 2–5 mg PO tid or qid, or an equivalent dosage of a similarly acting phenothiazine. A benzodiazepine (e.g., lorazepam [Ativan]) should be used as an alternative or in instances where the individual is also using drugs with strong anticholinergic side effects.

3. Dosage of the antipsychotic drug is gradually reduced over days or weeks as the patient's symptoms subside.

4. Intake of amphetamine or a similarly acting sympathomimetic should be discontinued immediately.

5. The depression that frequently follows the pronounced fatigue and apathy after cessation of sympathomimetic use is usually countered by administration of antidepressants for 1 or 2 months. If suicidal risk is significant, use of electroshock may be required.

6. Individuals should be allowed to sleep during the few days of hypersomnia that follow cessation of drug use.

7. Individuals should be evaluated for benefit from brief psychotherapy to explore reasons for sympathomimetic abuse if present. Patients should be alerted to the fact that the normal after-effect of sympathomimetic use is a period of decreased initiative, apathy, and depression, and that these symptoms tend to pass in 2 to 4 months. These symptoms are not necessarily an indicant of intrapsychic turmoil but rather the usual sequelum.

8. Remember that individuals who have been prescribed sympathomimetic substances for narcolepsy, minimal brain damage, and asthma may develop intoxication, delusions, and delirium and go through withdrawal symptoms upon cessation of use.

9. Attending physicians should not be induced into providing a new source of amphetamine or another sympathomimetic substance at times of stress. Individuals who have abused sympathomimetic substances should be continuously evaluated for the need of long-term antidepressant therapy or psychotherapy.

10. It may be necessary with a sociopathic patient to obtain serum or urine samples periodically to check for amphetamine content in order to maintain the patient free of drugs.

11. Group therapy with "speed freaks" may be of some value.

Quality Assurance Issues
1. Was the patient evaluated for suicide risk? If suicidal, were precautions taken?
2. Was the patient evaluated for an underlying psychiatric disorder (e.g., depression, schizophrenia)?

Ethical/Legal Issues
1. Was abuse of these substances induced by psychiatric treatment?

2. Was the psychiatrist sensitive to the abusing patient? Did the psychiatrist contribute to the abuse, intoxication, withdrawal, or adverse consequences?
3. Were appropriate actions taken to commit or otherwise handle the suicidal or dangerous patient in withdrawal?

AMPUTATION
(Acute)

Amputation may be anticipated (as in instances of patients with peripheral vascular disease and insulin-dependent diabetes) or sudden (as following a car, industrial, or airplane accident or diagnosis of a malignant osteogenic sarcoma). In both instances an emergency psychiatric clinician may be called for crisis intervention and evaluation of concurrent psychiatric disorders such as a post-traumatic stress disorder or affective illness.

Symptoms
1. Phantom limb phenomena.
2. Flashbacks to the accident.
3. Regrets over opportunities not taken.
4. Body image disturbances.
5. Game of ifs (e.g., What if I hadn't taken that plane?).
6. Anger.
7. Depression.
8. Diminished self-esteem.
9. Sense of helplessness.
10. Sexual dysfunction.
11. Grief.
12. Suicidal ideation.

Management
1. Grief counseling should be provided (Friersen and Lippman, 1990).
2. Diagnostic-specific psychopharmacotherapy (e.g., antidepressants for PTSD or depression).
3. Suicide evaluation and appropriate suicide precautions taken, if required.
4. Family therapy.
5. Pain medication, if required, with awareness that risk of addiction is enhanced in patients with a personal genetic predisposition to substance abuse disorders.
6. Peer-group support (Friersen and Lippmann, 1987).
7. Sexual counseling if dysfunction is present.
8. An excellent relationship between patient and caregiver is a requisite to successful community management and a return to near-normal functioning at home and work (Friersen and Lippmann, 1987).

Quality Assurance Issues
1. Was the patient evaluated for the acute sequelae anticipated from amputation?
2. What about the possibilities of depression, anger, and suicide ideation—were these anticipated?
3. What counseling was conducted for sexual dysfunction?

Ethical/Legal Issues
1. Was patient evaluated as to suicide potential?

ANALGESIC ABUSE
(Non-Narcotic)

Non-narcotic analgesic abuse is common but often goes unsuspected (Gallagher et al, 1988). The fact that it is often concurrent with medical and psychiatric disorders confuses diagnoses and complicates management. A careful physical examination, serum or urine drug screens, and other clinical studies (e.g., serum electrolytes, liver function studies) are essential to management. Salicylates, phenacetin, and acetaminophen are commonly abused. Abuse is five to six times more common in women. Estimated prevalence in Australia is 10% (Gallagher et al, 1988). Percentage of population abusing non-narcotic analgesics in the United States is generally found to be lower, but this may be due to lack of consideration of abuse of these drugs by evaluating clinicians. Headache is the common rationale for abuse. These headaches are often due to analgesic abuse and represent a rebound phenomenon initially worsening with cessation of the analgesic. One-third of all male and one-half of all female non-narcotic analgesic abusers are dually diagnosed (Gallagher et al, 1988). Comorbid psychiatric diagnoses include affective illness, hypochondriasis, personality disorders, and paranoia. Dementia has been reported with both aspirin and phenacetin abuse (Gallagher et al, 1988).

Management
Successful management entails treatment of both the comorbid medical and psychiatric disorders as well as specific management of the substance abuse disorders. Since there often is a family history of abuse, the clinician may find family members to be codependent and enabling. Denial is usual and, given the easy access to nonprescription drugs such as aspirin, relapse is common.

Quality Assurance Issues
1. Was a substance-abusing or psychiatric patient asked about non-narcotic analgesic substance abuse?
2. Did a clinician ascertain if there was concurrent medical/psychiatric illness?
3. Was a serum or urine drug screen performed?
4. Were other appropriate studies (e.g., serum electrolytes) obtained?

Ethical/Legal Issues
1. Given the high likelihood of dual diagnosis, was the patient evaluated to rule out an affective disorder, especially depression, which could be easily treated?
2. Was the patient evaluated to establish if he or she was a suicidal risk?
3. These substances can cause serious dementia. Was the patient's competency to enter informed consent to treatment established?

ANGEL'S TRUMPET INTOXICATION AND DELIRIUM

Angel's Trumpet (*Datura sauvealens*) is a poisonous plant that grows wildly in several Southeastern and Gulf states.

History
1. It is available for individuals interested in experimenting with hallucinogens, as a legal source of a drug with atropine-like qualities.
2. The flowers of Angel's Trumpet are either directly eaten or brewed in a tea to produce a central nervous system anticholinergic psychosis.
3. Hyoscine (scopolamine) is the principal and most toxic alkaloid found. Lesser amounts of atropine and hyoscyamine are also present.
4. Individuals who have taken the drug because of its hallucinogenic properties or have inadvertently ingested the substance may present intoxicated or delirious.

Symptoms and Signs
1. Symptoms and signs of intoxication are comparable to those seen with intoxication from other strongly anticholinergic substances.
2. Individuals present agitated, confused, and hallucinating.
3. Pulse pressure is widened; the skin is hot, dry, and flushed.
4. Sensorium is usually clouded and patients have persistent memory disturbance.
5. Severe intoxication results in convulsions, flaccid paralysis, and death.
6. Elevation of body temperature is the combined result of inhibition of sweating and a hyperthermic response.
7. Scopolamine further elevates temperature by increasing the basal metabolic rate.
8. Skin is flushed because of the dilation of the cutaneous blood vessels.

Management
1. In addition to supportive measures to prevent patients from harming themselves or others, gastric lavage is coupled with physostigmine to reverse the effect of the alkaloids found in Angel's Trumpet. The usual dosage is 1–4 mg intramuscularly.
2. Phenothiazines and other antipsychotic drugs that have strong anticholinergic properties should not be given because they potentiate the anticholinergic effects of the alkaloids. The alpha-blocking effects may precipitate cardiovascular collapse and death.

Quality Assurance Issues

1. Was the medical seriousness of the intoxicated patient recognized and appropriate treatment instituted?
2. Was the cause of delirium established?
3. Was counseling initiated to prevent chronic ingestion?

Ethical/Legal Issues

1. Were the drugs legally obtained?
2. Is it illegal to grow "Angel's Trumpet?"
3. What other sources (illegal) could explain the individual's use of these drugs?

ANOREXIA NERVOSA

Few psychiatric disorders are fatal. Extreme manic states and catatonic excitement accompanied by psychomotor excitation can lead to death from exhaustion. Individuals in catatonic stupor or profound depression requiring tube feeding may die from inanition. Homocide and suicide are risks with profound depression, schizophrenia, and a number of toxic encephalopathies such as LSD-induced or amphetamine-induced psychosis. Finally, some individuals starve to death thinking they are overweight. This last group—patients with anorexia nervosa—is predominantly composed of young women, usually of middle-class background.

Some authors feel that there is no such illness as anorexia nervosa, but rather that the symptom complex seen in patients with anorexia nervosa is a symptom of diseases as varying as endocrinopathies, bipolar illness, and schizophrenia.

History

1. Incidence of anorexia nervosa appears to be increasing in industrialized nations. This increase is *not* due to the fact that anorectic patients are hospitalized earlier or that they are hospitalized for less severe illness (Willi and Grossman, 1983).
2. History is that of profound weight loss or self-imposed restriction of food intake ostensibly because of fear of being "overweight."
3. Weight loss may be aggravated by hyperactivity, self-induced vomiting, and purging with strong laxatives.
4. Bulimia is a poor prognostic sign. Bulimic patients (those who use laxatives and vomit) tend to have histories of weighing more and, more commonly, are premorbidly obese. Bulimic patients tend to display impulsive behaviors such as suicide attempts, self-mutilation, alcohol and other substance abuse, and stealing. There is a frequent history of obesity in patients with bulimia in addition to anorexia (Garfinkel PE et al, 1980).
5. Relatives of anorexics have increased incidence of major depressive and bipolar illness (Winokur A et al, 1980a).
6. Data in support of the hypothesis that anorexia nervosa is a unique illness rather than an atypical form of affective psychosis in young females includes the fact

that anorexia nervosa in young women differs from affective illness in the same group in age of onset of symptoms, marital status, patterns of psychiatric illness when in the family, and educational achievement (Eagles et al, 1990).

7. In follow-up studies, the majority of anorexics (about 75% in one study) have been shown to be improved in body weight. Improvement in menstrual function and psychiatric status is less satisfactory (Hsu, 1980).

8. Criteria of the diagnosis of anorexia include disturbed perception of body weight, intense fear of becoming obese, loss of at least 25% of original body weight, and refusal to maintain minimal normal body weight.

9. Abnormalities in growth hormone, thyrotropin-releasing hormone, and luteinizing and follicle-stimulating hormone have been reported (Gold et al, 1980).

10. Is is questionable whether criteria used for adults are appropriate for young children at average weight. Children have a smaller percentage total body fat than adolescent counterparts suggesting that the 25% total weight loss required for the diagnosis may be unrealistic. A prepubertal child with a 15% weight loss appears quite emaciated (Irwin, 1981).

11. Temporal lobe epilepsy has been associated with affective disorder and dysmorphic delusions contributing to the diagnosis of anorexia nervosa (Signer and Benson, 1990).

12. Late-onset anorexia nervosa is called "tardive" anorexia nervosa (Fenley et al, 1990).

Symptoms

1. Distortion of body image such that a patient insists that her weight is normal or that she is fat despite her emaciation and cachexia.
2. Anorexia.
3. Loss of self-esteem.
4. Increased self-consciousness about physical appearance.
5. Unreasonable fear of eating with pride in ability to lose weight (the "anorectic attitude") (Casper and Davis, 1977).
6. Restlessness.

Signs

1. Hypothermia.
2. Bradycardia.
3. Hypotension.
4. Malnutrition.
5. Edema.
6. Muscular wasting.
7. Hyperactivity.
8. Amenorrhea.
9. Weight loss such that weight is about 75% of that expected for height, age, sex, and bone structure.
10. Fatal cardiomyopathy may occur due to ipecac intoxication. Clues to ipecac tox-

icity include dysphagia, muscular weakness, and severe palpitations (Freidman E, 1984).

Clinical Studies

1. Hypoproteinemia.
2. Electrolyte disturbance.
3. Cortical atrophy with hypocephalus ex vacuo (Fenley et al, 1990).
4. Anemia.
5. Osteoporosis.
6. Impaired lower gastrointestinal motility (Fenley et al, 1990).
7. Leukopenia (from starvation-induced bone marrow hypoplasia).
8. Elevated 24-hour concentrations of plasma cortisol and significantly less cortisol suppression following dexamethasone (Walsh BR et al, 1987).

Differential Diagnosis

1. Anorexia nervosa.
2. Schizoaffective disorder.
3. Schizophrenia.
4. Major depressive disorder.
5. Bipolar disorder.
6. AIDS.
7. Hypopituitarism.
8. Hypothalamic neoplasm (Weller and Weller, 1982).
9. Superior mesenteric artery syndrome (Sours and Vorhaus, 1981).
10. Conversion disorder (Garfinkel PE et al, 1983).
11. Temporal lobe epilepsy (Signer and Benson, 1990).
12. Gastrointestinal disease.
13. Osteoporosis (Fenley et al, 1990).

Management

1. Many of these patients have endocrinopathies, particularly deficiencies in production of pituitary gonadotropins, that must be treated. In some patients, a functional anterior hypothalamic defect may be etiological (Rieger et al, 1978).
2. Amitriptyline (Elavil) produces a modest weight gain and rarely obesity in some cases of anorexia nervosa. This response supports the relationship of some cases of anorexia nervosa to affective illness (Moore DC, 1977; Kendler, 1978).
3. Some therapists have successfully employed paradoxical intention in the management of chronic anorexia nervosa (Hsu and Lieberman, 1982).
4. Traditional psychoanalysis with its emphasis on interpretation of unconscious process is rather ineffective. Active participation on the part of the patient in therapy and the experience of being listened to appear to be of utmost importance (Bruch, 1982).
5. Cardiac compensation during the nutritional rehabilitation phase of treatment is a danger. Abnormal electrocardiograms are found in the majority of anorectic patients seen. The increased demands created by re-feeding may predispose the

patient to such difficulty. Therefore, physical exercise should be kept to a minimum during the recovery phase to prevent increasing the patient's basal metabolic rate (Powers, 1982).

Prognosis
1. Impulsive patients tend to fare poorly in outcome studies (Sohlberg et al, 1989). The poor prognosis of impulsive patients may be due to cognitive impairment.
2. On long-term follow-up of adolescent girls with the disorder, weight has been found to more closely approximate the ideal, and menstruation has resumed. In one study, all patients who subsequently wished to become pregnant were successful in doing so (Kreipe et al, 1989).

Quality Assurance Issues
1. Were underlying psychiatric conditions—especially affective disorders and schizophrenia—ruled out?
2. Was HIV testing done to determine whether treatment for AIDS was required?
3. Was the patient medically managed during the rehabilitation phase?
4. Was cardiac consultation obtained?

Ethical/Legal Issues
1. In seriously decompensated anorexia, the patient's cognitive capacities may be affected. Was an evaluation done to establish competency for informed consent?
2. Would commitment ever be justified?

ANTICHOLINERGIC INTOXICATION, HALLUCINOSIS, AND DELUSIONAL STATES

Anticholinergic psychoses resemble those caused by atropine and are, therefore, often referred to as atropine psychoses. The symptoms and signs seen are the result of parasympathetic blockade.

History
1. Atropine psychosis develops from ingestion of a variety of drugs including atropine, hyoscine, belladonna, Jimson weed pods, scopolamine, henbane, stamonium, thorn apple pods, and hyoscyamine.
2. Cogentin, the tricyclic antidepressants, phenothiazines, antihistamines, and hypnotics such as glutethimide have prominent anticholinergic properties as do over-the-counter sedatives.
3. Some cough mixtures contain scopalamine.
4. Signs of toxicity may appear after intranasal use of solutions as well as after ingestion of plants containing belladonna alkaloids.
5. Scopolamine and atropine may be found in over-the-counter sleep medications, antispasmodics, eye-drop preparations, and nonprescription asthma remedies.

The latter may also contain belladonna and stramonium (Brizer and Manning, 1982).

6. Urine and serum screens must be obtained immediately in cases where anticholinergic intoxication is suspected, because of its rapid rate of excretion.

7. Most laboratories do not routinely screen for anticholinergics. Usually, a specific request must be made to identify their presence.

8. There is some suggestion that "temporary psychoses," thought to be due to anticholinergic agents, are increasing due to use of anticholinergic medications (e.g., eye-drop preparations containing either scopolamine or atropine) or beverages (Brizer and Manning, 1982).

9. Untreated, the psychosis caused by ingestion of a beverage containing anticholinergic agents clears within 24 to 48 hours. Results for urine and serum screen are usually negative.

10. Orally ingested belladonna alkaloids are rapidly absorbed from the gastrointestinal tract. They rapidly disappear from the bloodstream and are distributed throughout the body. Most are excreted in the urine within 12 hours of ingestion.

Symptoms

1. Dryness of mouth and other mucous membranes.
2. Hoarseness.
3. Urinary retention.
4. Dysphagia.
5. Intense thirst.
6. Burning of eyes and throat.
7. Strangury (slow and painful urinary discharge).
8. Restlessness.
9. Disorientation.
10. Visual hallucinations without perceptual distortion.
11. Double vision.
12. Memory impairment.
13. Poor concentrations.
14. Body image distortion.

Signs

1. Talkativeness.
2. Widely dilated and inactive pupils.
3. Hot, dry skin.
4. Flushed skin.
5. Rapid and weak pulse.
6. Terminal coma and circulatory collapse.
7. Hyperthermia (particularly if the weather is hot because of the inability to sweat).
8. Psychomotor excitement.
9. Normal or decreased blood pressure.

Scopalamine Toxicity

Scopolamine toxicity is said to differ from that of atropine toxicity by the presence of a slow pulse, lack of flushing of the skin, and central nervous system depression, with lethargy and somnolence rather than excitement. The Babinski sign may occur with scopolamine poisoning but not after atropine poisoning.

Management

1. Give the patient sips of water.
2. "Artificial tears" are used to moisten eyes, nose, and other mucous membranes.
3. Gastric lavage should be performed after oral ingestion.
4. Catheterization may be necessary.
5. With scopolamine toxicity, mild stimulation with caffeine or amphetamines combats depression.
6. If respiration is inadequate or appears to be failing, artificial respiration may be necessary.
7. Methacholine or pilocarpine relieves the peripheral symptoms. However, if there is a severe degree of block these parasympathomimetic drugs have little or no effect. If there is no response after the injection of 5–10 mg of methacholine subcutaneously, poisoning with belladonna alkaloids should be considered.
8. Anticholinergic, drug-induced delirium and coma is readily reversed by the anticholinesterase physostigmine. Unlike related substances such as neostigmine, this drug crosses the blood–brain barrier and thereby reverses both peripheral and central nervous system cholinergic blockade. By inhibiting the destructive action of cholinesterase, physostigmine prolongs and exaggerates the effect of acetylcholine. One to three milligrams of physostigmine given intramuscularly or intravenously will, in most cases, reverse CNS toxic effects of the tricyclic antidepressant drugs. Since there appears to be a complete breakdown of physostigmine in the body within $1\frac{1}{2}$ to 2 hours, doses should be repeated at 30 minutes if symptoms persist. The usual adult dosage of physostigmine salicylate is 0.5–2.0 mg intramuscularly or intravenously. Reversal of the anticholinergic effects of atropine sulfate or scopolamine hydrobromide given as a preanesthetic medication usually requires a dose of physostigmine that is twice that of the anticholinergic drug administered by injection. Due to the frequent occurrence of toxicity, physostigmine is decreasingly used.
9. Minor tranquilizers such as alprazolam (Xanax), diazepam (Valium), and lorazepam (Ativan) may be prescribed for management of agitation and combativeness.
10. Neuroleptics enhance the delirium because of their anticholinergic properties and therefore are contraindicated.

Side-Effects of Physostigmine

1. Nausea.
2. Vomiting.
3. Excessive sweating.
4. Pupillary contraction.
5. Increased intestinal muscular tone.

6. Salivary secretion.
7. Bronchial construction.

Management of Side-Effects of Physostigmine
1. Reduce the dosage of physostigmine.
2. Do not use in patients who are predisposed to toxicity due to age or concurrent medical illness.

Quality Assurance Issues
1. The etiology of the patient's symptoms need to be examined carefully, as the symptoms are diffuse. Is there a history of ingestion of an anticholinergic?
2. Were diagnostic studies such as urine/serum screens conducted in a timely fashion?
3. Was toxicity from physostigmine considered when this drug was used?

Ethical/Legal Issues
1. What are the medical justifications for prescriptions of drugs with high anticholinergic properties?
2. What is the suicide potential of the patient? What other causes of an organic mental disorder were considered?

ANTICONVULSANT INTOXICATION, DELUSIONAL STATES, AND DELIRIUM

Patients taking anticonvulsant medication may become psychotic or delirious at normal or elevated serum levels of the seizure medication.

History
1. Phenytoin (Dilantin), primidone (Mysoline), carbamazepine (Tegretol), and clonazepam (Klonapin), among others, have been implicated in alterations of thought, mood, and behavior resembling functional psychiatric disorders such as schizophrenia.
2. The usual physical signs of toxicity such a lethargy, dysarthria, nystagmus, and ataxia are not always present.
3. Inappropriate affect, bizarre behavior, and evidence of a thought disorder have been reported, as well as have clinical syndromes more organic in character with clouding of the sensorium, visual hallucinations, and decreased short-term memory.

Management
1. The serum level of the anticonvulsant should be obtained to document toxicity.
2. If the serum level is within normal range, a trial of lower drug dosage may be necessary to establish the diagnosis.

Quality Assurance Issues
1. Were different diagnostic conditions considered? Were serum studies conducted to rule out anticonvulsant intoxication?

ANTIMALARIAL TOXICITY

Antimalarial drugs such as amodiaquine, chloroquine, and hydroxychloroquine may cause alterations in mood, thought, and behavior resembling major psychiatric disturbance (Good and Shoder, 1977).

History
1. Therapeutic doses of these agents have been associated with depression, psychosis, delirium, and other personality changes.
2. Patients tend to have insight into their condition in the early stages of the change.
3. Moderately low doses of chloroquine can lead to state-dependent overdosage and death.
4. This is an increasing danger since chloroquine is both being used more commonly as Americans travel more frequently and is being used in rheumatology.
5. In one study, neurotic-like changes were reported in as many as 28% of patients on chloroquine.
6. Age and sex do not seem to play a role in determining who develops symptoms.

Management
1. Symptoms are usually reversible within 1 week of cessation of drug use and generally do not reappear after reinstitution of therapy.

Quality Assurance Issues
1. Does the patient exhibit psychiatric signs and symptoms of reactions to the antimalarial drugs?
2. Are there medical indications to substantiate keeping the patient on these drugs for periods of time?
3. Is a management plan constructed to handle their need for medication rationally and the need to prevent toxicity?

Ethical/Legal Issues
1. Has the patient been properly evaluated for suicide potential?
3. Has the patient been given a safe number of pills for the condition?

ANTISOCIAL BEHAVIOR

Antisocial behavior is more frequently seen in male adoptees (who have been raised by a psychiatrically ill adoptive family member or who have experienced a divorce between the adoptive parents) than in female adoptees (Cadoret and Cain, 1980). Having an antisocial or alcoholic relative is a genetic predictor of sociopathy in an adoptee.

History
1. Nonalcoholic petty criminals have an excess of biologic parents with histories of petty crime but not of alcohol abuse (Bohman et al, 1982).
2. Risk of criminality in alcohol abusers is not correlated with criminality in biologic or adopted parents but is correlated with severity of their own alcohol use (Bohman et al, 1982).
3. While low socioeconomic status alone is not sufficient to lead to criminality, it does increase risk in combination with specific genetic factors (Cloninger et al, 1982a).
4. Genetic antecedents of criminality are the same regardless of sex, but the genetic load must be greater for a woman to be affected (Sigvardsson et al, 1982).
5. Postnatal antecedents differ in their contribution to criminality between sexes. Low social status of adoptive homes and multiple temporary placements increase risk of criminality in men but not women. Urban rearing and prolonged institutional care, on the other hand, increase risk of criminality in women but not men (Sigvardsson et al, 1982).

Management
1. Psychiatry has very little to offer patients with character disorders characterized by criminal behavior. An evaluation should be undertaken to ascertain if a psychiatric disorder, other than a sociopathic character disorder, may be responsible for the criminal behavior. For instance, a depressed patient may hear the voice of God telling her to kill her child. An Alzheimer patient may steal and a manic patient may prostitute her- or himself.
2. Risk of suicide and risk of harm to others should be determined.
3. If an underlying substance abuse disorder or borderline personality disorder is responsible for the criminal behavior, it should be treated.

Quality Assurance Issues
1. Have treatable psychiatric conditions that may be responsible for sociopathic behavior been considered?
2. Does the patient have concurrent Axis I disorder (e.g., depression)?
3. Does the patient have a concurrent substance abuse problem?
4. Does the patient have adult attention deficit hyperactivity disorder?

Ethical/Legal Issues
1. If the patient plans to murder someone, is the third party warned or protected (Tarasoff, 1977)?
2. Is the patient spreading AIDS without informing contacts (e.g., female or male prostitutes)?
3. What is the obligation or duty of the therapist to inform the police if the patient has already committed a criminal act?

4. Can the prosecution in a case compel the disclosure of information obtained in a therapeutic relationship or in the context of an emergency treatment situation?

ANXIETY STATES

Everyone feels anxious at one time or another just as everyone is depressed at some time. The difference between anxiety that most of us feel and that experienced by patients who present to psychiatric clinicians is either the intensity of the feeling or the fact that the family and friends of the patient cannot tolerate it.

History

1. The first task in the evaluation of the etiology of anxiety is to carefully document the circumstances associated with the first and subsequent appearances of anxiety. What was happening in the patient's life at the time? Since its first appearance, has it gotten worse, better, or remained the same in intensity? What are the duration and frequency of the anxiety attacks? Do they vacillate in intensity? If they do, what makes them better or worse? What other psychological symptoms (e.g., phobias) or physical symptoms (e.g., tachycardia, headaches) are associated with them? Is the patient's appetite, sleep, or sexual potency affected by the anxiety attacks?

2. Medical conditions such as hyperthyroidism, pheochromocytoma, and temporal lobe epilepsy may present with constant or episodic anxiety. A careful medical history and physical examination may be needed to ascertain if significant medical disease is present.

3. Fear should be distinguished from anxiety and panic. Fear is an emotional response to something in the environment perceived as dangerous. This may be a person, a place, or an activity. Anxiety is subjective fear. The cause is not as readily apparent.

4. Anxiety is the most frequent psychiatric symptom reported in children and adolescents. The diagnostic subtype of anxiety varies with age (Kashani and Orvaschel, 1990).

5. There is a significant relationship between anxiety in parents and anxiety in their children. Parents of anxious children report more negative family relations than parents of nonanxious children. Severely anxious children report more dysthymia and negative life events (Kashani et al, 1990).

6. While there appears to be a clear distinction between specific affective disorders and specific anxiety disorders, there is a less clear separation between dysthymic disorder and generalized anxiety disorders (Holmberg, 1987).

7. Anxiety has many forms. It may be vaguely present at all times and be free floating. There may be times when it is nearly of panic proportions. Anxiety may be combined with phobias and depersonalization. It may accompany depression or substance abuse or be part of the clinical picture of an acute or chronic psychosis or a post-traumatic stress disorder.

8. At times, no precipitant may be found or there may be a clear link to a life event such as divorce, job promotion, impending graduation, death, or first sexual experience.

9. Individuals vary in their ability to tolerate anxiety. To some degree, social and personal histrionic factors determine how individuals handle anxiety.
10. Family studies (Noyes et al, 1980) indicate that risk for anxiety disorders is significantly greater for first-degree relatives of individuals with anxiety disorders than it is for controls. Relatives of patients with anxiety disorders are also at higher risk for the development of alcoholism. Female relatives are at greater risk for anxiety disorders than male relatives.
11. Secondary depression, reported in as many as 44% of individuals with anxiety disorders, is the most serious and most frequent complication (Noyes et al, 1980).
12. Six years after diagnoses, nearly two-thirds of patients diagnosed to have anxiety disorders are either recovered or only mildly impaired (Noyes et al, 1980).
13. In general, the lesser the duration of the illness, the more frequent the remissions and the fewer and less severe the symptoms at followup (Noyes et al, 1980).
14. Patients of lower socioeconomic status tend to have a less favorable prognosis (Noyes et al, 1980).
15. Suspicion of an organic cause for the anxiety symptoms should be raised when age of onset is greater than 35; when there is an absence of family history of anxiety disorders; when patient perceives the symptoms as ego-dystonic; when there are unexplained physical findings, laboratory abnormalities, or inadequately treated physical illness; when there is a history of substance abuse; and when there is a failure of a patient to identify a significant psychological conflict related to the onset of the symptoms (Mackenzie and Popkin, 1983).

Symptoms
1. Feeling of panic.
2. Feeling of impending danger.
3. Phobias.
4. Apprehension.
5. Loss of interest.
6. Difficulty concentrating.
7. Dryness of mouth.
8. Nausea.
9. Vomiting.
10. Tenseness.
11. Vague sinking feeling in abdomen.
12. Diarrhea.
13. Constipation.
14. Urinary frequency.
15. Light-headedness.
16. Sense of fullness in stomach.
17. Palpitations.
18. Unceasing worry.
19. Amenorrhea.
20. Sleep disturbance.
21. Lack of pleasure.

22. Dyspepsia.
23. Irritability.
24. Sense of pressure in the chest.
25. Impotence.
26. Nightmares.
27. Incapacity to relax.
28. Sense of choking or suffocating.
29. Decreased appetite.
30. Shortness of temper.
31. Episodic panic anxiety.
32. Restlessness.
33. Impatience.

Signs

1. Hyperactivity.
2. Hyperventilation.
3. Sweaty palms.
4. Dry mouth.
5. Tremor.
6. Tachycardia.
7. Increased muscle tone.
8. Fidgety movements of the hands.
9. Respiratory irregularity.
10. Facial tics or grimacing.

Differential Diagnosis

1. Normal anxiety.
2. Generalized anxiety disorder.
3. Incipient psychosis.
4. Major depressive disorder.
5. Hyperthyroidism.
6. Hypoglycemia.
7. Pheochromocytoma.
8. Caffeinism.
9. Borderline personality disorder.
10. Chronic schizophrenia.
11. Dysthymic disorder.
12. Psychomotor epilepsy.
13. Other temporal lobe disease.
14. Paroxysmal atrial tachycardia and other cardiac arrhythmias.
15. Internal hemorrhage.
16. Impending myocardial infarction.
17. Post-concussion syndrome.
18. Bipolar disorder.
19. Alcohol withdrawal.

20. Barbiturate and other drug withdrawal.
21. Essential hypertension.
22. Cerebral arteriosclerosis.
23. Phobias.
24. Amphetamine and other sympathomimetic psychoses.
25. Cocaine psychosis.
26. Homosexual panic.
27. Hypocalcemia.
28. Hypokalemia.
29. Mitral valve prolapse.
30. Hyperventilation syndrome.
31. Encephalitis.
32. Pulmonary embolism.
33. Subacute bacterial endocarditis.
34. Panic disorder.
35. Post-traumatic stress disorder.

Management

1. The first step in the management of anxiety is the identification of its underlying etiology. History, physical examination, and laboratory tests are required.
2. If the etiology is felt to be psychiatric in origin:

    a. Allow the patient to ventilate in a supportive psychotherapeutic setting.
    b. If the anxiety seems overwhelming, and ventilation fails to bring about sufficient amelioration of the symptoms, an anxiolytic agent may be given and prescribed as needed. Alprazolam (Xanax) 1 mg PO qid prn or lorazepam (Ativan) 0.50–1.0 mg qid prn is usually sufficient for a nonaddictive patient.
    c. Social engineering may be required to minimize the precipitant stresses in the environment.
    d. The disposition of the patient depends on the intensity of the patient's symptoms and his or her response to a crisis psychotherapeutic intervention and antianxiety agents, given either orally or intramuscularly. If there is a reduction of tension and the patient is obviously more relaxed, he or she may return home. If the anxiety appears to be unresponsive to crisis therapy or seems to be escalating, hospitalization may be necessary to get the patient away from intolerable situations and to allow some rest and relaxation.
    e. If the problem is one of long standing, the patient should be placed in long-term supportive psychotherapy. The patient should explore with the therapist those situations that are the most overwhelming and look at which alternatives may be available.
    f. If the anxiety is part of an affective or schizophrenic illness, antidepressants and antipsychotics are needed in addition to or in lieu of benzodiazepines. Benzodiazepines are primarily anxiolytic. They may be useful, however, for the anticipatory anxiety that accompanies some affective and schizophrenic disorders.

Anticipatory anxiety should be distinguished from psychotic anxiety. Antipsychotic medication is required for the management of psychotic anxiety.

g. Monoamine oxidase inhibitors, beta-blocking agents, tricyclic antidepressants, fluoxetine (Prozac), and sertraline (Zoloft) have been used with success in the treatment of panic disorder and certain phobic disorders. Patients with social anxiety usually respond to 60–120 mg of propranolol (Inderal) when used. If propranolol is used, care should be given to the usual contraindications such as asthma and congestive heart failure.

3. If the etiology is a medical disorder such as hyperthyroidism, the appropriate medical intervention is indicated. Psychotherapy or sociotherapy may be needed if a life event or interpersonal stress has precipitated the medical or surgical condition.

4. The incidence of sedation with the use of the triazolobenzodiazepine alprazolam is reported to be less than with diazepam (Rickels et al, 1983).

5. The beta-adrenergic blocking agent propranolol hydrochloride has been demonstrated to be particularly efficacious in reducing the somatic symptoms of chronic anxiety disorders. Its principal side effects (dizziness, fatigue, and insomnia) are difficult to distinguish from anxiety symptoms (Kathol et al, 1980).

6. Benzodiazepines must be given with extreme caution to patients with a family history of substance abuse. It is recommended that they be avoided completely in patients with a personal history of substance abuse including alcoholism. In all instances, a patient must be monitored carefully to ascertain if addiction may be a problem. Those who are addictive tend to report a high or euphoric feeling with use rather than simply relief from anxiety.

7. In rare instances where other treatments have failed, clonazepam (Klonapin) in small doses is used for patients with disabling anxiety even if there is a history of addiction.

8. The usual problem associated with use of benzodiazepines such alprazolam or lorazepam in patients who are not addictive is that they fail to comply with the dosage schedule required to make them anxiety-free.

9. Behavioral therapy such as desensitization and exposure to the source of the phobia are often used in concert with benzodiazepines, antidepressants, and beta blockers (Wardle, 1990).

10. Patients with anxiety disorders that are intensified by exercise should be alerted to this fact much as patients whose intensity of symptoms are increased with caffeine are alerted. In the former group, exercise should be monitored (Cameron and Hudson, 1986). In the latter group, caffeine-containing substances such as coffee, tea, and chocolate should be avoided.

11. Patients attempt suicide if anxiety symptoms become unbearable. Patients should be evaluated for risk of self-destructive behavior and appropriate precautions taken if required.

12. Patients seen by physicians other than psychiatrists are often not referred for management of their anxiety disorders (Schwartz GM et al, 1987). This results in undertreatment, no treatment, and at times, prescription of benzodiazepines for those at risk for addiction.

13. Buspirone (Buspar) is a nonaddicting anxiolytic that can reduce anxiety with less

fatigue, lethargy, and drowsiness than lorazepam or alprazolam and therefore is specifically useful in patients with a history of addiction (Cohn and Wilcox, 1986). Unfortunately, it may take as long as a month to impact and it is difficult to relieve symptoms in patients who have had prior exposure to a benzodiazepine.

14. Imipramine (Tofranil) and the MAOI phenelzine (Nardil) are particularly useful in the management of chronic anxiety disorders. Clomipramine (Anafranil) is specifically effective in managing the anxiety associated with obsessive–compulsive disorders (Modigh, 1987).

Quality Assurance Issues

1. Are patients warned of the addictive qualities of benzodiazepines?
2. Are patients on benzodiazepines monitored to ascertain if they are becoming addictive?
3. Are patients evaluated for suicide potential?
4. Was a differential diagnosis performed and diagnostic-specific treatment provided?
5. Were alternatives to benzodiazepines employed in patients with a personal or family history of substance abuse?
6. Has the clinician ruled out causes for the symptom of anxiety that represent illnesses that may be potentially life threatening to the patient such as cardiac arrhythmias, internal bleeding, pulmonary emboli, congestive heart failure, or toxicity from substances?

Ethical/Legal Issues

1. What would be the legal responsibility of the therapist/clinician to establish that the patient, in addition to an anxiety disorder, did not have a concomitant life-threatening medical condition? How would negligence be determined where such an evaluation had not been properly conducted?
2. In the patient whose anxiety had reached the level where he or she was potentially dangerous to third parties, how would the underlying condition be considered for mitigation of legal charges?
3. What are the clinician's obligations with regard to the patient potentially becoming addicted to benzodiazepines?
3. What obligation does the clinician have, in regards to the patient suffering from severe anxiety, to inform the Department of Motor Vehicles that the patient is on benzodiazepines and may be potentially dangerous as a driver?
4. In regards to the patient who suffers from severe anxiety and is on benzodiazepines, what obligation does the clinician have, in the face of minimizing broader societal risk, to protect the confidentiality of the patient?

ARRHYTHMIA-INDUCED DISORDERS

Cardiac arrhythmias may present as a psychiatric disorder (e.g., panic attack), may occur concomitantly with a psychiatic disorder complicating diagnosis (e.g., occurring concomitantly with schizophrenia with the predominant symptom being a feeling of impending doom), may be produced by the psychiatric disorder (e.g., cardiac arrhythmias associated with cocaine abuse), or may be caused by treatment (e.g., tricyclic-induced cardiac arrhythmia).

History

1. The patient often has a history of abusing drugs that may induce a cardiac arrhythmia such as PCP, cocaine, and amphetamines, or of being treated with drug with cardiotoxic effects (e.g., tricyclics, MAOIs).
2. While tricyclics can be used safely with many patients, including those with heart disease, and may in some instances suppress cardiac arrhythmias, some individuals will develop cardiac toxicity including congestive heart failure (Young RC et al, 1984).
3. Plasma concentrations of the metabolites of tricyclics, unlike the parent antidepressant, may vary as much as twenty-fold among individuals (Young RC et al, 1984).
4. Cardiac arrhythmias should be suspected whenever there is an acute psychiatric change in a patient with known cardiovascular disease.

Differential Diagnosis

1. Cardiac arrhythmias.
2. Pulmonary embolism.
3. Myocardial infarction.
4. Congestive heart failure.
5. Septic embolus.
6. Panic attack.
7. Panic disorder.
8. Generalized anxiety disorder.
9. Substance abuse.
10. Withdrawal from drugs.

Clinical Studies

1. Cardiac toxicity relates not only to a patient's age and premorbid medical condition but also to the plasma concentration of the tricyclic and its metabolites.
2. Electrocardiogram may reveal slowing of intracardiac conduction, decrease in measures showing left ventricular performance, and increased heart rate (Young RC et al, 1984).

Management

1. Cardiac arrhythmias are a medical emergency requiring medical consultation and diagnostic-specific antiarrhythmic therapy.
2. Patients who survive a malignant ventricular arrhythmia are particularly prone to psychiatric sequelae given the reality that there is a 30% recurrence rate within 1 year in patients successfully resuscitated (Fricchione and Vlay, 1986).
3. Alprazolam (Xanax) has been used to reduce the anxiety associated with chronic cocaine abuse.

Quality Assurance Issues
1. Has the condition that the patient is suffering from been properly diagnosed?
2. If the patient has an arrhythmia-induced disorder, has the appropriate medical treatment been provided for the arrhythmia?

Ethical/Legal Issues
1. How would standards of care be determined in assessing the appropriateness of diagnostic measures for ruling out arrhythmia-induced disorders? Would a psychiatrist be compared in his ability to do this with the competency of an internist or of a cardiologist?
2. What obligation does the clinician have to obtain appropriate consultation in the diagnosis of this condition?
3. What would be appropriate followup for treating a patient suffering from an arrhythmia-induced disorder?

ATASIA–ABASIA

Both men and women may present in the emergency room with psychogenic difficulty in walking (Sirois, 1990). Because the individuals cannot ambulate by themselves, they obviously cannot be sent home until they can walk again or until the cause has been determined and a viable homecare plan commenced.

History
1. Onset is usually sudden following a stressful event.
2. There is a history of previous somatic symptoms of psychogenic origin.
3. There is an indifference to the severity of the symptoms ("la belle indifference").
4. The same symptoms may have occurred in the past.

Symptoms
1. Inability to walk or stand with normal muscle tone, development, and reflexes.
2. Seeming lack of concern over severity of the symptoms.

Differential Diagnosis
1. Somatoform disorder.
2. Malingering.
3. Neurologic disorder of acute onset such as transverse myelitis.

Management
1. Remove relatives and friends who may be both stressing the patient as well as providing secondary gain while the patient is being examined and treated.
2. A careful physical examination is necessary to assure that there is no medical, surgical, or neurologic disease responsible for the impairment. If there is, the

patient must be evaluated immediately by a neurosurgeon to ascertain if the process is reversible if immediately treated.

3. Suggestion, hypnosis, ventilation, and sodium amytal interviews have all been successfully used in mobilizing a patient.

4. Suggestion and ventilation with gradually increased pressure to perform is the simplest approach. The patient is asked to move from the lying position to the sitting position. Then the patient is assisted to a chair. If a stool is present, that is used as an intermediate step prior to assisted ambulation. The final step is walking with the patient while discussing how to structure his or her life to avert another occurrence (e.g., reduce stress by minimizing contact with those who contribute to symptom formation; psychotherapy).

5. Hypnosis can be used to induce both light states as well as deep states with success in amelioration of symptoms.

6. Sodium amytal has been historically used to differentiate neurologic from psychogenic disorders. Unfortunately, if the patient receives too much sodium amytal, he or she falls asleep and cannot be aroused to walk or go home. Psychogenic symptoms tend to improve dramatically when the suggestion that the patient can walk is provided in the sedated state.

Quality Assurance Issues

1. Was a physical examination provided to assure there is no neurological process that acute intervention may be successful in reversing?

2. What are the appropriate diagnostic measures that should be used to rule out a neurologic, metabolic, or psychiatric basis for the atasia–abasia (e.g., hypnosis, sodium amytal interview etc.)?

Ethical/Legal Issues

1. Often the patient presenting with atasia–abasia develops the condition following some tortious action such as a car accident. What is the legal role of the psychiatrist in differentiating between organic and nonorganic bases for the patient's symptoms?

ATTENTION-DEFICIT HYPERACTIVITY DISORDER

The etiology of attention-deficit hyperactivity disorder (ADHD) often remains unclear. Cerebral trauma (perinatally or in utero), occult cerebral infections in early childhood, the fetal alcohol syndrome, and transient episodes of anoxia while the brain is developing are causes posited.

History

1. Children and adults with ADHD are found to be easily distractible. They have a limited attention span and great need for activity (hyperactivity).

2. These individuals are rarely seen first in the emergency room. When they are, however, it is usually because of some delinquent behavior, and clinicians find

that rather than a sociopathic or depressed child or adolescent, they have discovered an undiagnosed case of ADHD.

3. Hyperactive children are also seen when they develop a sympathomimetic psychosis from the drugs they are taking for ADHD.
4. ADHD in childhood and adulthood is associated with an increased risk for development of alcoholism and other drug abuse (Wood D et al, 1983).
5. There is a genetic relationship between ADHD and alcoholism, antisocial behavior, Briquet's syndrome, and personality and mood disorders (Goodwin and Guze, 1979; Wender et al, 1981).
6. When ADHD continues to adulthood, it is referred to as the residual type.
7. In one study of alcoholic patients, 33% gave a history of hyperactivity as children (Wood D et al, 1983).
8. Rate of institutionalization for delinquency and rates of single and multiple serious offenses are greater for individuals with ADHD when compared to normal controls. The rate for institutionalization in one study for those with ADHD was 19 times that of controls (Satterfield et al, 1982).
9. The diagnosis of ADHD in *DSM-III-R* is not contingent on any specific combination of symptoms but rather on the number of symptoms commonly associated with ADHD being present (Munoz-Millan and Casteel, 1989).
10. A significantly higher prevalence of restlessness, temper outbursts, impulsivity, and dysattention are reported in follow-up studies of hyperactive children in adulthood (Klee et al, 1986).
11. ADHD children have a higher incidence of parents who have and continue to suffer from ADHD symptoms (Klee et al, 1986).
12. There appears to be a subtype of alcoholic in whom ADHD symptoms play a role in the development of alcoholism (dual diagnosis) (MacNeill et al, 1987).
13. The diagnosis of ADHD in adults should be considered in patients who do not suffer mood disorders, schizophrenia, and schizotypal or borderline personality disorders but present with hot temper, restlessness, emotional lability, and impulsivity (Wender et al, 1985).
14. Recognition and appropriate treatment of juvenile ADHD may prevent the development of sociopathic traits that tend to persist into adulthood and are refractory to most therapeutic interventions.
15. There is no evidence that elimination of artificial food colorings and flavorings from the diet, the so-called "Feingold diet," alleviate symptoms of ADHD (Mattes and Gittelman, 1981).

Management

1. One of several agents that paradoxically have a calming effect on these individuals such as methylphenidate hydrochloride (Ritalin), dextroamphetamine sulfate (Dexedrine), and caffeine are successfully used to treat ADHD.
2. Side effects of methylphenidate *do not* consistently correlate with dosage.
3. Lack of a simple dose relationship of side effects to the amount of amphetamine-like drug taken has also been observed in adults who take the drug either therapeutically or recreationally.

4. The effect of dextroamphetamine is not unique in patients with ADHD. Normal men and both normal and hyperactive boys exhibit many similar responses to stimulants including improved cognitive performance, improved vigilance, and decreased motor activity during cognitive testing (with the exception of adults taking high doses). Men report euphoria while taking the drug, while boys reported feeling "tired" or "different" (Rappoport JL et al, 1980).

5. The effects of pemoline tend to sustain longer after drug withdrawal than methylphenidate (Ritalin) (Conners and Taylor, 1980).

6. Imipramine (Tofranil) and desipramine (Norpramin) have been successfully used in the management of selected patients with ADHD. The rationale for their use is based on the observation that many children who meet criteria for ADHD also reach criteria for separation anxiety disorder (Cox, 1982).

7. Maximal success is reported when individualized multimodal treatment commensurate with each child's unique constellation of disabilities is employed (Satterfield et al, 1980).

8. Adults with the residual form of ADHD treated with methylphenidate show significant improvement in impulsivity, affective lability, attention, and motor activity (Wender et al, 1985).

9. Desipramine is reported to be effective in adolescents with ADHD within 1 month with effect generally persisting 9 to 12 months later (Gastfriend et al, 1984). In some patients, there is a decrease in effectiveness and emergence of new symptoms such as temper outbursts and antagonistic behavior aggressiveness (Klein DF et al, 1980).

10. Bupropion (Wellbutrin) is an alternate to stimulants in treating some adults with ADHD (Wender and Reimherr, 1990).

11. Long-term outcome studies of patients treated for ADHD are fraught with the same methodologic problems that make outcome research with other diagnostic entities difficult (Hechtman, 1989).

Quality Assurance Issues

1. Were the patients who presented with alcoholism or other substance abuse evaluated for ADHD?

2. Were parents of patients with children with ADHD advised of the fact that they, the parents, may have ADHD?

3. Were other psychiatric conditions considered in the patient with ADHD? To what extent is a patient suffering from ADHD likely to have a dual diagnosis, particularly a bipolar disorder?

4. Were patients with ADHD in their families advised of the side effects of stimulants use including addiction, paranoia, and instability?

Ethical/Legal Issues

1. What is the obligation of the clinician to obtain a consulting or second opinion in patients with ADHD where drugs such as methylphenidate are considered?

2. Given that the side effects of stimulants such as methylphenidate may include paranoia and instability—which are conditions that are frequently associated

with potential injurious behavior to third parties—to what extent would these medications be the basis for exculpation for such tortious or criminal conduct?
3. What would be the role of the psychiatrist in assisting the patient who has engaged in such aberrant disorders secondary to stimulants in the patient's defense against legal actions?
4. Were the patients and their families informed of the benefits, risks, and alternatives to stimulants in the treatment of ADHD?

AUTISM

Autism is a relatively rare disorder that may be confused in the emergency room with depression, schizophrenia, and various neurologic illnesses including mental subnormality.

History
1. The prevalence of autism is estimated to be approximately 4 per 10,000 population (Ritvo et al, 1989).
2. Autism is not associated with parental race, religion, educational attainment, or occupation (Ritvo et al, 1989).
3. The fact that 10% of families have move than one autistic child suggests there may be a family subtype of autism (Ritvo et al, 1989).
4. Signs are usually manifested by 30 months of age and are due to underlying CNS dysfunction rather than psychological trauma (Ritvo et al, 1989).

Signs
1. Difficulty relating to people.
2. Impaired response to sensory stimuli.
3. Retarded language development.

Clinical Studies
1. As great as 66% of autistic subjects score below 70 on standardized I.Q. assessments (Ritvo et al, 1989).
2. Nonspecific EEG changes.
3. Mean glucose rates on PET scan were either equal to or greater than those of control subjects (Hoh et al, 1989).

Pathological Findings
1. Decreased Purkinje and granule cells in the cerebellum and vernal hypoplasia (Hoh et al, 1989).

Management
1. While many of these patients require life-long support and supervision, some with milder forms have managed and gone on to have children of their own (Ritvo et al, 1989).

2. Neuroleptics are successful, in some instances, in enhancing social functioning.

Quality Assurance Issues
1. Were treatable illnesses such as hypothyroidism and affective disorders ruled out in evaluation?
2. Were illnesses such as neurologic disorders (many of which may be untreatable) ruled out in the evaluation of autism?

Ethical/Legal Issues
1. In addressing the parents of a child suffering from autism, is the clinician implying that the parents may be responsible for the condition?
2. Where autism is associated with severe retardation and concomitant behavioral disorder, how would the competency for personal actions be assessed?
3. Where the retarded autistic child engages in a dyssocial action, what role should the therapist/clinician have in assuring proper treatment through the legal system?

AUTOIMMUNE THYROIDITIS

Autoimmune thyroiditis is in the differential diagnosis of depression.

History
1. Autoimmune mechanisms are responsible for 10% of clinically apparent thyroid disease (Volpe, 1984) and may present as depression.
2. Autoimmune thyroiditis is not generally associated with panic disorder but may play a role in some specific clinical circumstances (Stein and Uhde, 1989a).

Symptoms
1. Depression.
2. Anergia.
3. Hypersomnia.

Signs
1. Psychomotor retardation.

Clinical Studies
1. The magnitude of the change in thyroid-stimulating hormone (TSH) response induced by thyrotropin-releasing hormone (TRH) is exaggerated in patients with autoimmune thyroiditis (Gold et al, 1987; Gold et al, 1982).

Management
1. Patients found to be hypothyroid should be referred to an endocrinologist or internist for management.
2. Thyroid replacement therapy is associated with remission of symptoms.

Quality Assurance Issues

1. Are all depressed patients evaluated to rule out autoimmune thyroiditis?
2. Has the patient suffering from this condition been referred to the proper consultant—endocrinologist, internist—for evaluation and proper treatment of the condition?

Ethical/Legal Issues

1. Regarding the patient suffering from this condition, what should be the role of the clinician in protecting the safety of third parties who may be exposed to accidents induced by the compromising of motor skills in the patient?
2. What should be the role of the clinician in informing an employer that one of their employees is suffering from this condition and therefore should not be working with highly tooled equipment that requires quick responses and a high level of coordination?

BARBITURATE AND SIMILARLY ACTING SEDATIVE–HYPNOTIC AMNESIC SYNDROME

Heavy use of barbiturates or similarly acting sedative–hypnotics leads to disturbance in short-term, but not immediate, memory. Digit span on testing is normal but individuals cannot recall names of three objects after a lapse of 15 minutes. Prolonged use of barbiturates or a similarly acting sedative–hypnotic substance is necessary to develop the amnestic syndrome. Onset is usually in the twenties. Unlike with alcohol amnestic syndrome, recovery is usually complete.

Quality Assurance Issues

1. Has a proper differential diagnosis been conducted to rule out alternative medical conditions responsible for disturbances in short-term memory?
2. What management issues must be considered in treating the patient suffering from amnestic syndrome secondary to the use of barbiturates or similarly acting sedatives?

Ethical/Legal Issues

1. Does a patient in the amnestic state with short-term memory loss harm themselves or others accidentally?
2. What obligation would the clinician have, for example, to inform the Motor Vehicle Department that a patient with amnestic syndrome may be a hazard while driving a vehicle?

BARBITURATE AND SIMILARLY ACTING SEDATIVE–HYPNOTIC WITHDRAWAL AND INTOXICATION ORGANIC MENTAL DISORDERS

Barbiturates, hypnotics, and similarly acting minor tranquilizers cause alterations in mood, thought, and behavior both when taken in excess through intoxication and at times of sudden cessation from doses that were sufficient to cause addiction. Prolonged use of barbiturates is required to produce the withdrawal syndrome of barbiturates and similarly acting sedative–hypnotics.

History

1. Patients have histories, although they may deny it, of taking one of a number of long, intermediate, or short-acting barbiturates, or one of the sedative–hypnotics or minor tranquilizers. The sedative–hypnotics include methaqualone, meprobamate, ethchlorvynol, glutethimide, methyprylon, chloral hydrate, and paraldehyde. The minor tranquilizers include the benzodiazepines. These drugs are nearly always taken orally.
2. The most frequently abused barbiturates are short-acting ones such a amobarbital, pentobarbital, and secobarbital (Seconal). Phenobarbital abuse is rare.
3. It is generally difficult to get a good history of barbiturate abuse. A clinician may be fooled by a quite proper woman who, once placed in a situation where barbiturates are not available (e.g., hospitalization for depression or for emergency surgery following trauma) goes into withdrawal.
4. The various barbiturates, benzodiazepines, and sedative–hypnotics differ in rates of absorption, metabolism, and distribution, but are quite comparable in the signs and symptoms of intoxication and withdrawal. The severity of the symptoms and the duration of withdrawal, however, depends on the particular type of drug used, individual susceptibility, and the duration of use.
5. Untreated, withdrawal from several of these drugs can be fatal.
6. Individuals who take 400 mg or less a day of pentobarbital or secobarbital for 3 to 12 months are unlikely to have symptoms of withdrawal. Those taking 600 mg per day for 3 to 4 weeks or more exhibit minor withdrawal symptoms such as anxiety, weakness, tremor, insomnia, involuntary twitching, nausea, and vomiting. Individuals using 800 mg or more for the same period, in addition, experience delirium and grand mal seizures (Epstein, 1980).
7. Essential signs and symptoms of withdrawal from these drugs are similar to that of alcohol withdrawal with the exception that the coarse tremor that is seen with alcohol withdrawal may be absent. Similarly, barbiturate intoxication resembles alcohol intoxication. It is difficult to determine clinically which symptoms are due to use of alcohol and which are due to use of barbiturates or similarly acting drugs. Serum and urine toxicology screens are often necessary. Differences sometimes attributed to the drug used relate more to the setting or the personality of the user than to alcohol or barbiturates.
8. The initial clinical symptoms of barbiturate intoxication are those of disinhibition. Only with continued use is inhibition seen. If enough is taken, death results from CNS depression.
9. Clinical severe intoxication from barbiturates with depression can be differentiated from opioid intoxication by parenteral administration of naloxone or another opioid antagonist. Opioid antagonists have no effect on intoxication due to other drugs.

10. Serum and urine toxicology tests confirm the diagnosis of barbiturate or similarly acting drug intoxication.

Symptoms of Withdrawal
1. Anxiety.
2. Insomnia.
3. Nausea and vomiting.
4. Malaise.
5. Irritability.
6. Restlessness.
7. Dysattention.
8. Disturbances in goal-directed thought and behavior.
9. Illusions.
10. Depression.
11. Visual hallucinations.
12. Formication.
13. Paranoid ideation.
14. Confusion.

Signs of Withdrawal
1. Increased or decreased psychomotor activity.
2. Disinhibition of sexual and aggressive impulses.

Signs of Intoxication
1. Slurred speech.
2. Ataxia.
3. Incoordination.
4. Dysattention.
5. Memory impairment.
6. Poor judgement.
7. Interference with goal-directed behavior.

Management
1. The amount of barbiturate a patient is taking daily is estimated from history and use of the barbiturate tolerance test. The patient is then withdrawn slowly, using doses of a barbiturate that just produces toxic symptoms.
2. A short-acting barbiturate such as pentobarbital or long-acting phenobarbital may be substituted for the drug the patient is taking.
3. Those who support the use of phenobarbital for withdrawal reason that its longer duration of action produces smaller fluctuations in barbiturate blood levels, thereby producing protection against withdrawal symptoms. Furthermore, phenobarbital does not produce the euphoria or "high" seen with short-acting barbiturates. After the daily does is estimated (in terms of short-acting barbiturates) using the patient's history of use and data from the barbiturate tolerance test, the total initial daily amount of phenobarbital to be taken is calculated by substituting 30

mg of phenobarbital for each 100 mg of the short-acting barbiturate. After 2 days on this dose, withdrawal is begun. If there has been an overestimation of the daily dose, signs of toxicity such as slurred speech and ataxia appear. If withdrawal symptoms and signs appear, 200 mg of pentobarbital can be given, and there should be an increase in the daily dose of the phenobarbital. After the patient is stabilized, this daily dose is reduced by 30 mg each day as long as there are no remarkable withdrawal symptoms. The daily amount taken should be divided into 4 doses to allow the nurse or physician to check each time how the withdrawal is progressing. If there is evidence of toxicity, 1 of the daily doses (i.e., one-quarter of the total daily dose) can be omitted that day.

4. Those preferring short-acting barbiturates for withdrawal emphasize that the action of drugs like secobarbital and pentobarbital lasts only 4 to 6 hours, making withdrawal flexible. The initial dose to be given is estimated by history and the barbiturate tolerance test. If the addiction is mixed, consideration must be given to the other drugs taken. Approximately 3 to 4 ounces of whiskey is equivalent for withdrawal purposes to 100 mg of pentobarbital. Comparably, 400 mg of meprobamate is equivalent to 100 mg of pentobarbital. After the daily intake of barbiturates is estimated, the daily dose is given in 4 divided doses. If evidence of intoxication occurs, a dose may be omitted as with the long-acting drugs, and if withdrawal symptoms appear, 100 to 200 mg of pentobarbital may be given every 1 or 2 hours until intoxication occurs. The dose of pentobarbital is then reduced by 100 mg each day unless there is evidence of intoxication or withdrawal. The bedtime dose is the last to be withdrawn.

5. Because of the danger of the medical complications of barbiturate withdrawal and the hazard of the patient taking additional amounts, withdrawal from barbiturates should be performed in a hospital.

6. After withdrawal is complete there should be some exploration in psychotherapy as to why the patient abused the drug.

7. Barbiturates or similarly acting sedative–hypnotic drugs are frequently used in suicide attempts, quite often successfully. Management of these overdoses is discussed in handbooks of medical emergencies.

Quality Assurance Issues

1. Has the proper differential diagnosis been done to rule out other causes of disturbances in psychomotor activity?

2. Have other causes of sexual and aggressive acting-out behavior been considered and ruled out?

3. Have proper treatments been proposed and implemented for disturbances of psychomotor activity and potential disinhibition of sexual and aggressive impulses?

Ethical/Legal Issues

1. Regarding the patient suffering from a disinhibition of sexual and aggressive impulses, what is the obligation of the clinician to assure that third parties are protected from his or her behaviors?

2. What management issues must be considered, with regard to protection of patients and staff, in the hospitalization of a patient who has disinhibition of sexual and aggressive impulses?
3. What is the role of the clinician where actions are brought against a patient by a third party claiming either sexual or aggressive behavior?
4. Can the clinician be requested to assist the court in determining proper disposition of a patient who engages in such dyssocial acts secondary to barbiturate or similarly acting hypnotic or sedative withdrawal?

BEHÇET'S SYNDROME AND ORGANIC MENTAL DISORDER

The multisystem panvasculitis of undetermined etiology known as Behçet's syndrome is characterized by iritis, genital ulcers, and oral ulcers. In some instances, involvement of the CNS, large blood vessels, joints, and gastrointestinal tract may also occur and dominate the clinical course. Nervous system involvement occurs in about 20% of the cases (Shimizu, 1979).

History
1. The syndrome is most often observed in Japan, the Eastern Mediterranean, and the Middle East (Uhl et al, 1985).
2. The course is generally chronic and relapsing (Borson, 1982).

Symptoms
1. Anxiety.
2. Fearfulness.
3. Depression.
4. Dementia.
5. Psychosis.
6. Characterological changes.
7. Painful joints.

Signs
1. Oral ulcers.
2. Iritis.
3. Genital ulcers.
4. Epididymitis.
5. Thrombophlebitis.
6. Erythema nodosum.

Laboratory Tests
1. There is no diagnostic laboratory test.
2. Elevated white cell count.
3. Elevated erythrocyte sedimentation rate.

Management
1. Referral for medical or neurologic management.
2. Steroids are commonly used (e.g., prednisone and dexamethasone ophthalmic drops).

Quality Assurance Issues
1. Have alternative conditions that would explain generalized anxiety and fearfulness been considered?
2. Where dementia and psychosis are present, has a proper differential diagnosis been made to rule out conditions that would require a different course of treatment?
3. Given the variety of signs and symptoms and the fact that some of these may be seen in AIDS, has this condition been considered?

Ethical/Legal Issues
1. Has the patient been referred to a proper medical or neurologic specialist?
2. What are the limits of psychiatric involvement in the diagnosis of Behçet's disease? Given the lack of specific diagnostic laboratory tests for this condition, how would one assess negligence in medical management?

BENZODIAZEPINE INTOXICATION AND WITHDRAWAL

Benzodiazepines can cause a toxic syndrome characterized by the signs and symptoms of alcohol intoxication and a withdrawal syndrome, which in the extreme resembles delirium tremens. The similarity of these states makes differential diagnoses difficult without serum and urine screens.

History
1. The patient may acknowledge or deny benzodiazepine and other drug and alcohol use.
2. Symptoms vary in intensity. Minor withdrawal symptoms include myalgia and insomnia, mild symptoms of intoxication, drowsiness, and dyscoordination.
3. Patients receiving benzodiazepines should be cautioned that they should ascertain the impact on their driving and on tasks requiring fine motor control before undertaking these tasks without supervision.
4. Patients must be alert to the fact that concurrent ingestion of alcohol may enhance lethargy and motor impairment.
5. Benzodiazepines are divided into the long-acting (diazepam [Valium], flurazepam [Dalmane], chlodiazepoxide [Librium]), intermediate-acting (clorazepate [Tranxene], oxazepam [Serax]), and short-acting (so-called second generation) (lorazepam [Ativan], alprazolam [Xanax], triazolam [Halcion]) types.
6. Long-acting benzodiazepines tend to accumulate in the body and are more associated with confusion, particularly in the elderly and brain damaged who have

cognitive deterioration or decreased ability to metabolize the drugs resulting in a decreasing tolerance to medication.

7. The shorter-acting benzodiazepines do not accumulate, allowing a dose to be tailored more easily to a patient's unique metabolic status (Salzman et al, 1983). It is also this fact that makes the short-acting benzodiazepines more likely to cause addiction.

8. Longer-acting benzodiazepines such as diazepam extensively accumulate with washout slow. Metabolites are present 2 weeks after discontinuation of the drug.

9. Symptoms of intoxication with short-acting benzodiazepines disappear within days of discontinuation of use. It may take as long as a week for symptoms of intoxication with a long-acting benzodiazepine to remit. Comparably, withdrawal symptoms appear within 1 day of cessation of a short-acting benzodiazepine while those from a longer-acting benzodiazepine take days to appear.

10. Benzodiazepines are the most common drug taken in overdose. Benzodiazepine overdose is associated with less disturbance of consciousness than with other drugs (Busto et al, 1981).

11. Flurazepam overdose is associated with more drowsiness than other benzodiazepines.

12. Serum levels of drugs such as benzodiazepines that are oxidatively metabolized are increased with long-term use of oral contraceptives (Abernethy et al, 1982).

13. Diazepam increases levels of estradiol resulting in gynecomastia (Bergman et al, 1981).

14. Younger and more anxious individuals have greater difficulty withdrawing than those older and less anxious (Cantopher et al, 1990).

15. Patients with a personal or family history of substance abuse are most likely to abuse benzodiazepines.

16. A clue that a person may abuse the drug is the fact that a patient does not only report remission of anxiety on the benzodiazepines but also experiences euphoria ("a high").

17. The problem with most patients prescribed alprazolam for an anxiety disorder is not addiction but rather failure to take the drug as prescribed, resulting in re-emergence of anxiety and an assumed lack of response to the drug.

18. The advent of triplicate prescribing procedures has resulted in greater use of alcohol by some patients, especially men with anxiety disorders, as well as prescription of more addictive drugs (Marks J, 1985).

19. It appears that panic disorder may be associated with a functional subsensitivity to benzodiazepines at a receptor level (Roy-Byrne et al, 1989).

20. Benzodiazepines are prescribed for anxiety, seizures, muscle spasms, and insomnia (Hammer et al, 1986).

21. The nonbenzodiazepine anxiolytic buspirone (Buspar) is not associated with withdrawal symptoms but patients appear less satisfied with it in the management of chronic anxiety (Rickels et al, 1988).

22. Previous discontinuous use of a benzodiazepine may predispose the user to withdrawal symptoms (Rickels et al, 1988).

23. Benzodiazepines vary in their potential for memory impairment (Scharf et al, 1984).

24. Use of benzodiazepines may cause the symptoms of psychoses in both adults and children (Pfefferbaum et al, 1987).
25. The amount of benzodiazepines prescribed, given the disorders they are indicated for, does not appear to be excessive (Nagy, 1987).
26. The side effects of all benzodiazepines are nearly identical. Differences in side effects and efficacy relate to the specific pharmacokinetics of each (Rifkin, 1990).
27. Panic or anxiety upon withdrawal of a benzodiazepine does not necessarily indicate addiction. It may simply mean that a patient has a chronic anxiety disorder requiring continued usage of the benzodiazepine (Talley, 1990).
28. Severity of withdrawal symptoms relates to dose, time of consumption, mode of withdrawal, and type of benzodiazepine (Wolf B et al, 1989).
29. Withdrawal symptoms occur with both long- and short-acting benzodiazepines (Berlin and Connell, 1983; Hollister, 1981; Winokur A et al, 1980b).

Symptoms of Withdrawal
1. Myalgia.
2. Anxiety.
3. Tearfulness.
4. Irritability.
5. Panic.
6. Rebound anxiety.
7. Insomnia.
8. Mood disturbance.
9. Psychoses.
10. Hallucinations.
11. Paranoia.

Symptoms of Intoxication
1. Drowsiness.
2. Ataxia.
3. Fatigue.
4. Depression.
5. Amnesia.
6. Pseudodementia.
7. Psychosis.
8. Diplopia.
9. Behavioral disinhibition.

Signs of Withdrawal
1. Tachycardia.
2. Tremors.
3. Seizures.
4. Delirium.
5. Myoclonus.
6. Bizarre involuntary muscle movement (Rapoport and Covington, 1989).

7. Urinary incontinence.
8. Muscle rigidity.

Signs of Intoxication
1. Ataxia.
2. Slurred speech.
3. Loss of fine motor coordination.
4. Urinary incontinence.

Differential Diagnosis
1. Benzodiazepine intoxication and withdrawal.
2. Alcohol intoxication and withdrawal.
3. Polysubstance intoxication and withdrawal.
4. Other drug intoxication and withdrawal.
5. Other neurologic causes of seizures, amnesia, cerebellar dysfunction, and the other symptoms and signs seen with benzodiazepine withdrawal and intoxication.
6. Conversion.
7. Malingering.

Laboratory Tests
1. Serum and urine drug screens.
2. Blood alcohol level.

Management
1. If a patient develops symptoms of withdrawal, return to the dose used without emergence of withdrawal symptoms and withdraw more slowly. Decrements as small as 0.125 or 0.25 mg per wk may be required to withdraw from alprazolam without symptoms.
2. If a patient develops symptoms of intoxication on a benzodiazepine, withhold the drug until symptoms abate and decrease the maintenance dosage.
3. Propranolol-assisted abrupt withdrawal is less effective than slow withdrawal without propranolol (Cantopher et al, 1990).
4. Clonazepam (Klonopin) allows a comfortable and smooth withdrawal in most instances due to its long duration of action.
5. Tapered benzodiazepine withdrawal does not appear to be more risky for older people than younger people (Schweizer et al, 1989).
6. Withdrawal symptoms persist for several days or weeks due to the presence of active metabolites that are slowly released. Half-lives of diazepam and flurazepam are 26–96 hours and 47–100 hours, respectively. Lorazepam's and oxazepam's half-lives are both, by comparison, approximately 8–20 hours with rapid elimination over 2 days. It is the rapid decline in serum levels that makes the short-acting benzodiazepines more addictive.
7. When rebound insomnia occurs after withdrawal of a benzodiazepine with a relatively short half-life, a nonbenzodiazepine sleep medication (e.g., diphenhydramine

[Benadryl]) or a benzodiazepine with a longer half-life such as flurazepam may be prescribed.

8. Symptoms that initially increase then decrease over time after abrupt cessation of a benzodiazepine may be assumed to relate to withdrawal while symptoms that steadily increase suggest re-emergence of the anxiety being treated (Winokur A et al, 1980b).

9. Clonidine has not been reported to be efficacious (in doses sufficient to markedly reduce blood pressure) for the reduction of symptoms of benzodiazepine withdrawal (Goodman WK et al, 1986) in contrast to the established efficacy of clonidine in opiate withdrawal.

10. Carbamazepine (Tegretol) has been demonstrated to facilitate rapid discontinuation of benzodiazepines without emergence of withdrawal symptoms (Ries et al, 1989).

11. It is recommended that alprazolam withdrawal be extremely gradual to minimize symptoms of anxiety and withdrawal (Roy-Byrne et al, 1989).

Quality Assurance Issues

1. Were patients evaluated to ascertain if there is a personal or family history of substance abuse? If there was, were they prescribed an alternative to a benzodiazepine? If prescribed a benzodiazepine, did the reason for doing so (given the history) justify its use?

2. Was the patient advised of the addictive potential of benzodiazepines?

3. Was the patient advised that abrupt cessation of use may lead to medical emergency (e.g., withdrawal seizures)?

4. Was use of the benzodiazepines carefully monitored and prescriptions limited?

5. Was the patient alerted to the fact that benzodiazepine use may present difficulty in driving or present a hazard if the patient is working with heavy machinery or machinery entailing fine motor skills?

6. Have patients been denied use of benzodiazepines for disorders for which benzodiazepines are appropriate and indicated with resultant undue prolonged suffering (Uhlenhuth et al, 1988)?

Ethical/Legal Issues

1. Does the potential benefit of benzodiazepine use to quality of life given other options outweigh the potential risk (Woods JH et al, 1988)?

2. What is the obligation of the psychiatrist in assessing the amount of benzodiazepines that are to be prescribed for a patient at any given time?

3. What is the role of the psychiatrist with respect to patients who may require long-term treatment with a benzodiazepine such as alprazolam to inform the Motor Vehicle Department of that patient's condition?

BEREAVEMENT

Following a loss—expected or unexpected—an individual must mourn. Eric Lindemann described, in 1944, the course of normal bereavement in relatives of those who died in the catastrophic Coconut Grove nightclub fire in Boston. He found that those individuals who were most stoic in their adjustment to death were eventually most affected by it. Mourning is a necessary and important part of psychological adjustment to loss. Encouragement of mourning and support of grief during the first 3 months following loss has been demonstrated empirically to lower post-bereavement morbidity (Raphael, 1977). Only when mourning becomes melancholia is grief pathological, and therefore, psychopharmacological, somatic (e.g., electroshock) or more specific psychotherapeutic approaches become necessary.

History

1. The first step in evaluation of individuals whose response to tragedy is interfering with their functioning is a determination of the nature of the loss as well as the circumstances surrounding it. If a friend or relative died, what was the cause of death (e.g., a car accident, suicide, cancer, AIDS, homicide)? Who was present when the patient died (e.g., spouse, children, lover as opposed to spouse)? What was the relationship of the patient to the deceased? How frequently did they see each other? Was there any sexual involvement? Did the patient argue with the deceased before his or her death?

2. The way an individual has managed loss in the past is a good predictor of how it will be handled in the present. If there is a past history of loss, how did the patient deal with it?

3. Information should be obtained as to the degree to which the loss will alter an individual's life. Will income decrease? Are there outstanding business obligations? Debts? Medical Bills? Funeral Costs? Is there a Will or will there be a delay in settlement of an estate because of absence of a Will? Will it be necessary to sell a family home or business? Is there tension among survivors over inheritance?

4. About 8% of deaths are reported to be "unnatural" (e.g., murder, suicide) (Rynearson, 1986). These deaths are likely to be associated with symptoms of post-traumatic stress disorder such as emergence of images of the event during the day (flashbacks), inability to concentrate, panic, and recurrent nightmares of the event (Slaby, 1990).

5. Having been married to the deceased and previous health problems are strong predictors of health care use and morbidity in those bereaved (Mor et al, 1986).

6. Over 800,000 men and women in the United States suffer loss of a spouse each year (Jacobs and Kim, 1990).

7. Symptoms that distinguish normal bereavement (mourning) from pathological grieving (melancholia) are that, in the latter case, one sees marked psychomotor retardation or agitation; suicide gestures or attempts; morbid preoccupation with feeling worthless, helpless, and hopeless; and marked functional impairment (Jacobs and Kim, 1990).

8. Response to bereavement varies tremendously. Some individuals actually mature and become more effective and well balanced. Others sustain permanent damage to their physical, social, psychological, and spiritual lives (Parkes, 1990).
9. Loss of spouse is ranked by individuals surveyed as the greatest stress of daily life and has been linked to increased susceptibility to medical illness, mortality, and affective illness, and a variety of life-threatening behaviors (Zisook et al, 1990).
10. In the Epidemiologic Catchment Area study in New Haven, Connecticut (Bruce et al, 1990), bereavement increased risk of a depressive episode more among respondents with no prior dysphoria than those who had reported such.
11. Absence of grieving at the time of a loss does not invariably mean that an individual will subsequently develop a pathological grief reaction, but many who do not express grief at the time of the death do later develop symptoms of pathological grief.
12. Normal grieving does not usually extend much beyond 4 to 6 weeks. Major depressive disorder, dysthymic disorder, and bipolar disorder of the depressed type usually does.

Symptoms of Normal Grief
1. Restlessness.
2. Guilt with feelings of not having done enough for the deceased.
3. Preoccupation with the image of the deceased.
4. Self-blame.
5. Inability to organize daily activities.
6. Hostility toward the doctors and other medical professionals who attended the deceased.
7. Insomnia.
8. Irritability.
9. Appetite loss.
10. Somatic symptoms such as headache and diarrhea.

Symptoms of Abnormal Grief
1. Panic attacks.
2. Taking on the symptoms of the last illness of the person who died.
3. Imprudent business transactions.
4. Apathy.
5. Personally destructive behavior.
6. Agitated to retarded depression.
7. Overactivity without a sense of loss.
8. Increased use of alcohol or drugs.

Management
1. Allow patients to ventilate their feelings of loss in a supportive atmosphere.
2. Help to identify and complete necessary tasks at the time of a death such as preparation for the funeral, burial, and the settling of the estate.

3. Relatives and friends should be encouraged to stay with the bereaved during the first few days after a loss. If indicated, suggest a relative or friend move in with the bereaved or that the bereaved stay at a relative's or friend's house for a few days.

4. Sleep medication may be required for the first few nights following a loss. A small dose of a benzodiazepine such as flurazepam hydrochloride (Dalmane), oxazepam (Serax), or triazolam (Halcion) is usually sufficient.

5. Assess suicide risk. If significant, and the patient is without social supports to reduce risk, he or she may have to be hospitalized.

6. Evaluate use of alcohol and other drugs. Some individuals first develop alcoholism or drug abuse in an attempt to self-medicate the pain of a loss and the anxiety of living alone and of redirecting the course of their life. A number of these become dually diagnosed.

7. If grieving extends beyond the usual course (i.e., 4 to 6 weeks), the need for antidepressant medication should be assessed.

8. Common sense is the best guide for care of individuals during the immediate few days following a loss. Friends, relatives, and familiar clergy should be encouraged to help take care of the patient and help to "people" the empty space created by the loss. The patient should be provided with good and tasty food and helped out with mundane household tasks.

9. Supportive brief psychotherapy is more suitable for patients with less motivation for therapy and lower organization of their self-concept. Better organized and more highly motivated patients benefit from more exploratory therapy (Horowitz et al, 1984).

Quality Assurance Issues

1. Was a differential diagnosis established to ascertain if a patient's mourning has become or is becoming pathological?

2. Was a proper history and evaluation of the patient's current life situation conducted to rule out other alternatives that may be responsible for some of the abnormal grief symptoms such as panic attacks, apathy, and substance abuse?

3. Was an effort made to rule out the possibility that substance abuse preceded the loss?

Ethical/Legal Issues

1. Was the patient properly assessed to determine suicide or homicide propensity?

2. Was the use of substances such as alcohol and other drugs anticipated prior to the prescribing of sleep or other medication? When is hospitalization indicated for the treatment of severe bereavement and what elements would enter into a determination of negligence in this regard?

BORDERLINE PERSONALITY DISORDER

There are a group of patients who, much like the fabled Richard Corey, look normal to all the world and one day go up to their room and kill themselves. These patients often talk about experiencing depression for as long as they can remember, anger as the strongest felt emotion, inconstant identity, and never feeling close to anyone. There is disagreement among clinicians and researchers as to whether or not what is observed is a real mental disorder or rather a psychodynamic constellation (Kroll et al, 1981). It is true that descriptions provided by various authors make it difficult to examine this group from an empirical basis. It is also true, however, that clinicians working in emergency settings are confronted with patients who do have these dynamics and find them, as a group, as difficult or more difficult than other patients to deal with. The crises these patients present involve:

1. Suicidal ideation.
2. Suicidal gesture.
3. Serious suicide attempt.
4. Homicidal ideation.
5. Homicidal gesture or attempt.
6. Drug abuse.
7. Other impulsive behavior.
8. Micropsychotic episodes.
9. Major psychotic decompensations.

History

1. These patients often look quite good clinically, even in a crisis. A careful history reveals the severity of illness. It is these patients about whom people comment, after the patient successfully dies by suicide, that "there never was any indication that anything was wrong." This, in fact, is what is most destructive to these patients. They themselves may be very supportive to others and never be given the opportunity to express how depressed and lonely they are. Never has anyone asked them if they view death as an arbitrary line to be drawn unexpectedly by them or someone else at a moment's notice. They may express the fact that although they do not feel suicidal now, when they do they will do it quickly and silently. No one will be notified. They commit suicide, often capriciously.
2. Patients with borderline personality disorders report significantly more childhood sexual and physical abuse and abuse by more than one person in childhood, with derealization and chronic dysphoria the greatest clues to abuse (Ogata et al, 1990).
3. These patients appear quite normal in appearance, manners, and social awareness and may do extremely well at school and work. This appearance in part is often due to a lack of a firm sense of identity with an extraordinary capacity to superficially and rapidly identify with others. At times this may take the form of conservative or radical politics and rapid and zealous religious conversions or interest in Satanism, witchcraft, and Satanic worship.
4. Interpersonal relationships are characterized by dependence, devaluation, demandingness, and manipulation.
5. Borderline personality-disordered patients are difficult to distinguish from antisocial and histrionic and other personality-disordered individuals (Pope et al, 1983b; Gunderson and Zanarini, 1987). The boundary with schizophrenia and

affective disorder is more clear. It is common for borderline personality disorder to be comorbid with affective disorder (so-called "double depression") or substance abuse disorders.

6. Borderline patients may do as poorly as schizophrenics, because of symptoms typical of borderline personality disorder and not from schizophrenic symptoms.

7. Depression, pathologic mood swings, and eccentric or peculiar behavior (but not schizophrenia) is increased among first-degree relatives of borderline patients (Soloff and Millward, 1983; Loranger et al, 1982).

8. While borderline patients often indicate that they have no immediate plans to kill themselves, they often report that their mood could change capriciously without their ability to seek help prior to another or initial attempt.

9. Borderline patients are often indifferent to sex. They may be abstinent for prolonged periods and then be hetero- and homosexually indulgent. They may report not being certain whether they are female or male even in the act of coitus.

10. Patients with borderline personality reflect baseline rates of occurrence of Axis I psychiatric disorders without any one specific disorder (e.g., major depression, schizophrenia) inherent to the disorder. It is a very heterogeneous disorder with unclear boundaries (Fyer MR et al, 1988b; Gunderson and Elliot, 1985) and cluster symptoms overlapping schizophrenia, affective disorder, and a number of other personality disorders.

11. Derealization, depersonalization, and drug-free hallucinations are the most common psychotic symptoms experienced by borderline patients (Chopra and Beatson, 1986).

12. In one study, homosexuality was ten times more common among men and six times more common among women with borderline personality disorder than in control groups of the general population and of depressed patients (Zubenko et al, 1987). This may relate to the great incidence of inconsistent identity in patients with this disorder.

Symptoms

1. Depression often as long as they can remember.
2. Polysubstance abuse.
3. Self-destructive and other-destructive behavior.
4. Derealization.
5. Depersonalization.
6. Absence of intimate relationships.
7. Loneliness.
8. Inconsistent identity.
9. Cutting or burning themselves, or masturbating to feel more real.
10. Readily adopting the identity of others (e.g., religiously, sexually, politically).
11. Polymorphous sexuality.
12. Intense anger often as the strongest emotion (as opposed to mood).
13. No commitment to an interpersonal relationship.
14. Impulsive behavior.
15. Promiscuity.

16. Drug and alcohol dependence.
17. Anhedonia.
18. A feeling of emptiness.
19. Paranoia.
20. Brief psychotic episodes.
21. Manipulativeness.
22. Devaluation.
23. Demandingness.
24. Dissociative phenomena.

Signs
1. Burn and cut marks on the body.

Differential Diagnosis
1. Borderline personality disorder.
2. Atypical depression.
3. Major depression.
4. Schizophrenia.
5. Temporal lobe epilepsy.
6. Obsessive–compulsive disorder.
7. Histrionic personality disorder.
8. Sociopathic personality disorder.
9. Narcissistic personality disorder.
10. Dysthymic disorder.
11. Cyclothymic disorder.
12. Panic disorder.
13. Somatization disorder.
14. Polysubstance abuse.

Management
1. These patients tend to get over-involved with their therapists. The slightest change in a clinician's affect may be a sufficient stimulus for self-destructive behavior. The best prophylaxes against the development of this "psychotic transference" is for the therapist to be real and to structure the interview. The tendency to regress should be countered. In reality, the therapist is not God but another real live human being with no more magical power than anyone else. These patients cannot tolerate silences. Therapists should take an active role in therapy. These patients have limited capacity to accept themselves and tend to see things in black or white. They are either all good or all bad. It is unfathomable to them that most of us are neither saints nor sinners but something in between. When they feel good, it seems nothing will ever go wrong again, but when they are down, it is hell, and suicide seems the only alternative.
2. Termination is extremely difficult for these people. All past endings of relationships are conjured up and like the concrete child, patients imagine that if therapists leave they may be dead, that the patient was the cause of their going, and

that they will not be able to survive without the therapist. They may, in fact, feel their anger killed the therapist. To avoid this, the therapy contract should be clear when it is set up and its duration indicated. Encouragement of outside relationships allows a dilution of the transference and mollifies termination. In some instances, concurrent therapy by two therapists reduces stress to patients and therapists alike, particularly at vacation time.

3. The patient's therapist should be called when the patient presents in the emergency room. This may be the single most valuable emergency psychotherapeutic ploy. A follow-up appointment soon after the emergency evaluation may negate a need for hospitalization even if the patient is mildly suicidal. They should feel that their therapists and the emergency room are readily available in times of crisis.

4. It is imperative to determine why a patient who is recurrently suicidal presents in the emergency room for evaluation. They may be having a micropsychotic episode, or some fantasy may have gotten out of hand. Such behavior might be controlled by a therapist's reassurance or an antipsychotic. Marijuana or another drug may have made the patient feel more unreal. A small dose of phenothiazine (e.g., 8–12 mg of perphenazine (Trilafon) PO) may reduce their anxiety. They may have a temporary stress-related sleep problem and may require a hypnotic such as diphenhydramine (Benadryl) 50–100 mg PO for the night. The emergency room psychiatrist should assess the patient's social and personal adaptive resources (i.e., "ego strengths"). If, in the past, they have made a serious suicide attempt, they may require hospitalization. If the precipitant is as uncomplex as their therapist going on holiday, all that may be needed is that the emergency room psychiatrist or the therapist's backup follow the patient until the therapist returns.

5. A subgroup of patients with borderline personality disorder respond to low doses of neuroleptic drugs, either antipsychotics or antidepressants. If antidepressants are to be used, however, they should never be started in an emergency situation. The response to antidepressants is too unpredictable and the potential for self-poisoning too great to use a potentially lethal medication. Antipsychotic, anti-anxiety, or hypnotic agents will suffice in emergency situations.

6. Borderline patients tend to decompensate at times of pressure and recompensate when the pressure is reduced. A discussion of what is going on in the patient's therapy may reveal that they are drawing "dangerously" close to their therapists, and are threatened by a loss of self and by personal annihilation. Reassurance and a single dose of medication may relieve the tension.

7. Patients should be evaluated for comorbid psychiatric disorders or of temporal lobe phenomena causing borderline symptoms (e.g., derealization, depersonalization, hallucinations, anxiety, depression). Once identified, these should be treated. The most commonly occurring comorbid diagnoses are primary major depression, secondary depression, bipolar disorder, dysthymic disorder, panic disorder, agoraphobia, somatization disorder, and alcohol and drug abuse (Prasad et al, 1990).

8. Therapy with borderline patients is complicated by the fact that threats of

separation or withdrawal of nurturing support gives genesis to hostile, devaluative, angry behavior accompanied by manipulative and self-destructive action in an attempt to gain contact with and control over the person who is withdrawing (Gunderson and Zanarini, 1987).

9. Alprazolam (Xanax) has been reported effective in treatment of borderline personality disorders that were resistant to treatment with other psychotrobes (Faltus, 1984). The addictive tendency of this diagnostic group by personal or family history is a consideration before prescribing a benzodiazepine. Alprazolam has also been reported to increase disinhibition in borderline patients (Psychopharmacology of Borderline Personality Disorder, 1987).

10. When hospitalization proves necessary to stabilize a patient, treatment is often complicated by regression, splitting, and self-destructive behavior. A structured therapeutic milieu, well-defined short-term goals, a focus on immediate problems with realistic expectations for resolution, and well-defined roles for the members of the treatment team minimizes problems (Sansone and Madakasira, 1990).

11. Antidepressants such as amitriptyline (Elavil) may paradoxically increase paranoid ideation, suicide threats, and demanding and assaultive behavior in some borderline patients (Soloff et al, 1986a).

12. There is some evidence to suggest that small doses of antipsychotics such as 4–10 mg of haloperidol (Haldol) may be more effective than antidepressants for treating symptoms of borderline personality such as depression, anxiety, psychotic thinking, paranoia, and hostility (Soloff et al, 1986b).

Quality Assurance Issues

1. Was the patient evaluated for concurrent psychiatric disorders including substance abuse and was diagnostic-specific treatment provided?
2. Was the patient evaluated for suicide and homicide potential?
3. If found to be other- or self-destructive, were appropriate precautions provided?

Ethical/Legal Issues

1. Was informed consent obtained from the patient before small doses of antipsychotic medication were used?
2. Given the risk of tardive dyskinesia and other side effects from antipsychotic medications, what would be the indications for using them in this population?
3. Would created and iatrogenically induced dependency on benzodiazepines (particularly alprazolam) be evidence of negligent medical management?
4. Given the caprice in the change of mood state in these patients, can the therapist be legally assured that a patient will not commit suicide or homicide?

BRIEF REACTIVE PSYCHOSIS

A number of psychotic symptoms may emerge briefly after a particularly stressful life event such as a rape or news that all of one's children and spouse were killed by a drunken driver. These symptoms abate with time but antipsychotics may be required for a few days or weeks to facilitate recompensation and reduce psychic pain.

History

1. There is considerable confusion regarding this diagnosis, as many patients who appear to suffer a psychosis less than 2 weeks later when re-evaluated are found to have another diagnosis that explains the symptoms (Munoz et al, 1987).
2. About three-quarters of patients with a first episode of schizophrenia, affective illness, or unspecified functional psychoses are in remission 1 year after. Predictors of poor outcome include premorbid asociality, longer duration of illness, and lack of maintenance medication (Rabiner et al, 1986).

Symptoms and Signs

1. All the symptoms and signs of psychoses are seen.

Differential Diagnosis

1. Brief reactive psychoses.
2. Bipolar disorder.
3. Schizophrenia.
4. Borderline personality disorder.
5. Temporal lobe dysfunction.
6. Alcohol and drug abuse disorders.
7. Other organic psychoses (e.g., migraine headaches).
8. Dissociative disorder.

Management

1. Patients should be carefully evaluated to ascertain whether what appears to be brief reactive psychosis may not be a brief manic episode, a micropsychotic attack of a borderline personality disorder, an organic condition such as migraine, temporal lobe epilepsy, hypoglycemia, or a substance-use toxic or withdrawal disorder. When an alternative diagnosis is substantiated, diagnostic-specific treatment is provided.
2. When heightened levels of anxiety appear to have led to psychiatric symptoms such as paranoia or depersonalization or a dissociative disorder, non-neuroleptic psychopharmacotherapy (e.g., use of lorazepam [Ativan]) may be effective without the risk of the side effects associated with use of neuroleptics, which may be construed to be an exacerbation of the disorder (Cohen and Lipinski, 1986).
3. Neuroleptics appear to be equally effective in the management of acute psychoses. Side effects more than therapeutic efficacy impact choice of neuroleptic used (Bailine et al, 1990).
4. Monitoring of clinical symptoms is as effective as measurement of serum neuroleptic levels in the management of most acutely psychiatric patients (Zohar et al, 1986).
5. Brief psychiatric hospitalization may supplement neuroleptic use to enhance

self-esteem, improve cognitive abilities, and increase perception of the availability of other people (Lieberman and Strauss, 1986). Patients attribute these changes to the opportunity to reflect, to making a decision to change, and to the formation of relationships with others. Sometimes hospitalization is simply necessary to stabilize a patient and reduce risk of self or other harm in the acute phase.

Quality Assurance Issues
1. Was the patient and his or her family warned of the dangers of neuroleptic use?
2. Was the patient evaluated for potential harm to self or others and precautions initiated if present?
3. Was a differential diagnosis performed and diagnostic-specific treatment provided?

Ethical/Legal Issues
1. Since the characteristics of brief reactive psychosis are similar to psychosis in general, what prognosis can be provided to the patient and his or her family suffering from this condition?
2. The possibility of self-destructive behavior is enhanced during the brief reactive psychosis; what is the obligation of the therapist for protecting the patient against her- or himself? How would negligence be determined in a situation where the patient's symptoms and signs are ambiguous and the therapist has not elected to intervene to protect the patient against his or her own self-destructive or potentially other-destructive impulses?

BRIQUET'S SYNDROME

1. Briquet's syndrome is an alternate appellation for somatization disorder. It is a distinct diagnostic entity with unique genetic clinical characteristics.
2. The lifetime prevalence for women is approximately 1% (Maany, 1981). It is rarely diagnosed in men.
3. It is considered in the differential diagnosis of any complicated surgical or medical case where symptoms cannot be explained by a single disease process.
4. Depression is frequent with such patients and the depression responds to antidepressants.
5. Secondary depression, such as those seen with Briquet's disease, are associated with more psychotic symptoms and suicide attempts than primary depressions (Andreasen and Winokur, 1979).
6. There is a need for studies to ascertain if the core psychopathology of somatization disorder is masked depression or an entity in itself.
7. Surgeons, internists, and psychiatrists must work collaboratively with such patients so unnecessary invasive procedures and other medical interventions are not undertaken.

8. The symptoms, signs, and treatment of Briquet's disorder are found in the discussion of somatization disorder.

Quality Assurance Issues

1. Has a proper differential diagnosis been conducted to rule out other causes of somatic symptoms?
2. What measures have been instituted to prevent the unnecessary invasive procedures in this population?
3. Has concomitant depression been properly diagnosed and treated?

Ethical/Legal Issues

1. Has the patient been properly evaluated by other specialists to rule out the possibilities of a biologic basis for the symptoms that may exist?
2. Has the suicidal potential of the patient been properly assessed and the proper measures introduced to prevent self-destructive behavior?

BROMIDE INTOXICATION, AFFECTIVE AND DELUSIONAL ORGANIC MENTAL DISORDER

1. Acute bromide intoxication (bromism) is rare because bromide tends to irritate the gastrointestinal tract. It is difficult to retain much without vomiting.
2. Bromide is excreted slowly by the kidneys and, therefore, tends to accumulate if taken daily.
3. The incidence of bromide psychosis is greatly underestimated because physicians do not think of it and consequently fail to look for its signs, symptoms, and presence in the serum.
4. Over-the-counter sedatives containing bromides are available to the public without prescription.
5. The diagnosis of bromide intoxication is corroborated by a serum bromide level. Generally, symptoms are slow in developing and usually will not be manifested until the serum bromide level exceeds 50 mg/100 mL. Urine bromide levels are not a reliable guide to intoxication.
6. Bromism, like tuberculosis and syphilis, is a great masquerader. Individuals intoxicated from bromides present as delirious, demented, manic, depressed, and schizophrenic in addition to having symptoms suggestive of a number of other clinical syndromes. Symptoms do not necessarily correlate with serum bromide levels.
7. As with all drug psychoses, the clinical course and presentation is a function of the interaction of the patient's premorbid physical and psychological state, the environment, the dose of and duration of bromide use, and the number of other drugs taken.
8. Bromism may be mistaken for a number of neurologic disorders and should be

suspected whenever a diagnosis remains unclear after a thorough history and physical examination have been performed.

9. Patients may become quite terrified and violent during the withdrawal phase and require protection from harming themselves or others.

10. The serum half-life of bromide is about 12 days.

Symptoms

1. Delusions.
2. Lethargy.
3. Auditory and visual hallucinations.
4. Dizziness.
5. Impairment of thought and memory.
6. Emotional lability.
7. Irritability.
8. Photophobia.
9. Loss of memory.
10. Mania.
11. Irrelevant speech.
12. Headache.
13. Decreased libido.
14. Fabrication.
15. Vertigo.
16. Depression.
17. Confusion.
18. Blurred vision.
19. Anorexia.
20. Diplopia.
21. Gastric distress.
22. Constipation.

Signs

1. Dermatitis. (The classical bromide rash begins as an acneform eruption on the face or around the hair roots and later spreads to the entire body. A nodular type of lesion may appear on the legs, known as nodosa bromoderma.)
2. Delirium.
3. Coma.
4. Pupillary dilation.
5. Heavily furred tongue.
6. Foul breath.
7. Babinski's sign.
8. Mild conjunctivitis.
9. Cyanosis.
10. Tremor.
11. Ataxia.
12. Disorientation.

13. Reflex disturbances.
14. Papilledema.
15. Stupor.
16. Vacuous facies.
17. Muscular weakness.
18. Motor incoordination.
19. Decreased superficial reflexes.
20. Sluggishness of movement.
21. Thick, slurred speech.

Laboratory Studies
1. In severe cases the cerebrospinal pressure may be elevated.
2. At high plasma levels the electroencephalogram may show a diffuse slow wave pattern. At low plasma levels there may be a pattern of sustained fast wave activity.

Differential Diagnosis
1. Bromism.
2. Acute alcohol intoxication.
3. Acute and chronic schizophrenia.
4. Tabes dorsalis.
5. General paresis.
6. Uremia.
7. Cerebral neoplasm.
8. Multiple sclerosis.
9. Encephalitis.
10. Major depression.
11. Dysthymic disorder.
12. Mania.
13. Other toxic syndromes.

Management
1. Obtain a serum level to confirm the diagnosis. A patient is considered toxic if his level is greater than 50 mg/100 mL.
2. Discontinue all intake of bromide.
3. Specific treatment involves the administration of large quantities (up to 6–12 g daily) of sodium chloride orally in divided doses or intravenously in the form of physiologic saline. Ammonium chloride not only provides a chloride ion but also acts as a diuretic.
4. In severe cases, hemodialysis may be used.
5. The patient's food intake should be monitored to correct the malnutrition often encountered with bromism.
6. Sedation is contraindicated unless a patient is extremely agitated. Paraldehyde and neuroleptics have been used intramuscularly or orally when required. Intramuscular administration of paraldehyde may cause sterile abscesses and nerve damage and is avoided where possible. When given, the dosage of paraldehyde

is 10–15 mL orally every 4 to 6 hours or 4 mL intramuscularly in each buttock every 6 hours. Alternately, 50–75 mg IM of chlorpromazine (Thorazine), 5–10 mg of haloperidol (Haldol), or 5–10 mg of perphenazine (Trilafon) may be given intramuscularly every 4 hours while monitoring blood pressure.

7. Following treatment of the bromide psychosis, exploratory psychotherapy may be used to get at the origins of the bromide abuse. Symptoms may last as long as 2 to 6 weeks after cessation of bromide intake because of the long serum half life.

Quality Assurance Issues

1. Given the wide range of mental symptoms and signs found with bromism, a differential diagnosis with particular emphasis on the history is critical. Have all other causes of dementia, mania, depression, and psychotic-like symptoms been considered?

2. During the withdrawal phase, a patient may become violent; what other conditions have been properly ruled out before arriving at a diagnosis of bromism? Have the indications for the use of paraldehyde and neuroleptics been properly established?

Ethical/Legal Issues

1. Has the violence-proneness of the patient been properly assessed?

2. Would bromism be an acceptable basis for an insanity plea in the event of an afflicted person causing violence to a third party?

3. When is the clinician negligent in the assessment and treatment of a violence proneness? Has the patient been properly assessed as to his or her suicidal tendencies?

BULIMIA

Bulimia is characterized by episodes of rapid consumption of large quantities of food in discrete periods of time (usually less than 2 hours), so-called "binge eating." The prevalence rate among adolescent and young women is about 1% (Fairburn and Beglin, 1990).

History

1. This chaotic eating pattern is usually accompanied by awareness of the disordered pattern of eating with fear of not being able to stop eating voluntarily, self-deprecating thoughts, and depressive moods following the binges and attempts to lose or control weight through purging behavior such as self-induced vomiting, laxative abuse, enemas, and severely restricted diets (Johnson and Berndt, 1983).

2. Bulimia may be seen alone or together with other disorders, particularly anorexia nervosa and obesity. Often it is seen with women of normal weight.

3. The prevalence among college populations has variously been estimated to be 1.3% to 13% (Halmi et al, 1981; Strangler and Printz, 1980; Schotte and Stunkard, 1987).

4. The modal patient is a single, white, college-educated woman in her twenties without a history of extreme weight disorders.
5. Difficulty in handling emotions and restrictive dieting are the most frequently cited precipitants.
6. Bulimic patients do not appear as severely symptomatic as patients with anorexia nervosa but are, as a group, more vulnerable to depression, anxiety, and mood fluctuations. They are more preoccupied with weight and eating than women without eating disorders.
7. Bulimic patients prefer high caloric, easily ingested foods.
8. Casper et al (1980) reported 67% of bulimic patients with anorexia admitted to binge eating at least once a week and 16% at least every other day. The mean number of binges in one nonanorexic population was 11.7 per week (Mitchell JE et al, 1981).
9. Patients with this disorder tend to have histories of impairment in work, school, and social relationships.
10. Medical complications seen with these patients include gastric dilation, fluid and electrolyte imbalance, and rarely gastric rupture leading to death.
11. First-degree relatives of bulimic patients include higher rates of affective illness, alcoholism, and eating disorders than controls suggesting a common diathesis between bulimia nervosa and affective disorder (Kasset et al, 1989; Hudson et al, 1982; Levy AB et al, 1989).
12. Underweight anorexics have defects in peripheral osmoregulatory mechanisms accompanied with hypersecretion of cerebrospinal fluid vasopressin. In addition, cerebrospinal fluid oxytocin levels are altered subsequent to abnormal gastrointestinal function during the acute stages of anorexia nervosa (Demitivek et al, 1989).
13. Bulimic and anorexic patients are a diverse group in terms of both food-related behavioral symptoms and associated psychopathology requiring an evaluating clinician to be especially astute in diagnosis and treatment planning (McKenna MS, 1989).
14. Medical consequences of bulimic behavior include dental problems, salivary gland inflammation and swelling, metabolic changes (e.g., loss of sodium and potassium in the vomitus or as a result of laxative and diuretic use); and lacerations of the esophagus. Use of Ipecac can lead to cardiac irregularities and a generalized myopathy (Ferguson, 1985).
15. Common symptoms of bulimia are binge eating, self-induced vomiting, laxative and diuretic abuse, and chewing and spitting out food. In one study (Mitchell JE et al, 1985), one-third reported alcohol and/or other drug abuse.
16. Anorectic patients who are bulimic tend to be more extroverted, older, and tend to have greater appetites than anorectics who fast. The latter group are more introverted, deny hunger, and exhibit less overt psychic stress (Casper et al, 1980).
17. Anorectic patients with bulimia tend to have a longer duration of illness, more hospitalizations, and less successful social adjustment than fasting anorectics (Garfinkel PE et al, 1977).
18. Kleptomania and other indications of lessened impulse and self-control, such as alcoholism, are seen with bulimia (Casper et al, 1980).

19. Depression, guilt, anxiety, and self-deprecating behavior are frequent in bulimic patients (Pope et al, 1983a).
20. Neuroendocrine changes found with bulimia resemble those found with affective illness. In one study, 80% of bulimic patients exhibited blunted thyrotropin-releasing hormone (TRH) tests and 67% exhibited abnormalities of cortisol suppression (Gwirtsman et al, 1983) with the dexamethasone suppression test (DST).

Management

1. Antidepressant medication (e.g., imipramine, trazodone, fluoxetine, sertraline) has been found to reduce frequency of binge eating and to bring about improvement on several other measures of eating behavior. This may be due to a link between affective disorders and bulimia (Pope et al, 1983a).
2. If a patient does not respond to a tricyclic or tetracyclic antidepressant, a monoamine oxidase inhibitor or fluoxetine (Prozac) should be used (Walsh BT et al, 1979).
3. Sodium valproate, like other medications used to treat major affective illness, has been reported effective with patients' refractory bulimia and affective symptoms (Herridge and Pope, 1985).
4. The significantly higher rates of substance abuse reported among bulimics (Bulik, 1987) indicate the necessity for treatment plans that address both the eating disorder and the substance abuse disorder.
5. Fluoxetine in doses of 60 mg per day, coupled with behavior modification techniques, is reported to be significantly more effective in inducing weight loss (but not binge eating) than placebo and behavior modification alone (Marcus et al, 1990).
6. Group psychotherapy significantly enhances treatment outcome of patients treated with imipramine when compared to imipramine treatment alone (Pyle et al, 1990).

Quality Assurance Issues

1. Was the patient evaluated for medical and other psychiatric disorders that may present as bulimia and, if identified, was diagnostic-specific treatment provided?
2. Was the patient evaluated for substance abuse and, if found to be chemically dependent, provided concurrent treatment for chemical dependence?
3. Was the patient referred to a self-help group for eating disorders to complement other treatment provided?

Ethical/Legal Issues

1. Has the patient been appropriately referred for follow up of medical and non psychiatric symptoms?
2. Has the clinician avoided iatrogenically substance abuse which would be relatively easy in this patient population?
3. Has the suicidal potential of the patient been properly evaluated and measures introduced to protect the patient against her own self destructive impulses?

BUPROPION-INDUCED DISORDERS

Acute psychoses have been reported with patients treated with bupropion, a unicyclic aminoketone antidepressant (Golden RN et al, 1985).

History
1. The patient has a history of being treated with bupropion.
2. Symptom appearance appears to be dose related (Golden RN et al, 1985).
3. Mechanism of production of symptoms probably relates to aggravation of the dopaminergic systems. It is a weak inhibitor of dopamine uptake with little effect on serotonin, norepinephrine, or monoamine oxidase activity (Golden RN et al, 1985).
4. If a patient has a previous history of or currently has schizophrenia, mania, or schizoaffective disorder, an antidepressant therapy could induce exacerbation or precipitation of the illness.

Symptoms
1. Auditory and visual hallucinations.
2. Agitation.
3. Disorientation.

Differential Diagnosis
1. Bupropion-induced psychoses.
2. Other drug-induced psychoses.
3. Mania.
4. Schizophrenia.
5. Schizoaffective disorder.

Management
1. Symptoms remit gradually over 1 or 2 weeks with cessation of bupropion.

Quality Assurance Issues
1. Was the patient evaluated for history and symptoms of mania, schizoaffective disorder, and schizophrenia before bupropion was prescribed?

CAFFEINE INTOXICATION
(Caffeinism)

Acute or continuing anxiety may be due to intake of excessive amounts of coffee, tea, or cola drinks. Individuals unable to sleep because of emotional turmoil may drink cup after cup of coffee adding a physiological cause of anxiety to a psychological one.

History

1. There is a history of ingestion of large amounts of coffee and/or other caffeine-containing compounds such as tea, hot chocolate, cola drinks, and cocoa or caffeine-containing over-the- counter cold preparations, stimulants, and analgesics or prescription drugs.
2. Individual susceptibility to caffeine varies. Usually, 50–250 mg of caffeine is needed to produce the characteristic pharmacologic action of caffeine. One cup of brewed coffee contains about 100–150 mg of caffeine.
3. Many people consume enough caffeine daily to produce symptoms without realizing it. Tea contains about half the amount of caffeine of coffee, and cola contains about one third the amount. Instant coffee contains about 86–99 mg/cup of caffeine and APCs contain 32 mg/tablet of caffeine. The caffeine content of other commonly used medications are as follows:

Darvon Compound	32 mg/tablet
Excedrin	60 mg/tablet
Anacin	32 mg/tablet
Aspirin Compound	32 mg/tablet
Bromo Seltzer	32 mg/tablet

Over the counter stimulants and migraine medications contain about 100 mg/tablet.
4. Doses greater than 1000 mg/day can result in muscle twitchings, increased psychomotor activity, and cardiac arrhythmias. Higher doses result in ringing in the ears and doses in excess of 10 g of caffeine can result in grand mal seizures and death secondary to respiratory failure.
5. Children who are low consumers of caffeine, when given caffeine containing beverages, are more inattentive, emotional, and restless. Children who are high consumers of caffeine, when restricted from use, are more anxious and tend to have lower autonomic arousal. When given caffeine, high users show less apparent change (Rapoport JL et al, 1984).
6. Patients with anxiety disorders are particularly sensitive to the impact of caffeine (Lee et al, 1988; Boulenger et al, 1984). As little as one cup of coffee can exacerbate symptoms. Patients with major depression also show some sensitivity to the effects of caffeine but not to the same degree.
7. Patients failing to respond to the usual effective doses of psychopharmacologic agents or nighttime hypnotics should be suspected of caffeine intoxication. Absence of expected effects of antidepressant medication on sleep may relate to the fact that a depressed patient is drinking a considerable quantity of coffee at night.
8. Symptoms of caffeine intoxication may be superimposed upon symptoms of mania, depression, and anxiety disorder or schizophrenia. People in emotional turmoil naively may sit up and drink coffee because they are having difficulty sleeping.

9. Excessive amounts of caffeine endanger a patient's cardiac or gastrointestinal status. Extremely high doses of caffeine can cause hypertension, cardiac arrhythmias, and circulatory failure, and should therefore be avoided by patients with a history of recent myocardial infarction. Epigastric distress, nausea, vomiting, and diarrhea are usual concomitants of caffeinism. Rarely, large amounts of caffeine have been implicated in the production of hematemesis or peptic ulcer.

10. Moderate and high consumers of caffeine report significantly higher trait anxiety and depression, higher frequency of psychophysiological disorders and, when students, tend to have lower academic performance (Gilliland and Andress, 1981).

11. Many individuals with anorexia nervosa consume large quantities of caffeine-containing beverages such as coffee and cola drinks because of the small caloric content and the suppression of appetite while increasing energy (Sours, 1983).

Symptoms
1. Restlessness.
2. Frequent sleep interruption.
3. Delayed onset of sleep.
4. Palpitations.
5. Excitement.
6. Anxiety.
7. Flushing.
8. Diarrhea.
9. Irritability.
10. Epigastric pain.
11. Nausea.
12. Vomiting.
13. Rambling speech.
14. Periods of inexhaustability.
15. Visual flashes of light.
16. Ringing in the ears.
17. Diuresis.
18. Sensory disturbances.
19. Agitation.
20. Tremulousness.
21. Headaches.

Signs
1. Muscle twitching.
2. Cardiac arrhythmias.
3. Tachypnea.
4. Hyperesthesia.
5. Extrasystole.
6. Tachycardia.

Differential Diagnosis
1. Mania.
2. Hypomania.
3. Panic disorder.
4. Delirium.
5. Depression.
6. Generalized anxiety disorder.
7. Akathisia.
8. Schizophrenia.

Management
1. Patients should be encouraged to restrict caffeine intake. This may be difficult since many people are accustomed to having several cups of coffee a day and withdrawal symptoms appear as intake is cut down or ceased.
2. Benzodiazepines may be used if indicated by symptom intensity to treat the acute effects of a single episode of caffeine excess.
3. Symptoms of caffeine withdrawal include dysphoria, inability to work effectively, restlessness, headache, lethargy, irritability, and nervousness. These symptoms pass within 24 to 48 hours of cessation of caffeine intake.

CANCER CHEMOTHERAPY-INDUCED DISORDERS

Psychiatric clinicians are sought for emergency consultation regarding patients being treated for cancer. Behavioral alterations seen with patients who have cancer may be the result of a number of conditions, one of which may be a cancer chemotherapyinduced disorder.

History
1. Cancer chemotherapy is a major variable associated with cognitive impairment (Silberfarb et al, 1980a).
2. Specific chemotherapeutic agents have been identified as responsible for delirium.
3. Steroids are notorious for altering mood, thought, and behavior.
4. Age is felt to be a major factor in the development of cognitive changes with cancer chemotherapy (Silberfarb et al, 1980a).
5. Pseudohallucinations of tastes and odors have been observed in cancer chemotherapy patients. The pseudohallucinations are associated with pretreatment nausea and extensive chemotherapy (Nesse et al, 1983). Pretreatment nausea is felt to be an example of the Garcia effect (Wesse et al, 1980), which is explained as a classical conditioned response learned by repeated episodes of medication-induced nausea and vomiting and the clinic odor. Because the pseudohallucinations are seen only in patients who exhibit pretreatment nausea, they are considered a conditioned perception or a vivid intrusive memory.

6. Greater depression may be seen in patients treated with the vinca alkaloid vincristine because of vincristine's reported ability to block the transport of dopamine beta-hydroxylase, the terminal enzyme converting dopamine to norepinephrine (Silberfarb et al, 1983).
7. Delirium is estimated to occur in 10 to 40% of terminally ill cancer patients (Massie et al, 1983). Successful cessation entails ascertaining how different mechanisms may be acting synergistically to cause the alteration in cognition functioning.
8. Cancer patients as a group show less dysphoria, depression, impairment of social functioning, and disturbance of affect and cognitive functions than patients without cancer who have a history of depression or suicide attempts. Cancer patients most likely to suffer depression are those with a previous history of affective illness (Plumb and Holland, 1981).
9. Agoraphobia and panic attacks have been reported as a sequela to termination of treatment in patients who have been deemed cured of the cancer (Viswanathan and Kachur, 1986). The mechanism of panic is considered to be both separation anxiety and emergence of aggressive impulses.
10. Cancer may present as treatment-resistant depression prior to diagnosis of the neoplastic process. The mechanism of the affective disorder is felt to be due to immunological interference (Takrani, 1986).
11. Psychiatric patients have been reported to induce electrolyte abnormalities through compulsive water drinking. The syndrome of inappropriate antidiuretic hormone also can present as a result of pulmonary carcinoma with hyponatremic psychosis and water intoxication (Grant and Lindsay, 1986).
12. The diagnosis of major depression in cancer patients using diagnostic tools such as the Hamilton Rating Scale for Depression and the Beck Depression Inventory varies with the diagnostic tool, with patients without major depression by criteria-based diagnostic systems being frequently misclassified (Kathol et al, 1990).
13. Patients with paraneoplastic encephalopathy presenting as dementia may be misdiagnosed as having Alzheimer's disease or multi-infarct dementia and referred to a psychiatric facility (Van Sweden and Peteghem, 1986). The bases of the dementia are endocrine/metabolic disorders or nutritional dysfunction related to the cancer or metastatic carcinomatosis deposits.
14. Patients with pancreatic cancer report significantly more psychiatric symptoms than patients with other cancer. Pancreatic cancer patients have comparatively more fatigue, mood disturbance, tension, depression, anxiety, and confusion (Holland JC et al, 1986).

Symptoms and Signs

Symptoms of all major psychiatric disorders may be reported as a manifestation of cancer and its treatment.

Differential Diagnosis

1. Cancer chemotherapy-induced disorders.

2. Primary neoplasm of the brain.
3. Remote effects of cancer.
4. Behavioral changes induced by a secretion of the tumor.
5. Adjustment disorder due to cancer.
6. Mechanical changes due to a tumor's presence impairing the function of other organs.
7. Infections secondary to immunosuppression being given as part of cancer treatment.
8. Other psychiatric disorders.
9. Other medical disorders.

Clinical Studies
1. CBC and differential.
2. SMA-22.
3. X-rays and other radiographic studies of areas of suspected tumor infiltration.
4. CT scans of suspected areas of tumor invasions.
5. Electroencephalography.
6. MRI.

Management
1. Antidepressant medication should be prescribed as indicated when the basis of the depression does not appear to be a correctable medical disorder (Goldberg and Cullen, 1986).
2. Benzodiazepines should be prescribed as needed for patients with anxiety or sleep problems, but must be given cautiously to patients who suffer respiratory impairment.
3. Agitated delirium can be managed with low-dosage, high-potency neuroleptics (e.g., haloperidol), lorazepam, or both conjunctively (Adams et al, 1896).
4. In many instances of chemotherapy-induced disorders, a combination of factors are responsible for the behavioral changes seen. As indicated earlier in this section, the role of each one of these must be elevated and treated to allow as optimal functioning as possible.

CANCER AND DEMENTIA

The prevalence of organic mental disorders among patients with cancer is estimated to be between 9 and 40% (Davis BD et al, 1987). Many of these are indistinguishable from primary dementias such as Alzheimer's disease and multi-infarct dementia.

History
1. Patients who have been diagnosed to have cancer and appear with the symptoms of dementia should be suspected of dementia due to metabolic or other cancer-related causes of dementia.

2. Approximately 20% of patients evaluated for dementia have potentially reversible causes (Davis BD et al, 1990). What appears to be dementia in a patient with cancer may be due to a reversible cause such as a chemotherapy-induced mental disorders or electrolyte imbalance rather than an irreversible cerebral disorder, a primary cerebral neoplasm, or meningeal carcinomatosis.

Symptoms
1. Sensory impairment.
2. Disorientation.
3. Dyscalculia.

Signs
1. Spacial disorientation.
2. Motor impairment.
3. Sensory impairment.

Differential Diagnosis
1. The differential diagnosis includes all the causes of dementia.

Clinical Studies
1. Neuropsychological testing.
2. SMA-22.
3. CBC and differential.
4. EEG.
5. MRI.
6. CT scan.

Management
1. Potentially reversible causes of dementia should be sought, and diagnostic specific treatment provided.
2. Dementiform symptoms associated with reversible causes of cognitive impairment may be mollified but not reversed by neuroleptics and antidepressants. High-potency, low-dosage neuroleptics may reduce agitation without further confusion and antidepressants may reduce depression enhancing cognitive ability.

CANCER OF THE BREAST

Individuals with cancer of the breast may seek emergency psychiatric help for help in adaptation to the diagnosis of life-threatening illness and to the course of therapy that is selected (e.g., mutilative breast surgery, chemotherapy, radiation).

History
1. Breast cancer, the most common malignancy in women, occurs in 1 out of every 13 women. About 90,000 new cases are diagnosed yearly.

2. The usual response to the diagnosis of breast cancer in a woman is weeks to years of depression, thoughts of suicide, decreased sense of femininity, and lowered self-esteem. Anxiety over the mastectomy and loss of breast may be greater than the fear of cancer (Jamison et al, 1978).

3. Psychological disturbances pursuant to mastectomy are said to be less frequent among postclimacteric women, but some studies have indicated otherwise. In one study (Goin and Goin, 1981), outward response of the postclimacteric group was found to be different but inwardly traumatic with feelings of depression, loss, and shame over sexual feelings that they felt inappropriate to their age. A need of some women to pretend that the mastectomy was relatively unimportant compounded difficulty in coping with other anxieties appropriate to their age. Reconstructive surgery decreased mastectomized patients' sense of dependence and mutilation.

4. The most emotionally disturbing time for a patient with breast cancer is the first recurrence, and the most common disturbance (regardless whether the cancer is primary or a recurrence) is in mate role performance (Silberfarb et al, 1980b).

CANNABIS INTOXICATION AND DELUSIONAL DISORDER

Cannabis, usually referred to as marijuana, is more frequently used than alcohol in some circles.

History
1. Cannabis and related derivatives of the cannabis plant (hashish and delta-9-tetrahydrocannabinol [THC]) may be smoked (e.g., "reefers" or "joints") or taken orally with a number of substances including food (e.g., "Alice B. Toklas brownies," "space cakes").

2. It is variously known as pot, MJ, Mary Jane, grass, bhang, dope, and the weed.

3. Use ranges from brief experimental trials to chronic daily use.

4. Individuals' reaction to cannabis varies and relates to:

   a. Set (expectations as to what is to happen or has in the past);
   b. Setting (e.g., a response in a laboratory setting may be strikingly different from that in a room with incense, strobe light, and rap music);
   c. Personality (e.g., obsessive–compulsive people would be expected to respond differently than hysterics); and
   d. Dose (hashish is generally quite potent, but some "grass" is just that, with no tetrahydrocannabinol).

5. Most marijuana smokers, like alcohol users, have mild to moderate reactions and do not seek medical assistance.

6. Intoxication occurs nearly immediately after smoking cannabis and peaks in about $\frac{1}{2}$ hour. Nearly all symptoms disappear after 3 hours. Absorption of cannabis taken orally is slower with a lower peak level, but a more prolonged effect. Symptoms should be entirely gone 6 hours after ingestion.

7. The individual may have the characteristic sweet smell of cannabis on his clothing.
8. College student drug use has remarkably fallen over the past 20 years (Pope et al, 1990).
9. College student drug users are reported to differ from nondrug-using students in reporting more frequent visits to psychological counseling services and more sexual activity but do not differ in athletic and other college activities, grades, or feelings of alienation (Pope et al, 1990).
10. Marijuana, like cocaine, can increase both heart rate and arterial blood pressure. When they are used together, increases in blood pressure and heart rate are greater than that of either taken alone (Foltin et al, 1987).
11. Marijuana and other psychoactive drug use should be considered in the differential diagnosis of conditions contributing to insomnia, loss of energy, problem behavior, poor appetite, decreased drive and motivation, and academic underachievement (MacDonald and Czechowicz, 1986).
12. Chronic marijuana users can become severely dependent, necessitating medical intervention to assure successful withdrawal (Tennant, 1986). The greater the potency of the tetrahydrocannabinol taken, the greater the likelihood of withdrawal symptoms on cessation of use. Withdrawal symptoms include sweating, chills, increased appetite, disturbed sleep, hiccups, loose stools, irritability, restlessness, nausea, feverish feeling, muscle spasms, tremulousness, stuffy nose, and wild dreams (Mendelson JH et al, 1984). Withdrawal symptoms have been reported to occur with as little as 21 days of marijuana use with onset 10 hours after cessation of use and a duration of symptoms of 96 hours (Mendelson JH et al, 1984).
13. Marijuana intoxication can mimic a number of different psychiatric disorders indicating need for a high index of suspicion whenever psychiatric symptoms appear in groups at risk (Estroff and Gold, 1986a).
14. Impairment of coordination may lead to automobile, airplane, and motorcycle accidents, and to industrial accidents.
15. The task in an emergency evaluation is to ascertain from history:

    a. Whether or not the premorbid personality of the patient was stable and whether the symptoms can be presumed to be a toxic reaction of the drug.
    b. Whether the patient was having a psychotic decompensation and took the drug in an attempt to self-medicate or help organize the internal chaos, or to be part of a group that would accept him or her despite bizarre behavior.
    c. Whether the patient was basically unstable with a family history or psychiatric difficulty and marijuana was the sufficient stimulus to put him or her over the edge.

16. Depersonalization, a common experience during acute intoxication with marijuana use, may be prolonged in instances where external stressors and intrapsychic factors contribute to its continued use as a defense mechanism (Szymanski, 1981).

Symptoms

1. Sensation of slowed time and apathy.
2. Heightened sensory awareness.
3. Changes in thought, incoherence, and impaired associations.
4. Self-confidence.
5. Depersonalization and derealization.
6. Disinhibition.
7. Impairment of immediate memory.
8. Laughter, silliness, and light heartedness.
9. Sensation of floating.
10. Disorientation.
11. Altered reality testing.
12. Suggestibility.
13. Decreased attention and concentration span.
14. Elation, euphoria, and marked relaxation.
15. Rapid or impaired speech.
16. Feelings of detachment.
17. Fear of dying.
18. Delusions of persecution and paranoia.
19. Paresthesias.
20. Illusions.
21. Changed sense of self-identity and body image.
22. Anxiety and panic attacks.
23. Nausea.
24. Sleepiness.
25. Depression.
26. Suspiciousness and ideas of reference.
27. Emotional lability.
28. Auditory and visual hallucinations.
29. Dreamy state.
30. Feeling of a heavy or pressured head.
31. Feeling more insightful.
32. Changed sexual feeling.
33. Increased appetite and thirst.
34. Precordial distress.
35. Feeling that one is going crazy.
36. Impaired judgement.
37. Diarrhea.
38. Light headedness.
39. Confusion.

Signs

1. Tremor.
2. Tachycardia.

3. Dry mouth.
4. Increased sensitivity to touch and pain.
5. Nystagmus.
6. Profuse sweating.
7. Restlessness.
8. Conjunctival injection.
9. Ataxia.
10. Urinary frequency.
11. Interference with social or occupational functioning.

Differential Diagnosis
1. Cannabis intoxication or delusional disorder.
2. Schizophrenia.
3. Adolescent adjustment disorder.
4. Depressive disorder of psychotic or nonpsychotic proportions.
5. Bipolar disorder.
6. Panic disorder.
7. Generalized anxiety disorder.
8. Alcohol intoxication or delusional disorder.
9. Hallucinogenic intoxication or delusional disorder.

Clinical Studies
1. Urine screen.
2. Blood screen.

As polydrug use is common (Verebey et al, 1986), blood and urine screens help identify other substances that may be contributing to and complicating the clinical presentation.

Management
1. Assess the suicidal and homicidal potential of the patient and whether there is any psychiatric condition other than cannabis intoxication. If other major psychopathology is identified, diagnostic-specific treatment is initiated.
2. If the behavioral, mood, and thought changes are felt primarily due to marijuana, an attempt is made to "talk down" the patient in a supportive safe atmosphere with minimal distraction. It should be explained to the patient that what he or she is experiencing is attributed to the drug and that he or she will get better.
3. Medication may be needed for anxiety or psychotic symptoms. Effective antianxiety agents include chlordiazepoxide (Librium) 10–15 mg, diazepam (Valium) 5–20 mg orally or intramuscularly, alprazolam (Xanax) 2–4 mg, and lorazepam (Ativan) 2–8 mg. For psychotic symptoms, haloperidol (Haldol), thiothixene (Navane) 5–10 mg, or chlorpromazine (Thorazine) 25–50 mg PO or IM is used, as well as a number of other antipsychotic agents.
4. The patient should be scheduled for a return appointment in 1 week to ascertain if all symptoms have subsided. Flashbacks occur with marijuana as with other

psychotomimetic agents and are treated with the usual antianxiety and antipsychotic drugs. If re-evaluation suggests original symptoms were due to another condition or that another condition is present, it is treated accordingly.

5. Cannabis may be contaminated with other drugs such as phencyclidine. In such instances, it is necessary to treat the patient for mixed drug intoxication and to be alert to the complications due to contaminants. Drug and urine screens usually confirm the presence of polysubstance abuse.

CAPGRAS SYNDROME

Capgras syndrome (Illusion des Sosies) is a condition in which an individual is unable to identify others well-known to him or her.

1. There is a systematized delusion of misidentifying a person or persons, objects, or animals.
2. Capgras syndrome is not a disorder itself. It occurs in psychiatric disorders as well as in medical conditions (Ananth et al, 1990; Berson, 1983; Signer, 1987) and therefore an organic etiology must always be considered and ruled out.
3. The majority of cases described have been women.
4. Capgras syndrome is not a specific symptom but rather a symptom common to many psychogenic and medical conditions.
5. Organic etiologies reported include myxedema (Madakasira and Hall, 1981), pseudohypoparathyroidism (Hay et al, 1974), organic brain disease (Christodoulou, 1977), and metrizamide myelography (Fishbain and Rosomoff, 1986). Metrizamide is a nonionic water soluble contrast medium used in ventriculography, myelography, cisternography, and cerebrospinal fluid imaging.
6. Capgras syndrome has been reported to occur simultaneously with folie a deux (Ananth et al, 1990).
7. In one series of 212 patients with the disorder (Signer, 1987), 46% were found to have affective disorders.

Symptoms
1. Delusions that someone close to the patient is an imposter or double who looks and acts just like the real person.

Differential Diagnosis
1. The differential diagnosis includes all the psychiatric and medical conditions in which delusions may appear.

Management
1. Management entails the diagnostic-specific treatment of the disorder presenting with Capgras syndrome and any concurrent psychiatric (e.g., folie a deux) or medical conditions that may be contributing.

CARBAMAZEPINE-INDUCED DISORDERS

Carbamazepine (Tegretol) is an iminodibenzyl derivative that is used in the treatment of temporal lobe epilepsy, trigeminal neuralgia and other pain syndromes, diabetes insipidus, dystonic disorders, and episodic mood disorders.

1. Carbamazepine has been used successfully in the treatment of intractable bipolar disorder (Ballenger and Post, 1980).
2. It has been suggested for use in prophylaxis as well as in acute episodes of both phases of manic–depressive illness, as an alternate to valproic acid, in people who do not respond to lithium.
3. Patients with acute mania who respond poorly to carbamazepine or lithium alone may respond well to the combination of drugs (Lipinski and Pope, 1982).
4. Carbamazepine is reported to be especially efficacious in individuals with affective syndromes who also have CNS disorders (Falks et al, 1982).
5. Bipolar disorder has been shown to respond to carbamazepine at doses of 600–1600 mg/day (Warren and Steinbook, 1983). Dose is dependent on serum level achieved.
6. The hematologic changes seen with carbamazepine may be irreversible (Warren and Steinbook, 1983).
7. Concomitant use of carbamazepine and haloperidol (Haldol) can result, in 2 to 3 weeks, in a reduction of plasma haloperidol levels as great as 60% (Jann et al, 1985).
8. Lithium appears to prevent the carbamazepine-induced hyponatremia despite lithium's tendency to increase polyuria (Vieweg et al, 1987).

Symptoms
1. Dizziness.
2. Nausea.

Signs
1. Ataxia.
2. Aplastic anemia.
3. Leukopenia.
4. Reticulocytosis.

Clinical Studies
1. CBC and differential.
2. SMA-22.
3. Serum carbamazepine level.

Management
1. Immediately upon discovery of a significant leukopenia or anemia, carbamazepine is discontinued and a hematologist sought to direct treatment of aplastic anemia

2. The nausea, dizziness, and ataxia reported with carbamazepine use decrease as serum levels drop upon cessation of use of the drug.
3. If CBCs and differentials are carefully monitored, prompt cessation of carbamazepine usually results in remission of leukopenia.

Quality Assurance Issues
1. Are regular CBCs and differentials being performed on patients receiving carbamazepine?

CARDIAC-INDUCED DISORDERS

Patients with angina, congestive heart failure and cardiac myopathies, and those who have suffered a myocardial infarction or are scheduled for cardiac surgery can present with psychiatric disorders attendant to a disorder impacting on an organ as critical to life as the heart or as a result of the physiologic changes that occur with cardiac disease.

History
1. Patients who have suffered a heart attack may go into congestive heart failure with the presenting symptoms of anxiety and increased difficulty in breathing. If the myocardial infarction was silent, a patient may be misdiagnosed as a panic disorder or generalized anxiety disorder and diagnostic-specific treatment may be delayed.
2. Personality factors, psychogenetic and biogenetic endowment, previous experience with illness, social support, and type and stage of procedure all impact on individual adjustment to cardiac transplantation, coronary angioplasty, and bypass surgery (Kuhn et al, 1988).

Symptoms and Signs
1. The symptoms and signs of cardiac illness and of adjustment to cardiac procedures depend on individual defenses, genetic endowment, social support, previous experience with illness, concomitant psychiatric and medical disorders, medications used, and the nature of the procedure or cardiac disorder.

Management
1. Alprazolam (Xanax) and lorazepam (Ativan) are used for the anxiety attendant with cardiac disorders and procedures.
2. Electroshock is often safer in the treatment of depression in patients with cardiac problems than antidepressants. Catecholamine release under stress can result in death from ventricular fibrillation. The risk of fibrillation is increased by anything that increases the electrical instability of the myocardium (Jefferson, 1985).
3. Although doses as low as 1–2 mg of intravenous haloperidol (Haldol) every 2 to 4 hours have been advocated for management of severe confusion and agitation

of patients on coronary care units, doses as high as 100 mg have been reported as safe for use (Tesar et al, 1985).

4. Patients who are candidates for coronary transplantation or bypass surgery should not be pressured into premature acceptance of a procedure (Kuhn et al, 1988).

5. Social support and ability to ventilate is critical to reduction of the stress attendant to severe cardiac disease and acceptance of cardiac surgery.

6. Contact with other individuals who have suffered severe cardiac illness or who have undergone cardiac surgery reduces stress. Contact may be with individuals or in a self-help support group. Nothing helps one to understand as much as to be understood.

Quality Assurance Issues

1. Was consultation with a cardiologist sought before antidepressant medication was prescribed to a patient with cardiac disease?

CATATONIC SCHIZOPHRENIA

The critical feature of catatonic schizophrenia is a marked psychomotor disturbance coupled with other features of schizophrenia. The disturbance in motor activity may take the form of rigidity, stupor, and posturing or excitement. In some instances, stupor may alternate with excitement.

History

1. Catatonic schizophrenia, like schizoaffective disorder, has a relatively good prognosis. This is especially true if the onset is acute, if there exists a clear precipitating factor, and if the patient has functioned well socially and at work prior to the onset.

2. The usual age of onset is between 15 and 25 years of age.

3. Catatonic schizophrenia is now relatively uncommon.

4. If a patient has had several catatonic episodes, either of excitement or stupor, the course of the illness may take on the characteristics of other forms of schizophrenia with a more permanent alteration in psychosocial functioning. Sometimes one sees a spontaneous remission without any treatment. Remission, in fact, may occur overnight.

5. Before the introduction of electroshock therapy and widespread use of neuroleptics, catatonic stupor often lasted as long as several months. Without psychiatric intervention, catatonic excitement can result in death.

Signs

1. Waxy flexibility (flexibilitas cerea): This term refers to the tendency of mute catatonic schizophrenics to allow their bodies to be molded into position, sometimes positions that are extremely uncomfortable. It is important to remember that such patients retain awareness during this state despite their ostensible

"coma." Later they may recount all that was said by examining medical and psychiatric staff.

2. Catatonic excitement: Catatonic excitement occurs with or without alternating episodes of stuporous behavior. Excited behavior in catatonic schizophrenics is differentiated from mania in bipolar disorder by its more bizarre and regressed character. Self-destructive and assaultive behavior may be part of the clinical picture.

3. Stupor: Very difficult to distinguish from coma in the absence of a psychiatric history, catatonic stupor is characterized by the nearly total absence of any movement. Saliva may flow from the patient's mouth. They are often incontinent and unresponsive to most stimuli. It may be necessary in extreme cases to feed, dress, and take over the toilet and bathing care of such patients.

4. Mutism: Loss of speech may occur for days or months in catatonic schizophrenia. In some cases the mutism may be episodic. Some of these patients will respond only monosyllabically.

5. Characteristic schizophrenic thinking may also be observed especially in patients who have had several episodes or who have family histories of schizophrenia.

6. Stereotypes.

7. Negativism.

8. Mannerisms.

9. Staring into space.

10. Posturing.

11. Rigidity.

Differential Diagnosis

Physical examination serves to help rule out organic causes for the stupor or excited behavior. The differential diagnosis is that of other forms of schizophrenia. In particular, catatonic stupor may be confused with the numerous other causes of coma, all of which could occur in addition to schizophrenia. Catatonic excitement resembles toxic states. Both stupor and excitement can be part of an hysterical psychosis. Catatonic-like symptoms have been reported as a side effect of high-potency neuroleptics (Brenner and Rheubon, 1978). In this latter instance, cessation of the neuroleptic medication and use of amantadine alleviated the symptoms. Periodic catatonia, thought to be due to a rapid switch from a predominantly cholinergic state to an adrenergic state, is discussed elsewhere in this book. Neuroleptics can induce catatonia resembling psychogenic catatonia, which may lead to the neuroleptic malignant syndrome. Psychogenic catatonia can lead to lethal catatonia.

Clinical Studies

1. Chest film.
2. Skull film.
3. CT scan.
4. MRI.
5. CBC and differential.
6. SMA-22.

7. Blood alcohol level.
8. EKG.
9. Toxicology screen.

Management

1. Catatonic schizophrenics need careful supervision because of the risk of exhaustion, starvation, and self- or other-injury.
2. The treatment approach is identical to that for management of acute psychosis, with emphasis on differential diagnosis and diagnostic-specific treatment. In an emergency situation, treatment interventions such as electroshock, tube feeding, and personal care are not immediately relevant. In addition to appropriate doses of antipsychotic medication, these are part of a long-term treatment program. Some catatonic patients, both excited and mute, respond quite rapidly to intramuscular neuroleptics. If excited, chlorpromazine (Thorazine) 50 mg every $\frac{1}{2}$ to 1 hour may be required, but blood pressure and pulse rate should be carefully monitored. Alternatively 5–10 mg of haloperidol (Haldol) can be given at hourly intervals. Even though the risk of hypotension is significantly lower, blood pressure and pulse should still be monitored. Response to treatment is sometimes dramatic.
3. Catatonic patients are at risk for medical problems associated with stasis such as deep venous thrombosis, pulmonary emboli, aspiration, and pneumonia. Patients should be monitored for any changes suggestive of medical problems that may result from immobilization. Inadequate food and water intake leads to urinary retention, dehydration, and inanition.
4. Lithium combined with a neuroleptic has been used for patients with neuroleptic-resistant catatonic stupor (Climo, 1985). Some individuals with catatonia feel both the range of symptoms (i.e., mutism to excitement) and the periodicity (ie., rapid change from excitement to immobility and vice versa), suggesting either a relationship to affective illness or a "forme fruste" of it.
5. Catatonia accompanying a pituitary adenoma has been found to respond to oral diazepam (Valium). The adenoma itself requires endocrinological intervention (Sheline and Miller, 1986).
6. Carbamazepine (Tegretol) has been reported effective within 6 to 24 hours following use for catatonia occurring both with a schizophreniform disorder as well as with schizoaffective disorder (Rankel and Rankel, 1988).
7. Lorazepam (Ativan), a benzodiazepine with a half-life of 10 to 20 hours that is used in the management of acute psychoses and delirium, is also useful in successful resolution of psychogenic catatonia without concern for appearance of acute dystonic reactions (Salam et al, 1987). Lorazepam is a facilitator of the gamma-aminobutyric acid system and believed to act in the cerebral cortex and in the limbic system.
8. Diazepam, like lorazepam, has proven effective in bringing about remission of life-threatening catatonia. Like lorazepam, it can be given intramuscularly in the acute state, and orally thereafter to maintain remission (McEvoy and Lohr,

1984). The absorption of diazepam intramuscularly is less predictable than lorazepam.

9. Careful medical and neurologic examination must be performed to rule out causes of catatonia that are not psychogenic in origin (Mann SC et al, 1986).

10. Lethal catatonia is characterized by mounting fever, extreme hyperactivity, and progression to stuporous exhaustion. Patients must be carefully monitored for early identification of symptoms to obviate loss of life.

11. Careful nursing care is required to maintain caloric and food intake during the acute stage.

Quality Assurance Issues

1. Were medical and neurologic causes of catatonia sought and diagnostic-specific treatment provided?

2. Was care for caloric and water intake provided in the acute phase?

3. Were signs of lethal catatonia monitored?

CEREBROVASCULAR ACCIDENTS

Individuals with cerebrovascular accidents may appear in emergency psychiatric settings both as "forme frustes" of other psychiatric illnesses such as schizophrenia, conversion reactions, or bipolar disorder as well as because individuals with strokes respond to their illness in ways that their family and friends find difficult to manage without professional help. The differential diagnosis of catatonia, for example, includes bilateral infarctions of the parietal lobe as well as other focal lesions of the cerebral hemispheres such as hematomas or meningiomas (Tippin and Dunner, 1981; Woods SW, 1980).

1. Cerebrovascular accidents (CVAs, shocks, and strokes) kill an estimated 275,000 people per year in the United States and disable another 300,000. Approximately one-half of those admitted to hospitals died within the first 3 weeks. Of those who survive, approximately 70% are vocationally impaired and one-third are completely dependent on various support systems. In one follow-up study, one-third had a second stroke and nearly one-half died within 3 years (Lishman, 1978).

2. For individuals so affected, cerebrovascular accidents raise concern over the loss of physical function, disfigurement, loss of control, insanity, death, and sexual dysfunction.

3. Stroke victims and their families and friends are concerned about explosive recurrence, prolonged treatment away from home, exhaustion of retirement funds, and disorganized thoughts and emotion.

4. Mania has been described as a sequela to infarction in several parts of the brain (Wilson and McLaughlin, 1990). Causes of secondary mania include lesions in all areas involved with modulation of emotion and neurovegetative functioning including the thalamus, basal ganglia, and limbic parts of the temporal and frontal lobes.

5. Eastwood et al (1989) found depression as a sequela in 50% of a series of stroke victims with the best predictor of mood disturbance being a history of a previous stroke or previous psychiatric disorder. Left-frontal and right-hemispheric lesions have both been associated with depression.
6. In another study of 976 patients (Wade et al, 1987), 25 to 30% were found to be depressed at 3 weeks, 6 months, and 13 months, with over 60% of those depressed at 3 weeks still depressed after 1 year.
7. Impairment does not appear to produce depression, but once depression occurs, the presence of a depression interacts with impairment to impede recovery (Robinson RG et al, 1986).

Symptoms and Signs
1. Virtually all psychiatric signs and symptoms may appear as sequelae to a stroke. When they occur they are referred to as "secondary" (e.g., secondary mania).

Differential Diagnosis
1. All the disorders included in the specific differential diagnoses of a psychiatric disorder are included in the differential diagnosis when the symptom occurs with stroke (e.g., the differential diagnosis of mania).

Management
1. Management is eclectic, tailored to unique patient and family needs (Goodstein, 1983).
2. Treatment of the various psychiatric disorders accompanying a stroke (or those that are reactions to the stroke) is the same as for the psychiatric disorder occurring alone, with the exception that any individual with brain damage is more sensitive to medication.
3. Patients with recurrent mania and depression, especially if rapid cycling, may be more responsive to mood stabilizers with anticonvulsant properties such as valproic acid, carbamazepine (Tegretol), and clonazepam than they would be to lithium.
4. Nortriptyline has been recommended for stroke associated with left frontal lesions (Eastwood et al, 1989).

Quality Assurance Issues
1. Was a stroke patient evaluated for the development of a secondary psychiatric disorder?
2. If a secondary psychiatric disorder was present (e.g., secondary depression), was diagnostic-specific treatment provided?

CHILD PSYCHIATRIC DISORDERS

Children who present in the emergency room are usually accompanied by parents. Exceptions would be children found following a suicide or homicide attempt or physical assault, sexually abused children, run-aways, children who are acutely psychotic or have substance abuse disorders, and those brought in by the police for legal infractions. The management of these problems are discussed in sections of this book under the various topics, but some general points regarding child emergencies, which distinguish them from adult emergencies, will be made.

History

1. Children may attempt suicide in ways not as overtly recognizable as those by adults. They may walk in front of cars or trains, jump off buildings, or jump into reservoirs or lakes. In all these instances, it may appear they had an "accident" and, therefore, psychiatric assessment to ascertain if a child is suicidal is not sought.
2. Children are the most sensitive barometer of what transpires in their parents' marriage. A child may present, but the genesis of the problem may be marital conflict or a clandestine affair of one or both of the parents. The child unconsciously detects a change in the affectional bonding of the parents and becomes symptomatic. In these instances, couples therapy may be required to treat the child's problem.
3. Sexual and physical abuse should always be suspected even in affluent families. A child in fear of rejection or retaliation, or acting out of guilt for assumed compliance, may deny the abuse despite evidence of physical harm or symptoms suggesting incest, rape, or other sexual abuse. In some instances, the abuse may be totally repressed and out of conscious awareness.
4. Children may suffer depression requiring antidepressants. Failure to treat the depression aggressively in childhood can lead to an enduring dysphoria, that is, low self-esteem and learned helplessness that becomes an integral part of the developing personality leading to a depressed adult. When another episode of major depression occurs in adult life, it becomes superimposed on that of a depressive personality resulting in "double depression." Antidepressants in adult life may successfully treat the major depressive episode but fail to cause remission in the enduring depression that resulted from an untreated major depressive episode occurring during the child's development of his or her sense of identity.
5. Drug doses for a child differ from those for an adult and are usually based on weight.
6. Children may respond differently to a drug than an adult. For instance, methylphenidate (Ritalin) may calm a hyperactive child but, after puberty, agitate an adult.
7. All illnesses are family problems. Wherever possible, clinicians should work with family members either therapeutically or in psychoeducation to help them better understand the etiology and management of a disorder such as the attention deficit hyperactivity disorder.
8. Childhood presentations of psychiatric disorder sometimes differ from those of adults. While some children may show the decreased appetite and sleep disturbance attendant with major depression, others may evince depression by withdrawal, impulsive acting out, stealing, substance abuse, and poor school performance.

9. While death from natural causes is not increased in children who have been psychiatrically hospitalized, mortality from unnatural causes (e.g., suicide) has been found to be more than twice as high as expected based on age- and sex-matched comparisons with general population statistics (Kuperman et al, 1988).

10. Children, like adults, use denial as a major means of coping with disaster (Benedek, 1985) making both assessment and management of post-traumatic stress disorder difficult in the acute situation. Children may present with symptoms years later as a sequela to major trauma in childhood, adolescence, or adulthood. In some cases the symptoms will be physical, not psychiatric. The organs weep when the eyes cannot, as the French say. The heart has ways the mind does not know.

11. A knowledge of the psychiatric history of the parents provides clues to diagnosis and management of the child's problem. For example, the vast majority of mothers of children with over-anxious behavior or separation anxiety report a history of anxiety disorder themselves (Last et al, 1987a). If, in another family member, a specific pharmacological intervention has been successful or a medication has caused problems, a clinician may anticipate the same success or problems in the child.

12. CT scans of children with Tourette's disorder, attention deficit hyperactivity disorder, and childhood infantile autism have not been found to distinguish those affected from a control group of medical patients (Harcherik et al, 1985).

Quality Assurance Issues
1. Was the child evaluated for evidence of sexual or physical abuse?
2. Were children who presented in the emergency room following being hit by a car or train or having fallen into a body of water evaluated for depression?
3. Were children who presented with histories suggestive of a biologic depression provided with antidepressants?

CHRONIC FATIGUE SYNDROME

Patients with the chronic fatigue syndrome often have psychiatric illness, which may in some cases cause them to seek psychiatric help.

History
1. Psychiatric illness more often precedes the chronic fatigue syndrome than follows it (Kruesi et al, 1989).

Symptoms
1. Anergy.
2. Malaise.
3. Debilitating fatigue.
4. Headache.
5. Dysphoria.

6. Depression.
7. Allergies.
8. Dysattention.
9. Musculoskeletal pain.
10. Recurrent sore throat.

Signs
1. Low-grade fever.
2. Tender lymph nodes.

Differential Diagnosis
1. Major depression.
2. Dysthymic disorder.
3. Chronic Epstein–Barr viral infection.
4. Chronic mononucleosis.
5. Hepatitis.
6. Lyme disease.
7. AIDS.
8. Occult neoplasm.
9. Other organic and psychiatric disorders.

Management
1. Evaluation of the patient for all the medical and psychiatric causes of the chronic fatigue syndrome precedes diagnostic-specific treatment of the disorder by the appropriate specialist.
2. Even when it is clear that depression exists, a concurrent physical illness should be sought which may be concurrent with the psychiatric disorder.

CHRONIC OBSTRUCTIVE PULMONARY DISEASE

It is not unusual for psychiatric illness to be comorbid with chronic obstructive pulmonary disease (COPD).

History
1. Depression may occur with COPD independent of the COPD, as a response to it, or as a side effect of medication used to treat it.
2. Panic disorder and other anxiety disorders are particularly prevalent in patients with COPD (Karajgi et al, 1990).

Management
1. Lorazepam (Ativan) is rarely used in the management of patients with COPD because of the danger of respiratory depression.

CHRONIC ALCOHOLISM

Long-term side-effects of chronic alcohol abuse include Korsakov's psychosis, Wernicke's encephalopathy, delirium tremens, alcoholic hallucinosis, alcoholic jealousy, cerebellar degeneration, dementia, and peripheral neuropathies.

History

1. It is extremely difficult to obtain an accurate history of the exact amount of alcohol consumed by alcoholics, but it is generally underestimated by the patient. The patient's diet is also poor.
2. Alcoholics are prone to develop severe medical and surgical problems. Falls while intoxicated or head injuries incurred in muggings or during a seizure may result in a subdural hematoma. Alcoholics are prone to infections such as pneumonia and tuberculosis. Pancreatitis is common and gastrointestinal bleeding frequent.
3. When evaluating a patient who chronically uses alcohol, the clinician should carefully look for evidence of another disorder that the patient may be self-medicating, such as schizophrenia, an affective disorder, or panic disorder. When alcohol use or other substance abuse is comorbid with a psychiatric disorder, the patient is said to have a "dual diagnosis."
4. Examination of patients' relationships to their families may reveal much stress with markedly ambivalent feelings towards several family members. In some cases, the patient is not the only family member drinking.
5. Drinking may cause a patient to neglect chronic health problems, as well as contribute to the development of new ones. Family members should be used to help assure that the patient receives a thorough medical evaluation, including a proper physical examination, laboratory studies, and a chest x-ray.
6. Even if a patient's family history is riddled with alcoholism—suggesting a strong genetic predisposition—a careful longitudinal history should be obtained to see what factors increase or decrease the intake of alcohol.
7. It is common for alcoholism to be comorbid with other substance abuse. For instance, a patient may use alcohol to modulate cocaine or amphetamine highs. Urine and serum drug screens are performed to identify the presence of other drugs.

Symptoms and Signs

The symptoms and signs of chronic alcohol abuse are those of the various psychiatric and medical syndromes that occur in these patients.

Differential Diagnosis

Alcohol may be taken to self-medicate a number of conditions. These should be sought out and treated to improve the prognosis. Common disorders, of which alcoholism may be a symptom, include:

1. Schizophrenia.
2. Borderline personality disorder.
3. Bipolar disorder.
4. Dysthymia disorder.
5. Major depression.
6. Multi-infarct dementia.
7. AIDS.
8. Alzheimer's disease.
9. Panic disorder and other anxiety disorders.
10. Attention deficit hyperactivity disorder.
11. Other medical and psychiatric disorders.

Management

1. Acute medical problems, including delirium tremens, must be treated prior to diagnostic-specific treatment of a concurrent psychiatric disorder.
2. The patient should be withdrawn from alcohol, using the usual precautions.
3. An adequate diet with vitamin supplements, including thiamine (50 mg tid or qid), should be provided.
4. The patient should receive the best medical attention that can be provided. Good personal hygiene should be encouraged, and special attention paid to both minor medical problems (e.g., skin infections, bunions) and major problems. Regular physical examinations are a necessary part of good medical followup of an alcoholic.
5. Sleep should be assured. Hypnotics that are nonaddicting are preferred, because alcoholics are prone to addiction to any substance that is habit forming.
6. If alcohol has been used to medicate an underlying psychiatric disorder (such as schizophrenia, panic disorder, or depression or mania) an antipsychotic agent, an antianxiety agent, lithium carbonate, or an antidepressant will be needed for long-term management.
7. Place the patient in an appropriate psychotherapeutic or sociotherapeutic modality. In many instances, this may be Alcoholics Anonymous (AA) alone, with family members referred to the appropriate groups for spouses (Alanon) and teenage children (Alateen). In other instances, a different form of treatment may be indicated, alone or together with AA. Some alcoholics may need educative and supportive individual psychotherapy. For others, a group may be appropriate, especially for those who have difficulty asserting themselves, for those who can't get on with peers, and for those who suffer from an inability to relate to authority figures.
8. Employment is important. Every effort should be made to encourage a patient to secure and maintain a job within his or her realistic potential and one which contributes to a sense of self-esteem.
9. Some patients may be candidates for disulfiram (Antabuse) therapy or aversion therapy. Psychiatrists should provide these treatments if they are skilled at them, or refer appropriate patients to those who have had experience with them.

10. Relatives, friends, clergymen, other close associates of the patient, and organizations that are available in the community are part of a complete treatment program. This may demand that a psychiatrist serve, with the patient's permission, as a consultant to clergy, social workers, or general practitioners about the problems of treating alcoholics in general and the patient in particular.
11. When there appears to be no viable social matrix to support patients, it may be necessary to refer them to a halfway house, therapeutic farm, or other live-in program to help them maintain sobriety.

CHRONIC CRISES PATIENTS

A significant number of patients seen in an emergency psychiatric setting return within 6 months.

History
1. In various studies, repeaters have been found not to differ from nonrepeaters in demographic characteristics (Miller W, 1968).
2. Bassuk and Gerson (1980) have studied a group of chronic crises patients and found:

    a. Chronic crises patients do not differ from nonrepeater patients in symptom acuity;
    b. They are generally negativistic and have a long psychiatric history of multiple hospitalizations and current outpatient treatments; and
    c. They have difficulty establishing rapport with emergency room clinicians and evoke feelings of dislike.

Treatment
1. Hospitalization of chronic users of emergency psychiatric services appears to be more a reflection of the difficulty the caregivers have in developing contact with chronic crises patients than clinical need (Bassuk and Gerson, 1980).
2. Emergency clinicians should develop, in concert with social worker members of the team, alternative sources of social support as this group tends not to have available the traditional resources.
3. If the repeater is in treatment, the focus of crisis intervention should be on what is transpiring in therapy. Repeaters, particularly those with borderline or narcissistic personality disorders, tend to split, making the therapist "bad" and the emergency clinician "good." The patient's therapist should be informed of the emergency contact. When possible, the therapist should be contacted at the time of the visit to minimize splitting and facilitate integration of the crisis contact into ongoing therapy.
4. Every attempt should be made to engage the patient with a therapist in ongoing treatment. Short-term hospitalization may be needed to facilitate evaluation and treatment, which may necessitate the use of medications (e.g., long-acting phe-

nothiazines or mood stabilizers). The decision to hospitalize must always be considered with full knowledge of the fact that such a decision may be regressive.

5. All members of the emergency psychiatric team should be made aware of the identity of repeaters and their problems on contact to avoid splitting among emergency psychiatric team members and to allow an integrative team effort in directing the patient to a consistent definitive disposition.
6. Therapists must be aware that the difficulty repeaters have accepting care dates back to much earlier conflicts in the familial constellation, in order to minimize the depression and rage that they, as therapists, may feel toward the abuse and uncooperativeness chronic repeaters exhibit toward them.

CHRONIC PAIN

Pain may occur without evidence of bodily damage or physiologic dysfunction and conversely, injury may be unattended by pain.

History
1. Differentiating psychogenic pain from pain of physical origin is difficult. Pain is always real unless a patient is malingering. Patients commit suicide from psychic pain more often than they do from pain of organic origin.
2. Regional pain may be hysterical (Weintraub, 1986). The diagnosis is not made on personality assessment or by exclusion but rather by documentation that the pain does not comport with known physiologic or anatomic patterns of enervation.
3. Several disorders present with pain that respond to antidepressant therapy. These are included together with major depression, panic disorder, obsessive-compulsive disorder, cataplexy, and attention deficit hyperactivity disorder, affective spectrum disorders, irritable bowel syndrome, migraine, atypical facial pain, and post-traumatic stress disorder (Hudson and Pope, 1990).
4. The number of conditions presenting with pain, more than severity of pain or pain persistence, is a predictor of major depression requiring antidepressant therapy (Dworkin SF et al, 1990).
5. Like anxiety and depression, pain is a subjective experience and its intensity can, therefore, only be corroborated by patient report and behavior (e.g., limping) and physiologic changes.
6. Patients will be referred for psychiatric consultation when nonpsychiatric clinicians are no longer able to alleviate pain in a manner consistent with their expertise or value systems (e.g., use of non-narcotic analgesics versus use of narcotic analgesics).

Management
1. The first step in the evaluation of pain is to obtain data from patients and their clinicians as to what has been used in the past and to what degree of success.
2. In some instances, a drug may not be given in sufficient dosage or at short-

enough intervals to impact on the pain. For instance, meperidine (Demerol) given at 3-hour intervals is a more effective analgesic than when it is given at 4-hour intervals.

3. Breaking the pain cycle may be necessary for effective pain management. This entails evaluating the patient to understand the maximal amount of pain medication that has been required and then prescribing a fraction more to totally diminish the pain. After this occurs, the patient is gradually withdrawn from the medication and monitored on the minimal amount of medication necessary to allow functioning.

4. Narcotic analgesia should not be prescribed for outpatient use without medical supervision (e.g., nurse administrator in the home). If a narcotic is needed for an occasion of cluster headache or migraine, it should be given in an emergency setting. Narcotic analgesia for a terminal cancer patient should be administered with a nurse or physician monitoring and with regular review.

5. Physicians should not prescribe narcotic analgesia for themselves or their families.

6. Operant conditioning has been successfully used with patients in a multidisciplinary setting when all else has failed (Latimer, 1982). The management involves systematic manipulation of the contingent consequences of pain behavior. This consists of giving attention and affection for well behavior and remaining neutral and undemonstrative in the face of pain behavior. Because this is easier to do in a controlled setting, it is more easily initiated in a hospital than in the natural environment. Medication is given on a time-contingent schedule rather than a pain-contingent schedule and is usually reduced or discontinued.

7. Antidepressant medication has been used successfully in some instances to manage chronic pain. A substantial proportion of patients without contributory medical pathology (30% in one study) demonstrate notable clinical depression and a positive family history of depressive spectrum disorder (Schaffer et al, 1980). A substantial number of pain patients with depression (90% in one study) exhibit resolution of the depression without medication (Kramlinger et al, 1983).

8. Concurrent use of antidepressant or anxiolytic medication may reduce the amount of other pain medication required.

CHRONIC SCHIZOPHRENIA IN EXACERBATION

Recognition of chronic schizophrenia in exacerbation is usually easier than identification of incipient schizophrenic break by the fact that patients usually have a history of psychiatric treatment and often of repeated hospitalizations. Their relatives may know the diagnosis, and a family history often includes members who are schizophrenic, have been hospitalized, have committed suicide, or were known for their "unusual ways." When asked what is meant by "unusual" the psychiatrist may be told, "Oh, he dropped out of college and went off to study mysticism in India and never returned." If there is a question of what a patient's previous diagnoses may have been, they should be asked, as should their relatives, as to what treatment was given. If the patient previously received high doses of phenothiazines, thioxanthenes, or butyrophenones, schizophrenia is suggested; although, if they have functioned extremely well between episodes and have a family history of affective disorder, they may have been given the drugs for mania or been misdiagnosed and treated inappropriately. Lithium carbonate suggests a cyclic mood disturbance that may have been part of the picture of bipolar disorder. However, lithium is also given for schizoaffective disorder or other disorders with a phasic pattern.

History

1. Sometimes a clear precipitant will be identified such as recent death, divorce, sexual encounter, drug experience, job loss, or change in social supports. Other times, patients may have simply stopped their medication. This may have represented an unconscious need to be hospitalized or they may have become psychotic at a time of stress. There is little evidence to support any notion that verbalization of this interpretation, however, will lead to acceptance of it by the patient and alteration of medication-taking behavior in the future.

2. Early signs of a psychotic decompensation include:

   a. Increasing sleep disturbance,
   b. Increasing social withdrawal,
   c. Increasing difficulty at work or school,
   d. A need for more medication such that patients begin to take one or more extra pills,
   e. Increasing paranoia with ideas of reference,
   f. Increasing concern with religious and philosophical problems, and
   g. Increasing grandiosity.

3. When patients decompensate, the pattern of breakdown frequently follows that of previous breaks. This is true of both recurrent schizophrenic episodes and recurrent depression or mania. If, with their first break, patients began to spend more time in empty churches while missing work, they may, as they relapse, begin to spend more time in empty churches or be absent from work again.

4. In other instances, patients who are obviously schizophrenic by history may have survived for years in a well-structured and minimally stressful environment. The intensity of their psychotic symptomatology may be due to an accumulation of a series of undesirable life events and losses in the face of minimal coping ability. This is frequently seen in patients from compromised socioeconomic circumstances who lack both the internal adaptive ability ("ego strength") and external economic, political, or social power to cope with stresses of their environment. These patients may have long histories of an inability to make or maintain friends, hold jobs over sustained periods of time, or even care for themselves in habits of personal hygiene. Their affect often appears blunted or flat. They appear to be without drive and incapable of emotionally investing in anything. They may be laborers, prostitutes, hustlers, or members of other marginal groups. Sexual life is impoverished for many and their hetero- or homosexual acts represent a futile attempt to make contact with the world rather than

represent any real closeness. Decision making is difficult, and if married, they seem to float in a role fairly well-defined by society.

5. Changes in clinical presentation of a chronic schizophrenic may be due to external factors such as deterioration of social supports, progression of disease, concomitant medical illness, or medication effect. There is some evidence to suggest that therapeutic doses of anticholinergics may cause impairment of cognitive functions (Tune et al, 1982).

6. Increased norepinephrine and 3-methoxy-4-hydroxyphenylglycol in the cerebrospinal fluid is correlated with, but does not necessarily cause, schizophrenic symptoms (van Kammen et al, 1990). There is some evidence (Reynolds GP, 1989) to suggest that there may be the loss of some neurons in temporal limbic regions in schizophrenia (leading to a disinhibition of dopamine neurons) providing the rationale for use of neuroleptics in its treatment.

7. Although incidence of schizophrenia worldwide in different cultures is found to be similar, there appears to be some decline in reported new cases (Der et al, 1990). This may be due to recognition and diagnostic-specific treatment of schizophreniform disorders.

8. Schizophrenics suffer more speech performance failure during distraction than do normal controls or even manic patients (Hotchkiss and Harvey, 1990).

9. Schizophrenics by history and measurement suffer more social and physical anhedonia than normal subjects (Kirkpatrick and Buchanan, 1990). The definition of schizophrenia has been narrowed in the past several years. The *DSM-III-R* requires chronicity, presence of psychotic features, exclusion of organic and affective features, and evidence of deterioration (Andreasen, 1989) for diagnosis, eliminating individuals with more time-limited psychoses (e.g., those with a course less than 6 months) and those with a strong element of depression or mania).

10. Schizophrenics with negative (deficit) symptoms (e.g., poverty of speech, withdrawal, blunted affect, anhedonia) are reported to be more likely to suffer greater neurologic impairment and have a poor premorbid adjustment than those with positive symptoms such as delusions or hallucinations (Buchanan RW et al, 1990). Severe delivery complications and impairment of autonomic responsivity during adolescence are more common in those with predominantly negative symptoms (Cannon et al, 1990). While there appear to be no sex differences in symptoms, men tend to be more likely to lack premorbid social competence and exhibit more asociality and withdrawal than women (Dworkin RH, 1990).

Symptoms
1. Hallucinations.
2. Disturbance of body image.
3. Delusions (especially somatic, nihilistic, and of influence).
4. Ideas of reference.
5. Fusion and loss of ego boundaries.
6. Hypochondriasis.
7. Ambivalence.

8. Depersonalization and derealization.
9. Thought broadcasting.
10. Thought withdrawal.
11. Thought insertion.
12. Delusions of being controlled.
13. Paranoia.
14. Impulse disturbances (e.g., suicidal and homicidal behavior).

Signs

1. Neologisms.
2. Concrete thinking.
3. Paralogical thinking.
4. Vagueness in thinking.
5. Withdrawal.
6. Magical thinking.
7. Preoccupation with mysticism and philosophy.
8. Incoherence.
9. Symbolism.
10. Blocking.
11. Overinclusive thinking.
12. Word salad.
13. Verbigeration.
14. Mutism.
15. Echopraxia and echolalia.
16. Suggestibility.
17. Fragmented speech.
18. Blunted or flat affect.
19. Inappropriate affect.
20. Negativism.
21. Stupor.
22. Waxy flexibility.
23. Mannerisms.
24. Catatonic excitement.
25. Stereotypes.
26. Deterioration of activity.

Differential Diagnosis

The differential diagnosis of schizophrenia is discussed elsewhere in this book.

Clinical Studies

1. CBC and differential.
2. SMA-22.
3. Protein electrophoresis.
4. Lupus test.
5. HIV studies.

6. Serology for syphilis.
7. EEG.
8. CT scan.
9. MRI.

Significantly higher ventricle brain ratio than normal for age and sex-matched controls has been found on CT scan of schizophrenics (Nasrallah et al, 1982) particularly those with negative symptoms.

Management

1. It is always important to remember that an original diagnosis may have been incorrect. A patient may have a degenerative disease such as Huntington's chorea or Schilder's disease presenting as schizophrenia. Also, another process may be active in addition to schizophrenia. A patient may have contracted syphilis that has gone untreated or AIDS. Schizophrenics in past times were more likely to contract tuberculosis in crowded state mental hospitals. A change in behavior of those so infected could have been due to a tuberculous meningitis or tuberculoma; just as today, the change may be due to asymptomatic HIV infection. Alcoholic or epileptic schizophrenics are more inclined to trauma and may have a subdural hematoma causing what appears to be an exacerbation of their schizophrenia. Finally, symptoms reported by schizophrenics are more likely to be written off as hypochondriacal. Thus a neoplastic process, either primary in the brain or metastatic, may be overlooked. The first step in treatment, therefore, of what appears to be an exacerbation of chronic schizophrenia is to ascertain if symptoms are due to the schizophrenia or to a superimposed organic process such as AIDS, syphilis, a subdural hematoma, or substance abuse requiring diagnostic-specific treatment.

2. Once it has been documented that the change in behavior is due to the schizophrenia, the treatment is the same as for an acute psychotic break of any nature. The quality of a patient's social supports should be assessed, and the risk of homicide or suicide evaluated. Initial response to medication should be observed to see if a patient can be managed outside the hospital.

3. If patients are in treatment, their therapists should be called. Calling therapists in the emergency situation serves several purposes:

   a. Therapists provide information as to what is transpiring in therapy (e.g., is termination being discussed?)

   b. Therapists are able to provide other information such as which and how much medication might be needed to manage the patient.

   c. Therapists are able to identify the precipitant from their knowledge of patients and their histories.

   d. Therapists may be aware of social manipulations that allow patients to be managed outside the hospital.

   e. Therapists have names and addresses of relatives or friends who may provide an alternate disposition if it is felt that a patient should not go home, but still is not disturbed enough for hospitalization.

    f. A therapist coming in or speaking to a patient on the phone may be sufficient to calm a patient down.

    g. Therapists should be alerted to any contemplated change in medication, and given an opportunity to participate in a decision to hospitalize.

    h. Therapists and their patients should set an appointment to meet together soon after the emergency room visit (if the patient is not hospitalized).

    i. Assessment of the real suicidal or homicidal potential may only be possible if a therapist who knows the patient well is given the opportunity to place a current threat in the context of the patient's history and what is known about previous attempts, gestures, and threats.

4. An evaluation should be made of why the patient is psychotic at this time. Is there an intolerable situation at home, work, or school that he or she wants to get out of? Was there a recent loss, move, job change, or other change in social matrix which has compromised the ability to cope? Is it an anniversary of a parent's death or other significant date (such as the time a woman would have given birth if she had not been aborted)? Is the exacerbation simply due to a reduction or discontinuation of medication by the patient or therapist? Has the patient just changed therapists or terminated therapy? Even something as ostensibly simple as discontinuation of medication may have been motivated by an unconscious need to be rehospitalized by an intolerable situation (such as completion of college and facing the job market, or a marriage).

5. Critical to outpatient management of chronic schizophrenics during a crisis or at other points during the trajectory of their illness is a knowledge of the efficacy of all the major groups of antipsychotic medications, the antidepressants, and the antianxiety agents. Schizophrenics in exacerbation usually need more medication during crisis as well as an increase in daily dosage for some time after. This is not to belittle the importance of sociotherapeutic interventions at times of crisis such as family or couples therapy. However, it is difficult to engage a grossly (or even moderately) psychotic patient in any meaningful therapy until the psychosis is under control. An acutely psychotic, chronic schizophrenic may be given liquid medication orally on an emergency basis such as 16 mg of perphenazine (Trilafon), 100–200 mg of chlorpromazine (Thorazine), 100–200 mg of thioridazine (Mellaril), 5–10 mg of haloperidol (Haldol) or thiothixene (Navane), or 5 mg of fluphenazine (Prolixin). If they are unwilling to take the medication, 5–10 mg of haloperidol or thiothixene can be given every hour intramuscularly up to about 60 mg without the fear of the hypotensive risk associated with chlorpromazine use. Chlorpromazine, 50 mg intramuscularly, may be given if sedation is desired, but blood pressure and pulse rate should be monitored carefully (i.e., recorded before it is given and at regular intervals after). This should be done with all intramuscular medications, but one should anticipate problems associated with chlorpromazine. In addition, perphenazine (5–10 mg) or fluphenazine (5 mg) may also be given intramuscularly. Additional medication should be given for sleep during the acute episode as with the first acute schizophrenic episode. For example:

    a. Chlorpromazine 100 mg PO every hour until asleep

    b. Perphenazine 8 mg PO every hour until asleep

    c. Thiothixene 10 mg PO every hour until asleep

    d. Thioridazine 25 mg PO every hour until asleep

6. Medication should be continually re-evaluated during the acute phase until the appropriate amount is arrived at, which then may be given in divided doses during the day and at bedtime. Alternately, the clinician may give all the medication at bedtime. Antidepressants may be added if there exists a strong depressive character to the illness, but this should be done by the patient's therapist, and not in any emergency situation. Whether or not an antiparkinsonian agent should be given concurrently with an antipsychotic agent depends on the amount and the particular agent given, as well as a patient's current and past history of need for these agents.

7. Psychiatric clinicians should discuss with patients and, when indicated, their families the importance of continued medication and involvement in therapy. If there exist particular signs that foreshadow a decompensation or give warning of increased risk of suicide or homicide, these should be identified and articulated, and the route to hospitalization outlined. Namely, who should be called? Where could the patient be hospitalized? A patient's insurance and eligibility for a veteran's hospital should be known. If violent or suicidal, and patients protest hospitalization, how can they be hospitalized? Ambulance crews cannot legally bring patients to the hospital by force when they have not been committed or are not under arrest. If a patient's family finds it impossible to bring a patient into the hospital themselves and he or she is grossly psychotic, suicidal, or homicidal, it will either be necessary for a physician to go to the patient's house with the permission of the patient's spouse or parents to evaluate them or the patient's relatives may need to have him or her arrested for destroying property or threatening to kill them. If either of these has happened, one can give the police information about the patient's psychiatric history so that they may be brought to the emergency room rather than to jail.

8. A patient's relatives and friends should be instructed as to the continuing need for medication. If a patient has had one psychotic episode, it is usually not good to discontinue medication after 1 year, although it may be possible to taper the dosage significantly. After two psychotic episodes, it is generally best to wait at least 2 years before discontinuation and if there have been three episodes, medication may have to be continued indefinitely.

9. Always use the rule of thumb of minimal dose of maximal functioning. Patients and their relatives must be made aware of both the need to keep down the undercurrent psychotic process to avoid regressive rehospitalization and of the possibility of tardive dyskinesias or the neuroleptic malignant syndrome from long-term antipsychotic therapy. Drug holidays with weekends off or 1 week a month off may help this. In addition, it may be necessary to switch to another agent if a patient becomes psychotic off medication, but also has developed a tardive dyskinesia with a particular drug.

10. If a patient is unreliable and cessation of medication quickly results in rehospitalization, a regimen of long-acting fluphenazine in the form of Prolixin decanoate or Prolixin enanthate or depot haloperidol may be needed. The dosage of Prolixin to be given every 2 weeks is determined by calculating the total amount that would be given orally over 14 days and then taking one-fourth to one-sixth that dose and giving it in the enanthate or decanoate form by deep intramuscular or subcutaneous injection. If a patient has not had the medication before, a test dose of 0.1 mL should be given subcutaneously while monitoring blood pressure and general reaction. This is to test both for allergy to the fluphenazine as well as to the vehicle. If there is no indication of sensitivity after $\frac{1}{2}$ hour, the calculated dose, usually between 25–75 mg, can be given intramuscularly or subcutaneously.

11. The long-term treatment approach to any patient with chronic schizophrenia involves an integration of psychotherapy, sociotherapy, and psychopharmacotherapy. This includes structuring the patient's environment, such as making sure they keep their job, pay their rent, and take care of other mundane activities such as eating and bathing. If they are not working and have discontinued medication, this alone may indicate a need for inpatient hospitalization. Such might allow the patient to obtain a job and recommence his or her medication. If he or she has had several exacerbations due to a failure to take medication, long-acting fluphenazine would be started and the patient's response monitored.

12. Family therapy should also be undertaken in an attempt to help the family become aware of the chronicity of the patient's illnesses and how the patient may respond in a way that will promote optimal functioning. Obviously, it is not infrequent to find a sibling or a parent with schizophrenia. This complicates matters for both the parents and the therapist. All the therapist can do is work with the reality of the family situation if no other disposition is possible, or if other dispositions have been tried, but are nonviable. If other members of the family are healthy, it may be possible to explain that despite the fact that the patient appears well on medication, a chronic psychotic process exists underneath. It may be explained that as little as 30 years ago, patients with even one schizophrenic episode often spent months to years in a state or private psychiatric hospital, acting bizarrely with great pain within them, and at great emotional and financial expense to their family. Only through the advent of the antipsychotic agents has it been possible to manage such patients outside a hospital. However, this is only symptomatic relief. If medication is stopped, the psychotic symptoms return and sometimes become more florid than before. At these times, neither psychotherapeutic nor sociotherapeutic interventions are successful. Only after a psychosis has run its course or is in remission, is it possible to reduce or discontinue medication. The potency of our antipsychotic agents is attested to by the extent to which psychotic thinking and behavior returns when they are discontinued.

13. It takes a long time for some families to face the reality that one among them is recurrently or chronically psychotic. A few families may never feel this reality. Most families, however, first respond with denial; a patient is seen as "eccentric"

or "going through a stage." Later, when denial is no longer possible, there is anger. This may be directed at a spouse, parents, or siblings. Each may blame the other, or a family may turn its anger toward the patient and extrude him or her from the family circle. Only in later stages, when a family is willing to acknowledge that a patient is ill and that they may have played some part in the genesis of the illness (or may be able to play some part in the healing process), is it possible to form a working relationship in which therapist, patient, and family work together to achieve the best milieu for the patient's continued functioning. Raymond et al (1975) have called this a "healing alliance." The therapist's awareness that the family (like the therapist) may at times feel frustration, anger, guilt, and hopelessness and want to deny the seriousness of a patient's illness, allows the therapist to work better with the reality of the family's dynamics. It is obviously impossible to make any realistic plans for the family to participate in the effort to keep the patient in therapy and take medication while they still deny the illness. At the stage of guilt, there may be such overwhelming self-flagellation that the family may need to be helped to look forward, rather than backward, as to what must now, and in the future, be done. It neither helps the family nor patient to recount a litany of psychological indiscretions from the past. To know the past will help a therapist to make realistically viable plans for the future and reduce a repetition of past mistakes by a knowledge of what has failed or made a patient worse or better. Unfortunately, there is little controlled evidence that intellectual insight in patients themselves necessarily leads to modification of maladaptive behavior.

14. A follow-up study of 119 chronic schizophrenics (Caton, 1982) revealed that length of inpatient stay bore no relationship to subsequent hospitalization, clinical or social functioning, or treatment compliance. Postdischarge experiences of a patient with significant others and treatment were critical in determining future use of hospitalization.

15. A structured milieu contributes to greater improvement than an open ward where patients have more freedom (Cohen and Khan, 1982).

16. Currently, the two strategies more frequently used to reduce risk of medication exposure are targeted or intermittent treatment and continuous low dose treatment (Schooler and Keith, 1989). Reduction of dose to 10 to 20% of a standard dose range appears to reduce side effects without increased risk of relapse for a year; reduction longer than 1 year or below this threshold leads to exacerbation of symptoms and of relapse. The intermittent concept of medication is predicated on the fact that a patient is very cautiously monitored off medication so that it is possible to rapidly detect an exacerbation of psychosis and focally medicate the episode. In some ways this latter approach is a version of the "drug holiday" method. The holidays are just longer and the need for careful monitoring greater to detect incipient relapse (Schooler and Keith, 1989).

17. Clozapine, a dibenzodiazepine derivative chemically related to the antipsychotic loxapine with unique adrenergic, serotonergic, and histaminergic effects, has been found to be especially effective in managing deficit or negative symptoms of schizophrenia. Agranulocytosis with fatalities due to secondary infection is a

risk requiring weekly monitoring of white cell count and differential. The hematopoeitic suppression appears to be reversible without physical sequelae if detected within about 2 weeks (Kane JM et al, 1988).

18. Combined neuroleptic–carbamazepine (Tegretol) therapy has been effective in excited or aggressive/violent states associated with schizophrenia or schizoaffective disorder when a neuroleptic alone has failed (Okuma et al, 1989). While carbamazepine does not reduce serum levels of lithium, when used concurrently with haloperidol it can reduce serum haloperidol levels, requiring monitoring of serum levels of the neuroleptic when combined with carbamazepine to reduce risk of symptom exacerbation (Kahn et al, 1990).

Quality Assurance Issues

1. Was evaluation performed to assure that the diagnosis of schizophrenia was valid and that the patient was not suffering a schizophreniform psychosis of a primary affective nature?
2. Was an evaluation performed to ascertain if what appeared to be an exacerbation of schizophrenia was not another comorbid illness such as substance abuse, AIDS, or syphilis?
3. Was an evaluation of suicide and homicide potential performed?
4. Was the least amount of neuroleptic that was clinically effective prescribed to minimize neuroleptic adverse effects?

CIMETIDINE PSYCHOSIS

Cimetidine, a competitive histamine H_2 receptor antagonist, is widely used as an inhibitor of gastric secretion in short-term management of duodenal ulcer, and in treatment of pathological hypersecretory syndromes such as multiple endocrine adenomas, systemic mastocytosis, and the Zollinger–Ellison syndrome.

History

1. Cimetidine is usually well tolerated. Cases are reported, however, of neuropsychiatric toxicity with severe acute confusional psychoses, lethargy, slurred speech, unsteadiness, depression, disorientation, restlessness, agitation, delirium, visual impairment, incontinence, and coma (Crowder and Pate, 1980).
2. In most of these instances, there has been coexisting psychiatric illness, a history of the concurrent use of psychotropic medication that has strong central anticholinergic effects, older age, decreased brain perfusion due to cerebrovascular disease, overdosage, or impaired renal function (Crowder and Pate, 1980).
3. Cimetidine can trigger a predominantly paranoid psychosis that must be distinguished from other organic and functional psychoses (Adler et al, 1980).
4. Cimetidine is reported to inhibit the metabolism of imipramine (Tofranil) leading to a prolonged half-life, elevated serum concentrations, and increased side effects (Miller and Macklin, 1983).

Management
1. Symptoms usually disappear upon reduction of dosage of or discontinuation of cimetidine.

CIRRHOSIS-INDUCED DISORDERS

Billiary and other forms of cirrhosis are associated with depression and cognitive impairment.

History
1. Billiary cirrhotic patients have been found to suffer attentional, visuospatial, and perceptual–motor dysfunction (Hegedus et al, 1984).

Management
1. Patients with cirrhosis of any type should be monitored for the development of cognitive affective or behavioral deficits that may be reversible and which compromise their ability to function. Subtle deficits may be identified through use of psychological and neuropsychological testing.
2. Treatment of psychological symptoms that remain after appropriate management of the cirrhoses has been provided is symptomatic. Antidepressants, albeit in smaller doses given impaired hepatic functioning, are used for depression. Plasma levels of the antidepressants serve to guide dosage level and minimize toxicity.

CLONIDINE WITHDRAWAL

The imidazoline antihypertensive clonidine hydrochloride has been used alone or in combination with naltrexone hydrochloride to suppress the signs and symptoms of opiate withdrawal (Charney et al, 1982).

History
1. Exacerbation of psychosis on withdrawal from clonidine has been observed when prescribed as an antipsychotic for schizophrenic and manic patients as well as in previously nonpsychiatric patients who abruptly discontinued clonidine prescribed for hypertension (Geller, 1982).
2. A low incidence of anxiety and irritability is reported when clonidine is withdrawn as an antihypertensive (Garbus et al, 1979).
3. Violent behavior has been reported when clonidine has been withdrawn from psychiatric patients (Geller, 1982; Tollefson, 1981).
4. The mechanism of induction of psychosis is not clear.

Management
1. Symptoms generally abate with time. As the incidence of violence, on clonidine

withdrawal, from patients who are psychotic is impressive, appropriate precautions should be taken.
2. Neuroleptics may be necessary to manage psychotic symptoms if severe.

Prevention
1. Gradual withdrawal may prevent symptoms and minimize the incidence of violence.

CLORGYLINE

Approximately 25% of patients with bipolar affective illness will show little or no response to traditional prophylactic treatment (Dunner et al, 1976). Patients with rapid cycles (four or more episodes a year) are particularly refractory. The selective MAO-A inhibitor clorgyline given in low doses lessens the severity of mood cycles (Potter et al, 1982).

CLOZAPINE-INDUCED DISORDERS

The antipsychotic clozapine impacts the dopamine, norepinephrine, and serotonin systems (Achenheil, 1989).

History
1. Clozapine has potent antipsychotic impact on treatment-resistant negative and positive symptoms without production of extrapyramidal side effects (Green and Salzman, 1990).
2. Side effects correlate with dosage of clozapine (Leppig et al, 1989). In one study of 387 patients treated with clozapine (Naber et al, 1989), 56% reported adverse effects. Two percent became delirious.
3. Risk of tardive dyskinesia with clozapine is either remarkably reduced or entirely absent (Lieberman J et al, 1989).
4. Whereas up to 75% of patients receiving traditional neuroleptics suffer extrapyramidal symptoms such as parkinsonism, akathisia, and dystonia, these are infrequently reported with clozapine (Casey DE, 1989). The clozapine is specifically used for schizophrenics with tardive dyskinesia.
5. Gaertner et al (1989) reported a 41 to 61% incidence of rise in liver enzymes in patients on clozapine. When only cases with a two-fold increase over normal values were counted, incidence was reduced to 20 to 31%. Leukopenia (white cell count less than 3,500) was found in 2% of cases. Adverse reactions such as fever, rise in liver enzymes, fatigue, or hypotension required change of medication in 17% of cases.
6. The combination of clozapine and benzodiazepines has been reported associated with severe respiratory and cardiovascular dysregulation (Grohmann et al, 1989).

7. Weight gain, a common side effect with many neuroleptics, is also reported with clozapine (Cohen S et al, 1990).

Symptoms
1. Sedation.
2. Fatigue.
3. Dizziness.
4. Constipation.

Signs
1. Hypotension.
2. Changes in white cell count.
3. EKG changes.
4. Increased weight gain.
5. Increase in liver enzymes (transaminases).
6. EEG changes.
7. Fever.
8. Hypersalivation.
9. Delirium.
10. Tachycardia.

Clinical Studies
1. CBC and differential.
2. SMA-22.
3. EEG.
4. EKG.

Management
1. Gradual increase in clozapine dosage minimizes side effects (Naber et al, 1989).
2. When side effects that are severe (e.g., delirium), life-threatening (e.g., agranulocytosis), or intolerable to the patient (e.g., weight gain, hypersalivation) appear, the drug is discontinued and another neuroleptic used.
3. When agranulocytosis appears, emergency medical intervention is required.

Quality Assurance Issues
1. Were CBCs and differentials performed weekly?
2. Are liver function studies monitored?

COCAINE INTOXICATION AND DELUSIONAL DISORDERS

Cocaine intoxication and delusional disorders resemble those of amphetamine and other sympathomimetic substances. Cocaine differs from amphetamines and most other sympathomimetic substances in dose and, therefore, availability. It is the recreational drug most frequently associated with use by people of circumstance. Professional men and women such as lawyers, physicians, business people, and those in the theater and art world reported using it. The advent of "crack" cocaine changed the entire picture and now virtually anyone can afford its use. This has contributed to the drug use epidemic here and abroad.

History

1. Cocaine is sold as crystalline flakes or powder (hence it is sometimes called "snow").
2. The usual routes of intake are application to the mucous membrane of the nose ("snorting coke"), intravenous administration, and smoking in the free-base or crack form. Nasal application may result in perforations of the nasal septum. In some instances, there may be some evidence of the white powdery substance in the nasal area.
3. The onset of symptoms and physical signs is more rapid than with amphetamine and related substances. Symptoms being within 1 hour after nasal administration and are usually entirely gone within 24 hours. Depression, fatigue, irritability, anxiety, and tremulousness may appear within the hour or following the subsiding of the psychological and behavioral manifestations of use. In instances of intravenous administration or smoking of cocaine, onset is rapid and the effect brief—lasting only minutes. The effects of intravenous administration of methamphetamine may be hours.
4. As with all drug intoxication states, the clinical presentation represents an interaction of the patient's premorbid personality; the environment in which the cocaine is taken; other physical and psychiatric illnesses the individual suffers; genetic constitution; the number, kind, and quantity of other drugs that the individual may also have taken; the dose of cocaine; and the route of administration.
5. Amphetamine and cocaine are sometimes taken with heroin and called a "speedball" or "croak."
6. The intake of a large dose of cocaine over a brief period can lead to seizures and even death from respiratory paralysis or cardiac arrhythmias.
7. Identification of the metabolites of cocaine in a urine specimen may be the only absolute way to differentiate cocaine from amphetamine intoxication. Unfortunately, detectable amounts of cocaine remain in the urine for only 4 to 6 hours after usage.
8. Cocaine is extremely addicting for susceptible persons.
9. Central nervous system complications associated with cocaine use include intracerebral and subarachnoid hemorrhage, seizures, psychosis, and ischemic stroke (Levine SR et al, 1987).
10. Medical and psychiatric complications of cocaine use relate to purity and sterility of the drug and the route of administration, with greater problems reported with free-base and intravenous use (Estroff and Gold, 1986b).

11. Specificity of the thyrotropin-releasing hormone (TRH) test for major depression is reduced significantly when cocaine abuse is present (Dackis et al, 1985).
12. There is some evidence (Griffin et al, 1989) to suggest that women cocaine users as a group are more depressed and the depression persists after cessation of use indicating dual diagnosis and need for diagnostic-specific treatment of the affective disorder.
13. Chest pain, even in young cocaine users, can be an indicant of cardiac damage and may be a harbinger of sudden death from a cocaine-induced cardiac arrhythmia (Decker et al, 1987).
14. Cocaine dependence appears based on neurophysiologic down-regulation of specific CNS processes that regulate hedonic (pleasure) responses and is not merely "psychological," in nature. (Gawin and Ellinwood, 1989).

Symptoms of Cocaine Intoxication and Delusional Disorder

1. Loose associations.
2. Euphoria and elation (the cocaine "rush").
3. Decreased sleep.
4. Paranoid ideation.
5. Ideas of reference.
6. Vivid auditory and visual hallucinations, which at times may be quite frightening ("Snow lights" may be present that resemble migraine hallucinations).
7. Grandiosity.
8. Feeling of mental agility.
9. Insomnia.
10. Loquacity.
11. Heightened awareness of sensory input.
12. Restlessness.
13. Sense of confidence.
14. Anorexia.
15. Impaired judgement.
16. Inability to meet social and occupational responsibility.
17. Confusion.
18. Anxiety and apprehension.
19. Ringing in the ears.
20. Sensations of seeing insects and feeling insects, small animals, and other vermin crawling up the skin (formication), which may lead to picking at the skin and subsequent excoriation of the skin.
21. Hostility.
22. Feeling of immunity to fatigue and great muscle power.
23. Illusions.
24. Dream-like states.
25. Broodiness.
26. Irritability.
27. Hypervigilance.

Physical Signs of Cocaine Intoxication and Delusional Disorder
1. Pupillary dilation.
2. Perforated nasal septum (sometimes seen with a whitish powder on it).
3. Seizures.
4. Perspiration or chills.
5. Vomiting.
6. Tachycardia.
7. Elevated blood pressure.
8. Psychomotor excitement.
9. Skin pallor.
10. Haggard look.
11. Elevation of body temperature.
12. Tremulousness.
13. Evidence of "skin popping" or needle marks.
14. Violent or assaultive behavior if the patient is paranoid.

Differential Diagnosis
1. Cocaine intoxication or delusional disorder.
2. Amphetamine or similarly acting sympathomimetic intoxication or delusional disorder.
3. Anxiety disorders.
4. Mania.
5. Acute psychosis.
6. Paranoid schizophrenia.
7. Chronic schizophrenia.
8. Delirium tremens.
9. Schizoaffective disorder.

Management
1. The management of cocaine intoxication and delusional disorder is comparable to that of sympathomimetic intoxication.
2. Cocaine intoxication is usually self-limited and an individual feels fully recovered within 24 hours.
3. If medication is needed, haloperidol (Haldol) or thiothixene (Navane) 2–5 mg or an equivalent dose of a similarly acting antipsychotic agent given orally or intramuscularly is usually sufficient. If an atropine-like substance has been taken together with the cocaine, a benzodiazepine such as 1–4 mg of lorazepam (Ativan) should be given to manage the psychomotor retardation rather than one of the antipsychotic agents that have anticholinergic properties.
4. There is no danger in immediately withdrawing the individual from cocaine.
5. An hour or so after the patient's symptoms have subsided, he or she may "crash" (i.e., feel depressed, anxious, irritable, and fatigued). The desire for more cocaine is great during this period and the individual may resort to robbery, burglary, or prostitution to obtain the money needed to purchase the drug.

6. The use of sympathomimetic substances, including amphetamines and cocaine, may precipitate a psychosis in predisposed individuals or be taken as "self-medication" as an individual is breaking down.

7. Chronic cocaine users may be self-medicating themselves for affective illness and require antidepressant or mood-stabilizing drugs for definitive treatment (Khantzian, 1983).

8. Chronic cocaine users may need to be referred for surgical or medical consultation. In addition to the expected complications, such as a perforated nasal septum, individuals who are involved in freebase or crack cocaine smoking may have a significant reduction in the carbon monoxide diffusing capacity of their lungs (Weiss RD et al, 1981).

9. A number of pharmacologic approaches to cocaine dependence have been tried with varying success (Taylor and Gold, 1990). Desipramine (Norpramin), for instance, is reported to reduce cocaine craving and is used in patients with histories of intravenous cocaine use (Kosten et al, 1987) as well as to reverse withdrawal symptoms (Baxter, 1983). Desipramine has comparably been reported successful in reduction of craving and use of cocaine in other studies (Gawin et al, 1989; Gawin and Kleber, 1984). Bromocriptine has also been reported effective in reduction of cocaine craving (Dackis et al, 1987).

10. Cocaine abuse is often comorbid with another *DSM-III-R* Axis I psychiatric disorder requiring diagnostic-specific treatment (Gawin and Kleber, 1986). Successful management entails diagnostic-specific treatment of the non-substance abuse disorder as well as of the substance abuse.

11. Plasma prolactin levels persist after cocaine withdrawal suggesting that chronic use of cocaine may result in derangement of the neural dopaminergic regulatory system (Mendelson JH et al, 1985).

COCAINE OVERDOSE

1. Large doses of cocaine may result in syncope, chest pains, delirium, tremulousness, and seizures with a temporal lobe discharge pattern.

2. Death may result from respiratory paralysis or cardiac arrhythmias.

3. The treatment is basically supportive. Intravenous barbiturates or intramuscular antipsychotic agents can be employed, but only with caution, because the respiratory depression that accompanies cocaine poisoning can be aggravated by large doses of sedating agents. Anticonvulsants are not felt to be effective in preventing seizures.

COLLAGEN DISEASE

Collagen disease may present with a plethora of changes in mood, thought, or behavior that may be mistakenly attributed to a psychogenic origin delaying diagnosis and specific treatment.

History

Twenty-five to 33% of all patients with systemic lupus erythematosus have CNS involvement (Gurland et al, 1972; Feinglass et al, 1976). Neuro-ophthalmic involvement due to optic neuritis, retinal vasculitis, occlusive retinal arterial disease, retinal vein occlusion, or optic nerve involvement anywhere along the optic tract may result in an initial diagnosis of hysterical blindness (Stoudemire et al, 1982).

Clinical Studies

1. Protein electrophoresis.
2. ESR.
3. Specific tests for collagen disease.

Management

1. Symptoms due specifically to the underlying collagen disease require diagnostic-specific treatment by an internist.
2. Any comorbid psychiatric illness is treated as dictated by the diagnosis (e.g., mania with mood stabilizers).

CORONARY BYPASS SURGERY

Psychological response to bypass surgery is dependent on the physiological changes contributing to delirium, social support, preoperative preparation (particularly speaking with those who have had bypass surgery), premorbid psychiatric status, medications the patient is on, biogenetic endowment, age, sex, religious belief, and concurrent life stressors.

History

1. Approximately 175,000 coronary artery bypass grafting procedures are performed each year (Sokol et al, 1987).
2. Evidence suggests that women either experience more psychological problems than men or problems are similar in frequency for both sexes (Sokol et al, 1987).

Management

1. The management of delirium, anxiety, and depression is diagnostic-specific (e.g., alprazolam [Xanax] or lorazepam [Ativan] for the acute anxiety attending the procedure).
2. Meeting with others who have successfully undergone bypass surgery prior to the procedure and involvement transiently in postsurgical support groups can facilitate coping by enhancing awareness of what problems may be anticipated and how they are managed.

COTARD'S SYNDROME

The delusion of death and nonexistence is referred to as Cotard's syndrome.

History
1. Cotard's syndrome is most frequently a symptom of schizophrenia or affective illness. It is rarely if ever a disorder of its own (Joseph, 1986).
2. The typical patient is a depressed female (Joseph, 1986).
3. In contrast, Capgras' syndrome (delusional hypoidentification) most frequently occurs in patients who suffer delusional disorder or paranoid schizophrenia.
4. Patients with frontotemporal lesions and seizures (Drake ME, 1988) and partial occipital and temporal pathology (Joseph, 1986) have been reported to suffer this syndrome.
5. It is possible that the syndrome represents an extreme form of depersonalization and nonreality associated with temporal lobe epilepsy (Drake ME, 1988).

Management
1. The management is diagnostic specific. Antidepressants and neuroleptics where required for depression, anticonvulsants for epilepsy, and neuroleptics for schizophrenia are employed.

Quality Assurance Issue
1. Was an EEG and CT scan performed to ascertain if nonpsychiatric cerebral pathology is present?

CRIMINALITY

Not everyone who presents with criminal behavior in a psychiatric emergency room has a psychiatric disorder. The role of the emergency clinician is to identify those whose legal infractions are a product of mental illness and provide diagnostic-specific treatment. Those who do not suffer psychiatric illness are the domain of the legal system.

History
1. Patients who are schizophrenic, have severe depressions, or who are toxic from drugs with sympathomimetic effects such as PCP, cocaine, and amphetamines may experience command hallucinations directing them to torture or to kill others or themselves. Those with hallucination-related delusions and hallucinatory voices they could identify are more likely to comply with the commands (Junginger, 1990).
2. In one study (Junginger, 1990), 69% of patients with command hallucinations were reported to be directed to commit suicide, murder, or injure themselves or others.

3. Criminal behavior appears correlated with decreased autonomic responsivity such that criminals tend to exhibit smaller skin conductance responses and smaller heart rate accelerating and deceleratory responses than noncriminals (Raine et al, 1990). This suggests that those who commit crimes may not be as responsive to the physiological correlates of guilt.
4. Conduct disorders impairing functioning at school and home (wherein children or adolescents demonstrate a range of antisocial behavior including lying, truancy, vandalism, theft, and firesetting) that cannot be managed by teachers or parents affects 2 to 6% of all children in the United States. Approximately one-third to one-half of all child and adolescent psychiatric clinic referrals are for conduct disorders (Kazdin, 1990).
5. The prevalence of major psychiatric illness and affective disorder, in particular among criminal offenders, is relatively small (Kunzukrishnan and Bradford, 1990).

Management
1. Evaluation of the emergency room referral is focused on identification of a psychiatric disorder responsible for the criminal behavior.
2. Those with a psychiatric disorder are referred for diagnostic-specific treatment. The others remain the purview of the forensic system.

CULTS

Individuals with psychiatric disorders are particularly prone to involvement in cults. A cult provides an external structure and identity when the internal sense of identity and structure is weakened or in chaos. While the majority of cult members are found to be normal, 30% to 50% are reported to suffer psychiatric problems (Langone, 1990).

History
1. Cult victims exhibit a wide variety of Axis I and Axis II disorders (Siskin and Wynne, 1990).
2. Some individuals who do not suffer psychiatric problems prior to involvement in a cult do so after becoming a member due to the intense group influence. (Galanter, 1990).
3. Charismatic groups with a strong social cohesiveness, professed influence on members' behavior, and an intensely held belief system can provide relief of some psychiatric symptoms as well as produce them (Galanter, 1990).
4. A potentially pathogenic characteristic of a cult is attack on the stability and quality of evaluations of self-contents to consent to control behavior and reform thought (Singer and Ofshe, 1990).
5. Individuals particularly prone to cult involvement are those with borderline and narcissistic character disorders and those who are depressed secondary to loss of a significant figure (Halperin, 1990).

6. Particularly attractive to individuals suffering vulnerability, low self-esteem, boredom, alienation, and impotence is the solidarity, community, and lofty goals promised by cult leaders (Hochman, 1990).

Management
1. The task of the emergency clinician confronted with a member of a cult seeking psychiatric help is to ascertain, when a psychiatric disorder is present, that the disorder either contributed to cult membership or resulted from it.
2. Some individuals become acutely suicidal during membership in a cult or when the cult disintegrates and require both protection from self-inflicted harm and a diagnostic-specific treatment.
3. Family members may be particularly upset when one among them joins a cult and may require an opportunity for ventilation and support around the time of a perceived loss of a child.

CUSHING'S SYNDROME

Increase in plasma steroids from Cushing's syndrome from adrenocortical tumors or ACTH-dependent Cushing's disease due to exogenous causes is associated with a plethora of psychiatric and medical signs and symptoms.

History
1. Eighty-three percent of patients in one series (Haskett, 1985) met strict diagnostic criteria for an affective illness sometime during the course of Cushing's syndrome. Approximately two-thirds were endogenously depressed; the other one-third were manic or hypomanic.
2. The symptoms of affective disturbance with Cushing's syndrome may be indistinguishable from that of major depression or bipolar illness. (Krystal et al, 1990).

Clinical Studies
1. Cushing's syndrome patients are more likely than patients with affective illness to have markedly increased 24-hour urinary free cortisol and cortisol nonsuppression after dexamethasone administration (Krystal et al, 1990).
2. Bedside cognitive tests (e.g., serial sevens, recall of three cites after 5 minutes) correlate significantly with nonverbal and verbal subtests of the neuropsychological battery administered to patients with Cushing's disease (Starkman et al, 1986).

Management
1. Patients with Cushing's syndrome are referred to an endocrinologist for diagnostic-specific treatment. The role of the psychiatric clinician may be concurrent management if the patient is suicidal or homicidal.

2. Stressors that may have led to the development of the disease should be sought and the patient provided assistance in managing them if present.
3. If the illness has led to problems in a marriage or family, couples or family therapy may be required.

DELINQUENCY

Delinquency is a term used for the behavior of minors which, if perpetrated by adults, would be considered criminal. The task for the emergency clinician is to identify those delinquents whose antisocial behavior is a symptom of a psychiatric disorder.

History
1. Delinquency, like substance abuse, is a symptom of conduct disorders as well as of childhood and adolescent depression.
2. In a 7-year follow-up study of 118 male and female subjects who had been incarcerated, 7 had died by their 25th birthday, giving them a mortality rate of 58 times the national average for their age group. All died of violent deaths, giving the group 76 times the national average for the group (Yeager and Lewis, 1990).
3. Delinquents are more likely to suffer illnesses, injuries, and accidents than nondelinquents (Yeager and Lewis, 1990).
4. Between the 1950s and 1980s there was a doubling of the homicide rate and tripling of the suicide rate for young people (Yeager and Lewis, 1990).

Management
1. The task of the emergency clinician is to ascertain whether the delinquent behavior observed is due to a treatable psychiatric illness and then to refer the patient for diagnostic-specific treatment be it medical or psychiatric.
2. Delinquency is often a symptom of profound depression and risk of suicide or homicide may be great. The patient should be evaluated for risk of self- or other-directed violence and safeguards against physical harm initiated if required.
3. Delinquency and other psychiatric symptoms of young people may be an indicant of family problems, particularly in the patient's relationship with his or her parents. Crisis intervention may entail long-term family or couples therapy with the parents to prevent further development of the delinquent behavior into a criminal life style.

Quality Assurance Issues
1. Have all delinquents been evaluated for medical/psychiatric/surgical causes of delinquency?

Ethical/Legal Issues
1. Have all delinquents with illness-based behavior problems been provided diagnostic-specific treatment?

DELIRIUM

Cognitive changes associated with delirium result from changes in cerebral metabolism secondary to toxic, metabolic, traumatic, vascular, neoplastic, and degenerative processes. The primary treatment is that of the etiologic process. Psychiatry offers sociotherapeutic and psychopharmacologic assistance to comfort these patients and facilitate management while they are receiving diagnostic examinations and treatment. Psychiatric clinicians should be able to recognize signs and symptoms of delirium and make recommendations for management.

History
1. Delirium occurs at any age. It is sometimes very difficult to detect in very young children.
2. Onset is rapid, usually over hours or days. Symptoms generally first appear at night when sensory input and environmental cues are reduced.
3. Patients may have histories of infections, recreational or prescription drug use, or other contributing illness such as recent surgery or trauma.
4. Cognitive impairment tends to fluctuate unpredictably and often rapidly. Lucid intervals in which a patient is more rational are interspersed with confusional states (more marked at night).
5. Duration is usually brief, lasting a few days to a week. Occasionally, delirium may last longer as with bromism.
6. Recovery is usually complete. Rarely the patient will go on to have more permanent cognitive deficits consistent with dementia or die.
7. Older people and those with pre-existing brain damage are more likely to develop delirium than younger people and those without brain damage.
8. Etiological factors include medical and surgical illnesses as well as substance intoxication and withdrawal.
9. Delirious patients present management problems both in and out of the hospital and are at risk for accidents and violent behavior including suicide.
10. Patients with delirium become worse at night when frightening dreams and hallucinations may be interpreted as actual events.
11. There is usually evidence on physical examination or laboratory tests of the etiology of the disorder.

Symptoms
1. Fear.
2. Anxiety, apprehension, and panic.
3. Vivid dreams and nightmares.
4. Irritability.

Signs
1. Clouding of the sensorium.
2. Fluctuating levels of consciousness.

3. Insomnia, reduced wakefulness, and reversal of sleep–wake cycle.
4. Agitation.
5. Inability to sustain attention to environmental stimuli.
6. Delusions.
7. Disorientation.
8. Dysgraphia.
9. Dysnomia.
10. Emotional lability.
11. Lack of cooperation with medical staff.
12. Hallucinations (predominantly visual).
13. Perceptual difficulty including illusions.
14. Difficulty performing simple calculations.
15. Outbursts of rage and anger.
16. Memory changes with difficulty in retention and recall (both antegrade and retrograde amnesia occurs).
17. Incoherent speech.
18. Denial of defects.
19. Difficulty in goal-directed behavior and thinking.
20. Fragmented and disjointed thinking (may be slowing of thinking in early stages).
21. Perseveration of speech and behavior.
22. Misidentification of people and places.
23. Dilated pupils.
24. Euphoria.
25. Apathy.
26. Coarse tremor.
27. Sweating.
28. Tachycardia.
29. Urinary and fecal frequency.
30. Hyperventilation.
31. Restlessness.
32. Slow response to questions.
33. Avoidance, denial, and inconsistent responses to questions.
34. Increased or decreased psychomotor activity (picking at bedclothes, attempting to get out of bed, and sudden changes in activity are common).
35. Catatonia with speech approximating mutism.
36. Flushed face.
37. Elevated systolic blood pressure.
38. Flapping tremor of extended hands (called asterixis and most common with hepatic encephalopathy, but also seen with other syndromes).

Differential Diagnosis
1. Cerebral and systemic infections.
2. Post-operative, post-traumatic, and puerperal states.
3. Hyperthyroidism.
4. Excessive use of alcohol.

5. Substance withdrawal following dependence.
6. Pernicious anemia.
7. Cerebral vascular insufficiency.
8. Cerebral neoplasia, especially focal lesions of the right cerebral hemisphere and undersurface of the occipital lobe.
9. Adrenal insufficiency.
10. Substance intoxication.
11. Congestive heart failure.
12. Hyperparathyroidism.
13. Postconvulsive states.
14. Bromism.
15. Hypoxia.
16. Hypercarbia.
17. Uremia.
18. Hepatic encephalopathy.
19. Ionic imbalance.
20. Hypoglycemia.
21. Brain trauma.
22. Seizures.
23. Other organic states.
24. Delirium.
25. Schizophrenia.
26. Other psychoses with delusions.
27. Sensory deprivation.
28. Disassociated disorders.
29. Conversion disorders.
30. Factitious illness (such as Ganser's syndrome, pseudostupidity, pseudodementia, or pseudopsychosis).
31. Dementia.

Management

1. Physical examination and appropriate laboratory studies aimed at identifying the etiology is the first step in management.
2. The primary focus of treatment is the appropriate medical and surgical treatment of the underlying disorder causing the delirium. These patients should be kept on a medical or surgical unit with a psychiatrist acting as a consultant.
3. Until the etiology of the delirium is found and treated, fluid and electrolyte balance should be maintained. Care should be taken to provide an appropriate diet for the patient, and certainty that he or she eats it. Blood pressure, heart rate, and temperature should be monitored. If infection, hyperthermia, or circulatory collapse occurs, these must be properly treated.
4. If patients remain somewhat alert, reassure them and explain to them in a way they can understand what is happening.
5. Structure and simplify the patient's environment. A small night light counters nighttime confusion. Placing a calendar and family pictures in the room helps by

day to orient the patient. It is best to have one familiar nurse tend the patient rather than a number of them. A relative at the bedside with restriction of less familiar visitors is helpful.

6. When a patient becomes unmanageable, low doses of antipsychotics may be helpful. These include haloperidol (Haldol) 0.5–1 mg, perphenazine (Trilafon) 1–2 mg, fluphenazine (Prolixin) 0.5–1 mg, chlorpromazine (Thorazine) 10–20 mg, thiothixene (Navane) 2 mg, and thioridazine (Mellaril) 25 mg PO. Lorazepam (Ativan) 1–2 mg may also be used but can further confuse some patients and is contraindicated if respiratory impairment is present.

7. Central nervous system depressants such as barbiturates are contraindicated as they may increase the confusion. In addition, barbiturates are specifically contraindicated in acute intermittent porphyria, and in severe renal or pulmonary disease. Chlorpromazine tends to cause hypotension and should not be used for patients with cerebrovascular and cardiovascular disease.

Quality Assurance Issues
1. Were appropriate precautions taken for self-destructive and other destructive behavior?
2. Is there continued documentation of the evolving extent of the delirium?
3. Has there been an evaluation of the multiple factors contributing to the etiology of the delirium to facilitate remission?

Ethical/Legal Issues
1. Have family, friends, and patients been advised of how delirium impacts judgment?
2. Have patients and families been advised both how to avoid delirium in the future and how to recognize early signs, especially if medication-induced?

DELUSIONAL DEPRESSION

In addition to the unipolar–bipolar dichotomy of affective illness based on the presence or absence of a history of mania and the primary–secondary dichotomy based on the presence or absence of pre-existing nonaffective psychiatric illness (Nelson and Charney, 1981), there is the delusional–nondelusional dichotomy of unipolar affective illness.

History
1. Delusional patients tend to exhibit more agitation, guilt, and ideas of reference than nondelusional patients.

Management
1. Patients with delusional depression tend to respond poorly to antidepressant therapy alone.
2. Delusional depression appears best managed by either a combination of antide-

pressant medication and antipsychotic medication or electroconvulsive therapy (Charney and Nelson, 1981).

Quality Assurance Issues
1. Has the patient received continuous evaluation for threat of harm to self and others?
2. Has the patient been provided precautions to prevent harm to self and others?

Ethical/Legal Issues
1. Have patients been provided diagnostic-specific treatment for their depression?

DELUSIONAL DISORDER

Delusional disorder at various times has been referred to as paranoia, paranoid state, paraphrenia, and paranoid psychosis.

History
1. Patients with delusional disorder constitute approximately 1 to 4% of all psychiatric first admissions (Kendler, 1982).
2. It is predominantly an illness of mid- to late-life.
3. Patients with the disorder usually have been married (Kendler, 1982).
4. Unlike affective illness, but like schizophrenia, delusional disorder occurs more frequently in lower socioeconomic subpopulations and is associated with a poor prognosis for full recovery.
5. Delusional disorder is reported more frequently than schizophrenia or affective illness among immigrants (Kendler, 1982).
6. The disorder does not closely resemble either affective illness or schizophrenia from a demographic perspective.
7. Despite the fact that delusional disorder may somewhat resemble alcoholic paranoia, alcohol does not appear etiological in most patients (Kendler, 1982).

Management
1. An antipsychotic such as thiothixine (Navane), haloperidol (Haldol), or fluphenazine (Prolixin) (1–10 mg PO bid or tid) is generally sufficient to control symptoms. In some instances considerably higher doses are required.
2. Patients with poor drug compliance should be given a trial of Prolixin decanoate or enanthate. Generally 12.5–50 mg every 3 to 4 weeks will provide symptom control.

DEMENTIA

Dementia, like epilepsy, is a symptom of a number of illnesses. The management of some patients with these diseases (e.g., Huntington's chorea, cerebral neoplasia) requires close collaboration between a psychiatrist and members of other medical specialties such as neurology and neurosurgery. In an emergency situation, usually all that is required is either the separation of patients with true dementia from the so-called "functional" psychoses, or consultation regarding the management of patients already identified as having a chronic organic mental disorder who are deteriorating. At all times it must be remembered that patients who are demented are sometimes quickly cast into the genre of the "incurables." This is not always the case. Normal pressure hydrocephalus, vitamin deficiencies, cerebral infections, and cerebral tumors are all examples of organic brain disorders that present with dementia, which in some cases show remarkable improvement with appropriate therapy.

History
1. The term "dementia" implies a deterioration of intellectual ability as a consequence of malfunctioning cerebral cortical or subcortical cells.
2. Symptoms of dementia include disorientation, difficulty with memory, alterations in personality, impairment of judgement, and deterioration of other intellectual functions such as the ability to calculate and to abstract.
3. The disorder may be detectable any time after the intellectual quotient is considered stable (usually after age 3 or 4).
4. About 5% of Americans over age 65 are considered demented with up to 20% of those over age 65 living in the community reported to have cognitive impairment on testing (Balster et al, 1990). Being bright and mentally active enhances septuagenarians, but nevertheless overall vocabulary decreases, particularly in the categories of family, health, and occupation (Shneidman, 1989). By age 90, upwards of 45% of the population exhibits cognitive impairment (Odenheimer, 1989).
5. Reported predictors of mental disability in older age are low forced vital capacity and low forced expiratory volume, hypertension in middle age, low educational level, low body mass index, low serum cholesterol, low hemoglobin, low alcohol or coffee consumption, and presence of transient ischemia or stroke (Lammi et al, 1989).
6. People with organic mental disorders in the Iowa Record-Linkage Study (Black et al, 1985b) were at risk for early death (especially those younger than 40 years) from cancer and heart disease in women and influenza and pneumonia in men. Men were also at greater risk for death from accidents and suicide.
7. Many demented patients have treatable mental disorders responsible for progression such as depression and delusions (Zubenko, 1990).
8. Passive symptoms are more common among patients with mild senile dementia of the Alzheimer type than agitation, self-centeredness, and suspiciousness (Rubin et al, 1987).
9. The ratio of primary degenerative dementia to multi-infarct dementia is variously reported at 6:1 to 2:1 (Barnes and Raskind, 1981; Maletta et al, 1982).
10. Relatives of individuals with Alzheimer's disease are more likely to have the illness themselves. Risk to relatives decreases sharply with a decrease in the se-

verity of the illness. Relatives also have a higher incidence of Down's syndrome, lymphonia, and immune diatheses (Heston et al, 1981).

11. Patients with Alzheimer's disease show a marked decrease in life expectancy (Schneck et al, 1982).

12. It is uncertain at this time whether depression seen with Alzheimer's disease is an independent disorder or a component of the disease itself. If it is a separate illness it could be assumed that patients with Alzheimer's disease and depression may benefit from aggressive management of the affective illness (Knesevich et al, 1983).

13. The physical signs seen when examining a demented patient depend upon the underlying pathology responsible for the cognitive and behavioral changes. These are as numerous and varied as the number of illnesses causing dementia. For instance, normal-pressure hydrocephalus commonly presents with the triad of symptoms of dementia, fecal or urinary incontinence, and ataxia. Cerebral neoplasia generally presents with focal signs and symptoms.

14. Most degenerative diseases accompanied by dementia present with a gradual progressive intellectual deterioration together with diffuse neurologic signs. Sometimes a presentation may be confusing. Well-localized signs are usually indicative of a neoplasm, a cerebral abscess, a syphilitic gumma, a tuberculoma, sarcoidosis, or a cerebral aneurysm.

15. Careful neurologic and physical examination is always an important part of the evaluation of these patients.

Symptoms
1. Confusion.
2. Disorientation (first to time, then to place, and last to person).
3. Dysmnesia (with impairment of recent memory greater than for past memory).

Signs
1. Changes in personality (those related to the premorbid personality, the stage of illness, the part of the brain affected, the sociocultural matrix, the psychological response to the organic changes, and other pathophysiologic changes due to alcohol, etc.).
2. Impairment of judgement.
3. Emotional lability.
4. Occupational delirium.
5. Catastrophic reactions. (When patients are confronted with tasks they cannot perform, they may show evidence of sudden autonomic arousal.)
6. Difficulty calculating.
7. Difficulty abstracting.
8. Lack of impulse control.

In the later stages:

1. Paranoia.
2. Global loss of memory.

3. Total disorientation.
4. Motor unrest.
5. Perseveration.
6. Verbigeration.
7. Stereotypies.
8. Intellectual dullness.
9. Loss of sphincter control.
10. Complete apathy.
11. Inability to feed and clothe oneself.

Clinical Studies

1. Brief bedside screening tests are more effective in identifying mild cognitive impairment than the usual components of the mental status examination such as serial sevens, orientation testing, and three object recall (Roca, 1987).

Differential Diagnosis

The differential diagnosis is complex and a variety of classifications have been devised for clinical purposes. Practically speaking, the most important step is to identify those forms of dementia that may be effectively treated with arrest or reversal of symptoms.

Treatable Forms of Dementia

1. Addison's disease.
2. Some angiomas of the cerebral vessels.
3. Anoxia secondary to chronic cardiac or respiratory disease.
4. Cerebral abscess.
5. Some cerebral neoplasias.
6. Chronic subdural hematomas.
7. Electrolyte imbalance.
8. Endogenous toxins (as with hepatic or renal failure).
9. Exogenous toxins such as carbon monoxide.
10. Hypothyroidism.
11. Hypoglycemia.
12. Cerebral infections such as tuberculosis, syphilis, parasites, or yeasts.
13. Intracranial aneurysms.
14. Normal pressure hydrocephalus.
15. Pseudodementia (e.g., schizophrenia or depression).
16. Vitamin deficiencies.
17. Wilson's disease.

Untreatable Forms of Dementia

1. Alcoholic encephalopathy.
2. Alzheimer's disease.
3. Arteriosclerosis.
4. Behçet's syndrome.

5. Cerebral metastases.
6. Some primary cerebral neoplasms.
7. Creutzfeldt–Jakob's disease.
8. Dementia pugilistica.
9. Familial myoclonus epilepsy.
10. Friedreich's ataxia.
11. Huntington's chorea.
12. Kuf's disease.
13. Marchiafava–Bignami disease.
14. Mongolism.
15. Multiple myeloma.
16. Multiple sclerosis.
17. Collagenoses.
18. Parkinsonism/dementia complex of Guam.
19. Pick's disease.
20. Postconcussion syndrome.
21. Presenile dementia with motor neuron disease.
22. Presenile glial dystrophy.
23. Primary parenchymatous cerebellar atrophy with dementia.
24. Primary subcortical gliosis.
25. Progressive supranuclear palsy.
26. Sarcoidosis.
27. Schilder's disease.
28. Senile dementia.
29. Trauma.
30. Simple presenile dementia.

Management

1. The first step in the management of dementia is to separate that group of patients for whom there is a specific treatment. This requires in addition to the history and mental status, physical, and neurological examinations, a complete battery of other tests ordered as indicated such as:

    a. Laboratory studies. (These include a CBC, serum B_{12} assay, bone marrow studies, serology HIV test, erythrocyte sedimentation rate, serum albumen–globulin ratio, BUN, glucose tolerance curve, serum cholesterol, T_3, T_4, T_7, serum enzymes, serum copper, and ceruloplasmin. Urinalysis should be performed for presence of red cells and the Bence–Jones protein.)
    b. Lumbar puncture. (Opening and closing pressures are recorded and samples sent off for cells, protein, serology, viral titres, and appropriate cultures where indicated.)
    c. Skull and chest films.
    d Echoencephalography.
    e. Electroencephalography.
    f. Brain scan.

    g. CT scan and MRI.

    h. Cerebral angiography (if indicated).

    i. Neuropsychological testing.

2. When patients with a treatable form of dementia have been isolated, the specific treatment is initiated. In the instance of cerebral neoplasm, this would usually mean surgical extirpation, and at times radiotherapy. Ventriculoatrial shunting is the treatment of choice for normal pressure hydrocephalus. In case of thyroid or vitamin deficiencies, replacement therapy is indicated.

3. For patients with untreatable forms of dementia, individual and family therapy can help both patients and families maximize their strengths as cognition deteriorates. Obviously, in the later stages, any individual work with a patient may be futile. Early in the course of the illness, when there is only a mild memory deficit, patients can be directed to areas of activity that will allow them to maximize their strengths. Family members can use therapy to ventilate their feelings. This is especially important when dementia occurs early in life as with Pick's or Alzheimer's disease and leaves the patient's spouse solely responsible for the economic welfare and child-raising of the family. A therapist can help with many practical everyday problems, from helping to guide family members in taking over financial responsibility for the family to restricting car driving by the patient. Explanations of how unfamiliar situations may result in a catastrophic reaction may help a family to minimize demands on a patient that result in confusion or intense adverse emotional responses.

4. Familiarity of environment is a key in maintaining patients' orientation. Changes in their physical surroundings should be minimized. If hospitalization or nursing home placement is necessary, objects that are familiar to them like a favorite lamp, family picture, or religious object should be placed in their new bedroom. A night lamp is important in reducing the confusion present when a demented patient awakens in a dark room.

5. Psychopharmacotherapy is often helpful in management of demented patients but doses should be scaled down, especially if there is evidence of renal or hepatic damage (Raskin et al, 1987). Both agitation and depression specifically respond to pharmacotherapy. Thioridazine (Mellaril) 25 mg PO bid or qid is often helpful both for agitation and depression. Amitriptyline (Elavil) or imipramine (Tofranil) 10–25 mg PO bid or qid are more specifically antidepressant in the elderly demented patient. For excitement, insomnia, or agitation small doses of the phenothiazines may be helpful. Patients in their senior years may already have some extrapyramidal disease and the phenothiazines aggravate this. Unfortunately, while the antiparkinsonian drugs can be used quite successfully, in many cases they can provoke an atropine psychosis, as can amitriptyline.

6. In all instances, the patient should be encouraged to do as much as they can for themselves. Regression is always a danger and is not only destructive to the patient's continued functioning but also further frustrates, depresses, and angers those close to them.

7. Food and vitamin intake should be monitored, sometimes with help of daily weighings, and supplementary vitamins provided. Patients who are mildly demented and neglect their diet or abuse alcohol can develop additional cognitive changes.
8. There are several other considerations in the management of patients who are demented and deteriorating. These include:

   a. Recommending soft diets or tube feedings in the latter stages when swallowing can be impaired.
   b. Physiotherapy to improve a patient's functional capacity.
   c. Recommending use of a writing pad to patients who are not aphasic but because of a process involving muscles find it difficult to speak.
   d. Supportive devices for weakness of feet, hands, neck, etc.
   e. Anticonvulsants for seizures.
   f. Antispasmodics for muscular spasms.
   g. Antiparkinsonian drugs for extrapyramidal dysfunction.
   h. Antibiotics for infection.
   i. Custodial care when the family can no longer care for the patient by themselves.

9. Physostigmine has been used with some success to enhance memory. The mechanism of action is felt to be acute augmentation of cholinergic activity (Davis and Mohs, 1982).
10. Patients with the most severe symptoms of dementia appear to benefit the most from the use of antipsychotic medication, particularly if excitement, anxiety, uncooperativeness, or emotional liability are present (Barnes R et al, 1982).
11. Electroshock may be effective in management of atypical depressions in patients with severe degenerative dementia (Demuth and Rand, 1980).
12. Pharmacologic agents that have been employed with varying success in addition to those mentioned above include neurotransmitters, neuropeptides, psychostimulants, Gerovital H3, lecithin, and hydergine (which is reported to increase cerebral blood flow) (Reisberg et al, 1981; Newhouse and Bridenbaugh, 1976).
13. In addition to increased intracranial pressure and endocrinopathy, vasculitides and inflammatory processes causing dementia may respond to steroid therapy (Paulson, 1983). If improvement is not apparent, steroids should not be continued.
14. No one neuroleptic has proven more effective in management of cognitively impaired patients than another (Salzman, 1987). Choice of neuroleptic as of antidepressant is contingent on side effects and differential toxicity. Imipramine, for instance, causes more orthostatic hypotension in the elderly than doxepin (Sinequan) (Neshkes et al, 1985).

Quality Assurance Issues

1. Was the demented patient evaluated for the role played by depression in causing cognitive changes?

2. Was the demented patient evaluated for reversible causes of dementia before a program of custodial care was initiated?

Ethical/Legal Issues
1. Has the patient been provided protection from self-harm due to depression or poor judgment?
2. Have efforts been made to use the least restrictive interventions to manage the patient?

DEPERSONALIZATION

Depersonalization (standing back and perceiving oneself as an actor on a stage) and derealization (feeling unreal) are common experiences in a number of pathologic and normal studies.

History
1. Depersonalization is commonly experienced in adolescence, under stress, and when one is burned out in marriage or work.
2. In pathologic states of depersonalization, a person may cut themselves and watch the blood flow, burn themselves, or masturbate to feel more real.
3. Chronic depersonalization and derealization referred to as the depersonalization disorder is rare (Stein and Uhde, 1989b).
4. Onset, when it occurs, tends to be adolescence or early adulthood.

Differential Diagnosis
1. Depersonalization disorder.
2. Schizophrenia.
3. Dysthymic disorder.
4. Bipolar disorder.
5. Substance abuse (e.g., marijuana, PCP).
6. Major depression.
7. Dissociative disorder.
8. Multiple personality disorder.
9. Post-traumatic stress disorder.
10. Temporal lobe epilepsy.
11. Panic disorder.
12. Borderline personality disorder.
13. Medication side effects (e.g., indomethacin)

Management
1. Management is diagnostic specific.
2. Depersonalization disorder may respond in some instances to anticonvulsants such as clonazepam (Klonopin) and carbamazepine (Tegretol) (Stein and Uhde, 1989b).

Quality Assurance Issues

1. Has the patient been evaluated for organic causes of depersonalization?

DEPRESSION

The essential feature of any disorder with depression is depressive mood coupled with a pervasive loss of interest and pleasure.

History

1. Depression as a mood is not in itself a disease entity. We all are depressed at one time or another and only a fraction of these depressions will cause an individual to seek psychiatric consultation.

2. Of those depressions seen by physicians, there will be a number of underlying etiologies with various degrees of social, biologic, and psychological causations. Some may be entirely due to physiologic changes and a history will give clues to causation such as use of diuretics resulting in hypokalemia or the use of reserpine as antihypertensive therapy. There may be a previous history of hypothyroidism with a recent cessation of thyroid replacement. Other depressions will follow a clearly defined stress or major life event such as death, divorce, or job advancement or loss.

3. Depression may be subdivided into those depressive syndromes of nonpsychotic proportions and those of psychotic proportions. Some of these depressions will have primarily medical bases (e.g., hepatitis) or surgical bases (e.g., carcinoma of the pancreas) and are called secondary depression. Others will be what is traditionally labeled psychogenic and appear in some instances to follow a life event and may present with a strong family history of recurrent affective disorder, suicide, or both.

4. Depressions of nonpsychotic proportions are distinguished from those of psychotic proportions qualitatively by the presence in the latter case of certain symptoms not seen in the former, such as delusions and hallucinations. The depression of a nonpsychotic person may in fact, in selected cases, be of greater intensity with the risk of suicide higher than in the psychotic patient. In both instances, there may be a family history of affective disorders, the presence of a recent life event that might have been a precipitant, and a past personal history of depressions of nonpsychotic proportions, hypomania, or mania. Both types may be recurrent or occur only once in a patient's life.

5. A carefully taken history may provide clues to appropriate treatment both during emergency and consultation as well as for long-term therapy. One important part of the evaluation is to determine whether the change in mood can be viewed as posture assumed by the patient in order to obtain some gain, or as having a strong biologic basis with neurovegetative signs. In the former instance, clinicians should try to identify the secondary gain. In the latter, they should document the chronology of sleep loss, appetite loss, weight loss, social dysfunction, etc.

Clinicians should obtain some understanding of the degree of guilt and how realistic it is as well as of denied guilt. If guilt is denied by the patient but should be present, what are the reasons for the patient's failure to acknowledge its presence?

6. Try to identify what brought the patient to seek psychiatric help at this time. Some people are somewhat depressed all their lives and the help-seeking behavior is more of an indicant of a life stress than the presence of depression per se. Was there a recent major life event? Was there a recent loss, be it real such as the death of a loved one or divorce, or a psychological one such as loss of self-esteem? Depression may also follow a gain such as a job promotion. While this may signal an increase in status and money, it also means the addition of personal responsibility, loss of a relatively more dependent relationship, or moving to a position of social status for which the patient has had no preparation from his past personal life experiences.

7. Some patients who present with the symptom picture of anorexia nervosa have underlying affective illness and respond to antidepressant medication.

8. Varying presentations in different sectors of medical care, differing clinical acumen, and factors impacting third-party reimbursement contribute to what appears to be over-diagnosis of depression by psychiatric clinicians and underdiagnosis by primary care clinicians when rates are compared to those derived from use of the Diagnostic Interview Schedule (Schulberg et al, 1985).

9. Depressed patients tend to report more severe life events in the 3 months prior to illness onset (Emmerson et al, 1989). Premorbid effective coping skills are associated with better outcome on treatment (Parker G et al, 1986).

10. Women presenting with pregnancy-related affective disorder tend to be younger at age of onset, exhibit more premorbid emotional instability and be more severely depressed at baseline (Frank et al, 1987). Bipolar women appear particularly prone to pueriperal depression (Brockington et al, 1988).

11. Age at onset of illness does not appear to differ in patients suffering delusional or nondelusional unipolar depressions over age 60 (Nelson et al, 1989).

12. Two-thirds of 260 patients studied with *DSM-III-R* depressive disorders were found to concurrently have one other Axis I disorder, most often an anxiety disorder that followed onset of depression in most instances (Sanderson et al, 1990). In other studies, anxiety disorders are found to be a precursor syndrome in some forms of depression, suggesting depression and anxiety may represent different phenotypic manifestations of the same genetic predisposition (Paul, 1988) explaining the good response of many anxiety disorders to antidepressants.

13. Factors associated with depressions in older people include lack of a confidant, urban residency, widowhood, financial difficulty (among urban people), physical impairment and disease, and poor education (Carpiniello et al, 1989).

14. Prognostically patients with depression and mania associated with schizoaffective disorder do worse than those with major depression (Coryell et al, 1990) particularly if the illness is the chronic subtype.

15. The circadian rhythms of physiologic variables are disturbed in affective illness (Tsujimoto et al, 1990).

16. An enduring personality trait of depressed mood (e.g., "life is a vale of tears") is considered by many to be a variant of normal personality affect rather than a personality disorder or attenuated form of affective illness (Phillips et al, 1990).
17. The more strict the defining criteria for major depression, the greater the likelihood of a family history (Klein DW, 1990).
18. Identification of childhood depression is somewhat more difficult than recognition of the syndrome in the adult (Carlson and Cantwell, 1980; Angold, 1988). Major depressive disorder and alcoholism are more common in first- and second-degree relatives of children with depression (Puig-Antich et al, 1989). Children without depression but with separation anxiety disorder are at greater risk for the development of depression as adults (Puig-Antich et al, 1989).
19. Adolescents and young adults born in the years after World War II show greater risk of depression, alcoholism, and other drug abuse and suicide (Klerman, 1988).
20. In a study (Kashani et al, 1983) of 9-year-old children where point prevalence of major and minor depressive disorder were found to be 1.8% and 2.5%, respectively, parents more than teachers were able to detect the behavioral problems and negative self-perceptions in the academic performance of children.
21. Depressed children, like depressed adults, frequently (as great as 41%) suffer comorbid anxiety disorders such as separation anxiety disorder and over-anxious disorder of childhood (Kovacs et al, 1989). In children the anxiety disorder often precedes the depression and remains after remission of depression.
22. Depression of mentally retarded individuals is often overlooked, but if identified and treated can significantly enhance performance (Kazdin et al, 1983).

Symptoms
1. Depression.
2. Hopelessness.
3. Sadness.
4. Neurasthenia.
5. Negative self-image.
6. Feeling "blue."
7. Apathy.
8. Preoccupation with thoughts of death, suicide, and wishing to be dead.
9. Decreased sexual drive.
10. Loneliness.
11. Despondency.
12. Self-blame.
13. Worry.
14. Constipation.
15. Fearfulness.
16. Discouragement.
17. Desire to escape or hide.
18. Irritability.
19. Anhedonia.

20. Sleep disturbance (difficulty falling asleep, awakening during the night, early morning awakening, or hypersomnia).
21. Hyperphagia.
22. Feeling worse in the morning.
23. Loss of energy.
24. Tiredness.
25. Slowness of thinking.
26. Decreased interest in usual activities.
27. Mixed-up thoughts.
28. Fatigability.
29. Pessimism.
30. Guilt.
31. Diminished ability to concentrate or think.
32. Increasing use of alcohol and other drugs.
33. Psychomotor retardation.
34. Hypochondriasis.
35. Depressive equivalent (e.g., chronic headache, atypical pain).

Signs
1. Weight loss or gain.
2. Reduced animation of facies.
3. Psychomotor retardation or agitation.
4. Decreased salivation.

Clinical Studies
1. Psychostimulants given in a brief trial have successfully predicted in some studies (but not all) subsequent response of depressive symptoms to tricyclic medication (Goff, 1986). Oral doses over an extended period of time are more predictive than a single intravenous challenge dose.
2. A positive dexamethasone suppression test (DST) (continued cortisol nonsuppression) on discharge from the hospital has been associated with high rates of relapse and poor clinical response (Nemeroff et al, 1984). The role of the DST in identifying major depression remains controversial (Balcon, 1989) with hypothalamic–pituitary–adrenal cortical hyperactivity before the test one of the best predictors of nonsuppression (Poland et al, 1987). Rates of DST nonsuppression are high among children with depression and those with separation anxiety disorder (Livingston et al, 1984), perhaps reflecting a relationship of the disorders to each other and their response to antidepressant medication.
3. Subcortical hyperintensity on MRI has been found to be more common in elderly patients referred for ECT than nondepressed older people (Coffey et al, 1990b).

Differential Diagnosis
1. Reactive depression.
2. Depressive character style.

3. Schizoaffective disorder.
4. Chronic schizophrenia.
5. Acute psychosis.
6. Bipolar disorder, depressed type.
7. Borderline personality disorder.
8. Major depression.
9. Hypokalemia.
10. Antihypertensive (e.g., reserpine, Aldomet, propranolol) toxicity.
11. Steroid psychosis.
12. Hypothyroidism.
13. Cerebral neoplasia.
14. General paresis.
15. Cessation of amphetamine or cocaine use.
16. Carcinoma of the pancreas.
17. Hepatitis.
18. Postviral infection syndrome.
19. Degenerative diseases of the nervous system (e.g., Huntington's chorea, Alzheimer's disease, Pick's disease).
20. Cirrhosis of the liver.
21. Arteriosclerosis.
22. Infectious mononucleosis.
23. Hyperthyroidism.
24. Occult malignancy.
25. AIDS.

Management

1. Assess the suicidability along with other parameters. In addition to all those factors delineated in the section on suicide assessment (e.g., mental status, living situation, family history, previous attempts), overt hostility is highly correlated with suicide. Depressed patients who are argumentative, hostile, and irritable are at high risk. If patients are not psychotically depressed but grossly suicidal and impulsive, they will need hospitalization to protect them during the crisis.
2. If a patient is without any of the major neurovegetative signs of depression (indicating that an antidepressant may be appropriate) and without any evidence of a cyclic mood disturbance (suggesting that lithium carbonate may be efficacious), all that may be needed may be supportive psychotherapy around the crisis precipitating the depression, be it loss of self-esteem, job, lover, or something else. The task of the therapist in such instances is to help identify the loss and empathize with the patient around its significance. In an emergency room situation, some encouragement and direct advice may need to be given. A follow-up appointment may be scheduled to discuss what further treatment is necessary as well as the desire on the part of the patient to pursue it.
3. If the patient has sleep loss and is seen in the emergency room, a medication to guarantee sleep should be written. Diphenhydramine (Benadryl) 50–100 mg or flurazepam (Dalmane) 15–30 mg will usually suffice for the night. A more

definite plan can be worked out when the patient begins therapy where a clinician can monitor symptom response to medication.

4. As a general rule, antidepressants should not be dispensed in the emergency room. They take several days to weeks to impact and if taken in overdose can cause serious medical problems. Antidepressants, like lithium carbonate, should be commenced after physical examination and appropriate laboratory examination including an electrocardiogram. Patients on tricyclics, monoamine oxidase inhibitors, and lithium carbonate should always be under a physician's supervision.

5. The crisis intervention model of treatment is often applicable to the management of patients with depressive symptoms of a nonpsychotic nature in the emergency room setting. Patients may be significantly helped with a single interview in the resolution of a conflict and finding more choices available than they previously thought. This may entail social engineering such as referral to an abortion clinic if that is a patient's desire, or in other cases, referral to a variety of other social agencies that may assist the patient in financial, religious, or legal problems. All the patient may want is a home-maker to help out during a particularly rough time, a clergy person, or a lawyer to initiate divorce proceedings.

6. Once the need for hospitalization has been ruled out, the essential goals in the emergency room management of a patient with a depressive syndrome of nonpsychotic proportions is assurance of sleep, the instillation of hope that things will get better, and the sense that benefit can come from the psychiatric care the patient has plans to seek.

7. Combined psychopharmacotherapy and psychotherapy (Bellak and Siegel, 1983) has been found to be more effective in the treatment of major depressions and the delay the return of symptoms than either treatment alone (Kupfer and Frank, 1987). Early intervention in the depressive episode of a patient with recurrent affective illness has been shown to significantly reduce overall length of an episode (Kupfer et al, 1989).

8. Major depression in the elderly responds both to acute treatment and to prophylaxis, reducing both morbidity and mortality (Young RC, 1990).

9. Successful management of a depressive episode entails compliance with medication provided over the course of months and sometimes years (Abou-Salek and Coppen, 1987; Consensus Development Panel, 1985; WHO Mental Health Collaborating Centers, 1989; Paykel, 1989).

10. Melancholic patients are more likely to respond to drug treatment than to hospitalization alone (Nelson et al, 1990).

11. Follow up studies indicate that more than 20% of patients develop chronic depression after an index episode. Partial recovery occurs in 15 to 20% of patients, and 15 to 25% of those who recover relapse within 1 year. Only a minority of patients maintain complete recovery (Sargeant et al, 1990).

12. Monoamine oxidase inhibitors coupled with lithium have proven effective in treating some refractory depressions (Price LH et al, 1985). Central serotonergic pathways are assumed to mediate this response. Lithium augmentation has also proved effective with other antidepressants (Nierenberg et al, 1990).

13. Electroshock and/or antidepressants coupled with neuroleptics appear more effective in management of psychotic depressions than antidepressants alone (Kocsis et al, 1990; Spiker et al, 1985).

14. Tricyclic antidepressants with significant anticholinergic activity can adversely impact cognitive thinking and memory. Nontricyclic antidepressants such as fluoxetine and trazadone do not appear to do so (Fudge et al, 1990).

15. Serum levels of nortriptyline are increased with concurrent use of chlorpromazine (Thorazine) requiring less of the antidepressant to achieve therapeutic plasma levels (Geller et al, 1985).

16. Electroshock is a safe, effective, rapid-acting therapeutic modality for major depression (Coffey and Weiner, 1990).

17. The accelerating frequency of recurrence of successive episodes of affective illness suggesting an electrophysiologic kindling has been the basis for use of carbamazepine (Tegretol) (Post, 1990) and other anticonvulsants (i.e., valproic acid, clonazepam) in their management. Weight gain seen with carbamazepine use is believed due to improvement in depression and not a drug effect per se (Joffe et al, 1986a).

18. The dysfunctional attitude (Perelow et al, 1990) or learned helplessness seen with depressed patients requires sociotherapeutic and psychotherapeutic intervention to counter.

19. Alprazolam (Xanax) has not been demonstrated to be as efficacious as antidepressants in the management of depression (Hubain et al, 1990).

20. Monoamine oxidase inhibitors such as isocarboxazid are particularly effective in management of atypical depression (Zisook et al, 1985).

Quality Assurance Issues

1. Was the depressed patient evaluated for suicidal and homicidal risk?
2. Were antipsychotics used together with antidepressants in management of psychotic or delusional depressions?
3. Was a differential diagnosis developed to identify and appropriately treat non-affective psychotic and medical illnesses presenting with depression?
4. Was the patient evaluated to see if he or she had dementia presenting as pseudodepression?
5. Were antidepressants or ECT recommended for all patients with major depressive disorder?
6. Was risk of recurrence due to lack of compliance with treatment explained to patients and their families?

Ethical/Legal Issues

1. Was the patient evaluated for risk of harm to self or others before discharge from the emergency room/crisis unit/hospital?
2. If a patient was suicidal, were the least restrictive means consistent with the severity of the patient's suicidality provided to prevent self-harm or harm to others?

DERMATOSES
(Self-Inflicted)

Patients may be referred for emergency psychiatric evaluation who have been found to have dermatologic lesions suggestive of self-mutilation (such as the excoriations common to cocaine users who have dug into their skin to find "cocaine bugs" or the burn and cut marks of a borderline personality disordered person).

History
1. Patients with trichotillomania dermatitis artefacta and neurotic excoriations often deny they have any psychiatric problems (Gupta et al, 1987).
2. Suicide has been associated with psychogenic dermatologic disorders (Gupta et al, 1987).

Management
The management of the dermatologic disorder is the diagnostic-specific management of the underlying psychotic disorder. For instance, if trichotillomania occurs in a schizophrenic adolescent, it abates with successful management of the thought disorder.

Quality Assurance Issues
1. Has the patient been provided diagnostic-specific treatment?
2. Have appropriate precautions been taken to prevent self-harm?

DIABETES MELLITUS

Diabetes mellitus may produce psychiatric symptoms with hyperglycemia and, when treated in excess, with hypoglycemia. In addition, patients may develop psychiatric symptoms in response to having a serious chronic illness when stressors impact on the course of the illness.

History
1. Psychiatric diagnoses assigned to patients with early onset diabetes do not differ significantly from those assigned to other medical/surgical disorders (Popkin and Callies, 1987).
2. A number of neurochemical changes that result in enhanced hormonal and behavioral responsiveness to stress occur in insulin-dependent diabetes. In animal models, these changes appear to result from reduction in metabolism of dopamine norepinephrine and serotonin in the CNS (Rowland and Bellush, 1989).

Management
The management of the psychiatric symptoms entails both successful management of the diabetes by an internist or endocrinologist and management of the stress

and specific associated psychologic responses and psychiatric disorders by a psychiatrist.

Quality Assurance Issues
1. Are patients and families advised of means of support such as self-help groups in order to reduce the stress of managing diabetes?

DIGITALIS TOXICITY

Digitalis preparations are widely prescribed for congestive heart failure and other cardiac conditions. Psychiatric symptoms are side effects of their use and appear to be dose related.

History
1. Patients on digoxin and related compounds are frequently found to have toxic levels of the drug in their serum.
2. Cardiac arrhythmias are the most serious side effect. Anorexia, nausea, vomiting, diarrhea, and visual and other CNS disturbances are also frequently found.
3. Visual disturbances include chromatopsia (i.e., objects appear to have yellow-green edges or tints), scotomas, hazy vision, and flickering halos.
4. Psychiatric complications are seen more frequently in the elderly.
5. Chronic obstructive pulmonary disease (COPD), pneumonia, and congestive heart failure may also cause an organic mental disorder and either confuse or complicate the picture.
6. On admission, approximately 20% of patients taking digitalis preparations show signs and symptoms of digitalis toxicity (Wamboldt et al, 1986).
7. Depression is a frequent presentation of digitalis toxicity (Wamboldt et al, 1986).
8. Psychiatric symptoms can occur at therapeutic (not toxic) levels of digoxin and remit when the drug is discontinued (Eisendrath and Sweeney, 1987).

Symptoms
1. Anorexia.
2. Nausea.
3. Chromatopsia.
4. Restlessness.
5. Agitation.
6. Malaise.
7. Fatigue.
8. Hallucinations.
9. Illusions.
10. Delusions.
11. Irritability.
12. Labile mood.
13. Distractibility.

Signs
1. Vomiting
2. Diarrhea.
3. Delirium.

Clinical Studies
1. Serum level of digitalis confirms the diagnosis of digitalis toxicity.
2. Characteristic changes occur on the electrocardiogram as digitalis levels increase.

Management
1. Reduction or discontinuation of the digitalis preparation brings remission of symptoms.
2. Digitalis delirium is often a harbinger of more serious and potentially lethal side effects of digitalis. Cardiac consultation, with monitoring of the electrocardiogram, is sought to ascertain whether emergency coronary care is indicated in the acute toxic phase.

Quality Assurance Issues
1. Are all patients on digitalis advised of the potential for depression and delirium?

DISSOCIATIVE PHENOMENA AND TEMPORAL LOBE EPILEPSY

1. Patients with temporal lobe epilepsy may experience dissociative episodes as a forme fruste of the form of epilepsy or together with other temporal lobe epileptic phenomena.
2. Dissociative phenomena reported with temporal lobe etiology include alterations in speech patterns, handedness, and altered sense of personal identity, creating a clinical picture of multiple personality (Schenk and Bear, 1978).
3. In some instances, ego-alien behavior will be attributed to demons or alternative personalities.
4. Patients generally claim amnesia for the episodes.
5. In one study (Schenk and Bear, 1978), 33% of clinic patients with temporal lobe epilepsy exhibited some dissociative phenomena.
6. Dissociative phenomena occur in other psychiatric disorders and dissociative disorder may be misdiagnosed as temporal lobe epilepsy, bipolar disorder, or another psychiatric illness (Steingard and Frankel, 1985).

Management
1. The management is that of the specific disorder.
2. When dissociative phenomena occurs without other symptoms, signs, or clinical

evidence of a specific psychiatric or medical disorder, a trial of carbamazepine (Tegretol), valproic acid, or clonazepam (Klonopin) may prove beneficial.

Quality Assurance Issues
1. Have all patients with dissociative phenomena been evaluated for medical/surgical causes of the symptom?

DISULFIRAM AND ALCOHOL

Disulfiram (Antabuse) interferes with the metabolism of alcohol in the body. As a result of its interaction, the level of blood acetaldehyde begins to rise.

History
1. Symptoms of the disulfiram reaction appear within 15 minutes to $1\frac{1}{2}$ hours after ingestion of alcohol.
2. Individual response to alcohol varies among people taking disulfiram. Some show very little response to the ingestion of a considerable amount of alcohol, while others respond dramatically to very little.
3. The typical response after a small amount of alcohol is ingested is unpleasant. High doses of alcohol may lead to coma and death.
4. Some individuals on disulfiram are so sensitive that exposure to fumes of substances containing alcohol (e.g., rubbing alcohol) may set off a reaction.
5. The usual maintenance dose of disulfiram is 0.25–0.50 g daily.
6. Its use is contraindicated in patients with psychoses, cardiac disease, diabetes, cirrhosis, epilepsy, organic mental disorders, nephritis, psychosis, and in pregnancy.
7. Those who advocate the use of disulfiram feel that the unpleasant symptoms that follow alcohol ingestion will reduce the amount of impulsive drinking.
8. A single 500 mg dose of disulfiram results in a gradual increase in plasma disulfiram and its metabolites, with peak levels generally occurring 8 hours after dosing (Jensen et al, 1982).

Symptoms
1. Sensation of heat over the face.
2. Throbbing headache.
3. Nausea.
4. Dyspnea.
5. Apprehension.
6. Hyperventilation.
7. Sleepiness.

Signs
1. Sweating.
2 Facial flushing.

3. Bloodshot eyes.
4. Tachycardia.
5. Vomiting.
6. Hypotension.

Management
1. The treatment of a disulfiram reaction involves antihistamines and having the patient lie down if hypotensive.
2. If shock is present, the usual means of treating circulatory collapse, including administration of intravenous fluids, are used.

Quality Assurance Issues
1. Have all patients been advised of the signs and symptoms of the disulfiram reaction and how to manage it?

DISULFIRAM TOXICITY

Disulfiram (Antabuse) is used in the management of well-motivated patients with alcohol dependence to prevent sporadic unconsidered drinking. The disulfiram alcohol reaction consists of the rapid onset of diaphoresis, facial flushing, hypotension, and tachycardia after an individual who is on disulfiram drinks or is otherwise exposed to alcohol. Disulfiram alone, however, has a toxicity that is due to its biochemical and histopathologic effects and the effects of its three major metabolites: diethyldithiocarbamate, diethylamine, and carbon disulfide.

History
Clinicians should be aware of these symptoms and signs so that they are not confused with other clinical syndromes such as schizophrenia (Weddington et al, 1980). Hypomania has been reported when marijuana is used simultaneously with disulfiram suggesting an adverse interaction between the two drugs (Lacoursiere and Swatek, 1983).

Symptoms
1. Delirium.
2. Lethargy.
3. Loss of libido.
4. Psychosis.
5. Depression.
6. Mutism.
7. Negativism.
8. Stereotypies.
9. Staring.
10. Combativeness.

Signs
1. Unilateral weakness.
2. Meningeal signs.
3. Peripheral neuropathy.
4. Optic neuritis.

Differential Diagnosis
1. Disulfiram toxicity.
2. Bipolar disorder.
3. Schizophrenia.
4. Other neurologic and psychiatric illness.

Management
Reduction of the dose or complete cessation of the disulfiram will usually bring about amelioration of the symptoms.

Quality Assurance Issues
1. Have all patients been advised of the symptoms of disulfiram toxicity?

DUAL DIAGNOSIS

Dual diagnosis is the term used when two psychiatric illnesses exist comorbidly. Treatment of only one leads to either the appearance of a "treatment refractory" disorder or to rapid exacerbation of the illness. Obviously, in reality there can be triple or quadruple diagnosis. An anxiety disorder may be comorbid with major depression and both may be self-medicated with alcohol creating an alcohol abuse disorder. Psychiatric illness may be comorbid with physical illness such as panic disorder associated with mitral valve prolapse or AIDS associated with schizophrenia. In most instances, however, dual diagnosis refers to the coexistence of a psychiatric disorder and a substance abuse disorder.

History
1. Successful treatment of patients who are dually diagnosed entails careful evaluation to ascertain to what degree the substance abuse represents self-medication of a psychiatric illness, to ascertain whether the substance abuse itself has become an autonomous illness requiring substance abuse treatment, and to ascertain to what degree the two disorders may be occurring concurrently in a person biogenetically predisposed (Lehman et al, 1989). In some instances, it may be difficult to ascertain which symptoms are due to substance abuse and which are due to a concurrent psychotic disorder, as in the instance of a cocaine or amphetamine-addicted schizophrenic (Kulick and Ahmed, 1986).
2. Comorbid substance abuse disorders play major roles in the etiology and

prognosis of affective illness, conduct disorder, anxiety disorder, and attention deficit hyperactivity disorder in adolescents (Bukstein et al, 1989).

3. More than one substance may be abused in addition to whatever psychiatric disorder exists. For instance, it is common for cocaine users to "come down" with alcohol. This may lead to triple diagnosis if a patient is bipolar: alcohol abuse disorder, cocaine abuse disorder, and bipolar disorder.

4. Percentages of Americans surveyed who have ever used cigarettes, alcohol, or marijuana are 75, 86, and 31% respectively. Those using in the last month before the survey were 35, 55, and 11% respectively (Kreek, 1987).

5. Clues to dual diagnosis are presence of psychiatric symptoms before commencement of substance abuse, intensification rather than amelioration of symptoms after substance abuse ceases, and family history of psychiatric disorder rather than substance abuse disorder (Weiss and Mirin, 1989).

6. Age of risk for onset of alcoholism for those with genetic loading is as young as 15 years (Miller and Mirin, 1989).

7. The majority of violent offenders and fire setters have been found to have alcohol abuse disorders (Linnoila et al, 1989).

8. Fire setters and violent offenders who are alcoholic and have alcoholic fathers have lower 5-hydroxyindoleacetic acid concentration in their cerebrospinal fluid and are more impulsive, providing more corroborating evidence for the relationship between impulsivity, violence, and low serotonin (Linnoila et al, 1989). This suggests that serotonin agonists such as fluoxetine (Prozac) sertraline (Zoloft), paroxeline (Paxel), and trazadone (Desyrel) may be effective in their management.

9. A survey of patients with *DSM-III-R* borderline personality disorder indicated 67% had concurrent *DSM-III-R* substance abuse disorders, most likely of sedative–hypnotics or alcohol (Dulit et al, 1990). Other personality disorders associated with substance abuse are narcissistic and antisocial personality disorders. Personality disorder features commonly occur secondary to substance abuse, and successful management of the substance abuse disorder forebodes positively for the prognosis of the personality disorder (Nace, 1989).

10. Substance abuse and major depression are independent and interactive risk factors for suicide ideation and attempts in adolescents. The greatest concern for lethality is among older adolescents with suicide ideation who suffer both major depression and substance abuse (Levy and Deykin, 1989).

11. Repeated relapse occurs when substance-abusing patients who are depressed do not receive concurrent treatment of the affective disorder. Cocaine addicts in particular are more likely to have bipolar disorder (Sternberg, 1989) which, if unmanaged, can easily lead to relapse.

12. Prevalence of substance abuse among schizophrenics appears similar to that of the general population with the exception that hallucinogen and stimulant use may be greater in schizophrenics (Mueser et al, 1990). Cocaine and amphetamines are among the drugs most frequently used, probably due both to the nature of the illness and to treatment side effects that induce patients to use drugs with dopamine agonist properties (Lieberman and Bowers, 1990).

13. Concurrent psychoactive drug abuse impacts the course and outcome of schizo-

phrenia by contributing to both early onset of the illness as well as to exacerbations of the illness and treatment resistance (Turner and Tsuang, 1990). In some instances, also ironically, drug abuse is reported to produce symptom reduction in subgroups of schizophrenics who report feeling more energetic and less anxious and dysphoric while intoxicated (Dixon L et al, 1990; Lieberman and Bowers, 1990).

14. Comorbid alcohol abuse disorders and schizophrenia are associated with poor treatment response and adjustment (Duke et al, 1990).
15. Neuroleptic refractoriness is contributed to, even in the early stages of schizophrenia, by previous use of psychotogenic drugs. Treatment resistance and development of the psychosis may be due to the psychotomimetic impact on the dopaminergic system (Bowers et al, 1990).
16. Anxiety disorders, particularly adjustment disorder with anxiety or mixed emotional features, are seen in excess in chemically dependent populations (Goggans et al, 1990). Panic attacks were found to precede use of alcohol in 50% of cases in one study (Johannessen et al, 1989) of a series of 154 male alcoholics where 13% give a lifetime history of panic attacks, with 45% of those with a panic history suffering current panic disorder.
17. Self-medication with alcohol is more common with social phobias and agoraphobia. Generalized anxiety disorder and panic disorder are more likely to be sequelum of pathologic intoxication. Simple phobias do not appear related to alcohol consumption (Kushner et al, 1990).
18. Chronic lung disease has been found to be related to increased rates of both affective illness and substance abuse (Wells et al, 1989).

Symptoms and Signs

The symptoms and signs of dual diagnosis vary with the nature of the concurrent drug use and medical and psychiatric disorders, are dependent on whether the person is intoxicated or withdrawing from recreational substance abuse, and are dependent on the drugs concurrently prescribed and taken for psychiatric or medical disorders (if recognized and treated).

Management

1. The first step in management of dually diagnosed patients is withdrawal from the recreational drugs used so that symptoms and signs of concurrent psychiatric and medical disorders may be identified and diagnostic-specific treatment initiated.
2. Specific twelve-step and other substance abuse treatment must be provided concurrently with diagnostic-specific psychiatric and medical treatment after withdrawal is complete.
3. Patients must master non-substance abuse methods of managing stress of work and interpersonal relationships and suffering psychiatric or medical illness.
4. Patients must be able to say "no to drugs" and to drug pushers. This may entail a change in environment if a user was a lucrative source of income for a drug pusher or if the patient him- or herself was a dealer and made a considerable income as a drug entrepreneur.

5. Hospitalization or rehospitalization may be required to break the cycle of drug use and stabilize compliance with treatment of the primary psychiatric disorder.
6. Patients should be evaluated for potential for violence to self and others. Suicidal or homicidal behavior may result from drug use (e.g., from use of PCP, crack, or amphetamines), drug withdrawal (e.g., "crashing" upon cessation of cocaine use), and from a concurrent psychiatric disorder (e.g., major depression, panic disorder).
7. Obtaining funding for care of dual diagnosis is complicated by the naive belief that all depression and other psychiatric symptoms seen with substance abuse are due to the fact that a drug-using person's behavior is out of control or that a person who self-medicated a depression with alcohol or cocaine will not need concurrent substance abuse treatment if the primary psychiatric disorder is treated. Lack of providing reimbursement for appropriate care for the dually diagnosed leads to overutilization of emergency and inpatient services (Ridgely et al, 1990).
8. Adolescents who abuse drugs, if concurrently depressed, are at particular risk of more lethal suicide attempts, greater frequency and repetitiveness of suicide attempts, greater suicidal ideation, and measured seriousness of intention with a specific documented relationship between suicide by firearms and alcohol intoxication (Crumley, 1990).
9. Exacerbation of substance abuse during treatment results in increased severity and frequency of psychotic exacerbations. Psychostimulant use in particular complicates the course and outcome of treatment of schizophrenics (Sirois, 1990).
10. While both desipramine (Norpramin) and bromocriptine (Parlodel) have been used to reduce exacerbation of cocaine use, lithium carbonate has not been demonstrated to impact cocaine use (Nunes et al, 1990).
11. Alcohol-abusing schizophrenic patients are at greater risk for developing psychosis when taking disulfiram (Antabuse). Two reasons are posited for this observation: First, dopamine may increase as a result of blockade of dopamine beta-hydroxylase (the enzyme that catalyzes conversion of dopamine to norepinephrine) by disulfiram thereby enhancing the psychosis and contributing to treatment resistance. In addition, disulfiram interferes with monoamine oxidase activity and mixed-oxidative hepatic metabolism (Kingsbury and Salzman, 1990).

Quality Assurance Issues

1. Is every patient presenting with substance abuse evaluated for concurrent psychiatric and medical disorders that may have contributed to onset of substance abuse or been induced by substance abuse?
2. Are all dually diagnosed patients treated for both the psychiatric disorder and the substance abuse disorder?
3. Are any concurrent medical disorders identified and provided diagnostic-specific treatment (e.g., intravenous cocaine and/or heroin use and AIDS)?
4. Are dually diagnosed patients evaluated for suicide and homicide potential and appropriate precautions taken where indicated?

Ethical/Legal Issues

1. Are all substance-abusing patients evaluated for concurrent psychiatric/medical/surgical illness and provided diagnostic-specific treatment both for the substance abuse disorder and the concomitant illness(es)?

DYSPHAGIA
(Drug Induced)

Both tardive dyskinesia and Parkinson's disease are associated with difficulty in eating and swallowing. Malnutrition, aspiration, and sudden choking may result.

History

1. All problems with swallowing in patients should be evaluated to see to what degree tardive dyskinesia, parkinsonism, or another drug-induced phenomenon may be contributing and to what degree the impairment may result in a life-threatening problem.
2. Dysphagia is seen in 50% of patients with Parkinson's disease (Weiden and Harrigan, 1986).
3. Neuroleptic drugs are believed to induce dysphagia through blockade of dopaminergic transmission in the proximal pharyngeal and esophageal musculature, which are under central dopaminergic control (Weiden and Harrigan, 1986).
4. Postsynaptic dopaminergic supersensitivity contributes to the choreiform movements seen in tardive dyskinesia that disrupt swallowing by the hyperkinetic movements of the tongue and upper esophagus (Weiden and Harrigan, 1986).
5. Anticholinergics concurrently used with neuroleptics further contribute to dysphagia and choking deaths by impairment of the gag reflex (Weiden and Harrigan, 1986).

Management

1. The simplest approach to management of drug-induced dysphagia is reduction or cessation of the offending neuroleptic or anticholinergic drug. In some instances an alternative drug with less anticholinergic or dopamine antagonist properties is prescribed.
2. Patients who suffer severe tardive dyskinesia when off medication may necessitate being given instruction in cutting food into very small pieces before eating and swallowing.

Quality Assurance Issues

1. Are all patients who present with dysphagia evaluated for the role neuroleptics and anticholinergic medication may be contributing?

DYSTONIA
(Drug Induced)

Neuroleptic-induced dystonias have been reported to occur in 21 to 94% of patients on neuroleptics unattended by anticholinergics (Arana GW et al, 1988).

History

1. Drug-induced dystonias are especially common in patients taking high-potency, low-dosage neuroleptics, particularly with commencement of psychopharmacotherapy.
2. The muscles most effected are those of the head and neck. Oculogyric crises, torticollis, grimaces, opisthotonus, and posturing may be seen (Winslow et al, 1986).
3. Women and younger patients are more likely to suffer acute dystonic reactions. Twice as many women as men suffer these reactions (Winslow et al, 1986).
4. Patients receiving intravenous haloperidol (Haldol) seem at lower risk for extrapyramidal side effects than those receiving the oral form (Menza et al, 1987).

Management

1. In a review of data from nine studies (Arana GW et al, 1988), concurrent use of anticholinergic agents produce nearly a two-fold decrease in all neuroleptic-induced dystonias and a five- to eight-fold reduction in patients on high-potency, low-dosage neuroleptics with incidence and efficacy of anticholinergic prophylaxis inversely related to age. Young male patients were most benefitted.
2. Initial prophylaxis with benztropine serves to significantly reduce drug-induced dystonia and enhance compliance with neuroleptic therapy, with little risk (Winslow et al, 1986).

Quality Assurance Issues

1. Were patients at high risk for neuroleptic-induced dystonia provided anticholinergic drug prophylaxis?

Ethical/Legal Issues

1. Were all patients prescribed neuroleptics advised of the possibility of dystonic side effects?

ELECTROCONVULSIVE THERAPY
AND ORGANIC MENTAL DISORDERS

Intensity of electrical stimulation, placement of electrodes, age, diagnosis, concurrent medical illness and medication, and number and interval of electroconvulsive therapy (ECT) treatments impact occurrence and duration of cognitive changes with ECT (Mondimore et al, 1983).

History

1. ECT has been and continues to be a treatment for drug-resistant depressions, drug-resistant schizophrenia, and certain organic affective disorders.
2. A generalized tonic–clonic seizure is necessary for an optimal therapeutic effect (d'Elia et al, 1983).
3. Despite the fact that the use of unilateral (as opposed to bilateral) ECT reduces amnesia, more than two-thirds of British and U.S. practitioners use bilateral ECT (Fink, 1983). The reason pointed out for this preference is that induction of seizures is more difficult with the unilateral approach, particularly if benzodiazepines are used for sedation and anesthesia is deep.
4. ECT can initially impair memory of events occurring years earlier but recall is virtually complete by 7 months. Recall of information acquired a few days prior to treatment may be permanent and recall for information acquired 2 years prior to treatment may not be complete (Squire et al, 1981). Depression itself can impair registration of new information (and therefore recall) in the euthymic state.
5. ECT can cause an increase in blood glucose level as high as 20% for each successive treatment and therefore should be used cautiously in patients with diabetes mellitus (Yudofsky and Rosenthal, 1980).
6. Steroid-resistant depression caused by the collagenoses such as lupus cerebritis may respond to ECT (Douglas and Schwartz, 1982).
7. ECT may be used to reduce or eliminate psychotic self-injurious behavior in patients with severe mental retardation (Bates and Smeltzer, 1982).
8. Major depression with melancholia or psychotic features is the main indication for use of ECT in the elderly. In addiction patients with impaired renal, hepatic, or cardiac functioning (enhancing the risk of using antidepressants) should be given ECT prior to thymoleptic use to minimize both distress to the patient from the affective illness and harm from antidepressant side effects (Greenberg and Fink, 1990).
9. Patients with higher anticholinergic levels after ECT are at greater risk for development of post-ECT confusional states than those with low levels of anticholinergics (Mondimore et al, 1983).
10. During ECT, only a minimum amount of electricity reaches the heart because of the high resistance of body tissues and, therefore, ECT is safer for the management of depression in patients with cardiac disease than are tricyclic or tetracyclic antidepressants.
11. ECT is relatively safe for patients with pacemakers if a clinician is aware of the nature of a patients' heart disease and the properties of his or her pacemaker, if radiologic and ECT studies indicate that the insulation of the electrodes is intact and the placement of electrodes is proper, if a magnet is available to convert demand pacemakers to fixed mode if necessary, if medication with atropine is

avoided where possible, and if the patients' heart rate is monitored (Alexopoulos and Frances, 1980).

12. There is evidence that the combination of ECT and lithium carbonate use is associated with a severe acute organic mental disorder even in patients who can tolerate either treatment well when administered separately (Weiner RD et al, 1980).

13. Malignant hyperthermia, a rare hypermetabolic state, has been reported to occur more frequently after administration of certain drugs, particularly succinylcholine and anesthetics (Yacoub and Morrow, 1986). It is transmitted as an autosomal-dominant trait and is heralded by isolated masseter spasm after induction of anesthesia.

Management

1. Organic mental changes, including retrograde and anterograde dysmnesia, are aggravated by supraliminal stimulation. Induction of a seizure with minimum electrical energy is recommended to minimize confusion.

2. Unilateral stimulation of the nondominant lobe minimizes confusion (Daniel WF et al, 1983). It should be noted, however, that patients given unilateral ECT tend to show less improvement than those given bilateral ECT and tend to receive more total treatments independent of severity of illness, sedative drug administration, or age (Abrams et al, 1983).

3. Caffeine pretreatment intravenously has been demonstrated to effectively maintain seizure duration without any increase in mean stimulus intensity in contrast to electrical stimulus intensity dosing without caffeine-induced side effects (Coffey et al, 1990a).

4. Adjustment of muscle relaxant and anesthetic doses lessens ECTs amnestic effects. Doses of succinylcholine and methohexital are inversely related to seizure duration (Miller AL et al, 1985).

5. Intravenous dantrolene therapy is used for malignant hyperthermia with ECT (Yacoub and Morrow 1986).

Quality Assurance Issues

1. Was the patient's mental status evaluated before and after each ECT treatment?

Ethical/Legal Issues

1. Are patients provided the option of electroshock who are appropriate for it and may benefit from it?

ENCEPHALITIDES

Psychiatric symptoms with absence of sensory and motor findings on neurologic examination can lead to misdiagnosis of encephalitides as a psychiatric disorder.

History

1. It is probable that a number of patients with transient psychoses (or what is perceived to be a single episode of schizophrenia) were cases of encephalitides without sequelae. Obviously, if you don't think of it, you can't diagnosis it (Deaton et al, 1986).
2. Psychiatric symptoms (in addition to organic symptoms) can endure as a sequela to encephalitis (Deaton et al, 1986).
3. Clues to encephalitis are elevated temperature, delirium, slowing on the EEG, and increased white cells in the cerebrum spinal fluid.
4. Patients with the childhood exanthems often experience concurrent encephalitis or carditis that goes undetected if an EEG or EKG is not performed during the course of the illness.

Clinical Studies

1. EEG.
2. Lumbar tap.
3. CBC and differential.

Management

1. The patient is referred to a neurologist or specialist in infectious disease for diagnostic-specific treatment.
2. In addition to proper diagnosis and referral for diagnostic-specific treatment, a psychiatrist may provide concurrent treatment of the psychoses, as in instances where patients with AIDS encephalitis receive small doses of antipsychotics to manage the agitation and psychotic thought processes.

EPISODIC DYSCONTROL SYNDROME

Individuals with the episodic dyscontrol syndrome precipitously and impulsively exhibit violence (under little or no stress) toward themselves, other people, or property.

History

1. Increasing tension frequently precedes the dyscontrol act.
2. Episodes are repetitive, short in duration (lasting minutes to hours) and end abruptly.
3. Partial amnesia and relief of tension and guilt follow the act.
4. The dyscontrol acts include drug or alcohol abuse, acts of violence, traffic violations, job or school failures, and suicide attempts.
5. A childhood history of hyperactivity, learning disabilities, and head trauma, and a family history of violence, sociopathy, and alcoholism are usually described.
6 Electroencephalography frequently reveals nonspecific frontal lobe abnormalities, slow or sharp wave activity in the posterior quadrant, or 14 per second or 6 per second positive spiking in the temporal lobes.

7. Soft neurologic signs are usually found.
8. The temporal lobe/limbic system has been etiologically implicated.
9. Anger attacks that are uncharacteristic of an individual and occurring inappropriately to a situation have been posited to be a variant of panic attacks and of major depressive disorder because of their response to antidepressants (Fava et al, 1990).

Differential Diagnosis
1. Conduct disorder.
2. Borderline personality disorder.
3. Organic personality disorder.
4. Attention deficit hyperactivity disorder.
5. Panic disorders.
6. Major depression.
7. Alzheimer's disease and other degenerative dementias.
8. Schizoaffective disorder.
9. Schizophrenia.
10. Psychoactive substance intoxication.
11. Psychoactive substance withdrawal.
12. Paranoid disorders.
13. Dysthymic disorder.
14. Epilepsy.
15. Mental retardation.
16. Encephalitis.
17. Cerebral vascular disease.
18. Head trauma.
19. AIDS dementia.
20. Endocrine disorders.
21. Metabolic disorders.
22. Cerebral tumors.
23. Mania.
24. Intermittent explosive disorder.
25. Other neurologic illness.

Management
1. The first step is evaluation of the disorder to determine if a diagnostic-specific treatment is available.
2. Acts of dyscontrol tend to be managed by the spectrum of drugs used for periodic behavioral aberrations such as lithium, beta-blockers, valproic acid, carbamazepine (Tegretol), diphenylhydantoin (Dilantin), and clonazepam (Klonopin) and ethosuximide (Zarontin) (Andrulonis et al, 1980).
3. Episodic angry acts uncharacteristic of an individual have been reported to respond to antidepressants in some instances (Fava et al, 1990).
4. Low 5-hydroxy-indoleacetic acid has been reported in the cerebrospinal fluid of some patients with violent acts suggesting serotonin production is decreased. Therefore, serotonin agonists such as fluoxetine (Prozac), trazadone (Desyrel),

and buspirone (Buspar) should, in theory, play some role in mollifying violent behaviors.

Quality Assurance Issues
1. Have all patients with episodic dyscontrol syndrome been provided therapeutic trials of psychopharmacologic agents that will stabilize their episodic behavioral disturbance?

EPSTEIN–BARR VIRAL SYNDROMES

The Epstein-Barr virus has been found to cause a prolonged depression or fatigue syndrome (often lasting years) resembling neurosthenia.

History
1. Epstein–Barr antibodies have been found to be statistically significantly excessively present in patients diagnosed as unipolar depressives compared to schizophrenics, substance abusers, and controls (Dubner et al, 1987).
2. In the absence of signs (other than depression) of a chronic active Epstein–Barr infection, current data does not support determination of Epstein–Barr antibodies on a routine basis (Amsterdam et al, 1986).
3. Epstein–Barr virus may present as an acute mononucleosis (Amsterdam et al, 1986).
4. The most common presentation is that of a persistent fatigue syndrome.

Symptoms
1. The psychiatric symptoms of Epstein–Barr virus vary from those of a dysthymic disorder to a major depression with somewhat greater predominance of fatigue or neuroasthenia.
2. Myalgia.
3. Arthralgia.
4. Headache.
5. Sleep disturbance.
6. Dysattention.

Signs
1. Low-grade fever.
2. Lymphadenopathy.
3. Weight loss.

Clinical Studies
1. Epstein–Barr antibodies.
2. CBC and differential.

Management
1. Antidepressants are indicated for management of the depression in addition to

whatever care is prescribed by an infectious disease specialist for the chronic Epstein–Barr infection.

EROTOMANIA

Erotomania is the delusional belief that one is passionately loved by another.

History
1. Erotomania is a symptom seen with a number of psychiatric disorders.
2. Erotomanic patients as a group exhibit more manic and other affective symptoms (Rudden et al, 1990).
3. DeClerambault argued that erotomania was a discrete entity. If free of symptoms that comport the diagnosis with other disorders, delusional disorder is generally deemed the diagnosis (Rudden et al, 1990).
4. In general, the course is seen as chronic with symptoms being relatively treatment refractory (Rudden et al, 1990).

Differential Diagnosis
1. Delusional disorder.
2. Paranoid schizophrenia.
3. Affective illness.
4. Schizoaffective disorder.
5. Schizophrenia.

Management
1. Management is for that of the primary disorder. If the delusion of erotomania appears alone, neuroleptic medication is used.

Quality Assurance Issues
1. Was the patient evaluated for symptoms attending erotomania suggestive of a disorder other than delusional disorder, such as bipolar disorder?

ESTROGEN-INDUCED PANIC ATTACKS

Estrogen, like caffeine, marijuana, sodium lactate, yohimbine, cocaine, and isoproterenol, has been reported to induce panic attacks (Price and Heil, 1988).

History
1. Estrogen is a modulator of neurotransmitters in the CNS (Price and Heil, 1988).
2. Onset of anxiety and of panic attacks have been reported after the initiation of estrogen replacement therapy (Price and Heil, 1988).

Management

1. If estrogen therapy is needed and the dose cannot be diminished or discontinued with cessation of the panic attacks, management of the anxiety disorder is indicated in the same manner as when the anxiety disorder occurs alone.

FIRE SETTING

Fire setting is a symptom of many psychiatric disorders.

History

1. Fire setting (pyromania) is seldom if ever a disorder in its own right. In most instances it is a symptom of another disorder (Bradford and Dimock, 1986; Geller JL, 1987).
2. Hallucinations and delusions have been reported to be the motivation for arson in as great as one-third of the cases (Geller JL, 1987).
3. Among those affectively ill, manic patients are reported in particular to be prone to setting fires (Geller JL, 1987).
4. About 10% of both adult and adolescent fire setters are mentally retarded. Conduct disorders are common among adolescent fire setters and schizophrenia, alcoholism, and personality disorders are common among the adults (Bradford and Dimock, 1986).
5. Physical abuse and parental pathology are common in the homes of adolescent fire setters. In one study, alighting one's own home has been found in 50% of adolescent cases, with the primary motivation being revenge. In the same study, 50% of adults also set their own homes ablaze (Bradford and Dimock, 1986).
6. At least one-third of 10,000 fires in Canada considered of undetermined origin are believed due to arson and 15% of 900 Canadians who annually die from fire are considered arson-related deaths (Bradford and Dimock, 1986).

Differential Diagnosis

1. Mental retardation.
2. Organic mental disorder.
3. Schizophrenia.
4. Bipolar disorder.
5. Major depression.
6. Conduct disorder.
7. Personality disorder.
8. Alcoholism.
9. Substance abuse.

Management

1. Fire setters as a group have significant social deficits requiring a social learning model in the therapeutic intervention (Geller JL, 1987).

2. Psychopharmacotherapeutic, psychotherapeutic, and sociotherapeutic treatment of fire setting is for that of the primary disorder. Hospitalization is often required in the acute stage to avoid harm to property and person.

Ethical/Legal Issues
1. Have all patients with fire-setting behavior been evaluated for a medical/psychiatric/surgical illness and provided diagnostic-specific treatment?

FLUOXETINE-INDUCED DISORDERS

Although fluoxetine (Prozac) (a purely serotonergic agent), trazadone (Desyrel), and sertraline (Zoloft) are associated with fewer side effects than other currently used antidepressants, the changes in serotonin levels in the brain are associated with behavioral changes.

History
1. Common side effects associated with fluoxetine are agitation, sedation, diminished appetite, and headache.
2. There is no definitive evidence that fluoxetine induces suicide. Return of energy prior to amelioration of depressed mood and increased ability to concentrate associated with fluoxetine may lead to a perceived intensification of suicide ideation at a time energy is returning. This is seen with other antidepressants. As suicide ideation is a symptom of major depression, risk of suicide may increase in a depressed patient if energy returns prior to remission of the feelings of hopelessness, worthlessness, and helplessness (Teicher MH et al, 1990). Patients may also experience intensification of suicide ideation if they are treatment-resistant, as they experience lack of response to a fabled "miracle drug." This suicide ideation would be assumed to persist and worsen after discontinuation of fluoxetine as the depression worsens. Finally, in the period prior to a response, a patient may become anxious or even agitated. This coupled with hopelessness may lead to increased suicide ideation and risk.
3. Like other antidepressants, fluoxetine can evoke hypomania and mania in a biogenetically predisposed, depressed patient, (e.g., a latent bipolar) (Settle and Settle, 1984).
4. Fluoxetine is reported to reduce interest in alcohol consumption and to reduce body weight (Naranjo et al, 1990). These effects appear to occur unrelated to change in depression, anxiety, the alcohol sensitizing reaction, or side effects.

Management
1. If a patient is sedated with fluoxetine, it is given at bedtime.
2. Patients who cannot tolerate an increase in energy or who suffer sleep disturbance or agitation with fluoxetine are instructed to take the drug in the morning and trazadone (which is more sedating) at bedtime for sleep.

3. Mania and hypomania are treated with neuroleptics, lorazepam (Ativan), or both.
4. Patients who develop mania on fluoxetine should have the drug discontinued during treatment for the elevated mood. If depression recurs, either another antidepressant should be cautiously used or fluoxetine or another antidepressant concurrently used with lithium carbonate or another mood stabilizer.

Quality Assurance Issues
1. Have all patients on fluoxetine been advised of the side effects and monitored for their appearance?

FOLIC ACID DEFICIENCY AND EXCESS PSYCHIATRIC DISORDERS

Folic acid deficiency is associated with a variety of psychiatric symptoms including depression, fatigue, and organic mental syndromes.

History
Folic acid hypervitaminosis is comparably associated with alterations in mood, thought, and behavior including overactivity, excitability, euphoria, altered sleep patterns, psychosis, and irritability (Prakash and Petrie, 1982). The mechanism of changes seen with folic acid deficiency and excess are believed to be mediated by folic acid's impact on a neuronal level.

Clinical Studies
1. CBC and differential.
2. Serum folic acid level.

Management
1. Symptoms abate with restoration of normal serum folate levels.

FOLIE 'A FAMILLE

Folie 'a famille is a disorder where a persecutory delusion is shared among a family.

History
1. The most common shared persecutory delusion is that of *folie 'a deux*. Shared delusions beyond a dyad are uncommon with only approximately 20 cases reported of *folie 'a famille* (Glassman JN et al, 1987).
2. It is extremely rare that a psychotic belief of one family member is shared with another.

3. Glassman JN et al (1987) report six characteristics of families that develop *folie 'a famille*. These include repeated familial crises, an underlying threat or frank presence of violence, a dominant family member around whom the delusional belief evolves, relationships among family members that are ambivalent and mutually dependent, social isolation, and membership in the family being stable over time.
4. Family members who share in the delusion of the dominant figure tend to be female, passive, suggestible or histrionic, dependent, and less intelligent (Glassman JN et al, 1987).
5. The original delusion tends to be that a single person is persecuted. With time, the belief is expanded and the entire family is seen as the object of persecution.
6. As with other instances of paranoia, the individuals concerned do not tend to seek treatment because they do not see their belief of persecution as false. They are brought in by relatives, friends, or police when the belief impacts negatively on others' functioning or when their own physical health is beginning to be negatively impacted. Because of this, there are probably many families with the illness that do not seek help and therefore are not included in reported prevalence rates.

Differential Diagnosis
1. Delusional disorder.
2. Paranoid schizophrenia.

Management
1. Antipsychotic medication in doses appropriate to manage paranoid schizophrenia or delusional disorder is indicated.
2. In patients who are noncompliant, family members, friends, or clergy may need to be rallied to support the treatment program and insure compliance with psychopharmacotherapy.
3. In resistant cases, depot haloperidol (Haldol) or fluphenazine (Prolixin) may be needed.
4. Family therapy is required to enhance compliance with pharmacotherapy and insure reality testing is in tact.
5. If children are involved, it is advisable that child psychiatric consultation be sought and therapy initiated to prevent long-term deleterious effect on the reality testing of the developing child.

GAMBLING ADDICTION

Gambling can become an addiction and, like many other addictions, be quite intractable to treatment.

History
1. Gambling becomes a problem, causing people to seek emergency psychiatric

care, when losses exceed expendable income and when it is a pattern of spending sprees associated with another psychiatric disorder such as mania or substance abuse.

Management

1. When gambling is associated with another psychiatric disorder such as bipolar disorder or substance abuse, diagnostic-specific treatment is provided for the primary psychiatric disorder and group therapy or a self-help group for the gambling problem.
2. Financial and legal counseling may be required for patients to help reduce the stress of accumulated indebtedness.
3. In a study of 232 attendees at Gamblers Anonymous groups (Stewart and Brown, 1988), total abstinence was obtained by only 8% of all comers after 1 year and by 7% after 2 years from first attendance.

Quality Assurance Issues

1. Have all individuals addicted to gambling been evaluated for a mood disorder?

GERIATRIC EMERGENCIES

Adverse drug reactions appear more frequently in older people because of age-related body changes in absorption, distribution, excretion, and receptor site sensitivity.

History

1. Passive absorption of chlordiazepoxide (Librium) may be delayed in elderly patients taking anticholinergic drugs and antacids such as milk of magnesia (Salzman, 1982).
2. The increased fat-to-muscle ratio in older people leads to increased apparent volume of all psychiatric drugs with the exception of lithium (Salzman, 1982).
3. Hypoalbuminemia in the elderly is associated with increased drug toxicity (Salzman, 1982).
4. Alterations in hepatic metabolism with age resulting in decreased demethylation and decreased hydroxylation may be responsible for increased serum levels and prolonged excretion (Salzman, 1982).
5. The decrease in renal blood flow with age, with a reduction in drug clearance and decline in glomerular filtration rate and reabsorption capacity, leads to a decrease in lithium clearance and prolongation of time to reach steady-state lithium (Salzman, 1982).
6. Increase in CNS sensitivity to benzodiazepines and decrease in nigrostriatal dopamine and CNS cholinergic functioning results in an increase with age in sedation disinhibition; confusion with chlordiazepoxide, flurazepam (Dalmane), and nitrozepam, and an increase in extrapyramidal side-effects with neuroleptics and an increase in sensitivity to anticholinergic properties of psychiatric drugs leading to confusional states (Salzman, 1982).

7. Orthostatic hypotension is a frequent effect of psychiatric drugs in older people leading to strokes, heart attacks, and fractures (Blumentahl and Davie, 1980; Davie et al, 1981). The combination of tricyclics and other hypotension-inducing drugs is most frequently associated with falling. Underlying medical disease, particularly heart disease, enhances the likelihood that a patient will report such symptoms.

Quality Assurance Issues

1. Are all psychiatric patients seen with geriatric emergencies evaluated for occult or overt medical/surgical illness contributing to their problem?

GILLES DE LA TOURETTE'S SYNDROME

Gilles de la Tourette's disorder is described as a triad of explosive vocal utterances, tics, and imitative phenomena.

History

1. Patients with this rare disorder give a history of explosive involuntary utterances, either in the form of obscenities (coprolalia) or inarticulate noises such as yelps, grunts, coughs, and barks. These may be accompanied by sudden involuntary movements including vulgar gestures (copropraxia) and both verbal and behavioral imitative phenomena (echolalia and echopraxia).
2. Diagnosis is based on the presence of coprolalia or the more rarely occurring copropraxia.
3. The disorder occurs more frequently in males than in females.
4. Onset usually occurs before age 7 with an age range of 2 to 18 years. Onset is rare in adults but does occur (Burd et al, 1986; Marneros, 1983).
5. The course is usually progressive with waxing and waning of symptoms, but arrest may take place at any stage.
6. The disease is not believed to result in psychoses or any mental or neurologic deterioration.
7. Tourette's disorder has been reported after long-term neuroleptic administration (Stahl, 1980) and deemed a form of tardive dyskinesia. The pharmacology of both is considered similar with exacerbation by d-amphetamine and amelioration by haloperidol (Haldol) and physostigmine.
8. The pathophysiology of Tourette's disorder is comparable to that of tardive dyskinesia with both assumed to be characterized by dopamine–acetylcholine imbalance. Dopamine is assumed to be in relative excess and acetylcholine relatively deficient. Supersensitivity of postsymptomatic dopamine receptors, a possible cause of tardive dyskinesia, may also be a cause of Tourette's disorder (Stahl, 1980).
9. Multiple tics appear to be a mild form of the disorder (Pauls et al, 1983).
10. There is a high incidence of obsessive–compulsive disorder (OCD) with Tourette's disorder with a greater incidence of tics in both patients with OCD and their rela-

tives. Both OCD patients and Tourette's patients suffer a greater incidence of generalized anxiety disorders and unipolar depression (Pitman et al, 1987a).

11. Tourette's disorder has been reported to appear for the first time during pemoline (Cylert) therapy (Mitchell and Matthews, 1980) and not to remit after the drug was discontinued (Bachman, 1981). Pemoline has clinical indications similar to those of methylphenidate (Ritalin) and dextroamphetamine (Dexedrine) but does not appear to precipitate or significantly exacerbate the disorder to the degree the latter agents do.

12. Tourette's disorder and multiple tics appear to be diseases that are transmitted together in families with tics being a milder manifestation of Tourette's disorder. The severity difference appears to be a threshold phenomenon related to transmission. Female probands, although less common than male probands, had a higher proportion of affected relatives (Kidd et al, 1980).

13. The incidence of family cases may be underestimated because of the difficulty in ascertaining the true number of affected relatives (Hajal and Leach, 1981).

Symptoms

1. The first symptoms are usually uncontrolled, often explosive in the area of the head, neck, and shoulder girdle.
2. These may progress to include movements of the upper extremities, shoulder, and chest. Lastly, if at all, the lower extremities may be affected.
3. The movements tend to be brief and explosive.
4. After several months or even years, the vocal tics become apparent and consist of obscenities or inarticulate sounds.
5. Sometimes the coprolalia or verbal tics may be the presenting symptom.
6. Imitative phenomena are often seen such as echolalia or echopraxia.
7. Stress, anger, excitement, and fatigue may increase the intensity of symptoms while fever, relaxation, sleep, and drowsiness bring about improvement.

Signs

1. Sudden involuntary movements.
2. Explosive involuntary utterances and imitative phenomena.
3. The pathognomonic feature is the uncontrolled repetitive utterances of obscenities. The abnormal movements are *not* associated with a paroxysmal dysrhythmia on the electroencephalogram.

Differential Diagnosis

1. Tourette's disorder.
2. Syndeham's chorea.
3. Schizophrenia.
4. Encephalitides such as encephalitis lethargica.
5. Wilson's disease.
6. L-dopa toxicity.
7. Obsessive–compulsive disorder.
8. Tardive Tourette's syndrome.

Management

1. Haloperidol given in a dosage of 2–10 mg per day is effective in many cases. Dosage is regulated by disappearance of symptoms or greater occurrence of severe side effects of the drug. Doses greater than 10 mg may be required. Neuroleptics are reported to result in greater improvement across a range of symptoms in Tourette's than clonidine (Shapiro et al, 1983).
2. Antiparkinsonian medication should be given to counter the extrapyramidal side effects of haloperidol.
3. Symptoms and signs of Tourette's disorder resemble movement disorders seen as a side effect of L-dopa therapy. Interestingly, while its etiology still remains veiled in mystery, the disorder is treated by haloperidol, the most potent dopamine-blocking agent currently available.
4. Clonidine hydrochloride, a centrally active alpha-adrenergic agonist, has been found to ameliorate the disorder in patients who are unresponsive or can not tolerate haloperidol (Cohen DJ et al, 1980). Transdermal clonidine is reported to cause subjective (patients feel better) but not objective improvement in symptom severity in Tourette's disorder (Gancher et al, 1990). Abrupt withdrawal of clonidine hydrochloride leads to a rebound phenomenon with marked worsening of tics, increased blood pressure and pulse rate, and restlessness. Restoration of tic severity to prewithdrawal levels after reinitiation of clonidine therapy takes 2 weeks to 4 months (Leckman et al, 1986).
5. Motor and vocal tics have been reported to occur in adults treated for a minimum of 2 years with neuroleptics. Called tardive Tourette's syndrome, these tics are presumed to be a variant of tardive dyskinesia. Tardive Tourette's may remit after withdrawal of neuroleptics but usually requires haloperidol or clonidine (Munetz et al, 1985).
6. Calcium antagonists (such as verapamil) and nifedipine have shown some promise in the treatment of the disorder with fewer negative side effects and a sustained response (Walsh TL et al, 1986).
7. Pimozide is another option in the treatment (Walsh TL et al, 1986).
8. Akathisia due to increasing dosage of neuroleptics can result in worsening of symptoms of Tourette's disorder (Weiden and Bruun, 1987).

Ethical/Legal Issues

1. Are all Tourette's patients who are prescribed neuroleptics advised of the risk of tardive dyskinesia?
2. Are all patients on neuroleptics for Tourette's syndrome monitored for emergence of signs of tardive dyskinesia?

GLOBUS SYNDROME

Globus hystericus is a syndrome wherein afflicted patients report a fear of intermittently choking and being unable to breathe.

History

1. If untreated, patients with the globus syndrome may require aggressive medical care due to life-threatening weight loss or may become markedly disabled (Brown et al, 1986b). In others, dietary restrictions limit social activities.
2. Generally, patients with the globus syndrome report the sensation of "a lump in their throat."
3. Some patients recognize that the sensation remits with swallowing, others are phobic if eating solid or dry foods (Bishop and Riley, 1988).

Management

1. Patients with this disorder are reported to respond to antidepressant therapy (Brown et al, 1986b).
2. In addition to medication, psychotherapy is indicated to manage the stress precipitating the symptoms (Bishop and Riley, 1988).

Quality Assurance Issues

1. Was the patient evaluated to ascertain if a physical illness is present that may impact neuronal enervation of the esophageal tract or a muscle disease of the esophagus?

GLUTETHIMIDE ADDICTION AND HYPOCALCEMIC-INDUCED ORGANIC MENTAL DISORDERS

Drugs such as phenobarbital, diphenylhydantoin, and glutethimide are known to alter vitamin D metabolism. The mechanism is thought to be enhancement of vitamin D degradation following induction of hepatic enzymes as well as perhaps a direct cellular effect on the intestine (Hahn, 1980).

History

1. The changes in mood, thought, and behavior, such as depression and pseudo-dementia, characteristic of severe hypocalcemia, are seen (Rober et al, 1981).

Management

1. Management consists of cessation of the etiologic agent (e.g., glutethimide) and restoration of calcium balance using appropriate medical therapies.

GROUP HYSTERIA

After a personal or collective tragedy such as a death, rape, or fire, a number of individuals may present bereaved in an emergency room. It soon becomes apparent what has happened, but the evaluation and treatment of a group of stressed individuals is more difficult than that of a single individual in crisis. There may be much crying, anger, hostility, and hopelessness. At times some may give evidence of a psychophysiologic response such as fainting. The group may be composed of all members of one family, all tenants of one building that burned, or some other combination, such as two families—one of a murdered girl, the other the family of her murderer (who was also her husband). As the members of the group continue to interact, symptoms may spiral in intensity.

Symptoms and Signs

1. The symptoms predominating in the group are often those of one or two key persons. When the key person screams, others scream in a way in which one might assume there is competition to see who will be most vocal. When a key person cries, others may follow suit. If one faints, others comparably may faint.
2. The overt display of emotion seems to vary from one subculture to another. Some ethnic groups such as the Puerto Ricans allow a much greater display of grief than others such as Anglo Saxons who may be cautioned by a relative to keep a "stiff upper lip."
3. A significantly higher increase of previous loss (e.g., parental divorce, death within the family) have been found among children most vulnerable to mass hysteria (Small and Nicholi, 1982).

Management

1. The key figure or figures should be separated out from the rest of the group, evaluated, and treated using the crisis intervention approach to therapy.
2. Calmer supportive family members, friends, and community leaders, such as the family's clergy person (minister, priest, or rabbi), should be called upon both to help in the management of the acute crisis as well as to make them aware of the family or group's need for support during the critical period.
3. If an individual had died in the emergency room, friends and family members should be allowed to see the body before it is taken to the morgue. This is best done by having an aide take a few people at a time to view the body, then have them go on home, and another few brought in until all have seen the body.
4. Offering coffee or another beverage sometimes calms a family in crisis.
5. In some cases oral antianxiety agents may be necessary such as 1–2 mg of lorazepam (Ativan) PO or diazepam (Valium) 2–10 mg PO to take the edge off the anxiety.
6. Sleep and good food are simple considerations often neglected in the management of bereaved patients.
7. Those less directly involved with the deceased, but supportive and interested, such as friends of the bereaved individuals, should be encouraged to either stay with the bereaved if the bereaved live alone, or invite the bereaved over to their own home or prepare some food for them.
8. It may be necessary to prescribe a sleep medication such as Dalmane, Halcion, or Benadryl for 1 to 5 days.

HALLUCINOGEN FLASHBACKS

Flashbacks are recurrences of symptoms experienced by the hallucinogenic drug user long after the original experience or experiences.

History
1. Flashbacks are usually brief, lasting only minutes and significantly attenuated in intensity. When lasting longer or if they are more intense, they can be quite frightening and can be confused with the micropsychotic episodes experienced by some individuals of borderline personality disorder.
2. Flashbacks may occur after one or several episodes of hallucinogenic use.

Symptoms
1. Intense panic.
2. Intensification of colors.
3. Visual illusions.
4. Synesthesias.
5. Pseudohallucinations.
6. Paresthesia.
7. Depersonalization.
8. Derealization.
9. Intense loneliness.
10. Depression sometimes to near or actual suicide proportions.
11. Paranoia.

Physical Signs
None.

Management
1. Flashbacks are usually self-limited and do not require any treatment other than reassurance.
2. Ten to twenty milligrams of diazepam (Valium) or 2–4 mg of alprazolam ،Xanax) or the equivalent dosage of another benzodiazepine can be given if there is an excess of anxiety at the time of recurrence.
3. If there is considerable depersonalization or derealization or psychotic symptoms such as paranoia, an antipsychotic such as 5–10 mg of thiothixene (Navane) or 50–100 mg of chlorpromazine (Thorazine) should be given.
4. The patient should be instructed to avoid all further hallucinogen use, including marijuana.
5. Persistances of flashback or intensification of symptoms requires extended neuropsychiatric evaluation to rule out an insidious organic process or more severe psychopathology.

Quality Assurance Issues
1. Was the patient evaluated for a psychiatric disorder other than substance abuse or temporal lobe epilepsy?

HALLUCINOGEN HALLUCINOSIS, DELUSIONAL DISORDER, AND AFFECTIVE DISORDER

Hallucinogenic drugs include lysergic acid diethylamide (LSD), mescaline, 2,5 dimethoxy-4-ethyl-amphetamine (STP), diethyltryptamine (DET), psilocybin, and dimethyltryptamine (DMT). Phencyclidine (PCP), marijuana and its active ingredient tetrahydrocannabinol (THC), hashish, Jimpson pod, nutmeg, and atropine-like substances such as Angel's trumpet are also sometimes referred to as hallucinogens, but differ structurally from those discussed in this section and are, therefore, considered separately. Most hallucinogens are structurally related to catecholamines (e.g., mescaline) or to serotonin (e.g., lysergic acid diethylamide).

History
1. Frequently, but not always, individuals presenting with a hallucinogen hallucinosis will give a history of having taken a hallucinogen by name (e.g., mescaline, DMT); of "dropping acid"; of "taking dope", "blotter", "microdot" or "purple haze"; or of having eaten morning glory seeds, nutmeg, psilocybin (mushrooms), cactus buttons (peyote), Jimpson pod, or other substances with hallucinogenic properties.
2. The effects of many hallucinogens are difficult to distinguish clinically. Stimulants such as cocaine and methedrine may be added to provide a kick. Strychnine is also sometimes added and can result in serious medical consequences including death.
3. Morning glory seeds and nutmeg (myristica) are readily available in food stores and garden shops and produce symptoms of psychosis if ingested in sufficient quantities.
4. The symptoms of a hallucinogen hallucinosis generally occur in a state of full alertness.
5. The symptom picture represents an interaction of:
   a. A given drug,
   b. The dosage taken,
   c. The duration of action,
   d. The effects of other drugs the individual has taken concurrently or which adulterate the hallucinogen,
   e. The rate of onset of the drug,
   f. The user's premorbid personality and physical health,
   g. The expectations of the user, and
   h. The setting in which the drugs are taken.
6. Hallucinogen users, unlike most schizophrenics or individuals toxic with sympa-

thomimetic substances or atropine-like drugs, are frequently aware that what is happening to them is the effect of a drug.

7. Low doses of hallucinogens will create a clinical picture resembling cannabis intoxication and may be mistaken for it.

8. Prolonged psychosis following hallucinogen use may relate to a genetic vulnerability to schizophrenic or affective illness. The fact that several hallucinogens are indole derivatives (e.g., LSD, DMT, DET, and psilocybin) or catecholamine derivatives (e.g., mescaline) raises the possibility that the psychosis may reflect a particular vulnerability of central serotonergic or catechol neuronal systems to the biochemical stressor.

9. Onset of symptoms generally begins within 1 hour of ingestion. The typical hallucinogen hallucinosis resolves in 4 to 16 hours untreated, but may last as long as 2 to 3 days.

10. Organic delusional disorders or affective disorders that persist beyond the period of direct effect of the hallucinogen used are referred to as hallucinogen delusional disorder and hallucinogenic affective disorder.

11. Mania has been reported to follow ingestion of LSD or an LSD analogue (Lake et al, 1981).

Symptoms

1. Distortions of body image.
2. Kaleidoscopic and other visual hallucinations.
3. Synesthesia (e.g., a sound produces a sensation of color).
4. Increased vividness of both real and fantasized sensory perceptions.
5. Confusion.
6. Visual illusions.
7. Alteration of mood, often in the direction of euphoria, but depression may also occur.
8. Pseudohallucinations (appearance of geometric figures and forms that the patient knows are not real).
9. Increased distractibility.
10. Impaired judgement.
11. Paranoia.
12. Anxiety, sometimes of panic proportions.
13. Fear of going crazy.
14. Lability of mood.
15. Feeling of having special insights or religious experiences.
16. Blurring of vision.
17. Depersonalization.
18. Derealization.
19. Difficulty expressing thoughts.
20. Hyperacusis.
21. Distortion of time such that everything appears to be happening more slowly.
22. Over-attention to detail.
23. Auditory hallucinations (rare).

24. Tactile hallucinations (rare).
25. Palpitations.
26. Violence to self or others (rare).

Physical Signs
1. Dilated, reactive pupils.
2. Sweating.
3. "Gooseflesh."
4. Slight increase in body temperature.
5. Tremors.
6. Slight increase in blood pressure.
7. Tachycardia.
8. Incoordination.

Differential Diagnosis
1. Hallucinogen hallucinosis, delusional disorder, or affective disorder.
2. Atropine-like drug intoxication.
3. Sympathomimetic intoxication.
4. Other toxic organic states.
5. Schizophrenia.
6. Micropsychotic episode in a patient with borderline personality disorder.
7. Mania.

Management
1. The level of some hallucinations can be detected in the serum to guide treatment.
2. Patients should be placed in a well-lit, quiet, nondistracting room away from disturbing noises and intrusive people.
3. Reassure patients that they are not becoming insane, but that the alterations in perception are due to the drug they took.
4. Help orient patients by mentioning where they are, the day, and the time. This process may have to be repeated several times and is referred to as "talking down" the patient.
5. Have a close friend or relative, if available, stay with patient to support, to alert, and to keep patients from harming themselves or others.
6. If sedation is necessary, diazepam (Valium) 20–40 mg may be given followed by 10 mg every hour until calm. Alternately, an equivalent dose of another benzodiazepine may be utilized.
7. If a patient is particularly disturbed, haloperidol (Haldol) or thiothixene (Navane) may be given. There have been reports that administration of chlorpromazine (Thorazine) is not safe with STP and therefore a benzodiazepine is preferred, and any antipsychotic given only with caution.
8. If psychosis persists, the possibility that the patient was psychotic prior to hallucinogen use should be considered and the psychosis treated appropriately. Contaminant drugs and underlying predisposition to psychosis or hysterical character features may contribute to prolongation of psychotic symptoms. It is, of

course, also possible that an hallucinogen may cause biologic changes in the brain that result in a more enduring psychosis.

9. Lack of response to medication or "talking down" within 6 to 16 hours may necessitate hospitalization.
10. Even if a patient is medicated, symptoms may return after the effect of the medication wears off and patients may then present again as a risk to themselves or others. Therefore, if the patients are not hospitalized following a bad trip, care should be taken to assure that patients are with another person such as a family member, lover, or friend. This person should be charged with the task of staying with the patient for 24 hours and to provide the prescribed medication if symptoms re-emerge and to return the patient to the emergency room if needed.
11. L-5-hyroxytryptophan, the serotonin precursor, has been found to be effective in relieving the symptoms of LSD psychosis, suggesting that some LSD-induced psychotic disorders may be caused by relative differences of CNS serotonin (Abraham, 1983).

Quality Assurance Issues

1. Was the patient evaluated to ascertain if the patient has a concurrent psychiatric disorder (e.g., schizophrenia) together with acute hallucinogenic psychosis?
2. Have all patients with hallucinogen-induced disorders been evaluated for other psychiatric illnesses that they are self-medicating?
3. Have all patients with hallucinogen-induced disorders been evaluated for concomitant use of other recreational drugs?

Ethical/Legal Issues

1. Have all patients with hallucinogen-induced disorders been evaluated for risk of harm to self or others?

HANDICAPPED PATIENT EMERGENCIES

In addition to the spectrum of psychiatric disorders that occur with all individuals, handicapped patients suffer specific problems due to the unique stresses of being handicapped. Also, the fact that they suffer the pain of limited functioning and control places them at greater risk for certain psychiatric disorders.

History

1. Handicapped people as a group are at greater risk for alcohol-related and drug-related problems and depression. As a family history of substance abuse and alcohol abuse problems is also more frequently reported in this group, it is possible that, in addition to the stress of dysfunction contributing to the increased morbidity, in some instances accidents may have resulted from drug or alcohol abuse or depression contributing to guilt and anger over the resultant injury and subsequent handicap (Motet-Grigoras and Schuckit, 1986).

2. Specific problems of being handicapped include limited access to the environment, restriction of daily routine due to extra hours required for personal care, communication problems in the hearing- and speech-handicapped, mobility problems in the blind and in amputees, and stereotyped perceptions of how handicapped people act and feel (Motet-Grigoras and Schuckit, 1986).
3. The need for assistance contributes to feelings of isolation and dependency that are determined in part by the nature of the handicap, the degree of limitation of functioning, and the age of onset (Motet-Grigoras and Schuckit, 1986).
4. Deaf people are reported to exhibit more paranoia as a group.

Management
1. The management of the psychoactive illness is diagnostic-specific (e.g., antidepressants for major depressive disorder).
2. Self-help, handicap-specific support groups (often using an adaptation of the AA philosophy: e.g., "Lord grant me the serenity to accept that which I cannot change, the strength to change what I can, and the wisdom to know the difference," "One day at a time," "Easy does it") are an important adjunctive therapy for all.

HEADACHE

Patients may appear in the psychiatric emergency room with the complaint of headache when referred by another specialist who believes the basis of the pain to be psychogenic or for help in management of a patient with headache of documented organic etiology (e.g., amitriptyline [Elavil] for headache due to a cerebral tumor) and when the headache is a symptom of a psychiatric disorder (e.g., racing thoughts with the feeling one's head is exploding with mania).

History
1. Headache is a relatively common symptom in community surveys with four or more headaches in the preceding 4 weeks reported by 6.1% of men and 14.0% of females from ages 12 through 29 in one study (Linet MS et al, 1989). Three percent of the men and 7.4% of the women were diagnosed to suffer migraine.

Management
1. No matter how the clinical presentation of a headache is suggestive of a psychiatric disorder or how many internists or neurologists believe the headache to be without physical course, recurrent evaluation should be performed if the symptoms persist. A patient may have an occult cerebral aneurysm or episodic severe hypertension.
2. Management is diagnostic-specific after a differential diagnosis is enumerated and a presumptive diagnosis arrived at through history, clinical investigations, and physical examination.
3. In some instances concurrent treatment by another specialist and a psychiatrist

may be required if a symptom is found to have an organic origin (e.g., migraine) but the symptom is particularly severe.

Quality Assurance Issues

1. Was a differential diagnosis elaborated and nonpsychiatric causes sought?
2. Is a patient recurrently evaluated to ascertain if any new evidence has emerged to suggest a nonpsychiatric disorder?
3. Has care been provided to avert drug addiction with a patient at risk for substance abuse and chronic headache?

HEAD INJURY

Head injury may result in a number of neurologic and psychiatric complications that a psychiatrist may be called upon to manage.

History

1. The circumstances of a head injury may contribute to development of a posttraumatic stress disorder in addition to the symptoms of the injury itself.
2. Approximately 26% of all deaths due to injury are due to a head injury. Motor vehicles account for 57% of head injuries; falls, 13%; and firearms, 14%. Of head injuries from firearms, homicide attempts accounted for 29% and suicide attempts for 63% (Bell, 1989).
3. The problem of head injury is particularly great among young adults, accounting for as many as 15% of deaths in this age group in the United Kingdom (McClelland, 1988). The fact that the survivors of head injury are predominantly adolescents and young adults with normal life expectancies places an exceptional burden on families and friends in addition to the burden of the patient whose psychological pain must be minimized and functioning maximized.
4. Severe head injury is a risk factor for marital aggression. In addition there is a correlation between child abuse and head injury and a significant association with alcohol abuse (Rosenbaum and Hoge, 1989).

Management

1. The cause of a head injury may lead to exceptional stress for families, lovers, and friends as well as for the victim. Compassionate friends provide support for survivors of loss of a child regardless the cause. People who have lost someone to suicide or homicide may usually find the specific support of people who have suffered a homicide or suicide more supportive than that of those who suffered loss to more "natural causes." Nothing helps one to understand as much as to be understood.
2. Couples and family therapy may be required if aggression or other personality or cognitive changes impair couple and family functioning and threaten survival of the couple or family as a result.
3. Obsessive–compulsive disorder reported as a possible sequelum of head injury is

managed in the usual way (e.g., clomipramine [Anafranil], fluoxetine [Prozac]). The depression and anxiety accompanying the obsessive concerns regarding the head injury in most instances remits with amelioration of the obsessive ruminations. Compensation payment is a factor in both maintenance and remission of the symptoms (Drummond and Gravestock, 1988).

4. Childhood head trauma may be a risk factor for later psychosis especially of a schizophreniform nature (Wilcox and Nasrallah, 1987). The nonspecific delusions and hallucinations that may appear immediately or arise later, and which are assumed to be related, respond to neuroleptics.

5. Bipolar disorder can be precipitated by head injury. When cerebral trauma-precipitated bipolar disorder is unresponsive to other therapeutic interventions, valproate has been demonstrated to be effective in some instances (Pope et al, 1988).

Quality Assurance Issues
1. Have efforts been made to reduce the persistence of psychological morbidity due to unresolved legal matters?

HEART FAILURE

Psychological symptoms, both preceding and following a myocardial infarction or severe coronary disease, bring patients to seek emergency psychiatric help.

History
1. In the absence of a history of a myocardial infarction or other coronary heart disease, mounting or episodic anxiety to panic proportions may be mistaken for panic disorder or a generalized anxiety disorder.

2. Decreasing energy, malaise, and mild depression may precede a heart attack (Appels, 1990).

3. When present, chest pain or dyspnea can alert the clinician to the possibility of heart disease.

4. Malaise and decreased energy is estimated to be a premonitory symptom in 30 to 60% of instances of heart attack (Appels, 1990).

5. When premonitory symptoms of a myocardial infarction occur in a patient already diagnosed to have a major psychiatric illness of which anergia or anxiety are symptoms, diagnosis become especially difficult.

6. Sudden death, stroke, and myocardial infarctions—as well as fractures—can result from the hypotension associated with tricyclic use.

Management
1. Adverse cardiac effects of the tricyclic antidepressants and MAOIs has led to consideration of electroshock for treatment of depression when depression follows a myocardial infarction. The new generation antidepressants bupropion (Wellbutrin), fluoxetine (Prozac), trazadone (Desyrel), sertraline (Zoloft), and

paroxetine (Paxel) are generally considered safe for use in patients with cardiac disease.

2. While imipramine (Tofranil) does not negatively impact on the ejection fraction of patients with impaired ventricular function, the frequent occurrence of severe orthostatic hypotension does cause problems with use of the drug (Roose et al, 1987).

3. Because the cause of death in tricyclic overdose is cardiac arrhythmias or heart block, risk of death from overdose of an amount of the tricyclic that would not usually cause death is increased.

Quality Assurance Issues

1. Was a patient's cardiac history reviewed before a tricyclic or tetracyclic antidepressant was prescribed?

HEMODIALYSIS

A number of disorders of mood, thought, and behavior have been reported in patients on chronic hemodialysis. These may be due to so-called psychiatric illness (e.g., major depression, bipolar disorder, schizophrenia) or to medical complications such as organic mental disorders due to hyperkalemia, cerebral infections, nitrogen retention, and anemia.

History

1. Psychological issues confronting hemodialysis patients include fears of sexual impotence (Campbell and Sinha, 1980), disturbances of body image, fear of death, and depression.

2. Incidence of suicide among hemodialysis patients is increased significantly among hemodialysis patients.

3. Patients may withdraw and refuse further dialysis treatments and refuse to follow dietary restrictions (so-called "passive" or "covert" suicide).

4. Noncompliance to fluid restrictions tends to begin early in treatment and remain stable over time. In some patients this may be less due to psychiatric problems than to dysfunction of the homeostatic mechanisms that regulate water metabolism and abnormalities in the renin–aldosterone–angiotensin system (Streltzer and Hassell, 1988).

5. Studies indicate that 25 to 50% of dialysis patients are regular noncompliers with regard to fluid restrictions (Streltzer and Hassell, 1988).

6. Noncompliance with maintenance dialysis is greater among the young due to the developmental pressures of the young adult years coupled with the stresses of having to cope with a chronic illness (Gonsalves-Ebrahim et al, 1987).

Management

1. Success of dialysis depends on strict adherence to dietary restrictions and on limiting potassium and fluid intake.

2. While both individual and group therapy have been used for hemodialysis pa-

tients, the group approach appears to be favored in many renal units, involving both patients and their families. The group focuses on altruism, information dispersal, socialization techniques, ventilation, instillation of hope, universality, interpersonal learning, and demonstration of family dynamics (Campbell and Sinha, 1980).

3. Psychopharmacologic agents to manage psychoses and mood disorders must be used with caution particularly if, as in the case of lithium, a drug has a narrow therapeutic index and is excreted predominantly by the kidneys (Zetin et al, 1981).

4. Noncompliance with fluid intake, as indicated by excessive gains in body weight between sessions, is managed in a nonmoralistic way, intervening psychologically early in the process of dialysis and employing a flexible schedule of dialysis treatments (Streltzer and Hassell, 1988).

HEPATITIS

All liver disease can be associated with depression. In some the cause of the depression is evident because of associated jaundice and the patient presents with a yellow color. In others, such as a hepatoma (tumor of the liver) or mononucleosis, the fact the liver functioning is impaired may not be apparent to the observer.

History
1. Infections of the liver can present with depression and elevation of the liver enzymes without clinical jaundice.
2. The course of most infections of the liver are limited, even if viral, but death does occur in some cases. Other cases may be fulminating and a good number are chronic, leaving a patient feeling malaise and dysphoric.
3. Because hepatitis is both common among intravenous drug users and in a gay population that does not practice safe sex, the diagnostician must also consider AIDS, and if a patient is HIV positive, must consider a number of opportunistic infections in addition to affective disorders.
4. Any individuals with recent travel to countries with poor sanitation and potentially contaminated water should be evaluated for the presence of hepatitis A antibodies.
5. Hepatitis B antibodies found in a patient who denies intravenous drug use should lead the clinician to suspect that the patient is lying if they do not have another obvious explanation for the presence of the antibodies (e.g., transfusion, gay sex) (Estroff et al, 1986).

Clinical Studies
1. Serum direct and indirect bilirubin.
2. Liver enzymes (SGPT, SGOT).
3. Hepatitis A, Ab antigens and antibodies.
4. Hepatitis B surface and E antigens and antibodies.

5. HIV testing.

Management

1. Treatment is diagnostic-specific depending on the etiology of the hepatitis coupled with supportive care and appropriate precautions.
2. Mood disorders with liver disease may be treated by the usual methods with *specific caution* due to impairment of liver metabolism. Consultation with an internist and concurrent monitoring is generally required with psychopharmacotherapy to prevent further harm to the patient and to maximize therapeutic success.

Quality Assurance Issues

1. Were appropriate precautions taken with infectious hepatitis to prevent contamination and further spread?
2. Was consultation with an internist sought when hepatic dysfunction was present in a patient requiring psychopharmacotherapy?

HOMELESS PEOPLE

The homeless are a subpopulation that includes many poor and disinherited people, some of whom have major psychiatric problems, and who, if willing to comply with treatment, may find gainful employment or willingly accept living in a shelter. When medical or behavioral problems bring them to the emergency room, they often are referred to psychiatry for primary care or consultation.

History

1. In one study (Susser et al, 1989) of 233 men at first entry of a municipal men's shelter in New York City, the majority of men had a history of psychiatric disorder or heavy substance abuse. Seventeen percent had a definite or probable history of psychosis and another 8% a possible history. A diagnosis of schizophrenia was made in 8% and a diagnosis of substance abuse in 58%, using structured epidemiologic interviews (i.e., the Center for Epidemiologic Studies Depression scale, the short Michigan Alcohol Screening Test, and the Structured Clinical Interview for *DSM-III-R:* Psychotic Disorders). Seven percent on interview were suicidal.
2. Physical and sexual assault of psychiatric patients have been found to occur in as great as 70 to 80% of patients (Jacobsen A, 1989).

Management

1. Treatment of a homeless patient is diagnostic-specific with the added burden of providing food and shelter.
2. For many homeless, the emergency room serves as the primary care provider. Care must be flexible, tailored to patients' needs and erratic time schedule but, nevertheless as continuous as possible given the circumstances. Careful review

of a chart and use of the problem-oriented approach to record keeping facilitates review.

3. The more severely mentally ill homeless sadly do not seek or obtain the psychiatric care they need. This includes the majority of the chronic schizophrenics who are vulnerable to physical and sexual abuse (complicating their medical presentation) and substance abuse (creating the problems of treating dually diagnosed individuals with limited compliance with treatment) (Aranag JD, 1990).

Quality Assurance Issues
1. Are all homeless people evaluated for psychiatric/medical/surgical disorders?

Ethical/Legal Issues
1. Are efforts made to provide homeless people with the shelter and medical care and nourishment they need on a more consistent basis?

HOMICIDAL AND ASSAULTIVE BEHAVIOR

The term "violence" denotes a spectrum of self- and other-destructive behavior. Self-destructive behavior ranges from suicide to more subtle forms of damage to one's personal integrity, such as tendency to repeated accidents ("accident proneness"), drug abuse and alcohol addiction, and lack of concern for exposure to AIDS. Other-directed violent behavior spans from careless automobile driving to robbery, assault, rape, manslaughter, and homicide. On the whole, such behavior is extremely difficult to predict although there are some factors that have been identified that characterize those who behave violently. Violence occurs in all clinical settings and is more common than previously assumed (Thackrey and Bobbitt, 1990).

History
1. More than 1% of the deaths in the United States are due to criminal homicide (Tardiff, 1985).
2. Readmission rates to hospital are significantly higher for patients with a history of violent behavior (Rossi et al, 1985).
3. The majority of inpatient psychiatric patients report being victims of physical or sexual assault (Jacobson and Richardson, 1987).
4. Sexual violence is more common than believed in the physical torture of women and female adolescents (Goldfeld et al, 1988).
5. Most instances of filicide and patricide are the result of major psychiatric disorder with delusions or substance abuse (Cravens et al, 1985; Campion et al, 1988).
6. Causes of inpatient violence more commonly relate to external situations than the patient's internal psychiatric symptoms (Sheridan et al, 1990).
7. The staff's ability to predict which patients are weapon carriers is low (Anderson A et al, 1989).
8. Cerebrospinal fluid 5-hydroxyindoleacetic acid, the principal metabolite of sero-

tonin, is low among aggressive impulsive children and adults (Kruesi et al, 1990).

9. Patient violence is more likely to be directed to a family member (Gondolf et al, 1990).

10. Police officers often seek help from mental health clinicians regarding a patient's risk of violence and past history of such acts and also seek assistance in managing violent patients (Gillig et al, 1990).

11. Studies of individuals involved in suicide pacts suggest similarities between perpetrators of murder–suicide, noncriminal murderers, and instigators of suicide pacts (Rosenbaum M, 1983). Depression is the most common illness seen in all groups. In suicide pacts, the instigator tends likely to be a male and psychiatrically ill. The survivor, when one exists, is more likely female and not psychiatrically ill and has not exhibited prior suicidal behavior. The "homicide risk" as well as the "suicide risk" must be ascertained when evaluating survivors of suicide pacts.

Risk Factors of Other-Directed Violence

1. Age: Violent people tend to be younger. There is a significant positive correlation between suicide and homicide rates for 15 to 24-year-olds and the proportion of 15 to 24-year-olds in the U.S. population from 1933 to 1982 (Holinger and Kuenigsberg, 1985; Swanson et al, 1990).

2. Psychopathology: The greater the degree of psychopathology, the more likely the patient will be violent (Tardiff and Swillam, 1982). While manic and schizophrenic patients are more likely to be assaultive prior to hospitalization, manic patients are more assaultive in the hospital (Binder and McNiel, 1988). Children with conduct disorders are more likely to be violent and to set fires and hit with objects than neurotic children (Pfeffer et al, 1983) and adult patients who are violent are more likely to have a history of childhood or adolescent psychiatric disorders (Tardiff and Koenigsberg, 1985). Patients who are assaultive who provide clues (verbal threats) differ on the Brief Psychiatric Rating Scale from those who are assaultive without cues on the dimensions of thinking disorders, anxious depression, activation, hostile-suspiciousness, and withdrawal-retardation (Tanke and Yesavage, 1985). Approximately 7% of patients in a survey of the New York State Hospital system were assaultive in a 3-month period, and other studies have indicated 10 to 40% of patients entering inpatient care have been violent or have exhibited fear-producing behavior prior to hospitalization (Silver and Yudofsky, 1987).

3. Command Hallucinations: If a patient has auditory hallucinations commanding them to harm someone, they are at greater risk for violence (particularly if the voice commanding is that of God).

4. Suspiciousness and hostility: Patients who exhibit suspiciousness and hostility on admission are more likely to become violent (Lowenstein et al, 1990).

5. Agitation: Emotional turmoil as evinced by agitation and anger tends to be a harbinger of violence among schizophrenics, diabetics, and those with organic brain disorders (Craig TJ, 1982; Lowenstein et al, 1990).

6. Antisocial personality: The most common diagnosis among female first offenders age 17 to 39 was antisocial personality. Those aged 40 to 54 had a greater frequency of other medical and psychiatric disorders.
7. Parental violence: Homicidal children are more likely to have had fathers who were physically abusive or homicidal, who had attempted suicide, or who had a seizure disorder (Lewis DO et al, 1983; Fenn, 1990).
8. Emotional relationships with victim: The majority of murders are committed by a relative of the victim or a person acquainted with the victim and the majority of aggravated assaults occur within a family, among neighbors, or among acquaintances.
9. Previous criminal behavior: Those with a number of previous arrests, juvenile police records, and histories of conviction for violent crimes are more likely to be violent. The more severe the original offense, the greater the likelihood of future violence.
10. Self-mutilation and other self-destructive behavior: Violent adults have a higher incidence of self-mutilation and other self-destructive behavior.
11. Fire setting and cruelty to animals as children: Violent adults, as children, tended to be impulsive and stimulus-seeking with a history of fire setting and/or cruelty to animals.
12. Violent environments: Those who live in subcultures characterized by violence tend to be more violent.
13. Weapons: Patients who have access to weapons can cause even greater harm than those without resources. A search for weapons not only is risky, but in addition it mollifies staff anxiety (Privitera et al, 1986).
14. Sex: Males are more likely (Tardiff and Koenigsberg, 1985; Swanson et al, 1990; Delga et al, 1989; Van Londen et al, 1990) to be violent and to die by homicide or accidents (especially if alcoholic or schizophrenic where increased risk is as great as two and one-half fold for accidental death and two-fold for homicide) (Hillard et al, 1985).
15. Previous history: Patients who have an immediate past history of violence in the community are more likely to be violent early in the course of hospitalization (McNiel et al, 1988b). In one study (Blomhoff et al, 1990), a history of violence successfully identified 80% of patients who acted out violently.
16. Substance abuse: Substance abusers are more likely to be violent (Swanson et al, 1990).
17. Neurologic impairment: Schizophrenics who are violent evince more neurologic and neuropsychological abnormalities (Krakowski et al, 1989).
18. Fantasy: Serial sexual murderers have been found to be driven by intrusive fantasies of organized crime scenes, paraphilias, and violence (Prentky et al, 1989).

Signs

1. Shouting.
2. Display of weapons.
3. Threatening talk.
4. Pacing.

5. Shaking fists.
6. Shooting.
7. Knifing.
8. Chair swinging.
9. Acid throwing.
10. Pounding fists.
11. Slamming door.
12. Agitation.
13. Anger.

Diagnosis

The first task of a psychiatrist evaluating a potentially violent person is to obtain some indication of its cause. Etiology directs treatment. If patients have a thought disorder characterized by command hallucinations telling them to kill their mother, they require psychiatric hospitalization and antipsychotic medication. If they do not accept this plan, medical commitment is necessary both to protect relatives as well as patients. Those who take extreme civil libertarian views often fail to recognize that medical commitment not only has evolved legally to protect society from the violent patient, but also to protect patients from consequences of their own uncontrollable behavior. Patients who, while psychotic, destroy their family's and friend's property, as well as threaten them with, or actually commit, violent assault, destroy the social supports that may be needed to help them function after their aberrant mood swings or delusional ideation is corrected with appropriate antipsychotic agents.

Differential Diagnosis

1. Temporal lobe epilepsy.
2. Delusional disorder.
3. Acute organic mental disorder secondary to drug intoxication such as PCP, amphetamine-induced psychoses, and LSD- and cocaine-induced psychoses.
4. Major depression.
5. Temporal lobe and other cerebral neoplasms.
6. Bipolar disorder.
7. Hypoglycemia.
8. Delirium.
9. Episodic dyscontrol disorder.
10. Sympathomimetic-induced psychoses (e.g., epinephrine-induced psychoses).
11. Borderline personality disorder.
12. Post-traumatic stress disorder.
13. Hysterical psychosis.
14. Idiopathic alcohol intoxication.
15. Alcoholic paranoia.
16. Alcoholic hallucinosis.
17. Chronic organic mental disorder.
18. Paranoid personality disorder.
19. Schizophrenia, especially paranoid schizophrenia.

20. Catatonic excitement.
21. Alcoholic intoxication.
22. Antisocial personality disorder.
23. Uncontrollable violence secondary to interpersonal stress (e.g., domestic quarreling).
24. Other organic states (e.g., encephalitis).
25. Decompensating obsessive–compulsive disorder.
26. Dissociative disorder.
27. Homosexual panic.
28. Side effects of barbiturate, tricyclic, tetracyclic, monoamine oxidase inhibitor, or benzodiazepine therapy.
29. Social maladjustment without manifest psychiatric disorder.

Management

The approach to treatment of all patients with other-destructive behavior is analogous to that of suicidal behavior after initial diagnosis.

1. Does the patient need to be hospitalized? If he or she needs to be hospitalized, will he or she go voluntarily, or does he or she require medical certification? What type of milieu will be necessary to contain his or her behavior? Will he or she need a locked ward or individual 24-hour surveillance? The answers to all these questions rest on a clinical judgment as to what the evaluating psychiatrist feels the patients are likely to do (given their past medical and psychiatric history), what patients say they will do, what patients have done recently, patients' moods and quality of thoughts and perceptions, and the patients' social situations.
2. If the decision is not to hospitalize, appropriate family members and friends should be made aware of the risk to their lives. Those at whom violent behavior might be directed, or who know a violent patient well, should be made aware of what behavior changes will necessitate immediate hospitalization. For example, a mother plagued by obsessive homicidal thoughts toward her child, which cause her anxiety, may be managed outside the hospital as long as she has good impulse control. But if the anxiety begins to diminish and her control begins to disintegrate, she will need to be hospitalized.
3. Medication should be given when indicated. If patients have clear-cut thought disorders with command hallucinations telling them to kill their own brother, they should be given antipsychotic medication just as should any patient with paranoid ideation. If they are in catatonic excitement, tranquilization will be needed. Episodic outbursts of violence may respond to a trial of lithium carbonate. If the history is more suggestive of seizure disorder, an evaluation should be performed on an inpatient or outpatient basis dependent upon the nature of the violence. If studies prove positive, anticonvulsants should be commenced. Treatment of other organic states may involve other medications, or as in the case of PCP and amphetamine-induced psychoses, simple conservative measures may lead to resolution of behavior aberrations. Typical medications used as chemical

restraints are sodium amytal (125–375 mg IM), diazepam (Valium) (15–45 mg PO or 5–15 mg IV), paraldehyde (10 mL IM or 8–12 mL PO), haloperidol (Haldol) (5–10 mg IM or 5–20 mg PO), thiothixene (Navane) (10–20 mg IM or 15–60 mg PO), chlorpromazine (Thorazine) (50 mg IM or 100–200 mg PO), and lorazepam (Ativan) (2–4 mg PO or IM).

4. Patients' social supports are assessed as well as the nature of their home environment. Individuals who become violent with their spouses may only require a change in living arrangements (e.g., move in with a friend or relative). A person who is paranoid and suspicious may be more inclined to act out in a neighborhood characterized by violence and muggings than in one where most individuals are quiet, law-abiding, and keep to themselves.

5. The great majority of patients who perpetrate violent acts, especially homicide, do not have a psychiatric or medical condition (strictly defined) as the basis for these acts. Some of the individuals have personalities that may be characterized as sociopathic or antisocial. This means that they appear unsocialized and repeatedly come in conflict with the values of society. They are callous, grossly selfish, impulsive, and unable to feel guilt or to learn from experience and punishment. Their frustration tolerance is low, and they are incapable of significant loyalty to groups, individuals, or to social values. It is unclear at this time whether psychiatry has anything to offer these people which will significantly alter their behavior. In fact, it can be seriously argued that while, as with all human behavior, genetic or early environmental factors play significant roles in the genesis of this behavior, this is not an illness but a style of life or pattern of personality. It may be necessary to protect society as well as these individuals themselves from abuse and fatal consequences by protective confinement. Social factors that contribute to this behavior cannot be dealt with by a psychiatrist engaged in treating psychiatric emergencies any more than it can by psychiatry as a profession. It is a challenge facing all contemporary society and one that will not readily yield a simple solution.

6. Violent outbursts should be prevented whenever possible. Staff should be aware of issues and problems and work to minimize the need for chemical or physical restraints. Written policies and procedures should be understood and have been practiced by the staff. Patients should be seen in areas that have adequate space, appropriate lighting, an alarm system, and ready accessibility to security officers. Self-defense courses may be in order for clinicians working in areas of high crime and predictable violence. The interviewing room should have multiple exits and a minimum of dangerous materials and furnishings that can be used as weapons.

7. If the violence has occurred, the clinician should document any personal or bystander injuries as well as damage to furnishings and equipment. The waiting room attendants and other patients should be approached as to what happened. Staff should meet to review the events in order to see what steps may be taken to avoid future occurrences.

8. Lithium carbonate, anticonvulsants (e.g., Dilantin, Tegretol, valproate, Klonapin), or beta blockers (e.g., propranolol) may be effective in patients with

chronic mental disorders when violent behavior is unresponsive to major tranquilizers. The associated memory impairment, disorientation, and psychotic thought processes are not altered by propranolol (Yudofsky et al, 1981).

9. Judicial concern that psychotropic medications are overused in patients who are violent has not been supported by research. Appelbaum et al (1983) found no significant differences in dose and type of medication used between nonviolent and control patients and violent patients before or after a violent act. Violent patients, however, tended to be on somewhat greater doses of psychotropic drugs on discharge.

10. Evaluation for head injury and neuropsychological sequelae should be made in all patients who have suffered torture (Goldfeld et al, 1988).

11. Evidence suggests that training staff in the clinical management of violence reduces staff injury and number of violent incidences (Carmel and Hunter, 1990; Infantino and Musingo, 1985). Regular inservice training of staff role models in handling violence, and awareness of how countertransference and staff psychological defenses may trigger violence is essential (Dubin, 1989; Dubin, 1981). Milieu factors can enhance or diminish violent acting out (Campbell and Simpson, 1986).

12. Patients who were violent within 2 weeks of admission should be considered at high risk for violent acting out (McNiel and Binder, 1989). Although ability to predict who will be violent is limited (Monahan, 1984), the best prediction of future behavior is past behavior.

13. Violence itself is not an important predictor of length of hospital stay but the diagnosis of schizophrenia coupled with violence is (Greenfield et al, 1989).

14. Anxiety and aggression often occur together (Kiroy, 1989). Benzodiazepines alone or together with neuroleptics are often used today to manage violence (Salzman et al, 1986; Sheard, 1988). This reduces risk of NMS and tardive dyskinesia by reducing exposure to neuroleptics.

15. Loxapine works more rapidly intramuscularly than equivalent doses of thiothixene (Dubin and Wells, 1986).

16. Both carbamazepine (Tegretol) and propranolol (Inderal) have been demonstrated effective in management of rage outbursts with carbamazepine more effective for intermittent explosive disorder and propranolol more effective for attention deficit hyperactivity disorder (Mattes, 1990).

17. Propranolol is used successfully to treat aggressiveness in mentally retarded and brain-damaged patients (Ratey et al, 1983).

18. Droperidol is seen as superior to other neuroleptics in management of violence. Unfortunately, it can only be given intrathecally. It is a safe butyrophenone that works more rapidly and effectively than haloperidol (Haldol) (Keshick and Burton, 1984).

19. Therapeutic holding, a technique whereby a violent patient is physically contained by people instead of chemical or mechanical restraints, is effective in more rapidly securing behavioral control than seclusion (Miller D et al, 1989).

20. Midazolam, a benzodiazepine derivative used as a parenteral anesthetic agent, is a seldom used but effective alternative for management of aggressive behavior (Bond WS et al, 1989).

21. Patients found resistant to all other modes of therapy for violence have been found to be controlled by a form of hydrotherapy in which cold, wet sheet packs are applied to self-destructive patients (Singh, 1986). Use in other-directed violence is not as impressive.

22. Loss of a friend or relative to homicide, as with suicide, differs in its impact on those who survive from loss by death of so-called natural causes. Group and individual therapy focus in on cognitive, behavioral, and affective responses unique to loss by homicide and best understood by others who have suffered similar loss (Rynearson, 1984).

23. Patients who kill someone create unique responses in those who provide care that impact on how care may be given. One sees a similar ambivalent response when a patient survives a gunshot wound in a suicide attempt (Conn et al, 1984).

24. Low cerebrospinal fluid 5-hydroxyindoleacetic acid, the principle metabolite of serotonin, and homovanillic acid, the metabolite of dopamine, are significantly lower among recidivistic violent offenders and fire setters (Virkkunen et al, 1989b).

Quality Assurance Issues

1. Was the least restrictive means employed to manage a violent patient?
2. If seclusion was employed, was care given to patient needs for food, water, and toilet?
3. If restrained, was restraint limited to the time it was essential to protect the patient and others?
4. Was every patient who presented in the emergency room evaluated for the potential of violence?
5. If a patient was considered violent, were precautions taken to prevent harm to the patient, family, friends, others in the community, and to caregivers?

Ethical/Legal Issues

1. Was an intended victim informed of the immediate danger to his or her life?

HOMOSEXUAL PANIC

Many of us have a component to our personality that is homosexual. For some it is quite small and only evoked under circumstances of deprivation from opportunity for heterosexual contact such as with men in prison or long voyages at sea without women. For others, a close, same-sex relationship will evoke love and love in turn a desire for intimacy of a sexual nature. Women tend to be able to tolerate these feelings better than men. When a sexual feeling toward a same-sex person cannot be accepted consciously a person may panic and/or project the feeling onto the person arousing it and become paranoid. In the paranoia, the person in homosexual panic can actually seriously harm or kill another innocent person without any sexual attraction toward the person who attacks him or her. In most instances those in homosexual panic are men. In instances such as "gay bashing," a number of men with unstable sexual identity will defend against their own homosexual drive by collectively beating known homosexuals in an attempt to keep their own homosexuality in check. Contrary to popular belief, homosexual panic does not usually involve individuals who are acknowledged to be same-sex oriented but rather individuals who are ostensibly heterosexual who have difficulty integrating their homosexual feelings or activity.

History

1. Homosexual panic usually occurs when an individual with strong, latent homosexual drive is placed in a situation such as dormitory or barracks where there is much visual stimulation of homoerotic fantasies such as seeing men naked or masturbating or is subjected to physical encounters common to these situations such as playful wrestling or hugging. It also may occur when a predominantly heterosexual man is "seduced" or "raped" or finds himself impotent in a heterosexual encounter and feels a desperate need to prove himself to be heterosexual or bisexual. Rarely do women experience this in the extreme.

2. Individuals in homosexual panic feel extremely anxious, agitated, fearful, and paranoid. They are intensely fearful of members of the same sex. They may panic and attack if touched and threaten any same-sex person's life who dares to take advantage of them.

3. They may appear to be decompensating and disintegrate into a paranoid psychosis.

4. The psychodynamic basis of the fear and panic is thought to be the emergence of repressed homosexual feelings that are consciously intolerable to the individual. They, therefore, are projected onto other same-sex people. Ideas of reference may develop and the individual feels that others, rather than themselves, are accusing them of "being homosexual." The individual defends against acting out their feelings by avoiding same-sex people or by actually being hostile to them.

5. There appears to be a significant family component to homosexuality (Pillard and Weinrich, 1986). If feelings emerge in an environment, familial or community, that is unaccepting or frankly hostile, the likelihood of development of homosexual panic or "gay bashing" to defend against homosexuality may be more likely to emerge. Anything that distinguishes a man as potentially homosexual, such as extreme good looks or sensitivity or behaviors such as having a greater emphasis on thinness (Yager et al, 1988), may serve to make a man a potential stimulus of panic in those predisposed.

Management

1. Patients in homosexual panic should preferably be (although this is not always possible) interviewed by someone of the opposite sex in the acute phase. The clinician should be particularly attuned to the intensity of patients' fear and the threat of violence (either self or other) created by the emergence of strong latent homosexual drives.

2. The patient should not be touched other than for routine procedures such as vital signs or a physical examination, which should be performed in the presence of

another person if done by a same-sex physician. A gentle slap on the thigh can give genesis to a physical attack. Examination of the genitals or rectum should be deferred until a patient has become more integrated.

3. Patients should be reassured and allowed to ventilate about their experience and fears in a supportive and accepting environment.
4. Exceptionally anxious patients should be given a minor tranquilizer such as 0.5–1.0 mg of alprazolam (Xanax) or lorazepam (Ativan) orally. Intramuscular injection may be seen by a male patient as a further attack, but if it is required, it should be given.
5. Particularly paranoid or psychotic patients (e.g., those with delusional thinking or hallucinations) should be given an antipsychotic such as 100 mg of chlorpromazine (Thorazine) or 5–10 mg of haloperidol (Haldol) or thiothixene (Navane) orally.
6. Crisis-oriented therapy and medication may not be sufficient for particularly violent patients who may try to defend themselves from a fantasized sexual assault. These patients may need to be hospitalized for a brief period until their potential for violence is diminished and their paranoia and ideas of reference subside.
7. If a young person presents in panic, simply sharing (if a clinician feels comfortable saying so) that not all of us are that "straight" including the clinician, may serve to assuage the anxiety of the patient over being a little bit "bent."

Quality Assurance Issues
1. Have all patients appearing with acute panic been evaluated for homosexual panic?

HUNTINGTON'S DISEASE

Huntington's disease is a fully penetrant genetic disorder that is diagnosed today with considerable certainty.

History
1. Diagnosis is made when an individual with a positive family history presents with the characteristic movement disorder. Laboratory studies confirm the diagnosis.
2. Individuals with the disease tend to maintain relatively preserved language function until late in the disease.
3. Patients with Huntington's chorea exhibit a panoply of behavioral signs and symptoms that evolve over time. These are often associated with marked apathy. Psychiatric changes reflect both pathologic and environmental factors.
4. In addition to the organic mental disorder the clinical symptom constellations seen with patients with Huntington's disease include major and minor depressive disorders, schizophrenia, paranoia, dysthymic personality disorders, atypical psychoses, paranoid personality disorder, anxiety disorders, antisocial

personality disorders, somatizations and intermittent explosive personality disorders (Caine and Showlson, 1983).

Management
1. Modest symptomatic impairment may be observed with psychopharmacotherapy. However, the course of deterioration, unfortunately, proceeds inexorably to death.

Quality Assurance Issues
1. Was psychoeducation and support provided the patient and family?

HWA-BYUNG

Hwa-Byung is a Korean folk illness term for patients who suffer from suppressed or repressed anger of long duration.

History
1. The illness is manifested by epigastric discomfort and a morbid fear of impending death.
2. The somatic preoccupations are very resistant to medical reassurance.
3. The delusion of an abdominal mass may lead to surgical intervention (Lin, 1983).
4. The term Hwa-Byung comes from the Korean *hwa* meaning "anger" or "fire" and *byung* denoting "sickness."
5. It is unclear whether Hwa-Byung is a culture-bound illness or a forme fruste of another disorder such as major depression or delusional disorder.

Symptoms
1. Indigestion.
2. Anorexia.
3. Insomnia.
4. Dyspnea.
5. Acute panic.
6. Palpitations.
7. Excessive fatigue.
8. Generalized aches and pains.
9. Morbid fear of impending death.
10. Feeling of a mass in the epigastric region.

Signs
1. Dysphoria.

Management
1. Some patients with Hwa-Byung respond well to antidepressant therapy (Lin, 1983).

HYPERKALEMIC PERIODIC PARALYSIS

Patients with hyperkalemic periodic paralysis can present with psychosis (Jenkins and Shaw, 1990).

Management
1. The psychotic symptoms remit with restoration of serum potassium to a normal value with medical treatment.

HYPERPROLACTINEMIA

Some patients with major depressive disorder are reported to have elevated serum prolactin levels with circadian fluctuations. Depression has been associated with remarkably high serum prolactin levels suggesting a possible etiologic relationship (Thionhaus and Hartford, 1986).

HYPERSOMNIA

Feeling excessively tired or sleepy is a common complaint. The cause is usually apparent. Individuals with active lives such as college students and those working two jobs are more tired and require more sleep. Individuals who are depressed (especially if the depression is part of bipolar disorder) may be hypersomnic and sleep 12 to 16 hours a day rather than be insomnic. Finally, there are a number of physical illnesses in which increased sleep may be a symptom. These include narcolepsy, sleep apnea, hypothyroidism, encephalitis, and the Pickwickian syndrome.

History
1. Individuals complain of some form of increased sleep or sleepiness. For some these are isolated episodes. An individual is overcome with an intense irresistible desire to sleep. For others, there is an increased number of total hours of sleep at night. For instance, a patient will report sleeping 14 hours, whereas, 5 months ago he or she only slept 7 to 8 hours. Still others complain of a constant feeling of exhaustion with a need for napping. The character of the need for increased sleep provides a clue to diagnosis.
2. The setting of the onset of the increased desire to sleep is important. Narcoleptics can fall asleep during activity while Pickwickians do not. A person who is depressed or has functional hypersomnia is generally tired and "washed-out" all of the time.
3. Associated symptoms and changes in behavior should be ascertained. A narcoleptic classically complains of sleep paralysis (episodes either just before falling asleep or awakening at which time the individual feels awake but unable to move), hypnogogic or hypnopompic hallucinations (vivid visual or auditory

hallucinations just before falling asleep or on awakening that seem so real the individual may act on them), and cataplexy (attacks at which time an individual becomes akinetic and falls down while remaining fully awake) in addition to sleep paralysis. Patients with sleep apnea characteristically do not feel rested at night because of airway obstruction and recurrent awakening. Their snoring and sonorous breathing may be commented upon by those who live with the patient. Attacks of sleep with sleep apnea occur at times when a patient is inactive, which differs from those of narcolepsy. Pickwickians are usually quite large (in excess of 300 lbs. in weight) and have compliance problems with resultant hypercapnia.

4. In the Kleine–Levin syndrome, personality changes are coupled with hyperphagia and hypersomnia. In all instances of hypersomnia, organic causes for increased sleep should be considered. Only in the absence of some intercurrent physical illness or obvious major psychopathology such as bipolar disorder should a diagnosis of functional hypersomnia be made.

5. Young depressed patients are reported to suffer prolonged rather than shortened sleep with duration of REM periods comparable to older patients (Hawkins et al, 1985).

Differential Diagnosis

1. Narcolepsy.
2. Sleep apnea.
3. Cerebral neoplasia.
4. Functional hypersomnia.
5. Pickwickian syndrome.
6. Seizure disorder.
7. Encephalitis.
8. Side effects of medication or illicit drug use (e.g., tranquilizers, barbiturates).
9. Hypoglycemia.
10. Hypothyroidism.
11. Kleine-Levin syndrome.
12. Sequela to cerebral trauma.
13. Major depression.
14. Bipolar disorder.
15. Dysthymic disorder.

Management

1. The first step in management of an individual presenting with hypersomnia is taking a careful history and performing a physical examination.
2. In some instances electroencephalograms will be helpful. A patient with a seizure disorder may show a dysrhythmic pattern or even an epileptogenic focus. The sleep EEG of a narcoleptic shows REM sleep as a patient falls asleep and increased REM activity throughout natural sleep.
3. After a diagnosis is made, disposition should be made to the appropriate specialty for treatment. Obviously, an individual found to have a cerebral tumor

should be referred to neurosurgery. Most other sleep disorders are treated by neurologists except when increased sleep is seen as part of an identifiable psychiatric disturbance. An exception is the treatment of narcolepsy for which both psychiatrists and neurologists are qualified to manage. Methylphenidate (Ritalin), dextroamphetamine (Dexedrine), imipramine (Tofranil), and protriptyline (Vivactil) have all been used to manage patients with the narcoleptic tetrad.

4. Individuals with functional hypersomnia usually have histories of rapid sleep onset, prolonged deep sleep (more than 9 or 10 hours), irritability, daytime sleepiness, and postdormital confusion. A tendency to worry and depression are also part of this syndrome. Excess stress may lead to the disorder. Methylphenidate or d-amphetamine administered about $\frac{1}{2}$ hour after awakening is usually significant to manage well-motivated patients or patients with conscientious family members or roommates who will monitor medication intake. Alternately, imipramine may be used for functional hypersomnia and given at the usual times.

5. CNS stimulants and imipramine have been found to have REM-suppressing properties and, therefore, are useful in the management of a number of other sleep disorders such as pavor nocturnus (night terrors), somnambulism (sleep walking), and enuresis (bed wetting).

Quality Assurance Issues

1. Have all patients with hypersomnia been evaluated for medical/psychiatric/surgical disorders which may cause the symptom?

HYPERVENTILATION

Hyperventilation may present as panic disorder or be part of it.

History

1. Patients with both panic disorder and hyperventilation are posited to share a biogenetically determined hypersensitive alarm system.

Management

1. Appropriate psychopharmacotherapy of patients with panic disorder leads to remission of hyperventilation.
2. In the acute situation, patients presenting with hyperventilation may breathe into a paper bag. Rebreathing of air rich in carbon dioxide reduces the panic.
3. Administration of either alprazolam (Xanax) or lorazepam (Ativan) leads to reduction of anxiety and restoration of normal breathing.
4. Breathing retraining such that a patient learns that breathing slowly reduces panic is critical to long-term management of patients who chronically hyperventilate.

HYPNOTICS

Use of hypnotics to induce sleep is fraught with problems. Patients may present in the emergency room both to seek renewal of a prescription when they have become addicted to those with habit-forming characteristics and when use leads to toxic symptoms suggesting a psychiatric disorder.

History

1. Any patient seeking renewal of an addictive hypnotic drug in the emergency room should be asked the name of his or her physician and the physician should be contacted to assure that the request is valid and that the attending physician be aware of the drug use and amount prescribed in the emergency room.
2. Patients who appear intoxicated (especially if older) without and sometimes even with the odor of alcohol on their breath, should be suspected of hypnotic intoxication alone or of a combination of hypnotic and alcohol intoxication (a common combination). The clinical symptoms may suggest a schizophreniform process. Serum drug and alcohol screens serve to confirm the diagnosis.
3. Patients who are chronic users of some hypnotics may go in and out of withdrawal and intoxication creating a oeneroid or dreamlike state. Total abstinence leads to delirium tremens with some hypnotics if taken in sufficient dosage over a period of time.
4. In all instances a patient who is on hypnotics should be continually evaluated to ascertain if there is a primary psychiatric disorder that is being masked.
5. Sleep is one of the most sensitive indicants of the emotional life of an individual. Sleep is an indica of the onset of a number of psychiatric maladies. Individuals who suffer from unipolar affective illness frequently have difficulty falling asleep, awakening in the middle of the night, and awakening early in the morning without an alarm clock, or, as frequently seen in the case of depressions associated with bipolar illness, they are hypersomnic. Individuals undergoing an acute schizophrenic break talk of their thoughts racing so fast that they cannot sleep. Patients in a manic state may go so many nights without sleeping that they develop hallucinations from lack of sleep causing a clinician to confuse them clinically with individuals who are undergoing a schizophrenic decompensation.
6. Tricyclic antidepressants, the monoamine inhibitors, and fluoxetine (Prozac) may disturb sleep. In such instances, giving all of the medication before 4:00 PM may negate the need for a hypnotic for sleep. At other times, the addition of a hypnotic is necessary. Trazadone (Desyrel) is often used with fluoxetine for sleep as it is more sedating and also a serotonin agonist.
7. Benzodiazepines are the drugs of choice for sleep (Roth et al, 1981). Short-activity benzodiazepines with a half-life of less than 12 hours such as triazolam (Halcion) are particularly useful. The half-life of triazolam is 1.5 to 5.0 hours (Kroboth and Juhl, 1983).
8. Triazolam (0.125 mgm and 0.25 mg), flurazepam (Dalmane) (30 mg), and nitra-

zepam (10 mg) have sleep-inducing and sleep maintenance properties. Flurazepam and nitrazepam have been shown to have residual effects during the following day; triazolam does not (Ogura et al, 1980).

9. Patients taking triazolam fall asleep faster and wake less often than those who take flurazepam (Keighley et al, 1980) suggesting that triazolam may be particularly useful as a hypnotic before elective major surgery.

10. Alprazolam (Xanax) is a short-activity benzodiazepine that may have antidepressant properties making it particularly useful as an adjunctive drug for sleep induction in patients with anxiety and depression (Feighner et al, 1983; Greenblatt et al, 1983).

Management

1. Withdrawal from hypnotics for patients who are chronic users and/or abusers can be quite difficult. In some instances very slow withdrawal on an outpatient basis is effective. In other instances, to facilitate compliance with a withdrawal regimen, inpatient detoxification is necessary.

2. Patients who present intoxicated with documented serum level by assay generally become asymptomatic when the serum level returns to normal or the patient is withdrawn from the drug.

Quality Assurance Issues

1. Have all patients who have been prescribed addictive hypnotics been advised of the risk of addiction?

2. Have the attending physicians of all patients who have been prescribed an addictive hypnotic in the emergency room been contacted to verify the prescriptions and to be advised of the amount prescribed in the emergency room?

3. If a patient's attending physician has not been contacted, is the amount of an addictive hypnotic prescribed only sufficient for one or two nights?

4. Are all patients on hypnotics continually evaluated for presence of an emergency psychiatric disorder with sleep disturbance that a hypnotic may be masking?

Ethical/Legal Issues

1. Have all patients on hypnotics been advised of the risk of their use with driving and machinery?

2. Have all patients prescribed addicting hypnotics been advised of their habit-forming potential?

3. Has care been provided to minimize management of patients with a substance abuse history with habit forming hypnotics?

HYPOGLYCEMIA

Hypoglycemia is associated with irritability, anxiety, depression, and other behavioral changes

History
1. Symptoms classically occur 2 to 4 hours after a meal, after excessive insulin has been taken, or when a diabetic has not sufficiently balanced food intake with insulin dose.

Clinical Studies
1. Diagnosis is confirmed with a 5 hour glucose tolerance curve demonstrating hypoglycemia.
2. Patients who believe hypoglycemia is at the basis of their panic attacks can have an attack induced by sodium lactate and a blood glucose drawn at the time of symptoms to ascertain if the patient is concurrently hypoglycemic (Gorman et al, 1984).

Management
1. Readjustment of insulin dose and dietary habits will reduce symptoms induced by exogenous insulin.
2. If a patient is found to suffer negative hypoglycemia, a consultation with a dietician for a diet to reduce the occurrence of low blood sugar is indicated.

HYSTERICAL FAINTING

Hysterical fainting is distinguished from vasovagal fainting because vasovagal fainting is associated with brachycardia, hypotension, EEG slowing, and prompt return of consciousness on lowering the head or lying down.

History
1. No known physiologic changes accompany hysterical fainting (Curtis and Thyer, 1983).
2. Hysterical fainting persists after the individual lies down or lowers his or her head.
3. Vasovagal fainting may occur during or upon cessation of great anxiety (Curtis and Thyer, 1983).

Management
1. Vasovagal fainting to phobic stimuli and subjective fear and behavioral avoidance (associated with both vasovagal fainting and hysterical fainting) may be reduced or eliminated by exposure therapy (Curtis and Thyer, 1983), ventilation, or hypnosis.

Quality Assurance Issues
1. Have organic causes of fainting been ruled out before the diagnosis of hysterical fainting was made?

HYSTERICAL PSYCHOSIS

Hysterical psychosis is distinguished from an acute schizophrenic episode by suddenness of onset and by the dramatic array of hallucinations, derealization, delusions, and bizarre behavior. Hallucinations tend to be visual rather than auditory as seen with schizophrenia. Affect tends to be expansive and effervescent rather than flat or blunted. If there appears to be a disturbance of thought processes, it does not resemble the loosening of associations seen with schizophrenia. The delusions and hallucinations, when present, are less like that of a schizophrenic adult than like the disturbance of a fearful, angry child.

History
1. Hysterical psychosis tends to be a response in an individual with the appropriate psychodynamics to an affect-laden situation.
2. As anxiety mounts, patients become overwhelmed, distraught, and unable to mobilize themselves in an integrated manner.
3. After the psychosis runs its course, no chronic disability remains.
4. Hysterical psychosis most frequently occurs in people described as having hysterical personality traits such as suggestibility, seductiveness, emotional lability, self-centeredness, and vanity who tend to be excitable, attention-seeking, and dramatic. These people are often quite dependent, shallow, and superficial.
5. Hysterical psychosis tends to occur suddenly and dramatically following a stressful life event accompanied by delusions, hallucinations, and bizarre behavior or depersonalization (Gift et al, 1985).
6. There is either no evidence of a thought disorder or the thought disturbance is transient and circumscribed with an affect that, rather than flat, is characterized as volatile (Gift et al, 1985).
7. The psychosis, if left untreated, would last 1 to 3 weeks (Gift et al, 1985).

Management
1. Hysterical psychoses are usually ameliorated by judicious use of benzodiaze pines, ventilation, and crisis-oriented therapy.
2. A sodium amytal interview may be helpful if the psychosis is precipitated by a traumatic event that the individual has difficulty discussing and integrating

IDIOT SAVANT

Idiot savants combine remarkable cognitive ability with a mental handicap They confuse an evaluating physician who is unfamiliar with the syndrome by presenting a mosaic of remarkable intellectual ability and profound limitations (Treffert, 1988).

History

1. All the psychiatric disorders that are seen with other organic disorders are seen with idiot savants including suicidal behavior, violence, and substance abuse.
2. The peculiar clinical presentation can confuse a psychiatric emergency clinician without previous exposure to idiot savants. In some instances, such a patient may be misdiagnosed as schizophrenic because of the extreme intellectual ability against a background of modulated or even flat affect.
3. Common skills include calendar calculations and musical talent.
4. There is a 6:1 male-to-female ratio (Treffert, 1988).
5. A common triad of symptoms of an idiot savant is blindness, musical genius, and mental subnormality (Treffert, 1988).
6. The syndrome is more frequently seen with infantile autism than other disabilities, further confusing the clinical picture.

Management

1. In addition to recognizing and diagnosing the condition of being an idiot savant, acute care includes evaluation for other psychiatric and medical disorders altering mood, thought, or behavior and providing diagnostic-specific treatment.

INCEST

Reported occurrence of incest among psychiatric patients ranges from 38 to 33% for outpatients (Rosenfeld, 1979), and up to 37.5% for hospitalized adolescents and children (Emslie and Rosenfield, 1983).

History

1. Incest involving male children appears less common than with female children.
2. In one study, 10% of psychotic girls and 8% of all psychiatrically hospitalized boys reported incest (Emslie and Rosenfield, 1983).
3. A comparison of nonpsychotic girls who reported incest and those without known history of incest demonstrated no specific effect of incest. The severe psychotic syndromes seen in some patients with incest does not appear to be the product of incest itself but of the severe family disorganization and resultant ego-impairment in instances where the incest occurred (Emslie and Rosenfield, 1983).
4. In a study of 437 adolescent girls admitted to a psychiatric hospital, 61 of whom reported incest, the mean age of first incestuous experiences was 11.9 years. Fathers were as often sexual partners as stepfathers. Other perpetrators of incest were brothers-in-law, brothers, uncles, grandfathers, half-brothers, and adopted fathers (Husain and Chapel, 1983).
5. Women reporting a history of incest often describe their fathers as violent and their mothers as chronically ill, battered, and disabled (Herman and Hirschman, 1981). Adolescent psychosis, repeated involuntary childbearing, and untreated depression are listed as causes of maternal inpairment.

6. Girls who have experienced incest have a higher rate of suicide attempts, running away, and adolescent pregnancy (Herman and Hirschman,1981).
7. Father-son incest is more common than mother-son incest (Dixon KN et al, 1978).
8. Post-traumatic stress disorder symptoms (e.g., nightmares, flashbacks to rape experience, depression, sexual dysfunction, anxiety, anger) are common sequelae to incest (Goodwin et al JM, 1990).
9. In an intensive study by Goodwin and her group (1990) of 10 women reporting incest, at least 7 of the following 11 problems were reported by each woman: rape victimization, somatic symptoms, battering by their sexual partner, borderline personality disorder, eating disorder, alcohol and substance abuse, three or more hospitalizations, affective disorder, dissociative symptoms, loss of child, arrests for antisocial behavior, and two or more suicide attempts.
10. Women most likely to suffer long-term adverse effects from incest are those who sustained prolonged, forceful, or highly intrusive sexual abuse or were abused by their fathers or stepfathers (Herman et al, 1986).

Management
1. The management of a patient reporting incest includes diagnostic social and medical working of both the offending relatives and the victim.
2. Social service should be employed in evaluation of the home situation when necessary and in planning disposition.
3. Treatment of victim and offender is diagnostic-specific and includes appropriate individual and family therapy and psychopharmacotherapy where indicated.
4. Support groups of women who all have suffered sexual abuse as children serve to mollify long-term negative effects by combining abreaction, support, and the understanding only other victims can provide.
5. Antidepressants have proven helpful in the management of the intrusive memories of the incident and recurrent nightmares that are part of post-traumatic stress disorders.

Quality Assurance Issues
1. Have relatives responsible for incest been evaluated for a psychiatric disorder and provided, where indicated, diagnostic-specific treatment?

Ethical/Legal Issues
1. Have all victims of incest been provided protection when indicated?
2. Has family therapy been provided for all families with incest?

INFECTIOUS MONONUCLEOSIS

Patients with infectious mononucleosis may present in the emergency room with depression with or without delusions and with a postviral fatigue associated with emotional distress (White and Lewis, 1987)

History

1. Patients present with depression and serological evidence consistent with infectious mononucleosis. Electroencephalography and cerebrospinal fluid studies are consistent with an encephalopathy.

Management

1. Management of the mood change is that of management of the primary illness coupled with use of antidepressants.
2. Suicide risk should be evaluated.

INSOMNIA

Prevalence of insomnia is thought to exceed 25% of the adult population (Walsh and Fillingim, 1990). Only a fraction of patients complaining of insomnia have objective difficulty inducing or maintaining sleep. However, the majority show polysomnographic evidence of some sleep disorder (Zorick et al, 1981).

History

1. Diagnostic categories of sleep disturbance are distinguished by polysomnography, psychological measures, and medical examination.
2. If a sleep disorder is a symptom of a medical disorder, this, rather than the sleep disorder, should be treated.
3. Significance of psychological factors in sleep disturbance is substantiated by the fact that anxiety and depression are more frequently reported by insomniacs than by good sleepers (Lugaresi et al, 1987).

Management

1. Muscle relaxants are indicated for the restless legs syndrome and nocturnal myoclonus (Ashtroy and Vigayam, 1980).
2. Atypical polysomnographic features such as alpha-delta sleep respond to tricyclic antidepressants (Zorick et al, 1981). The impact may be assessed by polysomnography as well as by subjective experience.
3. Only when insomnia persists without evidence of a specific primary disorder should sedative hypnotics be considered.
4. Evaluation for use of a hypnotic in an elderly patient includes assessment of safety, tolerance and efficacy (Gottlieb, 1990).
5. Transient sleep disturbance is common to many stressful situations and will usually remit over days without use of psychopharmacology (Kales and Kales, 1987).

Quality Assurance Issues

1 Have all patients with insomnia been evaluated for medical/psychiatric/surgical causes of symptoms?

2. Have patients with insomnia been provided diagnostic-specific rather than symptomatic treatment?

Ethical/Legal Issues
1. Has care been taken not to prescribe addicting hypnotics to a patient with a substance abuse history?

INSULIN-INDUCED DISORDERS

Hypoglycemia secondary to excess endogenous (as in the instance of an insulinoma) or exogenous insulin or oral hypoglycemic agents can present with anxiety and other symptoms characteristic of stress. Hypoglycemia can induce mood and behavioral changes suggestive of adrenergic hyperactivity but hypoglycemic-induced panic attacks are rare or nonexistent (Schweizer et al, 1986). Insulin-induced factitious hypoglycemia coma is rare despite the fact that hypoglycemia secondary to ingestion of oral hypoglycemic agents or injection of insulin is a common way for factitious disorder to present in the emergency room (Price et al, 1986).

Management
1. Management includes both restoration of serum glucose to normal as well as treatment of either the psychiatric disorder (when present) that led to induction of hypoglycemia or of the medical/surgical disorder (e.g., insulinoma).

INTERMITTENT ACUTE PORPHYRIA

Intermittent acute porphyria is rarely sought as a cause of behavioral disturbance but is more prevalent among psychiatric populations than among the population at large.

History
1. The overall incidence of intermittent acute porphyria was 0.21% among 3867 psychiatric patients given the spot test to detect diminished activity of the erythrocyte enzyme porphobilinogen deaminase (Tishler et al, 1985).
2. Patients with porphyria tend to be apathetic, have periods of agitated psychoses, or show depressive withdrawal with signs of neuropsychological impairment (Tishler et al, 1985).
3. Neurologic symptoms and signs are not always present

Management
1 Management of intermittent acute porphyria is both medical and psychiatric

INTERMITTENT EXPLOSIVE DISORDER

Intermittent explosive disorder is a rare disorder that replaces the *DSM-II* diagnosis of explosive personality.

History
1. Intermittent explosive disorder is one of several impulse control disorders. Others include kleptomania, isolated explosive disorder, atypical impulse control disorder, and pathologic gambling.
2. In field trials of the *DSM-III,* these diagnoses constituted approximately 1.8% of adult cases and 2.8% of cases under 18 years (Monopolis and Lion, 1983).

Management
1. All the medications that have been used for intermittent or cyclic behavioral disorder have been suggested for management of intermittent explosive disorder. These include lithium carbonate, diphenylhydantoin sodium (Dilantin), carbamazepine (Tegretol), and valproic acid.
2. There is mounting evidence that serotonin agonists such as fluoxetine (Prozac), sertraline (Zoloft), paroxetine (Paxel) and trazodone (Desyrel) may reduce impulsivity. Use of these agents is predicated on the observation that the principle metabolite of serotonin, 5-hydroxy-indoleacetic acid is reduced in the cerebrospinal fluid of those who impulsively attempt suicide or commit homicide and in other disorders characterized by impulsivity.
3. Metoprolol, a selective beta-adrenoreceptor blocker, is reported to bring about rapid remission of the symptoms (Mattes, 1985). Other beta blockers have also been reported to be efficacious.

IRRITABLE BOWEL SYNDROME

Patients with recurrent episodes of the irritable bowel syndrome may be referred for psychiatric consultation in an emergency room both to enhance compliance with treatment and to reduce the stress that exacerbates the illness.

History
1. Irritable bowel syndrome is the most frequently encountered gastrointestinal disorder by primary clinicians and constitutes 13 to 52% of new referrals to gastroenterologists (Walker et al, 1990).
2. Fifty-four to 100% of patients with irritable bowel syndrome have been reported to suffer concurrent psychiatric illness (Walker et al, 1990).

Management
1. If irritable bowel symptoms appear to be part of the symptom picture of another

primary psychiatric disorder, management entails treatment of the primary disorder (e.g., major depressive disorder, generalized anxiety disorder).
2. If irritable bowel syndrome has precipitated another psychiatric disorder due to the stress, irritable bowel syndrome is managed by combining medical therapy with individual or group psychotherapy and diagnostic-specific treatment for the concurrent psychiatric disorder.

Quality Assurance Issues
1. Have all patients with irritable bowel syndrome been evaluated for a concurrent psychiatric disorder and the concurrent psychiatric disorder, when present, treated appropriately?

ISOCARBOXAZID-INDUCED DISORDERS

Both use of and cessation of use of monoamine oxidase inhibitors can cause psychiatric syndromes.

History
1. Isocarboxazid, like other monoamine oxidase inhibitors, can precipitate mania and psychoses in those predisposed.
2. Cessation of isocarboxazid has been reported to result in mania much as cessation of tricyclic therapy has been reported to do so (Rothschild, 1985).

Management
1. Management of mania or psychosis is diagnostic-specific (e.g., lithium and neuroleptics or minor tranquilizers for mania).

KETAMINE-INDUCED DISORDERS

Ketamine, a congener of phencyclidine (PCP, angel dust), is an arylcycloalkylamine. Like PCP, it has a number of behavioral effects.

History
1. Ketamine is an anesthetic agent used with poor-risk and aged patients, patients with thermal injuries, and with some obstetrical patients. It is also used in emergency field work (Ghoneim et al, 1985).
2. Like PCP, it causes a dissociative hallucination state that makes it of interest to those using recreational drugs.
3. Even small doses (i.e., subanesthetic) impair immediate and delayed recall. The incidence of adverse reactions is high (Ghoneim et al, 1985).

Management
1. Benzodiazepines mollify or ameliorate symptoms associated with ketamine used recreationally or as an anesthetic agent.

LEAD TOXICITY AND ORGANIC MENTAL DISORDERS

The exact blood level of lead capable of producing an organic mental disorder is of considerable controversy. Levels capable of producing symptoms in some people are not found in others, suggesting varying levels of biologic CNS vulnerability (host resistance).

History
1. Minimally elevated levels affect susceptible individuals and result in mental retardation (David et al, 1982) and other mood, thought, and behavioral symptoms.

Management
1. Treatment of minimally elevated lead levels in the context of CNS dysfunction is currently experimental but of great public health importance as lead encephalopathy is preventable (David et al, 1982).
2. Early detection and prevention is the best approach to managing lead toxic disorders.

L-DOPA INTOXICATION, DELUSIONAL STATES, AND DELIRIUM

L-dopa, a precursor of dopamine, is used in the treatment of patients with idiopathic Parkinson's disease.

History
1. The amelioration of symptoms of Parkinson's disease with L-dopa is thought to be mediated by an increase in dopamine synthesis in the CNS.
2. Alterations in mood, thought, and behavior resulting from use of this drug resemble a number of clinical states.
3. Mania, depression, and schizophreniform psychoses have all been reported. Psychological changes include hallucinations, vivid dreams, illusions, and nonconfusional as well as confusional states.
4. L-dopa may induce rapid mood cycling in patients with bipolar mood disorder suggesting that a dopaminergic mechanism is involved in the frequency of cycling between mania and depression.

Management
1. Cessation of the drug or lowering its dosage where possible will generally bring about remission of symptoms.

2. If the dosage cannot be reasonably altered without considerable detriment to the patient, lithium carbonate may be of benefit.

LIDOCAINE-INDUCED DISORDER

Lidocaine causes mood and thought changes that may be misconstrued to reflect real concerns about the medical condition the drug was used for.

History
1. Lidocaine is a widely used antiarrhythmic agent.
2. Neurologic side effects may occur in as many as 6 to 20% of patients (Saravay et al, 1987).
3. Because the drug is used for the management of heart disease, the delusion that death has occurred or the fear of impending doom reported as a side effect of use of the drugs may be mistakenly believed by the patient, and are related to realistic fears about heart disease (Saravay et al, 1987).

Symptoms
1. Hallucinations.
2. Confusion.
3. Agitation.
4. Delusions.
5. Anxiety.
6. Depression.
7. Disorientation.

Signs
1. Diplopia.
2. Coma.
3. Dizziness.
4. Muscle twitching.
5. Paresthesias.
6. Dysarthria.
7. Drowsiness.
8. Obtundation.
9. Respiratory arrest.

Management
1. Other causes of psychiatric symptoms such as toxic metabolic imbalance or primary psychiatric disorder should be ruled out.
2. If dose of drug may be reduced or the drug discontinued, symptoms tend to diminish as serum level of the drug falls.

3. If a patient must be maintained on the drug, concurrent antidepressants or anti-psychotics may be administered to treat behavioral changes.

LITHIUM-INDUCED DISORDERS

Lithium is effective in mood stabilization, particularly of hypomanic and manic episodes, in augmentation of the action of some antidepressants, and in treating episodic behavioral disturbances. However, it can also cause changes in mood, thought, and behavior of its own, particularly at toxic levels. It is also associated with a number of medical side effects.

History
1. Lithium is administered orally in tablet, capsule, or liquid form. Lithium tablets are scored, which allows for a finer titration of dosage. The usual daily dosage range of lithium carbonate is 600–1800 mg.
2. Prior to initiating lithium, a complete medical history should be obtained with special emphasis on cardiopulmonary disease, thyroid disease, and kidney disease. Patients with neurologic illnesses appear to be particularly prone to lithium toxicity. Hypertensive patients who are taking diuretics and are salt-restricted are prime candidates for lithium toxicity.
3. The pretreatment lithium workup includes thyroid function studies, serum creatinine, serum electrolytes, urinalysis, complete blood count, and an electrocardiogram.
4. There is little evidence to suggest any adverse interactions between lithium carbonate and imipramine (Tofranil). Manic-prone patients and women are especially at risk for the development of mania when prescribed imipramine (Quitkin et al, 1981).
5. While lithium treatment is often felt to be contraindicated in patients with organic brain disorders, it has been proven efficacious in symptomatic control of hypomania and recurrent depression in patients with brain damage (Ozewumi and Lapiene, 1981).
6. Studies of healthy, conditioned athletes have demonstrated that under some circumstances heavy sweating may lead to lithium loss rather than (as popularly believed) always an increase in serum lithium, increasing risk of lithium intoxication (Jefferson et al, 1982).
7. Serum lithium levels are a rough guide to lithium's efficacy. Lithium can cause toxicity at "therapeutic" levels and be clinically efficacious at "subtherapeutic" levels (Jefferson and Greist, 1981).
8. Prophylactic lithium therapy does appear to provide a reversible memory dysfunction in patients with recurrent affected illness (Christodoulou et al, 1981).
9. Choreoathetosis, when a sign of lithium toxicity, is usually accompanied by delirium and cerebellar dysfunction. In some instances, particularly when neuroleptics are used concomitantly, the choreoathetosis may be a permanent sequela of lithium use (Reed SM et al, 1989).
10. Contraceptive and ovarian steroids do not appear to influence lithium levels over the course of the menstrual cycle (Chamberlain et al, 1990).

11. Lithium may impact serotonin function presynaptically with secondary postsynaptic effects impacting mood and behavior (Price LH et al, 1990).
12. Lithium must be used with special caution in patients with respiratory, renal, thyroid, cardiovascular, and dermatologic disease and those with disorders of calcium and glucose metabolism (Das Gupta and Jefferson, 1990).
13. Combined use of carbamazepine (Tegretol) and lithium carbonate for treatment-refractory psychiatric disorders results in reversal of carbamazepine-induced leucopenia increasing the white cell count, particularly that of neutrophils, but serves to act additively in producing antithyroid effects resulting in greater decreases in T-4 and free T-4 than is associated with carbamazepine alone (Kramlinger and Post, 1990).
14. Patients on a combination of neuroleptics, particularly haloperidol (Haldol) and lithium, should be monitored for signs of symptoms of an evolving encephalopathic process (Karki and Holden, 1990).
15. Patients with a history of recurrent substance abuse cannot be relied upon to take lithium as prescribed, creating problems of combined toxic syndromes (Aagaard and Vestergaard, 1990).
16. Lithium poisoning may occur as a consequence of faulty management (e.g., not warning a patient about the necessity of salt intake), by accident (e.g., a patient takes 1800 mg in one dose rather than in divided doses because he or she ran out of lithium and is trying to catch up), or as a consequence of a deliberate overdose.
17. Medical causes contributing to toxicity include salt restriction, use of diuretics, dehydration, illness, and childbirth.
18. Severe toxicity rarely develops at levels under 2.0 mEq/L, but toxicity can occur in susceptible individuals at ordinary therapeutic or even subtherapeutic levels.
19. Death may supervene from intercurrent infection, cardiovascular collapse, or CNS depression at high levels of toxicity.

Symptoms
1. Polyuria.
2. Polydipsia.
3. Anorexia.
4. Nausea.
5. Abdominal cramps or pain
6. Weakness.
7. Fatigue.
8. Dysattention.
9. Memory disturbance
10. Confusion
11. Somnolence.
12. Hallucinations

Signs
1. Interstitial fibrosis
2. Choreoathetosis.
3. Delirium.

4. Cerebellar dysfunction.
5. Goiterous hypothyroidism.
6. Weight gain.
7. Hypercalcemia.
8. Hyperparathyroidism.
9. Provocation of diabetic ketoacidosis.
10. Arrhythmias.
11. Benign reversible T wave changes on electrocardiogram.
12. Dermatitis.
13. Exacerbation of psoriasis.
14. Vomiting.
15. Loose stools and diarrhea.
16. Reversible mild leucocytosis.
17. Aplastic anemia.
18. Edema.
19. Hypokalemia.
20. Coarse tremors.
21. Cogwheeling.
22. Convulsions.
23. Ataxia.
24. Dysarthria.
25. Muscle twitching.
26. Muscular flaccidity
27. Delirium.
28. Coma.
29. Hypotension.
30. Shock.
31. Oliguria.
32. Anemia.
33. Electrolyte imbalance

Clinical Studies
1. Serum lithium level.
2. SMA-22.
3. CBC and differential.
4. Thyroid studies.
5. Electroencephalogram.
6. Electrocardiogram.

Management
1. Patients who show signs of severe toxicity are admitted to an intensive care facility. A toxicology screen is obtained to rule out ingestion of other drugs when an overdose is suspected. Severity of intoxication is related to serum lithium concentration and duration of the toxic level. Removal of unabsorbed lithium is accomplished, provided the patient is conscious, by inducing emesis or by endotracheal intubation and gastric la-

vage when the patient's level of consciousness has been compromised. Renal clearance of lithium is often reduced in cases of toxicity. If this is due to a negative sodium balance, sodium chloride should provide improvement. If lithium clearance has not been reduced, sodium chloride will not induce a significant increase in lithium excretion and may further aggravate fluid and electrolyte overload. This differential cannot be assessed in advance and all patients should receive approximately 150–300 mEq/L of sodium chloride over the first 6 hours.

2. Peritoneal and hemodialysis are helpful in promoting lithium loss. Dialysis should be instituted based on clinical condition, duration of poisoning, lithium level, and rate of renal lithium excretion. The following schedule for dialysis has been recommended:

   a. Dialyze immediately if the serum lithium level is above 4.0 mEq/L.
   b. Dialyze immediately if the serum lithium level is between 2.0 and 4.0 mEq/L and the clinical condition is poor.
   c. In other patients the rate of renal excretion should be monitored along with the clinical condition and the decision to dialyze based on these parameters.

3. Osmotic diuretics, aminophylline, acetazolamide, and sodium bicarbonate may be of benefit when dialysis facilities are not available. Correction of fluid and electrolyte balance is of vital importance. General measures include monitoring vital signs, cardiac and pulmonary support, and prevention of infection and seizures.

4. Delirium has been reported in association with hypothyroidism in a patient receiving both lithium and thioridazine. Symptoms abate when both drugs are discontinued and thyroid replacement therapy commenced (Norris et al, 1983).

5. Sialorrhea associated with salivary gland enlargement is reversed with discontinuation of lithium. Concomitant probantheline bromide treatment provides symptomatic relief (Donaldson, 1982).

6. The increase in parathyroid hormone production (Davis et al, 1981) and in some instances hyperparathyroidism (Franks et al, 1982) reported with lithium use reverts to normal on cessation of use of the drug. Patients on lithium show higher serum levels of total calcium and ionized calcium. The hyperthyroidism observed may be a direct result of the action of lithium or in the instance of the patients with lithium-induced nephrotoxicity, secondary hyperthyroidism.

7. Lithium has several adverse effects on the kidney including chronic tubulointerstitial nephropathy associated with long-term therapy, vasopressin-resistant diabetes insipidus, the nephrotic syndrome (Moskovitz R et al, 1981), and oliguric renal failure associated with lithium intoxication. Lithium-induced nephrogenic diabetic insipidus may present for years (Ramsey and Cox, 1981). In most instances only mild renal impairment is seen with lithium use (Colt et al, 1981) and its effects on renal electrolyte and water transport are readily reversible with cessation of lithium.

8. Pure-word deafness reported during recovery from lithium-induced delirium re verses as serum levels of lithium fall.

9. Lithium in combination with neuroleptics has been implicated in producing organic mental disorders with changes in mental status examination, neuropsychological testing, and on EEG (Fetzer et al, 1981). The encephalopathy

and changes on mental status exam clear with lithium withdrawal. Hyperpyrexia, mutism, severe rigidity, and development of an irreversible tardive dyskinesia have been reported in patients on combined haloperidol (Haldol) and lithium therapy (Spring and Frankel, 1981). The question has been raised as to whether this may represent neuroleptic malignant syndrome.

10. Patients on lithium with aggression associated with complex partial seizures and with personality features described as part of temporal lobe epilepsy (such as hyper-religiosity, hyposexuality, and hypergraphlia showing exacerbation of interictal aggression) (Schiff et al, 1982) show remission of the symptoms when the drug is discontinued.

11. Lithium-induced nephrogenic diabetes insipidus responds to thiazide diuretics. These, however, are associated with hypokalemia and reduced lithium excretion predisposing patients to lithium toxicity. Amiloride, provided to patients who have become hypokalemic while being treated with hydrochlorothiazide for lithium-induced nephrogenic diabetes insipidus, increases renal concentrating ability and reduces polyuria suggesting a role in the management of severe lithium-induced polyuria (Kosten and Forrest, 1986).

Quality Assurance Issues

1. Are patients' thyroid, kidney, cardiovascular, CNS, electrolyte, metabolic, and hematologic functioning monitored while on lithium?
2. Are all patients on lithium warned of potential side effects?
3. Have all patients with a recurrent mood disorder been afforded the option of a mood stabilizer?
4. Have patients on lithium been advised of potential toxicity when placed on low-salt diets or sodium is lost in perspiration when in hot weather?

LIVER TRANSPLANTATION

Patients undergoing liver transplant are at high risk of psychiatric disorders both due to the condition requiring liver transplantation as well as due to the stress of the illness and the procedure.

History

1. Delirium and adjustment disorders are the most common psychiatric disorders seen in patients undergoing liver transplantation (Trzepacz et al, 1986).
2. Delirium when seen is associated with a serum albumin less than 3.0 g/dL, grade 1 to 3 electroencephalographic dysrhythmia, a Mini Mental State score of less than 24, or impairment on the Trailmaking Tests (Trzepacz et al, 1986).

Management

1. Management of cognitive and behavioral changes entails conjoint medical psychiatric management of the pathophysiologic changes attendant with hepatic problems and diagnostic-specific treatment of psychiatric disorders.

Quality Assurance Issues

1. Have all patients who are going to have or have had a liver transplant been evaluated for psychiatric complications of liver disease or of transplant?

MALINGERING

It is very difficult at times to ascertain if a patient is malingering when seen in emergency psychiatric consultation.

History

1. Some patients will explicitly seek emergency consultation knowing that the constructed data base from which a clinician works within the crisis situation may lead to obtaining drugs or deferment from work or school due to an assumed psychiatric illness.
2. The severe personality disturbance that leads a person to feign psychosis is frequently a harbinger of severe psychiatric disorder including schizophrenia (Greenfeld, 1987).

Management

1. No matter how much it may appear that a patient is malingering, every effort should be made to ascertain whether a family or personal history coupled with a confusing clinical picture may represent a forme fruste of true psychiatric illness.
2. Patients who are malingering should be monitored for development of signs and symptoms of an evolving major psychiatric disorder given the high frequency of feigned psychosis being followed by true psychoses.

Quality Assurance Issues

1. Are all patients suspected of malingering evaluated for bonified medical/psychiatric/surgical illness?
2. Are records sufficient to document, for medico-legal and workmen's compensation purposes, that a patient is malingering and that all bonified illnesses have been ruled out?
3. Have all patients who are malingers been evaluated for concurrent medical/psychiatric/surgical illness?

Ethical/Legal Issues

1. If a patient suspected of malingering has a bonified medical/psychiatric/surgical disorder, has he or she been provided sufficient consultation to obviate any ensuant problems?

MANIA

A history of phasic disturbance in mood or behavior and a positive family history for affective disorder suggests bipolar disorder even if the presenting symptomatology is floridly psychotic. Manic–depressive psychoses occur in childhood and adolescence. Clinicians should be very careful not to automatically diagnose schizophrenia in a young person with florid, psychotic symptoms.

History

1. Manic–depressive illness may present with mania or depression or an admixture of both and will usually follow a course of recurrent episodes of either mood elevation or depression or both.
2. Interepisodic functioning of patients with this disorder is usually quite good and these patients often maintain employment in high standing and are responsible members of a family.
3. Lithium carbonate in most instances can sufficiently regulate the fluctuations in mood so that hospitalization may be avoided.
4. The depressions that occur in patients with this illness are characteristically of the hypersomnic, hyperlethargic, and hyperphagic type.
5. Many patients with bipolar disorder abuse alcohol or sedative medications such as barbiturates or benzodiazepines. Intoxication with these agents or withdrawal from them will frequently cloud the clinical presentation. These patients are referred to as dually diagnosed.
6. Depression, irritability, and anxiety are common correlates of a manic state. These individuals, referred to as dysphoric manics, tend to show less-rapid cycling and a greater number of hospitalizations than nondysphoric manics. Dysphoric manics have a poorer prognosis and less predictably respond to lithium. They may be the ones more likely to respond to carbamazepine (Tegretol) (Post et al, 1989).
7. Twenty to twenty-five percent of manics have the onset of their illness prior to age 20 (Hsu and Starzynski, 1986). This group is commonly misdiagnosed as schizophrenic. Failure to diagnose and treat major psychiatric illness at a time of evolving identity can lead to chronic impairment of psychosocial functioning and low self-esteem. The fact that manic adolescents present with more psychotic symptoms contributes to errors in diagnosis (McGlashan, 1988). Frequently, manic adolescents are mistakenly diagnosed as schizophrenic.
8. Mania has a differential diagnosis like headache, depression, fever, and anxiety. Organic affective disorder (Shukla et al, 1988) is common with secondary mania occurring with dysfunction of both the left and right hemisphere (Jampala and Abrams, 1983) as well as with many drugs including those used for medical indications (such as isoetharine for chronic obstructive pulmonary disease) (Goldman and Tiller, 1987).
9. Risk for development of persistent tardive dyskinesia in manic patients who have been treated with neuroleptics in the course of their illness is significant (Mukherjee et al, 1986).
10. Deprivation of sleep is believed to be a mechanism by which diverse pharmacologic psychological, environmental and, interpersonal factors induce onset of mania (Wehr et al, 1987a). The reduction of sleep that is a symptom of mania itself could serve to further self-perpetuate the manic state after being initiated by external factors.

11. The amount of lithium that is successful in managing inter-episode manic symptoms varies considerably among patients (Goodnick et al, 1987).

12. While episodes of mania and depression occur independently of stressful life events, those patients who have more recently become unstable are more likely to suffer an episode with a catastrophic event (Aronson and Shukla, 1987).

13. The dexamethasone test and the thyroid releasing hormone test has been reported to successfully discriminate patients with endogenous depression from those who are nonendogenous. Abnormal DST also discriminated patients with endogenous delusional depression from those without delusions (Levy and Stern, 1987).

14. Thought disorder occurs in some manic patients in the acute phase and in a subpopulation persists after treatment on followup (Harrow et al, 1987). Impairment of abstract ability is also reported with depression (Clark et al, 1985).

15. MRI studies of the frontal and temporal lobes of depressed bipolar patients indicate significantly higher proton T_{-1} relaxation times of red blood cells. These times tend to decrease with lithium treatment (Rosenthal J et al, 1986).

16. Rapid cycling is more common among bipolar patients than unipolar patients (Wolpert et al, 1990). Hypothyroidism during bipolar illness is a risk factor for rapid cycling, suggesting a relative central thyroid hormone deficit predisposes to a rapid cycling course in bipolar patients (Bauer et al, 1990).

17. There is no fixed pattern; a patient, after a series of manic episodes, may become depressed. A mild depression may, in fact, precede a manic episode. These periods may not always be remembered by a patient, but their relatives may remark that the patient seemed "blue" or "down" just before he became manic.

18. Family studies have revealed a strong genetic component, and when attempting to distinguish a schizophrenic episode with a strong affective component from an episode of mania or depression, a history of either schizophrenia or manic–depressive illness in the family should incline the therapist toward the disorder suggested by family inheritance.

19. Juvenile manic–depressive disorder is often associated with an early tendency for a cyclothymic mood with increasing severity and length of mood swings and delirious manic or depressive outbursts during febrile illness.

20. Amitriptyline (Elavil), imipramine (Tofranil), and other antidepressants are associated with a switch into mania in unipolar depressed patients. This phenomenon is believed to be due to the psychopharmacologic effect of the drugs on the activity of central dopamine and serotonin systems. Comparably, maintenance of tricyclic antidepressant therapy can induce rapid cycling between mania and depression in bipolar patients even while on lithium carbonate. In these instances, it is felt that the tricyclics accelerate the natural cyclic course of the illness in all its phases.

21. In a study by Winokur (1979), about 10% of hospitalized unipolar depressed patients ultimately became bipolar. Unipolar and bipolar probands have more affective illness in their families.

22. Research Diagnostic Criteria (RDC) appear useful in distinguishing schizoaffective manic patients from effectively ill manic patients. Schizoaffective patients show more paranoid and schizophrenic symptoms, have more manic episodes, and have a poor social outcome (Brockington et al, 1983).

23. Females are more affected by affective illness than males. The ratio of unipolar to bipolar illness for males and females is 1:1 and 2:1, respectively (Winokur and Crowe, 1983).
24. Individuals with late-onset bipolar illness report significantly more life events prior to onset than patients with early-onset bipolar illness (Glassner and Haldipur, 1983).
25. Adolescent patients with mania report more schizophreniform symptoms (e.g., delusion and ideas of reference) than those with episodes occurring later in life (Ballenger et al, 1982).
26. Bipolar patients and their spouses report more marital conflict than non-bipolar patients (Hoover and Fitzgerald, 1981). This is probably due to the instability that is attendant to the illness.
27. Early-onset probands have a greater morbidity risk for bipolar illness in first-degree relatives and a greater proportion of relatives with the more severe form than late-onset patients (Taylor and Abrams, 1977).
28. Untreated manic patients may progress to an intermittent or continuous delirious state simulating an organic mental disorder (Bond TC, 1980; Swartz et al, 1982).

Symptoms
1. Flight of ideas.
2. Hyperactivity.
3. Racing thoughts.
4. Euphoria.
5. Grandiosity.
6. Insomnia.
7. Irritability.
8. Hypersexuality.

Patients feel that the world is at their command and they appear to have boundless energy. Their demandingness, egocentricity, and inability to tolerate criticism sometimes serve to alienate those about them. Although uncommon, hallucinations occur secondary to sleep deprivation. There is frequently a festive air about the patient and an infectiousness about their enthusiasm. Clinicians usually feel that they can empathize more with manic patients than with those who have schizoaffective disorder. Delusions, when present, are often fascinatingly grandiose in nature. Not infrequently, a premonitory symptom or the predominant present symptom is paranoia. Other warning symptoms are: increase in social and motor activity, grandiose ideas and plans, extravagant spending, increased use of telephone, an increase in letter writing, litigiousness, increased sexual drive, decreased appetite, and decreased need for sleep. Some patients with bipolar disorder will begin to use or increase their intake of alcohol or sedatives in an attempt to calm themselves or get some sleep. Catatonia has been reported as a part of mania, and as great as 28% of patients presenting with mania have it; when present, it does not of itself forbode poor treatment response (Taylor and Abrams, 1977).

Signs

Physical examination is important to rule out organic disorders such as drug toxicity or encephalitis that may be accompanied by psychomotor agitation.

Differential Diagnosis

1. Bipolar disorder.
2. Schizophrenia.
3. Schizoaffective disorder.
4. Alcoholic excited states.
5. Catatonic excitement.
6. Delirium secondary to cerebral infection.
7. Hyperthyroidism.
8. Postencephalitic syndrome.
9. Steroid-induced mania.
10. Antidepressant-induced mania (Lewis and Winokur, 1982).
11. Decongestant-induced mania (Waters and Lapierre, 1981).
12. Amphetamine-induced mania.
13. L-dopa-induced mania.
14. Bronchodilator-induced mania (Waters and Lapierre, 1981).
15. Phencyclidine-induced mania.
16. Cocaine-induced mania.

Management

1. When patients present with mania or hypomania, the first questions that would be asked if patients are known to be manic–depressive is: "Is the patient on lithium carbonate?" If so, have they been taking their medication and what was the most recent serum lithium level? Patients who had been well-maintained at a serum level of 0.9 mEq/L may report that their recent level was 0.6 mEq/L and that they have been faithfully taking their medication. A temporary increment in dosage plus a few weeks of closer surveillance with family support may be all that is necessary. Adjunctive treatment with haloperidol (Haldol), thiothixene (Navane), or another neuroleptic or minor tranquilizer such as lorazepam (Ativan) may also be required. Some social engineering may be necessary.
2. If the patient has not been on lithium carbonate, then the first task becomes that of management of the acute episode. If patients are truly manic, their judgement may be so impaired and they may be so sleep-deprived that hospitalization is necessary for management with the appropriate psychotropic agents and lithium carbonate. If they are only hypomanic, it may be possible to control the derangement of mood with a drug such as haloperidol 2–20 mg daily and to arrange a workup for the institution of lithium carbonate maintenance (Janicak and Boshes, 1987). Adequate sleep is essential for bringing about a resolution of the acute symptomatology. Sufficient tranquilization is provided during the evening to insure restful sleep. A cooperative and knowledgeable family member can be of great help in establishing a viable treatment plan.

3. A careful history should be taken to determine if there are any clear precipitants such as recent loss, an anniversary, etc. which may be responsible for the change in mood occurring at this time. Frequently, none can be identified.

4. Family members may need some support and guidance, particularly if it is decided that it may be possible to manage the patient as an outpatient. Firm limit setting and restriction of activities is usually necessary during the acute phase when judgement is impaired.

5. Patients in a manic or hypomanic exacerbation are particularly sensitive to external and internal stimuli. Every effort should be made to interview the patient and begin medication in a quiet and controlled setting to insure that extraneous stimuli (e.g., television, radio, telephone) are kept to a minimum once the patient returns home.

6. Use of antidepressant medication in bipolar patients who have low serum lithium levels may result in a "switch" to mania (Jann et al, 1982; Wehr et al, 1988). Reported incidence of lithium noncompliance is as great as 45% (Shaw, 1986). Early relapse among lithium-treated patients is associated with greater risk of relapsing again (Strober et al, 1990). Substance abuse and many earlier admissions predict nonadherence to treatment (Aagaard and Vestergaard, 1990).

7. Because of bipolar patients' frequent desire to remain at a somewhat hypomanic state, titration of lithium levels to a stable state of hypomania may elicit greater cooperation in treatment (Burten and Ballard, 1981).

8. Hypermetabolic doses of levothyroxine sodium has been found to produce remissions in patients with intractable bipolar disorder who did not respond to treatment with neuroleptics, antidepressants, or lithium carbonate (Stancer and Persud, 1982; Bauer and Whybrow, 1990).

9. Patients presenting with mixed mania, where symptoms of depression are found together with those of clinical mania, respond more slowly and less predictably to lithium carbonate (Secunda et al, 1987).

10. Lorazepam is rapid and effective in the control of manic symptoms while serum levels of lithium are being built up without the risk of tardive dyskinesia, hypotension, and other neuroleptic side effects or of prolongation of the acute illness (Modell et al, 1985; Lenox et al, 1986).

11. Clinicians should be prepared for switches of patients from mania to depression or vice versa regardless of treatment states (Solomon et al, 1990; Thomas et al, 1990; Lucas et al, 1989; Coryell et al, 1987). Depression following a manic episode may be so profound as to require electroshock to reduce risk of suicide.

12. Suicide risk is great during both the manic and depressed phases of bipolar illness, requiring continuing reassessment of a patient's self-destructive potential.

13. The anticonvulsants carbamazepine (Tegretol) (Stoppaeck et al, 1990), valproate (Calabrese and Delucchi, 1990) and clonazepam (Clonopin) (Chouinard, 1985; Sachs et al, 1990) have all been found to be effective in lithium-resistant bipolar patients. Impact is best on mania and on cycling. Any antidepressant effect is generally reported to be considerably less.

14. Clonazepam, an alpha 2-adrenergic agonist, has been found to be efficacious in the treatment of manic patients, especially those who were nonresponsive to neuroleptics and those without a family history of affective disorder. Early response

predicted final result (Hardy et al, 1986). Clonazepam may be used alone or together with antidepressants and neuroleptics in mixed bipolar disorder (Kontaxakis et al, 1989).

15. Verapamil, an antiarrhythmic agent that blocks calcium and inhibits neurosecretory processes including excitation–secretion coupling at cholinergic and adrenergic synapses, has antimanic properties without any major side effects in most instances (Giannini et al, 1984c).

16. Mania comorbid with nonaffective psychiatric disorders or medical illness is less responsive to lithium and overall treatment than uncomplicated mania (Black et al, 1988). Patients who concurrently develop neuroleptic malignant syndrome are especially difficult to manage (Frances and Susman, 1986).

17. Additional support is required in the management of patient with bipolar disorder when confronted with stressful life events to minimize risk of exacerbation of the illness (Lieberman and Strauss, 1984).

18. Post-hospital prognosis of manic patients, even those maintained on lithium therapy, is less favorable than that of unipolar depressives (Harrow et al, 1990).

Quality Assurance Issues

1. Were all manic patients evaluated for an organic basis for their mood change?
2. Were all manic patients evaluated for suicidal and homicidal potential?
3. Were appropriate baseline studies obtained on all patients given lithium, valproate, or carbamazepine?

MARITAL CRISES

Crises within and around dissolution of marriages are one of the most common situations confronting psychiatric clinicians in emergency psychiatric services.

History

1. There are a number of questions that should be asked when one or both members of a couple appear in domestic crises. Is this the first emergency room visit of the couple?
2. What events led up to presentation in the emergency room?
3. Does either have a past psychiatric history?
4. Is there a personal or family history of divorce?
5. Are there any children? If so, what are their ages? When did the children leave home, or are any planning to leave or to marry?
6. Is either individual contemplating divorce?
7. Is a third party involved? Has, or is, either partner having an extramarital (heterosexual or homosexual) affair? (Questions regarding affairs should be asked each spouse privately as some who protest vehemently that they would *never* "wander" or experiment with homosexuality outside of a marriage will be found, on tactful questioning, to be involved in extramarital liaisons of some duration or to have deceived both spouse and clinician).

8. Does either use drugs or alcohol?
9. Has either attempted or threatened suicide? Are there fantasies of such? And, if so, how strongly are they defended against?
10. Is the spouse who appears the sicker of the two a symptom "cover" for the other? (e.g., a wife may take an overdose while acting out the suicidal preoccupations of her husband or his covert or overt homicidal messages).
11. Does it seem that the latent issue is that one spouse desires hospitalization or commitment for the other? If so, are there clinical indications for this or is it a maneuver to get rid of the spouse temporarily or permanently?
12. Be alert to the usual conflict areas in every marriage. Are the in-laws alive? How many children does the couple want and when? Are there arguments over religious, ethnic, or socio-economic class differences? How are finances regulated and are they balanced to each other's satisfaction? Has there been a recent loss or attainment of financial security or wealth? Has or is either about to retire? How is discipline of children handled? Is there child abuse? Have there been recent entrances or exits from the family system? Are they sexually satisfied with each other?
13. Inquire about physical health and attitude toward age. Has either just turned 50? Is the wife menopausal? Is either seriously ill? Has either had any recent operations? Mastectomy? Prostatectomy? Hysterectomy? Vasectomy? Is the husband impotent? Has either lost interest in sex?
14. Is help being sought for a crisis when one member of union has already independently decided to divorce the other? Have lawyers already been contacted and alternate living arrangements made?

Management

1. After obtaining a good history, observe the couple interact. If possible, interview them together as well as independently.
2. Obtain additional information from children, the family physician, or clergy as needed.
3. Consider hospitalization for one if he or she is homicidal, suicidal, or overtly psychotic. In rare instances it may be necessary or advisable to hospitalize both, either on the same treatment unit or different units.
4. Attempt to clarify the key issue, but be alert to deceptions, half truths, and family secrets when assessing the couple and planning disposition. More than one interview may be necessary to determine the appropriateness of a disposition. Trust may have to be firmly established before the real issues emerge.
5. Gauge the therapeutic intervention to the flexibility of the family system. In some cases ventilation at the time of crisis may be all that is needed. Other situations may require a variety of other approaches, including medication, referral to family agencies, referral to AA, and separation (at least during the crisis). One party may be advised to return home while the other stays with a friend or relative. If there has been a heated row and the couple has been brought in by the police but now seems to have calmed down enough to return home, the police may be willing to check on them in a couple of hours to see if the truce has continued.
6. Medication may be needed for sleep or anxiety.

7. If either has been drinking, risk of homicide or suicide increases as judgment becomes impaired and the person disinhibited. If they are truly hostile to each other, help arrange alternate living arrangements.

8. Long-term disposition depends on motivation, diagnosis, and resources. Private psychotherapy, family services, private marital counselors, legal aid, and community mental health center services are all possibilities.

9. If one party is depressed and divorce is being contemplated, crisis clinicians should be firm in the recommendation that lawyers be involved early so that one party is not exploited by the other. This is particularly important if children are involved and decisions are being made regarding both their living arrangements and support.

10. Principles of management of marital cases are not limited to conventional marriages but are also applicable to crisis work with individuals living together in a variety of alternate lifestyles such as a man and woman who do not wish to marry but live together (with or without children) or homosexual lovers living together with or without children from a previous marriage, an affair, or from adoption.

Quality Assurance Issues

1. Have both spouses been evaluated for a psychiatric disorder?

2. Has an assessment been made of possible spouse or child abuse?

3. Have both parties been interviewed alone to see if they are heterosexually or homosexually involved outside the marriage? Many people have very active sex lives outside the marriage but deny affairs because they either pay prostitutes or hustlers or have anonymous sex.

MENINGIOMA

Meningiomas may solely present behaviorally without evidence of a space-occupying lesion on physical exam. Radiographic studies of the brain corroborate diagnosis.

History

1. Meningiomas may present as seizures with psychiatric symptoms such as a feeling of impending doom or present purely behaviorally without seizure activity.

2. Symptoms seen relate to location of the meningioma. A tumor up the right temporal lobe, for instance, may present with anxiety attacks and depersonalization before the tumor itself is identified (Ghadirian et al, 1986).

3. Unexplained fear, irritation and depression that is found to be refractory to treatment may be due to unrecognized cerebral pathology involving the temporal lobes (Ghadirian et al, 1986).

Clinical Studies

1. EEG.
2. Brain scan
3 MRI

Management

1. The management of psychiatric disorders presenting as symptoms of a meningioma is that of a neurosurgeon (i.e. surgical extirpation of the tumor).
2. Psychiatric care may be required postoperatively to help repair damaged social relations due to the behavioral changes associated with the tumor that led to the crisis.

Quality Assurance Issues

1. Have all patients with meningioma been evaluated for and treated for psychiatric complications?

MENTAL SUBNORMALITY

Individuals with subnormal intelligence manifest the full spectrum of psychiatric illnesses that cause people to seek emergency psychiatric care.

History

1. Subnormal intelligence and social factors influence clinical presentation but not etiology (Sovner and Hurley, 1983).
2. For mildly and moderately retarded individuals, diagnoses can usually be made using *DSM-III-R* diagnoses. For the severely retarded it is necessary to base diagnoses on changes in vegetative functioning and changes in behavior (Sovner and Hurley, 1983).
3. The high incidence of associated CNS impairment with mental subnormality and low overall coping capacity increases the risk of associated psychiatric disorders (Eaton and Menolascino, 1982).
4. Self-injurious behavior occurs in about 10% of institutionalized mentally re tarded subjects (Kars et al, 1990).

Management

1. Mentally subnormal individuals with psychiatric illness are candidates for the full range of treatments specific to their illnesses (e.g., lithium carbonate, tricyclics, tetracyclics).
2. There is a trend toward decreased institutionalization of mentally subnormal individuals and greater normalization (Eaton and Menolascino, 1982).
3. Self-injurious behavior among the mentally subnormal is reported to respond to both naltrexone (Trexan) (Kars et al, 1990) and buspirone (Buspar).

Quality Assurance Issues

1. Are all mentally subnormal patients evaluated for a concurrent psychiatric disor der?

MEPERIDINE-INDUCED DISORDERS

Meperidine (Demerol) causes both agitation and confusion if its renal clearance is decreased as suggested by elevated serum creatinine levels.

History
1. Disorientation, hallucinations, visual disturbances, and dysphoria have been reported with meperidine use.
2. Meperidine-induced disorders occur more frequently when meperidine is used with cimetidine (Tagamet) or drugs having anticholinergic activity (Eisendrath et al, 1987).

Management
1. Physostigmine also has been reported to reverse meperidine-induced delirium suggesting that delirium, when it occurs, may be due to excessive anticholinergic activity of meperidine or normeperidine, its only active metabolite (Eisendrath et al, 1987).

METHYLPHENIDATE-INDUCED DISORDERS

Methylphenidate (Ritalin) produces psychiatric syndromes comparable to those induced by dextroamphetamine and other sympathomimetic substances as well as has psychiatric effects of own.

History
1. Patients generally present in the emergency room with a history of having taken methylphenidate for attention deficit hyperactivity disorder (ADHD) or another medical condition.
2. Individuals, including children, with a family history of bipolar disorder are particularly prone to development of mania (Koehler-Troy et al, 1986).
3. All substances that produce a hypervigilant state may provoke paranoid ideation and agitation regardless of whether or not that was present before.
4. Growth inhibition has been reported in children given methylphenrdate for ADHD but deviation from expected weight and height velocities does not appear to be significant in adolescence (Vincent et al, 1990).

Management
1. Methylphenidate should be used with caution in children, given the potential for impairment of growth. Other means of managing ADHD such as desipramine (Norpramin) should be considered in consultation with the child's attending pediatrician.
2 In most instances paranoia, agitation, and mania abate with cessation of methyl

phenidate. If they persist, as they may in a patient genetically predisposed to paranoid disorder or bipolar disorder, diagnostic-specific treatment is needed.

Quality Assurance Issues

1. Have all patients and families been advised of methylphenidate as a risk factor for growth retardation, mania and paranoia?

METOCLOPRAMIDE-INDUCED DISORDERS

Metoclopramide, used for stimulation of gastric mobility, management of reflux esophagitis, and as an antiemetic, is a dopamine-blocking agent with some side effects similar to antipsychotics.

History

1. Patients, particularly the elderly and those with renal insufficiency, should be prescribed this drug with caution as both tardive dyskinesia and acute extrapyramidal reactions have been reported (Lazzara et al, 1986).

Management

1. The same precautions should be taken with use of metoclopramide that are taken with any other dopamine-blocking agents.
2. Antiparkinson agents are used in the emergency situation to treat an acute dystonic reaction.
3. If evidence of a tardive dyskinesia is apparent, an alternate drug should be sought to manage the gastrointestinal disorder.
4. Concurrent use of antiparkinson agents may be required if a Parkinsonian tremor or akathisia is present at therapeutic doses without evidence of tardive dyskinesia.

Quality Assurance Issues

1. Are all patients informed of the risk of tardive dyskinesia and acute extrapyramidal reactions?
2. Are patients monitored for early signs of tardive dyskinesia?

METRIZAMIDE MYELOGRAPHY-INDUCED DISORDERS

Psychiatric disorders not only result from medical and surgical illness but may also be consequent to a diagnostic procedure.

History

1. The water-soluble contrast agent metrizamide is believed to have minimal neurotoxic potential but, nevertheless, has been associated with a number of psychi-

atric symptoms. These include mania, an organic affective disorder, anxiety, depression, and delirium (Kwentus et al, 1984).

Symptoms
1. Visual hallucinations.
2. Auditory hallucinations.
3. Psychosis.
4. Depression.
5. Memory impairment.
6. Delirium.

Management
1. Management is diagnostic- or symptom-specific.
2. Symptoms tend to pass as the dye is absorbed and excreted.

Quality Assurance Issues
1. Are metrizamide myelography-induced disorders included in the differential diagnosis for patients with myelography who develop psychiatric symptoms during or subsequent to the procedure?

MIGRAINE HEADACHES

Migraine is associated with transient visual disturbances, transient hemiparesis, and transient psychosis.

History
1. Vascular and neurochemical changes in the brain associated with migraine and its treatment are associated with a number of behavioral, thought, and affect disturbances.
2. Depressed men are reported to have a greater incidence of migraine than men in the general population. The same is not true of women (Garvey et al, 1984).
3. Changes in serotonin metabolism are probably responsible both for the headaches and psychiatric disorders.
4. Patients with migraine as well as with depression experience hypersomnia, fatigue, irritability, anorexia, and insomnia (Garvey et al, 1984).

Management
1. Management of psychiatric disturbances with migraine is diagnostic-specific.
2. Serotonin reuptake blockers appear to be useful both in the management of migraine alone as well as depressions that are felt due to serotonin depletion.
3. Drugs that deplete monoamines such as reserpine precipitate migraine.

MITRAL VALVE PROLAPSE

A significant number of agoraphobic patients have the mitral valve prolapse (MVP) syndrome as indicated by cardiac examination, echocardiography, phonocardiography, and electrocardiography (Kantor et al, 1980).

History
1. The dyspnea and palpitation associated with MVP may result in panic attacks and, in vulnerable individuals, agoraphobia.
2. The MVP symptoms may lead to fear and associated sympathetic response and aggravate symptoms by a feedback loop.
3. Presence or absence of MVP has no influence on indication of panic by sodium lactate (Gorman et al, 1981b).
4. In a controlled study of patients with MVP, the prevalence of anxiety disorders was interestingly no greater in patients with MVP than controls (Mazza et al, 1986). This finding was confirmed by another study comparing the incidence of anxiety disorders in MVP patients, patients with innocent murmurs, and patients without heart disease. No difference in prevalence of anxiety disorders was found (Bowen et al, 1985).

Management
1. Explaining that palpitations occur frequently with MVP and are rarely harmful alleviates the panic in selected individuals (Kantor et al, 1980).
2. Patients should be encouraged not to reduce their activities.
3. Imipramine (Tofranil) blocks the panic attacks in some individuals without curing the MVP (the mechanism of action is felt to be that either imipramine impacts a central autonomic abnormality common to both panic disorder and MVP or it alleviates the presenting of panic triggered by MVP) (Gorman et al, 1981a).
4. In susceptible individuals, cardiac arrhythmias may be produced with use of antidepressants such as desipramine (Pariser et al, 1978), enhancing panic.

Quality Assurance Issues
1. Have all patients with panic been evaluated for cardiac disease or arrhythmias triggered by medication that may enhance panic symptoms?

MOLINDONE-INDUCED DISORDERS

Massive rhabdomyolysis with subsequent acute renal failure has been reported with molindone administration (Johnson et al, 1986). Patients present with weakness, muscle pain, red or brown urine, and elevated serum creatine phosphokinase values. The symptoms and signs are similar to those seen with the neuroleptic malignant syndrome. This disorder is described as a consequence of molindone use in addition to the other typical side effects of neuroleptic drugs such as acute dystonic reactions and tardive dyskinesia.

Management

1. The management of the disorders associated with molindone use are diagnostic specific. Rhabdomyolysis is a medical emergency requiring acute intervention by specialists in internal medicine.

MONOAMINE-OXIDASE INHIBITOR (MAOI)-INDUCED DISORDERS

MAOIs are known to cause a number of reactions that range from their use alone (such as hypotension and mania) to disorders due to interactions with other drugs (such as hypertensive crises when used together with tricyclic antidepressants or tyramine producing substances) (Cooper, 1989).

History

1. A number of psychiatric disorders have been found to relate to changes in monoamine metabolism in the brain. Plasma 3-methoxy-4-hydroxy-phenoglyclol (MHPG) and homovanillic acid (HVA) concentrations, for instance, are elevated in a number of psychiatric disorders (Bowers, 1977). The principal metabolite of serotonin, 5-hydroxy-indoleacetic acid, is decreased in patients who are both suicidal and homicidal, especially in those who make the most severe suicide attempts and commit the host heinous murders (e.g., murder of spouse, child, or lover).
2. Efforts are being made to reduce the incidence of hypertensive crises. These include use of new selective MAOIs, use of new reversible MAOIs, and combining current (irreversible and nonselective) MAOIs with tricyclic antidepressants (Simpson and DeLeon, 1989).
3. The tyramine-provoked hypertension can largely be avoided by use of dietary and medication precautions through a pharmacy or by a consulting psychiatrist. Currently, second generation MAOIs are being developed with specific monoamine oxidase A and B inhibition that may eliminate need for dietary precautions (Cooper, 1989).
4. Parkinson-like tremors have been described in the elderly when given MAOIs (Teusink et al, 1984).
5. MAOI hypertensive crises have been described to occur without dietary indiscretions or use of contraindicated medications (Linet LS, 1986). The mechanism underlying this occurrence is not understood.
6. MAOIs, like tricyclic and tetracyclic antidepressants, have been reported to cause speech blockage. Explanations for this phenomenon range from relative decrease in cholinergic activity (secondary to increased noradrenergic activity) to a central anticholinergic effect (Goldstein and Goldberg, 1986).

Management

1. Management of the various MAOI-induced disorders is diagnostic and severity specific. Obviously a remarkable rise in blood pressure on an MAOI, with or without ingestion of an offending agent, is a medical crisis. Without reduction in blood pressure, the patient could sustain a cerebral hemorrhage. Less severe rise in blood pressure may be managed by withholding the MAOI and having the patient lie down and take chlorpromazine (Thorazine) or diazepam (Valium).
2. If a hypertensive crisis occurs without taking an offending agent and the crisis recurs in resumption of use of the MAOI, further medication with the MAOI should be ceased and an alternative antidepressant employed.
3. Speech blockage on any antidepressant tends to disappear with lowering of dosage of or discontinuation of the MAOI, tetracyclic, or tricyclic.

Quality Assurance Issues

1. Were all patients prescribed MAOIs provided a list of medications and foods to avoid?
2. Were all patients on MAOIs warned of the risk of an MAOI-induced hypertensive crisis, the signs and symptoms of its occurrence, and the course of action to take for treatment?
3. Were all patients on MAOIs advised to wear Medalert bracelets or necklaces indicating the fact that they are on MAOI?

MULTI-INFARCT DEMENTIA

Twenty to thirty-five percent of severe dementia is estimated due to infarctions (Cummings, 1987).

History

1. Multi-infarct dementia (MID) is characterized by a history of abrupt stepwise behavioral and cognitive deterioration coupled with a history of cardiovascular disease and the presence of focal neurologic signs and symptoms.
2. Organic affective syndromes are common to MID and include emotional lability, depression, and psychoses.
3. Underlying etiology includes atherosclerosis, collagen vascular disease, diabetes, hypertension, and embolic disease

Clinical Studies

1. MRI.
2. EEG.
3. CT scan.

Management

1 Treatment includes both diagnostic-specific management of the underlying dis-

order (e.g., hypertension) and generalized measures to minimize disability due to dementia and the impact of managing a demented patient on the family.

2. The organic mental disorders are managed by diagnostic specific interventions (e.g., antidepressants for an organic affective disorder, lithium and beta-blockers, or anticonvulsants for violent outbursts).

Quality Assurance Issues

1. Have all patients with multiinfarct dementia been evaluated for a depression causing pseudodementia superimposed on the multiinfarct dementia?

MULTIPLE MYELOMA

Multiple myeloma is an uncommon cancer. This neoplastic disease of plasma cells is the most common lymphoreticular malignancy in nonwhites and third most common in whites (Blattner et al, 1981).

History

1. Delirium is a common complication of multiple myeloma.
2. The etiology of the delirium seen may be due to (Silberfarb and Bates, 1983):

   a. Analgesics,
   b. Radiation therapy,
   c. Chemotherapeutic agents (particularly prednisone),
   d. Renal failure,
   e. Electrolyte imbalance,
   f. Anemia,
   g. Fever,
   h. Hepatic failure,
   i. Septicemia, and
   j. Affective disorders.

3. The delirium seen appears to be that of cerebral insufficiency (Lipowski, 1980).

Management

1. Amelioration of the delirium occurs to the degree it is possible to restore any of the contributing factors to normal (e.g., lowering or discontinuing the dose of prednisone, restoration of electrolyte balance, selection of an alternative analgesic).
2. Psychotherapeutically, it is important to give patients as much control as possible when they feel their body cells are out of control (and in reality they are) by allowing them to participate actively in treatment decisions.

Quality Assurance Issues

1. Have all patients been evaluated for psychiatric effects of the disorder and of the impact of the disorder on the family?

MULTIPLE PERSONALITIES

The etiology of multiple personality disorder (MPD) is felt to be due to unrecognized abuse of self-hypnosis by which a person creates various personalities (Bliss, 1983).

History
1. The disorder frequently begins early in childhood (i.e., 4 to 5 years of age).
2. Self-hypnosis allows compartmentalization of an experience or personality function to an alternate ego through the amnesia of hypnosis (Bliss, 1983).
3. These individuals are sometimes misdiagnosed as schizophrenic because of the presence of what appears to be delusional thinking, paranoia, and hallucinations.
4. Most such patients qualify for the diagnosis of hysteria that today would be called Briquet's syndrome. Hysterical symptoms may be due to self-hypnotic induction of conversion and other symptoms (Bliss, 1983).
5. Skillful use of hypnosis allows emergence of the various personalities and allows a clinician to obtain more history to better understand the etiology of the problem.
6. Patients with a history of childhood physical and sexual abuse report a greater incidence of dissociative symptoms than those without an abuse history (Chu and Dill, 1990).
7. Prostitutes and exotic dancers report both more dissociative symptoms and abuse (Ross CA et al, 1989).
8. MPD patients are found to have a consistently stable set of features when using structured interviews including a history of childhood physical or sexual abuse (Ross CA et al, 1990).

Differential Diagnosis
1. Dissociative disorder.
2. Multiple personality disorder
3. Schizophrenia.
4. Complex partial seizures.
5. Borderline personality disorder

Management
1. Personalities of an MPD patient that may cause presentation in the emergency room may be managed by hypnotizing the patient and accessing a less disruptive personality
2. Great skill is needed in long-term management of patients with MPD. Referral to a therapist with considerable experience in managing these patients enhances the possibility of a good prognosis.
3. MPD patients can be distinguished from patients with complex partial seizures who exhibit dissociative phenomena. Use of electroencephalography and struc

tured interviews facilitates differentiating the two disorders (Ross CA et al, 1989).

4. Emergency clinicians as well as ongoing therapists should be aware that a personality may exist or emerge de novo in some patients who are suicidal, homicidal, or otherwise self-destructive (e.g., they may act out the role of a female or male prostitute and contract AIDS). Circumstances that serve to elicit this personality consultation should be defined and steps made to minimize such dissociation while therapeutic effort is made to integrate the various unacceptable components of the personality and while less self- or other-destructive means are used to manage depression, low self-esteem, and rage (Hall PE, 1988).

Ethical/Legal Issues

1. Patients with MPD may commit crimes, including murder, and not recall the event when another personality assumes dominance, creating need for therapists to skillfully employ hypnosis to allow testimony and to direct treatment.

MULTIPLE SCLEROSIS

It used to be thought that euphoria was commonly seen with multiple sclerosis, the basis of which was posited to be either due to denial of the seriousness of the illness, or attributed to a "functional lobotomy" due to multiple sclerotic plagues. Today, we are aware that depression and cognitive impairment are as common, or more common, with suicide due to concurrent affective illness in some a major risk.

History

1. Multiple sclerosis (MS) is the most common of the demyelinating diseases.
2. About one-quarter of MS patients report euphoria; another one-fourth report depression (Kwentus et al, 1986).
3. Mania has been reported with MS as the only manifestation of disease activity (Kwentus et al, 1986).
4. Both functional loss due to physical disability associated with the illness and the exacerbation and progression of symptoms are particular stressors for MS patients (Devins and Seland, 1987).
5. There is some evidence suggesting that bipolar disorder is more common among patients with MS (Schiffer et al, 1986).
6. Depression is found more commonly among MS patients with cerebral involvement than MS patients with spinal cord involvement predominating (Schiffer et al, 1983).

Management

1. Treatment consists of neurologic management of the MS with concomitant psychiatric management of psychiatric disorders with diagnostic-specific treatment

2. Depression may occur with MS, creating a picture of pseudodementia that remits with appropriate antidepressant therapy.

MUTISM

Mutism may be the presenting condition in the emergency room for a number of neurologic and psychiatric disorders.

History
1. Illnesses presenting with mutism include diseases of the basal ganglia, limbic system structures, and frontal lobes, and schizophrenia, dementias, dissociative disorders, affective illness, and conversion disorders (Altshuler et al, 1986).
2. As great as 25% of patients with catatonia and mutism are depressed (Altshuler et al, 1986).
3. Conditions and agents that produce mutism with catatonia include myxedema, herpes encephalitis, tertiary syphilis, AIDS, phencyclidine-induced psychoses, closed-head injuries, Addison's disease, diabetic ketoacidosis, hyperparathyroidism, alcohol-induced psychoses, aspirin intoxication, frontal lobe lesions, postictal phase of seizures, Wenicke's encephalopathy, akinetic mutism, and maprotiline (Altshuler et al, 1986).

Management
1. Treatment is diagnostic-specific after the etiology of the mutism is determined.

MYOCARDIAL INFARCTION

Psychiatric symptoms may precede, occur concurrently with, or be pursuant to a heart attack.

History
1. As a heart goes into failure due to coronary occlusive vascular disease, blood pressure may fall and congestive heart failure may occur due to decreased ability of the heart to pump blood. When this occurs, epinephrine may be released by the body creating a subjective feeling of impending doom.
2. As a heart goes into failure, breathing becomes more difficult. Subjective anxiety may evolve into frank panic as the severity of congestive heart failure increases.
3. Depression following a heart attack does not usually commence until the third day (Hackett, 1985). The first 1 or 2 days are more fraught with anxiety over having sustained a life-threatening illness, and over the presence of a strange environment and machines. Depression generally centers on the possibility of recurrence of a myocardial infarction and death and concern over ability of the patient to serve in the role of parent, spouse, and worker.

4. Depression and anxiety disorders are more likely to occur if a patient suffers chest pain or impairment of cardiac functioning (Vazquez-Barquero et al, 1985).

Management

1. In the acute stage, benzodiazepines such as alprazolam (Xanax) serve to reduce anxiety and facilitate rest and sleep.
2. Ventilation serves to reduce anxiety as well as to reduce depression as a patient assumes control over whatever he or she can in their life (e.g., return to work) in order to handle that which they cannot control (e.g., the fact they had a heart attack).
3. Self-help groups of others who have sustained a heart attack allow ventilation of specific concerns (e.g., will it occur again?). Nothing helps one to understand as much as to be understood.
4. Antidepressants are ill-advised in the first 3 weeks following an attack and usually should not be given at anytime without prior consultation with the patient's cardiologist.
5. If patients are profoundly depressed and psychopharmacotherapy with antidepressants is contraindicated, electroshock is generally deemed safe.
6. In some instances, delirium may persist for days due to medication, environment, and physiologic changes attendant with the myocardial infarction. In such instances, careful attention to multiple factors impairing cognitive functioning facilitates resolution (e.g., hydration, restoration of electrolyte balance, discontinuation of meperidine [Demerol]).

NALTREXONE-INDUCED DISORDERS

The opiate antagonist naltrexone (Trexan) has been successfully used in some patients to prevent relapse. Unfortunately, in 2 weeks about 30% are noncompliant, and by the eighth month, 90% are noncompliant (Crowley et al, 1985). Naltrexone has also been successfully used to reduce self-injurious behavior (Sandman et al, 1987) that appears related to elevated opiate levels.

History

1. Naltrexone prevents activation of the body's opiate receptors, thereby blocking the euphoric effects of opiates. There is some evidence that use of naltrexone may, by virtue of this blockade, lead to a dysphoria that contributes to noncompliance with its use (Crowley et al, 1985).

Management

1. Clonidine hydrochloride, the imidazoline antihypertensive, coupled with naltrexone allows successful withdrawal from methadone in as little as 4 to 5 days with symptoms of abstinence such as muscular aching, anxiety, restlessness, insomnia, and anorexia being mild to nonexistent at the fifth day (Charney

et al, 1986a). This is an indication that the combination of the two drugs may facilitate compliance with naltrexone treatment.

NARCISSISTIC PERSONALITY DISORDER

Narcissistic personality disorders are characterized by exaggeration of talents, boastful and pretentious behavior, a sense of superiority and uniqueness, self-referential and self-centered behavior, grandiose fantasies, arrogance, haughtiness, need for attention and admiration, and high achievement (Ronningstam and Gunderson, 1990).

These patients are difficult to manage both in psychotherapy as well as in the emergency room. Many of the comments made regarding acute treatment of the borderline personality disorder apply to management of this group.

NARCOLEPSY

The key characteristics of narcolepsy are attacks of intense sleep cataplexy (drop attacks), sleep paralysis and hypnagogic hallucinations.

History
1. Paranoid disorders can develop in the treatment of narcolepsy due to abuse of analeptics (e.g., dextroamphetamine, methylphenidate) prescribed to treat the disorder (Leong et al, 1989).
2. Polysomnography is used to document the diagnosis of narcolepsy by the occurrence with daytime drowsiness of two or more rapid eye movement onsets (Rosenthal LD et al, 1990).

Management
1. Withdrawal of analeptics when paranoia occurs may lead to worsening of sleep attacks while addition of neuroleptics may enhance drowsiness, cause depression, dysphoria, or extrapyramidal side effects, and increase risk of tardive dyskinesia. Tricyclic medication, on the other hand, when used may exacerbate psychosis (Leong et al, 1989).
2. If the analeptic can be reduced, causing remission of the paranoia without impact on the narcolepsy, it is the treatment of choice.
3. If reduction of the analeptic causes exacerbation of narcolepsy, management with a tricyclic should be attempted.
4. If approaches 2 and 3 fail, a high-potency, low-dosage neuroleptic may be given with minimal sedating effects to manage the paranoia.

Quality Assurance Issues
1. Have all patients diagnosed to have narcolepsy been evaluated for organic factors contributing to the disorder?

2. Have patients treated for narcolepsy been advised of the complications of the medication used in the management of the disorder?

Ethical/Legal Issues
1. Have patients with narcolepsy been advised of risks of suffering the attacks?

NEUROLEPTIC-INDUCED DISORDERS

Neuroleptic drugs must be used with extreme caution because of risk of the neuroleptic malignant syndrome, tardive dyskinesia, and other adverse side effects.

History
1. Patients with affective illness including mania appear more vulnerable than schizophrenic patients to the development of acute extrapyramidal symptoms when prescribed neuroleptics (Nasrallah et al, 1988; Blum, 1980).
2. Patients provided trihexyphenidyl hydrochloride concomitantly with chlorpromazine (Thorazine) do not appear to show differences in chlorpromazine serum levels (Simpen et al, 1980). Adjunctive use of anticholinergics prophylactically both enhances patient compliance with neuroleptic therapy as well as minimizes occurrence of extrapyramidal disturbances such as akathisia, which may mimic psychopathology leading to ill-advised increase in neuroleptic dose (WHO Consensus Statement, 1990).
3. While drug-induced laryngeal spasm leading to cardiac arrest via vagal reflexes may represent a mechanism of sudden death on haloperidol (Haldol) and other neuroleptics (Modestin et al, 1981), asymptomatic coronary heart disease, the leading cause of sudden, natural death in young adults, must be carefully ruled out at autopsy (Smith et al, 1980).
4. Concomitant use of the anticonvulsants phenobarbital or diphenylhydantoin (Dilantin) significantly lower serum levels of haloperidol (Linnoila et al, 1980).
5. The antiparkinsonian agent biperiden (Akineton) has not been shown to lower plasma levels of haloperidol (Linnoila et al, 1980).
6. Young, acutely psychotic inpatients with relatively good prognoses who were treated by high- and low-dose haloperidol using a rapid neuroleptization technique showed no difference as to degree of symptom alleviation, suggesting that low-dose haloperidol may be as efficacious as high-dose in the symptomatic management of patients in this group (Weborsky et al, 1981).
7. The symptoms of withdrawal from neuroleptics include insomnia, restlessness, agitation, diarrhea, rhinorrhea, myalgia, diaphoresis, anorexia, nausea, emesis, anxiety, and paraesthesias. These symptoms are distinguished from those of incipient psychotic exacerbation such as anxiety, agitation, and insomnia by the former occurring earlier and including nausea, emesis, rhinorrhea, and myalgias (Dilsaver and Coffman, 1988).
8. There is some evidence that alprazolam (Xanax) given with neuroleptics may enhance clinical improvement without necessitating increase in neuroleptic

levels and without significant increase in neuroleptic serum level (Douyon et al, 1989).

9. Consideration of potential side effects is a major concern, such as anticipating anticholinergic effects from thioridazine (Mellaril) in elderly patients, or the knowledge that haloperidol is rarely associated with hepatic damage. A hallucinating man with a history of premature ejaculation might especially profit from thioridazine while a hallucinating woman who has long fought a battle with obesity is a candidate for molindone (Moban).

10. There is a consistent correlation between 48-hour change in the clinical picture and the eventual degree of improvement at the end of drug treatment, suggesting that early change with medication is a predictor of therapeutic outcome (May et al, 1980).

11. Effective weight-standardized neuroleptic dosage is significantly lower for Asians than for Caucasian counterparts (Lin and Findler, 1983).

12. Intentional neuroleptic overdose produces serious complications including CNS depression, hypotension, cardiac arrhythmias, respiratory failure, tachycardia, and death (Allen MD et al, 1980). Cause of death when it occurs is usually attributed to a cardiac arrhythmia.

13 Some schizophrenics, as great as 68% of the patients in one study (Manos et al, 1981), require continuous use of antiparkinsonian agents such as trihexyphenidyl during neuroleptic management of chronic schizophrenia.

14. All neuroleptics administered in equivalent doses appear to produce the same degree of antipsychotic activity (Kessler and Waletzky, 1981).

15. The most common cause of relapse in treatment of psychosis is patient noncompliance (Kessler and Waletzky, 1981).

16. The most common cause of treatment failure of acute psychosis is inadequate neuroleptic dosage (Kessler and Waletzky, 1981).

17. Vomiting may also occur after abrupt removal of benztropine (Cogentin) treatment while antipsychotic medication is continued (Schaffer et al, 1981). Nausea, vomiting, and diaphoresis are seen with withdrawal of anticholinergic agents from patients treated for Parkinson's disease.

18. The symptoms of neuroleptic withdrawal are felt to occur more frequently with antipsychotics with strong anticholinergic activity.

19. Symptoms of withdrawal are not as great if antiparkinsonian agents are not simultaneously withdrawn.

20. The medical symptoms of neuroleptic withdrawal are believed to be due to rebound cholinergic hypersensitivity associated with the anticholinergic action of drugs rather than to their dopamine blocking activity (Luchins et al, 1980).

21. There is a high rate of clinical nonrecognition of extrapyramidal disorders—particularly tardive dyskinesia—indicating a need for education in identifying these disorders in order to prevent long-term problems associated with tardive dyskinesia as well as to prevent increase in neuroleptic dosage when extrapyramidal effects are mistaken for psychotic symptoms (Weiden PJ et al, 1987).

22. Meige's syndrome (oromandibular dystonia and blepharospasm) has been reported to result from long-term neuroleptic use. It may be a variant of tardive

dyskinesia for which prompt cessation of the neuroleptic may be therapeutic (Ananth et al, 1988).

Management

1. In most instances, prompt cessation of neuroleptics reduces the side effects of neuroleptic use.
2. When tardive dyskinesia is present, discontinuation of neuroleptic use may reverse or at least reduce intensity of symptoms in some cases. When the movement disorder persists, other measures described in the section on tardive dyskinesia are required.
3. Intravenous, intramuscular, or oral benztropine or Benadryl effectively treat acute dystonic reactions.
4. When withdrawal symptoms emerge, recommencement of the neuroleptic with gradual withdrawal generally reduces withdrawal symptoms. Alternately, continuation of antiparkinson agents for 1 or 2 weeks will suppress withdrawal phenomena.
5. Not everyone on neuroleptics or antiparkinson agents requires them, but for those who do, much discomfort can be avoided, and in many instances noncompliance minimized, when extrapyramidal side effects cause a patient to discontinue antipsychotic medication.

Quality Assurance Issues

1. Were all patients warned of the risk of extrapyramidal side effects and explicitly of the risk of tardive dyskinesia?
2. Have patients been monitored for emergence of signs of tardive dyskinesia?
3. Is the minimum amount of neuroleptic prescribed to suppress symptoms?
4. When neuroleptics are discontinued, has the process been gradual or have antiparkinson agents been continued for 1 or 2 weeks after?
5. Have antiparkinson agents been prescribed when needed (and not excessively, if not needed)?
6. Have patients been evaluated for evidence of neuroleptic side effect before neuroleptic dosage is increased, feeling a particular movement disorder is due to psychosis?

Ethical/Legal Issues

1. Has a patient been kept on the minimally effective dose of a neuroleptic to minimize occurrence of tardive dyskinesia?

NEUROLEPTIC MALIGNANT SYNDROME

Neuroleptics can cause dysregulation of hypothalamic control of the autonomic nervous system (Henderson and Wooten, 1981) and in the extreme the neuroleptic malignant syndrome (NMS). A link has been suggested of this syndrome to lethal catatonia.

History

1. Structural changes have not been identified in patients who die of this syndrome (Morris et al, 1980).
2. NMS is estimated to occur in about 1% of neuroleptically treated patients (Keck et al, 1987). If episodes of milder cases are included, estimates go as high as 12% (Velamoor et al, 1990). NMS is a spectrum disorder with milder variants (Addonizio et al, 1986; Addonizio et al, 1987).
3. Factors that increase risk of NMS include a greater number of intramuscular injections, greater psychomotor agitation, and higher doses of neuroleptics at greater rates of dose increase (Keck et al, 1989). Low-dose neuroleptic use reduces risk considerably (Gelenberg et al, 1988).
4. NMS patients are not at considerably greater risk than others for developing malignant hyperthermia during ECT or surgery (Hermesh et al, 1988).

Symptoms

1. Alterations of consciousness.
2. Mutism.
3. Apprehension.
4. Dysphagia.
5. Urinary incontinence.

Signs

1. Hyperthermia.
2. Hypertension.
3. Diaphoresis.
4. Tachycardia.
5. Dyskinesia.
6. Tachycardia.
7. Rigidity.
8. Akinesia.

Management

1. The finding of an excessive catecholamine secretion component in NMS, indicating hyperactivity of the sympathoadrenomedullary component of the autonomic nervous system, provides a basis for use of catecholamine-blocking agents to treat some patients with the syndrome (Feibel and Schiffer, 1981).
2. Dantrolene sodium has been associated with improvement (Coons DJ et al, 1982; Rosebush and Stewart, 1989).
3. Bromocriptine mesylate 2.5–4.5 mg/day in 3 divided doses for at least 10 days has been used to successfully treat NMS (Dhib-Jalbut et al, 1987). Improvement tends to occur in 1 to 3 days and is associated with a drop in serum CPK levels. It takes about 1 week for the resolution of extrapyramidal rigidity. Bromocriptine is a dopamine agonist (Zubenko and Pope, 1983).
4. The fact that complications of NMS include renal failure, rhabdomyolysis, car-

diopulmonary failure, dehydration, disseminated intravascular coagulation, infection, and shock indicate that intensive medical management in a general hospital is indicated when the symptoms and signs are severe (Lazarus, 1990).

Quality Assurance Issues
1. Are all patients on neuroleptics monitored for NMS?
2. When symptoms and signs of NMS occur, is diagnostic-specific treatment provided?

NEUROLEPTIC NONCOMPLIANCE

Neuroleptic noncompliance may relate to side effects of the medication, the nature of a patient's psychiatric illness, psychoses, a patient's personality and family, or social pressure. In all instances, noncompliance enhances risk of relapse and hospitalization, and in some instances of suicide and homicide (Weiden PJ et al, 1986).

Management
1. Given the fact that it is difficult to predict who will be noncompliant, it is important to attempt to prevent noncompliance in all patients by working with patients and families to understand the consequences of noncompliance and to be aware of side effects and how they may be managed (Kane JM, 1986b).

Quality Assurance Issues
1. Have all patients been informed of the need for compliance to prevent rehospitalization and exacerbation of symptoms?

Ethical/Legal Issues
1. Consent to treatment is critical to compliance and is to be obtained from adult patients and from parents if a patient is too young to provide consent to treatment themselves (Schwartz, 1989).

NEUROSYPHILIS

Syphilis and tuberculosis are great masqueraders of many different illnesses. Psychiatric presentations of both are myriad and may appear with or without neurologic signs and symptoms. Both are included in the differential diagnosis of most psychiatric disorders. Neurosyphilis is often forgotten these days because of the emphasis on AIDS, but it may occur comorbidly with AIDS or, in fact, imitate AIDS.

History
1. The incidence of primary syphilis has increased in the past 2 decades but the incidence of neurosyphilis has fallen. This is attributed to the early identification of the illness (Rundell and Wise, 1985).

2. Partial treatment of primary syphilis due to use of antibiotics for concurrent infections when syphilis itself goes unrecognized has resulted in the emergence of atypical and aberrant presentations (Rundell and Wise, 1985).
3. Affective symptoms in patients with neurologic illness resemble those of primary affective illness with decreased frequency of family members suffering the same illness (Berrios et al, 1987).
4. Chronic affective illness forebodes negatively on the prognosis of neurologic disease (Berrios et al, 1987).

Symptoms and Signs
1. Nearly all psychiatric symptoms and signs may appear with the various forms of syphilis. In many instances these will be concurrent general or focal neurologic signs.

Differential Diagnosis
1. Syphilis is included in the differential diagnosis of all psychiatric disorders.

Clinical Studies
1. Serological test for syphilis.

Management
1. The management of the primary disease (i.e., syphilis) is appropriate antibiosis (e.g., penicillin) in doses and duration sufficient to eliminate the infection.
2. Concurrent psychiatric symptoms require diagnostic-specific treatment (e.g., neuroleptics for paranoia).
3. After syphilis is treated, the psychosocial consequence on the family may require supportive family therapy.
4. Residual psychiatric and neurologic symptoms may require long-term psychopharmacotherapy and rehabilitative therapy.

Quality Assurance Issues
1. Was the serological test for syphilis performed on all individuals at risk?

NICOTINE-INDUCED DISORDERS

There has been considerable controversy over whether sudden cessation of tobacco smoking leads to withdrawal symptoms and, if so, how to manage them. Current consensus is that there is a nicotine withdrawal symptom that enhances addiction.

History
1. Dependent smokers seek nicotine supplements when their intake is arbitrarily reduced (Shiffman et al, 1990).
2. Cotinine is a long-lasting metabolite of nicotine that is measurable in the blood.
3 Nicotine gum can create the same dependence that smoking does. When nicotine

gum is stopped suddenly, some users commence smoking again or surreptitiously seek nicotine gum despite proscription (Hughes et al, 1986).
4. Individuals with more withdrawal discomfort are more tolerant to the cardiovascular effects of nicotine (Hughes and Hatsukami, 1986).
5. There appears to be little consensus among definitions of tobacco dependence and withdrawal (Hughes et al, 1987).

Symptoms of Nicotine Withdrawal
(Hughes and Hatsukami, 1986)
1. Irritability.
2. Difficulty concentrating.
3. Restlessness.
4. Impatience.
5. Craving for tobacco.
6. Somatic complaints.
7. Anxiety.
8. Increased hunger.

Signs of Nicotine Withdrawal
(Hughes and Hatsukami, 1986)
1. Increased eating.
2. Bradycardia.

Management
1. Individuals who have more withdrawal discomfort do not have a lower rate of smoking cessation.
2. Treatment of nicotine withdrawal is superior in effect to no treatment but still somewhat limited (Mann et al, 1986).
3. Behavioral techniques to deter nicotine craving may help to break the habit of smoking and chewing nicotine gum (Mann LS et al, 1986).
4. The new "patch" used to curb smoking has proven successful in some cases.

Quality Assurance Issues
1. Is nicotine withdrawn gradually and is nicotine gum withdrawn gradually to minimize risk of relapse?
2. Has the patient been offered the option of behavioral control or the "patch?"

Ethical/Legal Issues
1. Have all patients who smoke been advised of the damage to their health?
2. Have all patients who smoke been offered smoking cessation programs?
3. Have individuals who have successfully ceased smoking been provided a smoke-free environment when hospitalized?

NIGHTMARES

Nightmares may be a symptom of psychiatric illness such as schizophrenia, panic disorder, or major depression, or occur independently without pathologic significance.

History
1. Nightmares are a common sequela to childhood and adolescent sexual abuse. Common themes are being chased by someone, often the molester, with the person chased (the dreamer or a beloved character) being killed. These dreams differ from dreams of being chased by nonabused individuals by the fact the protagonist in the dream is less frequently directly attacked or killed in nonabused adolescents' dreams (Garfeld, 1987).
2. Frequent nightmare sufferers as a group are found to be more open and sensitive, more artistic and creative, have more first- and second-degree relatives with frequent nightmares, have more features of schizophrenic spectrum disorders, and have more psychiatric hospitalizations than individuals without them (Hartmann et al, 1987).
3. Nightmares differ from night terrors discussed in the next section.

Management
1. Management of nightmares, when they are part of a specific psychiatric illness, is that of the specific disorder.
2. Nightmares are a common sequela together with intrusive thoughts of the post-traumatic stress disorder (PTSD) in which group support by individuals who have suffered a similar experience, together with ventilation and antidepressant pharmacotherapy, is the recommended course of therapy.

Quality Assurance Issues
1. Have all children with nightmares been evaluated for the occurrence of treatment-responsive night terrors, affective illness, and post-traumatic stress disorders?

NIGHT TERRORS

Night terrors are episodes of extreme panic and terror with intense motility and vocalization and increased autonomic discharge occurring at night.

History
1. Episodes tend to be of short duration lasting 1 to several minutes.
2. Individuals experiencing night terrors tend to have little or no memory of the event immediately after or the morning that follows.
3 Night terrors, like sleep walking, is a disorder of impaired arousal

4. Night terrors should not be confused with nightmares. The latter is not associated with the same degree of autonomic arousal, impairment of memory for the event, anxiety, motility, and vocalization.
5. Compared with sleepwalkers, individuals with night terrors have a later age of onset, a greater frequency of events, and greater time of rate of occurrence (Kales JD et al, 1980). Both groups have high levels of psychopathology.
6. Although night terrors and sleepwalking in childhood appear related to genetic and developmental factors, their onset in adulthood is found related to psychological factors (Kales JD et al, 1980).
7. Night terrors occur in stages 3 and 4 of sleep while nightmares are related to rapid eye movement sleep.
8. Night terror events are often accompanied by sleepwalking activity.
9. Night terrors are also known as "pavor nocturnus" in children and "incubus" in adults.
10. Sleep walking (which occurs in approximately 2.5% of the population) and night terrors may result in life-threatening injuries (Kauch and Stern, 1990).

Management
1. Safety measures such as special bolts on windows and sleeping on the ground floor may be necessary.
2. Benzodiazepine tranquilizers or hypnotics that suppress stage 3 or 4 sleep may be used in adults but are discouraged in children (Kales JD et al, 1980).
3. Because of the frequently attendant psychological problems, psychotherapy is often required.
4. Bedpartners and live-companions should be alerted that forcible interruption of a night terror may result in greater fear and confusion aggravating a patient's condition.

Quality Assurance Issues
1. Have all children with night terrors been provided diagnostic-specific treatment for the disorder?

NITROUS OXIDE-INDUCED DISORDERS

Nitrous oxide or laughing gas is used by teenagers and health professionals such as dentists who have ready access to it to develop a mild euphoria high and light headedness.

History
Younger adolescents may obtain it by using the gas from aerosol cans of whipped cream (referred to as using "whippeds" in the drug culture). Holding the can upright without shaking and pressing the release may allow them as many as 5 to 6 hits.

Symptoms
1. Mild euphoria.
2. Light-headedness.

Management
1. The effect is mild and transient and tends not to require any acute intervention.

Quality Assurance Issues
1. Have all patients with nitrous oxide-induced disorder been evaluated for another psychiatric disorder contributing to use of nitrous oxide for recreational purposes?
2. Have all patients with nitrous oxide-induced disorder been evaluated for a substance abuse disorder?

NONBACTERIAL THROMBOTIC ENDOCARDITIS

An organic mental disorder may be an indicant of bacterial and non-bacterial endocarditis.

History
1. Nonbacterial thrombotic endocarditis occurs when fibrin-platelet vegetations form on one or more uninflamed valve leaflets.
2. Although the onset of symptoms is usually sudden, onset may be subacute when microemboli are present (Mackenzie and Popkin, 1980).
3. Computed tomography may be normal.
4. Electroencephalography usually shows a diffusely abnormal rhythm confirming the diagnosis of an organic mental disorder (Mackenzie and Popkin, 1980).

Symptoms and Signs
1. The symptoms and signs are those of delirium.

Management
1. The management of nonbacterial, thrombotic, endocarditis-induced organic mental disorders involves concurrent treatment of the endocarditis by a cardiologist and of the delirium by a psychiatrist.
2. Small doses of a high-potency, low-dose neuroleptic such as perphenazine (Trilafon) 2 mg PO tid is generally sufficient to manage the agitation.
3. If the patient does not suffer chronic obstructive lung disease or another respiratory ailment that a benzodiazepine may exacerbate or worsen, small doses of lorazepam (Ativan) may be used.

Quality Assurance Issues
1. Have all patients with endocarditis and sudden onset of change in mental status been evaluated for non-bacterial or bacterial thrombotic endocarditis?

NUTMEG INTOXICATION

Nutmeg, derived from the seeds of the aromatic evergreen *myristica fragrans* native to the Spice Islands, is one of the oldest spices in use.

History
1. The psychoactive substance myristicin is found both in the seed coat and in the oil of the seeds.
2. Individuals seeking an inexpensive hallucinogenic experience may purchase the drug at the spice counter of a grocery story and take it directly or mix it with food.
3. Hallucinations and agitation have been reported when inadvertently a naive person has used inappropriate proportions of nutmeg in preparation of a pie.
4. Death due to fatty degeneration of the liver has been reported in severe cases of poisoning (Faquet and Rowland, 1978).

Symptoms
1. Agitation.
2. Palpitations.
3. Numbness in the extremities.
4. Visual hallucinations.
5. Severe headache.
6. Alteration of time and space perception

Signs
1. Flushing.
2. Muscular excitement.

Management
1. Symptoms abate with time.
2. Small doses of lorazepam (Ativan) may be used for agitation.

Quality Assurance Issues
1. Are all patients with substance-induced disorder evaluated for less common causes, not necessarily recreational, of substance-induced disorders such as excessive nutmeg on a traditional pumpkin pie?

OBSESSIVE–COMPULSIVE DISORDER

Patients with symptoms of obsessive–compulsive disorder (OCD) present in the emergency room when the symptoms have served to defend against emerging psychosis or unacceptable suicidal, homicidal, or sexual feelings and the defenses are failing or when patients with OCD itself are severely incapacitated by the symptoms and desperately seek immediate help.

History

1. The patients generally have months or years of increasing rituals and obsessions which limit their ability to function.
2. Anxiety and depression may be part of the illness or have evolved as separate illness states in response to the stress of having such incapacitating and limiting symptoms such as rituals and recurrent thoughts.
3. The most frequently observed personality traits in people with OCD include passive–aggressiveness, dependence, and avoidance (Joffe et al, 1988b).

Symptoms

1. Recurrent intrusive thoughts.
2. Rituals.

Signs

1. The patient may exhibit extremely dry skin or even excoriations and bleeding due to repeated hand washing.

Management

1. The first step in the emergency situation is to ascertain whether there is significant risk of homicide or suicide, or of a patient's defenses deteriorating. If so, appropriate safeguards must be undertaken to manage self- or other-destructive impulses.
2. If a psychosis such as schizophrenia is emerging, the patient should be started on a neuroleptic in doses sufficient to obviate need for hospitalization if possible.
3. OCD symptoms may be a symptom of a sequela to a number of organic mental disorders such as encephalitis. These symptoms have a differential that includes most psychiatric and medical disorders as their occurrence in a patient who is biogenetically or psychologically predisposed to manifestation of OCD may give genesis to obsessions or compulsions.
4. Skin care is medically required when excoriations are present in addition to psychopharmacotherapy.
5. Clomipramine (Anafranil) is a tricyclic antidepressant that has been found to have specific impact in managing OCD at doses comparable to those used with imipramine (Tofranil) (100–300 mg). The antiobsessional effect of both clomipramine and imipramine appears to occur at least partially independent of their antidepressant effect (Mavissakalian et al, 1985).
6. Fluoxetine (Prozac) at doses generally greater than that used for depression (e.g., 40–100 mg per day for OCD) has been reported to be effective for management of both obsessiveness and compulsiveness and attendant depression in OCD (Turner SM et al, 1985).
7. Fluvoxamine has been demonstrated to reduce obsessive–compulsive symptoms

as well as anxiety and depression (Perse et al, 1987). Fluvoxamine, like clomipramine and fluoxetine is a serotonin agonist (Goodman WK et al, 1989).

8. Fluoxetine and fluvoxamine have been augmented respectively with buspirone (Buspar) and a neuroleptic for treatment of refractory OCD. The fact that buspirone coupled with fluoxetine is more potent than fluoxetine monotherapy suggests that the site of buspirone impact (i.e., the 5-HT postsynaptic receptor) is of importance in treating OCD (Markovitz et al, 1990). Addition of a neuroleptic is not effective when OCD is comorbid with tic spectrum disorders or schizotypal personality disorder indicating that brain dopamine as well as serotonin may be involved in a subtype of refractory OCD (McDougle et al, 1990).

9. Alprazolam (Xanax) alone has been reported effective when anxiety accompanies OCD in patients with a history of panic attacks (Tesar and Jenike, 1984).

10. Sertraline (Zoloft) has not been demonstrated effective in treating OCD despite its serotonin agonist properties (Jenike et al, 1990).

11. Electroshock has been used in successfully treating some refractory cases of OCD (Mellman and Gorman, 1984).

Quality Assurance Issues
1. Are all patients with OCD provided diagnostic-specific treatment?
2. Are all patients with suspected OCD evaluated for other psychiatric disorders such as depression or schizophrenia in which obsessive–compulsive symptoms may be the presenting symptom?

OLIGODIPSIA OF PSYCHOGENIC ORIGIN

Confusion, lethargy, stupor, coma, muscle sensitivity, and seizures are frequently seen with hypernatremia.

History
1. Nephrogenic diabetes insipidus, water deprivation, and hypothalamic and supraoptic-hypophysial tract lesions are causes of hypernatremia.
2. Psychosis is a situation in which a patient may restrict water intake because of altered thinking, mood, or behavior.
3. Drinking is one of the most primitive drives and voluntary restriction of oral fluid intake is an indicator of severe psychopathology.

Symptoms
1. Confusion.
2. Disorientation.

Signs
1. Agitation.
2. Exacerbation of psychotic symptoms.
3. Oligodipsia.

Clinical Studies
1. Examination of serum electrolytes indicate elevation of serum sodium above the normal range of 135 to 146 mEq/L.

Management
1. Restoration of normal serum sodium level by hydration, orally or intravenously, results in remission of symptoms.
2. Increase in psychotropic medication or electroshock may be needed to manage the psychosis.

Quality Assurance Issues
1. Have all patients with oligodipsia been evaluated for CNS and endocrinologic causes of the disorder?

OPIATE DEPENDENCE

The distribution of methadone is carefully governed by federal regulations. Practicing physicians should be aware of what these are as they are bound to obey them or suffer the penalties. Generally speaking, it is not legal to provide methadone on an outpatient basis without a license to maintain an addict. In an emergency situation, at the time of hospitalization, it may be necessary to provide a dose to avoid the painful withdrawal symptoms, but the patient must already be hospitalized. *The law is very strict.* The usual mistake made by the novice is providing a sociopathic addict, well aware of the federal laws, a dose on an outpatient basis. In so doing the physician breaks the law, opening themselves up to penalties. It is therefore incumbent upon physicians to learn what outpatient, inpatient, and other live-in drug treatment programs are available in their community so that when they are confronted with an addict who expresses interest in ending his or her habit, they may outline what is available and direct them to the appropriate agency.

History
1. When patients in early withdrawal present themselves it is usually best to explain the law and the fact that physicians themselves do not make it but are bound to obey it. The physician should then explain what is available, and if the patient wishes to be admitted for withdrawal, arrange hospitalization.
2. If the patient desires an outpatient program, it is good practice to phone the agency and make the contact for the patient by providing his or her name and some identifying data (with the patient's permission). If it is possible that patients may be seen the same day, they should be sent to the agency immediately to maximize the probability that they will follow through on the referral.
3. Opiate abuse generally follows or is part of a general pattern of polydrug abuse that includes use of alcohol, marijuana, hypnotic-sedatives, cigarettes, amphetamine-like substances, hallucinogens, and prescription or nonprescription cough syrups.

4. Untreated, most opiate-dependent individuals either die before age 40 as a result of their life style, "mature out" and cease opiate abuse, or become alcoholics.

5. In a follow-up study of 990 daily opioid users 6 years after admission to community based programs, it was found that only 61% had achieved abstinence from opioid drugs for a year or longer (Simpson et al, 1982). Individuals who achieved abstinence, when compared to those who continued to use opiates or who had problems with non-opiate drugs or alcohol, were less involved criminally and were more productive socially.

6. In a study of 533 opiate addicts using a structured interview (the Schedule for Affective Disorders and Schizophrenia, Lifetime Version) and the Research Diagnostic Criteria, most individuals received one diagnosis in addition to opiate addiction (Rounsaville et al, 1982). The most common diagnoses assigned were alcoholism, major depression, and antisocial personality. The diagnoses of anxiety disorder and dysthymic disorder are used more frequently in a community population. Rates of mania and schizophrenia, however, were low and did not exceed those of the general population.

7. Examination of readmission patterns of treatment outcome measures in a national follow-up study of patients admitted to treatment in the Drug Abuse Reporting Program indicate the beneficial effect of a variety of treatment modalities including residence in therapeutic communities, outpatient drug-free programs, outpatient detoxification treatment, and methadone maintenance (Simpson and Savage, 1980).

8. Opiate addicts seeking help when compared to those not doing so in the community have less adequate social functioning, more drug-related legal problems, and higher rates of depressive disorders (Rounsaville and Kleber, 1985).

9. Opiate addicts on the whole have depression or personality disorders in addition to their drug abuse (Khantzian and Treece, 1985).

Quality Assurance Issues

1. Have all patients with opiate dependence been evaluated for other substance abuse disorders?

2. Have all patients with opiate dependence been evaluated for a psychiatric disorder for which opiates were being used in an effort of self-medication?

3. Have all patients with opiate dependence been evaluated for an HIV-related disorder contracted from either sharing needles or from prostitution to obtain opiates to satisfy the habit?

OPIATE INTOXICATION

Indicants of opiate intoxication include a number of psychological and neurologic signs and symptoms.

History

1. In the extreme, opiate intoxication leads to coma and death.

2. The effect of a single dose of intravenous or subcutaneous morphine peaks at about 20 minutes and 1 hour respectively and is nearly entirely diminished in 4 to 6 hours. There is usually a "down" feeling after the effect wears off.
3. For those who have never had opiates before, nausea may accompany the first dose.

Symptoms
1. Euphoria or dysphoria.
2. Apathy.
3. Drowsiness.
4. Reduced visual acuity.
5. Constipation.
6. Analgesia.
7. Nausea.

Signs
1. Flushing.
2. Hypertension.
3. Decreased heart rate.
4. Decreased body temperature.
5. Pupillary constriction (pupillary dilation may result from severe overdose).
6. Psychomotor retardation.
7. Slurred speech.
8. Dysattention.
9. Memory defect.
10. Impaired judgement.
11. Doses of meperidine (Demerol) exceeding 1,200 mg/day can cause psychosis, muscle twitching, and seizures.

Differential Diagnosis
1. Opiate intoxication.
2. Barbiturate intoxication.
3. Alcohol intoxication.
4. Hallucinogen hallucinosis.

Management
1. The signs and symptoms of opiate intoxication can be reversed by intravenous administration of a narcotic antagonist if irreversible cerebral anoxia has not occurred.
2. Narcotic antagonists include nalorphine, naloxone, and levallorphan.

Quality Assurance Issues
1. Have all patients with opiate intoxication been evaluated for opiate dependence or another substance abuse disorder?

OPIATE WITHDRAWAL

The prognosis for successful permanent cessation of opiate abuse in young people is guarded. Many young addicts who present for withdrawal either have been coerced by legal authorities, relatives, or friends, or wish to reduce the amount needed to give them a high by withdrawing and recommencing their drug use at lower and less costly doses.

History

1. Physicians who are used to working with addicted populations should be aware that many users of heroin are quite sociopathic and will lie about their symptoms and the extent of their habit in an attempt to obtain drugs.

2. In taking a history the physician should ascertain the type of drugs used, the amount used, the time of the last dose, and duration of use. Additional information should be obtained about the frequency of use, routes used, source, and cost. Symptoms and signs of opiate withdrawal are seen in withdrawal from codeine, morphine, Dilaudid, Demerol, Darvon, methadone, and Talwin.

3. Individuals addicted to drugs are prone to certain medical problems that may become apparent during history or physical examination. These include psychiatric illnesses such as schizophrenia or affective disorder, hepatitis, tuberculosis, and other infections.

4. When a patient has been admitted to an inpatient facility, physical examination should include a pelvic and rectal exam for the presence of hidden drugs. Arms should be carefully examined for evidence of needle marks, tracks (i.e., scarring along the veins of the arms), tatooing over veins, ulcers, and abscesses. The nasal mucosa should be checked for erosion and the presence of perforations of the nasal septum. Examination of the needle marks may give a clue to the time of the last injection.

5. Opiate withdrawal may be precipitated by either abrupt cessation of opiate administration after a 1- or 2-week period of continuous use or by administration of an opiate antagonist such as naloxone or nalorphine after therapeutic doses for as little as 3 or 4 days.

6. It is uncommon for opiate craving to occur after opiate administration for pain associated with physical disorders.

7. Usual withdrawal symptoms from morphine or heroin commence within 6 to 8 hours following the previous dose and peak within 2 or 3 days. In 7 to 10 days they have run their course. Withdrawal from meperidine commences within hours after the last dose, peaks within 8 to 12 hours, and is over within 4 to 5 days, while withdrawal symptoms from methadone may not begin for 1 to 3 days and continue for as long as 10 to 14 days.

8. Death rarely occurs from opiate withdrawal unless there are attendant medical problems such as coronary heart disease.

9. History and blood and urine analysis should be used to distinguish opiate withdrawal from other substance withdrawal.

Symptoms
1. Anxiety.
2. Panic.
3. Craving for opiates.
4. Myalgia.
5. Joint pains.
6. Decreased appetite.
7. Hot and cold flashes.
8. Nausea.
9. Irritability.
10. Depression.
11. Weakness.
12. Aggressiveness.

Signs
1. Yawning.
2. Perspiration.
3. Lacrimation.
4. Rhinorrhea.
5. Pupillary dilation.
6. Decreased pupillary reaction to light.
7. Pilomotor erection ("gooseflesh," "cold turkey," "kicking the habit").
8. Muscle twitches.
9. Fever.
10. Increased blood pressure.
11. Vomiting.
12. Weight loss.
13. Insomnia.
14. Orgasm.
15. Diarrhea.
16. Restlessness.
17. Tachycardia.
18. Increased respiratory rate and depth.
19. Tremor.

Differential Diagnosis
1. Opiate withdrawal.
2. Influenza.
3. Barbiturate and other hypnotic withdrawal.

Management
1. Because of its cross-tolerance with a number of opiates, methadone (a long, acting oral synthetic narcotic) is substituted for the opiate. The patient is then slowly withdrawn from methadone over 1 or 2 weeks.

2. The general basis of this approach is to provide a sufficient amount of methadone in the beginning to control the symptoms of abstinence. Sufficient time is then allowed for detoxification so that there is a gradual reduction in the patient's physical dependence.

3. The minimum time to allow for detoxification of a heroin addict is about 1 week. If detoxification is attempted more rapidly, signs of abstinence such as muscle and joint pains, insomnia, malaise, gastrointestinal disturbance, and sweating occur.

4. Typically, in the absence of any serious medical problems, the physician usually should wait for signs of withdrawal and then give methadone. Usually 10 mg either bid. or qid. will suffice. Then after giving the same dose for 2 days, the physician begins to cut the dose by 5–10 mg daily. For instance, 30 mg may be given for the first 2 days, 25 mg on the third, 15 mg on the fourth, 10 mg on the fifth, and 5 mg on the sixth and last day.

5. Acute inflammatory or febrile illnesses increase opiate tolerance and the severity of withdrawal symptoms, thus requiring higher initial doses, a longer period of withdrawal, and a greater number of doses (e.g., qid.).

6. Because of the general discomfort occasioned by medical or surgical problems, withdrawal may be of longer duration to minimize any additional stress for the patient.

7. The nurse and physician should check daily for signs and symptoms of toxicity or withdrawal and adjust the doses properly. In no instance should the rate of withdrawal be greater than 20% of the daily dose above 20 mg of methadone per day.

8. Seizures are not usual with opiate withdrawal, unless the patient is addicted to meperidine. If they do occur, the physician should suspect that the patient either has a mixed addiction and the withdrawal seizures are due to cessation of another drug such as barbiturates or alcohol, that the patient is epileptic, or that the seizures are hysterical or feigned. The barbiturate tolerance test may be used to corroborate the diagnosis. If there is no evidence of mixed addiction, seizures should be worked up to ascertain their etiology and then appropriately treated.

9. Patients who are intoxicated should not be allowed to smoke in bed unless attended and if they are able to get about, they should have a staff member assigned to accompany them to protect them from injuring themselves.

10. Antipsychotic agents are usually not required to control patients unless they are psychotic in addition to being addicted.

11. Vomiting is a symptom of withdrawal. However, some patients adequately covered with opiates for withdrawal experience nausea and vomiting coupled with fantasies of getting the "poison" out of the system. Intramuscular trimethobenzamide (Tigan) or hydroxyzine (Vistaril) can be used to manage this.

12. A 6- to 7-year followup of admissions to two high-dose, long-retention policy methadone hydrochloride maintenance programs and one low-dose program with a relatively strict policy regarding involuntary termination for program violations indicated that retention was much longer for clients in the high-dose programs and those clients had significantly fewer arrests and less incarcerations,

addiction, and self-reported criminal behaviors. These advantages existed for periods with and without methadone (McGlothin and Anglin, 1981).

13. Comparison of withdrawal from heroin in the 3 or 6 week periods with either methadone hydrochloride or methadyle acetate did not indicate the advantage of one agent over the other in terms of satisfaction, retention to the end of the dosing schedule, subjective discomfort, staff rating of global progress, use of illicit drugs during treatment, or durability of change at 3-month followup. Six-week withdrawal showed some temporary advantages over the 3-week withdrawal (Sorensen et al, 1982).

14. An evaluation of the use of short-term interpersonal psychotherapy (weekly individual psychotherapy) and low-contact treatment consisting of one brief treatment a month of methadone-maintained opiate addicts did not reveal any particular benefit of one approach over the other (Rounsaville et al, 1983).

15. A 2-year followup of 99 methadone clients enrolled in a Bakersfield (California) clinic at the time it closed, of whom 88 did not continue to receive methadone, revealed that 54% became readdicted to heroin (McGlothlin and Anglin, 1981). Arrest and incarceration rates were approximately double that of the comparison sample.

16. Most measures indicate that methadone hydrochloride is more effective than propoxyphene napsylate (Darvon-N) as a maintenance drug. Clients receiving propoxyphene reported more withdrawal-related symptoms early in treatment, tended to dropout sooner than patients receiving methadone, and were more likely to abuse heroin (Woody et al, 1981).

17. Naloxone, the opiate receptor-antagonist, has been used with small doses of clonidine during detoxification of opiate addicts. The rationale for the use of naloxone in detoxification is that the provocation of withdrawal symptoms by its use, while suppressing them with a drug such as clonidine, reduces the time of detoxification even though the half-life of the opiate is not affected (Loimer et al, 1989).

18. If a patient is dually addicted to a benzodiazepine, specific attention should be provided for specific withdrawal requirements for the benzodiazepine. Buspirone (Buspar) is uneffective in lessening intensity of benzodiazepine withdrawal indicating that it has no significant benzodiazepine receptor activity (Schweizer and Rickels, 1986).

Quality Assurance Issues

1. Have all patients experiencing opiate withdrawal been provided sufficient medication to minimize withdrawal discomfort?

2. Have all patients experiencing opiate withdrawal been evaluated for other substance abuse disorders?

3. Have all patients suffering opiate withdrawal been evaluated for a psychiatric disorder for which they are using opiates as self-medication?

4. Have all patients who have become dependent upon opiates for pain relief been provided a sufficient alternative?

5. Have all patients suffering opiate withdrawal been evaluated for HIV infection due to either prostitution to buy drugs or sharing needles?

ORGANIC DUST TOXIC SYNDROME

Symptoms (including muscle aches, low-grade fever, and cough) of an organic dust toxic syndrome have been reported among students following a party where there was straw on the floor. Serological and other tests did not demonstrate either a viral or allergic basis to the syndrome. Inhalation of molds growing in silage, hay, and other agricultural products are assumed the basis of the disease (Brinton et al, 1987). This syndrome alone or coupled with other syndromes (e.g., acute drug toxic syndrome) should be considered when symptoms appear in people following hay rides or dances in barns or other areas where air-borne molds may be present.

ORGAN TRANSPLANTATION

Psychiatrists on a consultation liaison service may be called upon for emergency evaluation of patients who have undergone organ transplantation. Current procedures are relatively safe and even patients with preoperative major psychiatric disorders do quite well. The usual changes in mood, behavior, or thought precipitating need for consultation represent a complex interplay of the premorbid personality, psychiatric disorders in patients who are predisposed, organic brain dysfunction, pre- and post-operative anxiety and depression, and the underlying medical/surgical illnesses that necessitated need for a transplant (Surman, 1989). Muromonab-CD3 and cyclosporine and technological advancement has enhanced the success of such operations increasing frequency of consultations of this nature (Surman, 1989).

PAIN

Patients with intractable pain due to documented medical or surgical illness or assumed to be of psychogenic origin may be referred for psychiatric evaluation in an emergency room or more likely for emergency consultation on a medical or surgical unit. In most instances one finds that either pain medication is not being given in doses sufficient to manage pain intensity or at frequent enough intervals given the half-life of the analgesic. It is unusual for a person with *acute* pain to become addicted if he or she is not genetically or psychologically predisposed to do so when analgesia is provided in hospital. In some instances combination of psychopharmacologic agents such as amitriptyline (Elavil) or behavioral techniques (e.g., self-hypnosis, muscle relaxation, imaging) coupled with standard analgesia will reduce pain (Wain, 1986). Some psychogenic pain is due to a primary Axis I psychiatric disorder such as major depression, which must be adequately treated to eliminate the discomfort. Profound depression occurring with an illness such as cancer may present with the predominant symptom of pain (Reich J et al, 1983).

Quality Assurance Issues
1. Have all patients with pain been afforded means of relief that are minimally dependent on drugs that are addicting and, therefore, with time may lose their ability to relieve pain?

PANCREATIC CANCER

Depression may be the initial or only symptom of pancreatic cancer *before* the illness itself is diagnosed. This is not true of gastric carcinoma (Joffe et al, 1986b). Characteristic symptoms include anxiety, depression, weight loss and insomnia.

PANIC DISORDER

Many patients with panic disorder or with panic associated with other psychiatric illnesses appear for the first time in the emergency room. They are generally quite frightened and imagine that they may be experiencing a number of life-threatening conditions that may first present with extreme anxiety such as pulmonary embolis, cardiac arrhythmia, or heart attack.

History
1. Characteristics and management of generalized and more specific anxiety disorders such as panic disorder are discussed in the section on anxiety.
2. Patients with panic attacks should be delineated from patients with other anxiety disorders as course of illness and response to treatment is different.
3. Panic attacks are best managed by antidepressants (Raskin et al, 1982), propranolol (Inderal), alprazolam (Xanax), or lorazepam (Ativan). Generalized anxiety tends best to respond to short- or long-acting benzodiazepines alone.
4. Patients with panic disorder, when compared to those with generalized anxiety disorder, do not have a greater evidence of early loss, separation disorder in childhood, or exacerbation of symptoms with separation, but do report a higher incidence of major depressive episodes and grossly disturbed early childhood involvements (Raskin et al, 1982).
5. Family members with or without mitral valve prolapse had a greater prevalence of panic disorder (Hartman et al, 1982; Weissman & Merikangas, 1986; Crowe et al, 1981).
6. Patients with panic disorder have significantly greater excess mortality when compared to age- and sex-specific comparison populations. Secondary depression and alcoholism appear to play roles in the excess death rates. Suicide accounts for about 20% of the deaths in 113 former inpatients with panic disorders studied 35 years after the initial admission (Coryell et al, 1982).

7. Naloxone infusions alone or with sodium lactate do not produce panic attacks, suggesting endogenous opiates do not play a role in the disorder (Liebowitz et al, 1984b).

8. Long-term substantial cocaine use, even in the absence of first degree relatives with the disorder, has been associated with atypical panic disorder unresponsive to usual modes of treatment, which suggests an acquired form of the disorder involving limbic neuronal hyperexcitability induced by cocaine use through a kindling mechanism (Louis et al, 1989).

9. Panic disorder occurs in children prior to puberty and may be comorbid with separation anxiety disorders or depressive disorders (Alessie and Magen, 1988). Symptoms resemble those of the adult disorder (Moreau et al, 1989).

10. Panic disorder, like depression, is a biologic disorder. The putative site of the acute panic attack is felt to be in the brainstem; the anticipatory anxiety, in the limbic system; and the phobic avoidance, in the prefrontal cortex (Gorman et al, 1989).

11. A number of antecedents of panic have been identified. These include more generalized anxiety, depression, and agoraphobia. The most frequent site of the agoraphobic patients first panic attack is a public place (Lelliott et al, 1989). Major depressive episodes are also reported to occur after the onset of the panic disorder. Alprazolam has been reported to be effective in reducing both depressive symptoms and panic symptoms in some of these patients (Lesser IM et al, 1988).

12. Panic disorder has been reported to improve during pregnancy. This may be due to improvement in psychological well being, pregnancy's attenuation of the sympathoadrenal response to simple physiologic stimuli, or its effect on barbiturate receptors (George et al, 1987).

13. Marijuana and cocaine use may precipitate panic disorder that endures years despite no further use of cocaine or marijuana.

14. There are pervasive health and social consequences of panic disorder that are similar to or greater than those associated with depression, including alcohol and drug abuse, increased suicide attempts, poor physical and emotional health, increased use of health services and psychopharmacologic agents, and financial dependence (Markowitz JS et al, 1989). Panic disorder is frequently comorbid with affective illness and substance abuse disorders (Weissman and Merikangas, 1986). The increased risk of a suicide attempt by a patient with panic disorder highlights the need for successful management of the symptoms of a panic disorder in the emergency situation (Reich P, 1989).

15. Panic attacks occur during sleep and can be quite disabling (Mellman and Uhde, 1989).

16. Reports vary on the role of the number of and type of life events in the precipitation of panic attacks but those who develop panic consistently see life events as having a significantly greater negative impact and have more difficulty adjusting to the change than those without panic (Rapee et al, 1990; Roy-Byrne et al, 1986). Unresolved response to traumatic life events may lead to development of atypical panic disorder characterized by intrusive visual images coupled with panic resembling post-traumatic stress disorder (Zeanah, 1988).

17. Patients with both obsessive–compulsive symptoms and panic are found as a group to suffer earlier onset, to be more likely to have family and personal histories of substance abuse and depression, and to experience a poorer outcome from treatment (Mellman and Uhde, 1987).
18. Hyperventilation with hypocapnia occurs more frequently in patients with panic disorder (Rose SP et al, 1987) and patients with chest pain who hyperventilate are more likely to experience panic (Bass et al, 1988).
19. Sinus tachycardia is a common concomitant of a panic attack (Taylor CB et al, 1986) alone or together with a greater frequency of ventricular premature complexes (Shear et al, 1987). The reported greater incidence of mitral valve prolapse in patients with panic disorders is not found in all studies (Shear et al, 1984).
20. Focal neurologic symptoms have been reported as a manifestation of panic attacks (Coyle and Sterman, 1986) and their presence should not exclude the diagnosis.
21. Patients with panic disorder have been found to surreptitiously use anxiolytic agents confounding both diagnosis and treatment outcome (Clark et al, 1990).

Symptoms and Signs

The symptoms and signs of panic disorder are provided in the earlier section on anxiety disorder.

Differential Diagnosis

The differential diagnosis of anxiety disorder and of panic disorder in particular includes a greater number of acute life-threatening disorders than other acute psychiatric emergencies (Lesser and Rubin, 1986; Stein MB, 1986; Dunner, 1985; Raj and Sheehan, 1987). The boundaries of the various subtypes of anxiety disorders and normal anxiety associated with physical illness and a number of major physical illnesses are sometimes ambiguous. Particular consideration in the differential diagnosis should be given to the following medical disorders (Raj and Sheehan, 1987):

1. Alcohol withdrawal.
2. Anticholinergic intoxication.
3. Asthmatic attack.
4. Cardiac arrhythmias.
5. Carcinoid syndrome.
6. Chronic obstructive pulmonary disease.
7. Congestive heart failure.
8. Coronary insufficiency.
9. Cushing's disease.
10. Delirium.
11. Epilepsy.
12. Hallucinogenic intoxication.
13. Hypertension.
14. Hyperthyroidism.
15. Hypoglycemia.
16. Hyperparathyroidism.

17. Myocardial infarction.
18. Narcotic withdrawal.
19. Pheochromocytoma.
20. Premenstrual tension.
21. Pulmonary embolism.
22. Sedative/hypnotic withdrawal.
23. Vestibular disease.

Clinical Studies

1. Sodium lactate infusions have been demonstrated to induce panic attacks in individuals with panic attacks but not in normal controls and are used by some as a diagnostic tool (Hollander et al, 1989). This response is seen in some but not all patients with panic disorder. The basis is believed to involve central noradrenergic arousal with inconsistent peripheral manifestations (Liebowitz et al, 1985b). After treatment, the patient's response to lactate infusion does not differ from normal controls (Liebowitz et al, 1984a).
2. Positron emission tomography (PET)-scans indicate that, in individuals prone to lactate-induced panic attacks, there is an abnormal hemispheric asymmetry of parahippocampal bloodflow, abnormally high whole-brain metabolism, and abnormal susceptibility to episodic hyperventilation in the resting state. This suggests that the neurobiology of panic disorder may involve the parahippocampal region (Reiman et al, 1986).
3. The dexamethasone suppression test (DST) is not of use in the diagnosis of panic disordered (Sheehan et al, 1983).

Management

1. Given the increased risk of suicide attempts with both panic disorder and with panic without symptoms conforming to criteria for the disorder, the acute treatment should be aggressive with the goal of allowing patients to be aware that they need not fear an episode in the future because acute symptoms can be aborted with alprazolam or lorazepam. Long-term management may entail benzodiazepines, antidepressants, and/or beta-blockers with or without psychotherapy and behavioral techniques such as progressive relaxation, self-hypnosis, or imaging.
2. In patients without a history of substance abuse, alprazolam has been demonstrated to be effective in both the acute and long-term management of panic disorder. When failure to control symptoms occurs it is frequently due to underdosing or failure to take the medication on a schedule consistent with the known half-life. Doses as high as 12 mg per day of alprazolam have been given on a qid. schedule. If a patient is not prone to addiction, a common problem is not to take the required dose to control symptoms (Ballenger et al, 1988; Noyes et al, 1988; Charney et al, 1986b). Symptom improvement is reported by end of the first week of treatment. Sedation is the most common side effect. This tends to subside with dose reduction or continued use.
3. Relapse and withdrawal are important considerations in the use of alprazolam. The two states are easily confused (Fyer AJ et al, 1987). Even in nonsubstance

abusing patients, the withdrawal schedule may be as little as 0.25 mg of alprazolam per week to minimize withdrawal symptoms such as dizziness, malaise, weakness, anxiety, insomnia, tachycardia, and lightheadedness. For many people, panic disorder is a chronic illness and may necessitate years of treatment (Pecknold et al, 1988).

4. Panic disorder patients who become depressed while on alprazolam require either addition of an antidepressant to the benzodiazepine or may respond better to use of an antidepressant alone, such as imipramine (Tofranil), to manage both the panic disorder and the major depression (Lydiard et al, 1987).

5. Clonazepam, (Klonopin) a longer-acting benzodiazepine used for the treatment of minor motor epilepsy, has been used effectively both to manage panic attacks not responsive to other modes of therapy as well as to manage symptoms of withdrawal from alprazolam (Fontaine, 1985; Spier et al, 1986). Half-life is approximately twice that of alprazolam. Initial dose is 0.25–0.5 mg bid.

6. While buspirone (Buspar), the nonaddicting anxiolytic agent, has not been demonstrated to be effective in management of panic, it does have adjunctive value when added to benzodiazepines to manage persistent baseline anxiety that is nonresponsive to the benzodiazepines (Gastfriend and Rosenbaum, 1989).

7. Parnate (e.g., 5–20 mg) and imipramine (e.g., 10–100 mg) in smaller doses than that used for management of depression may sufficiently control symptoms of panic (Garakani et al, 1984). Clomipramine (Anafranil), usually used for management of obsessive–compulsive disorder, has also been proven efficacious in management of agoraphobia with panic attacks (Ballenger, 1986).

8. Patients with panic disorder should avoid caffeine use as they as a group are more susceptible to symptoms of caffeinism such as anxiety, palpitations, restlessness, fear, nausea, nervousness, and tremors (Charney et al, 1985).

9. Inderal (20–80 mg/day) is often successful in managing a patient's tachycardia but is less effective in management of panic itself.

10. Patients with panic disorder and major depressive disorder may obtain relief of the symptoms of the panic disorder without relief from the depressive symptoms requiring adjunctive use of antidepressants and mood stabilizing agents (Nurnberg and Coccaro, 1982).

Quality Assurance Issues

1. Have all patients with panic been evaluated for medical/psychiatric/surgical disorders (e.g., pulmonary embolus, depression, complex partial seizures), which may, in part or completely, account for the symptom of panic?

2. Are all patients who have a personal or family history of substance abuse disorders provided a non-benzodiazedpine for management of their panic?

PARANOID SCHIZOPHRENIA

Few psychiatric emergencies are as frightening or as frustrating as managing a paranoid patient. While most are relatively benign there are a few who feel God or another force has empowered them to kill someone and that someone may be nonspecific enough to include the evaluating clinician. These patients must at times be either interviewed with another person present or in the lobby so a clinician does not expose him- or herself to undue harm. In addition, even if benign, a patient may refuse to take medication because they fear the therapist and others are trying to control—which of course is not entirely untrue as the medication is used to control the symptoms and self- or other-destructive behavior. Fortunately, use of long-acting depot neuroleptics and home visits when patients do not appear for their injection has made management of this group of patients somewhat easier.

History

1. Paranoid schizophrenia has a later age of onset than other forms of schizophrenia and has greater stability over time. Paranoid schizophrenics tend to be less disorganized and less acutely psychotic than chronic schizophrenics.
2. Paranoid schizophrenics may have a history of being in treatment, although if their delusions are well compartmentalized, they have often remained outside psychiatric care for months or even years. If they have been in treatment, history often reveals that they have stopped their medication and become psychotic.
3. Frequently, the delusion of paranoid patients revolves around the idea that someone is trying to control them. Insistence that they continue to take medication obviously corroborates this delusion.
4. The onset of the illness is usually in the fourth decade.
5. Paranoid patients often seem more intelligent than patients with other subtypes of schizophrenia. The complexity of their delusional systems frequently reveals how they brought their intelligence to bear on the problem of organizing their world as the chaos in their mind increases.
6. Deterioration may occur over time although it is usually not as severe as in forms such as the hebephrenic.
7. While such patients have a poor prognosis as to complete permanent remission of symptoms, they often can maintain some level of functioning in the community and are more in contact with reality than are the dementia praecox type of schizophrenics.
8. Premorbid personality is often one of coldness, suspiciousness, aloofness, resentfulness, and distrust. They seldom have had close or intimate friends.
9. While paranoia understandably has been reported to be greater among deaf patients, hearing loss has not been found to be greater in midlife paranoid patients (Watt, 1985) without schizophrenia.
10. Paranoid disorder independent of schizophrenia has not been found to be associated with a family history of schizophrenia (Watt, 1985).

Signs

Physical examination is necessary to rule out symptomatic schizophrenia associated with syphilis, AIDS, and cocaine, amphetamine, and PCP toxicity. In AIDS, tuberculosis, and syphilis there may be a variety of other diffuse and localizing neurologic signs including the classic pupillary changes with syphilis (i.e., a pupil that accommodates but does not respond to light). In the drug toxic states, one may observe tachycardia and pupillary dilation. In a study by Freedman and Schwab (1978) only one-half of those who were admitted to a general hospital psychiatric ward with paranoid delusions were found to have paranoid schizophrenia. A significant number had affective illness or organic mental disorders. A clinical sign of paranoid schizophrenia frequently mentioned by seasoned clinicians are patients' tendency to wear dark glasses. This supposedly seems to mask their own identity and allows them to watch others who may be "talking about" them or "plotting" to seduce or otherwise harm them. It is unwise for a male physician to perform a rectal examination or to examine the genitals of a paranoid schizophrenic male without proper precautions because of homosexual fears. Such action may be misconstrued as a homosexual attack and the patient might take violent action to counter the attack.

Differential Diagnosis

The differential diagnosis of schizophrenia in general is presented in an earlier section. Obviously, a change in mental status could be due to physiologic dysfunctioning. Both psychiatrists and internists may forget that schizophrenics are more prone to physical injury as well as to drug or alcohol abuse. Therefore, a change in a chronic paranoid schizophrenic's clinical status could be due to a physical injury such as subdural hematoma. Paranoia can also result from a transient decrease in blood flow to the brain secondary to a cardiac arrhythmia. Alcoholic paranoia and hallucinosis may be mistaken for paranoid schizophrenia. Some authors, in fact, feel that those with a genetic or psychological predisposition to schizophrenia are more prone to develop these states with chronic alcohol abuse. Amphetamine and PCP-induced psychosis may perfectly simulate paranoid schizophrenia and occur after as little as one large dose. The physiologic signs of sympathetic hyperactivity (e.g., tachycardia, pupillary dilation) are not always present. Cocaine toxicity is very comparable in its presentation to amphetamine psychoses. Nasal perforations in some instances may be present from "snorting" cocaine.

Management

1. The treatment is as outlined in the section on schizophrenia. The first consideration is whether or not the patient needs to be hospitalized. If patients are suicidal or homicidal, have an acute toxic psychosis superimposed, or lack sufficient social supports, they should be hospitalized. A toxic psychosis can in some circumstances be treated in an emergency room. In addition, an emergency room setting allows a 4 to 6 hour trial of aggressive medication. If patients respond to medication, it may be possible to follow them on an outpatient basis, at first by brief daily contacts, and then by the initiation or resumption of a weekly treatment appointment. If response to medication is equivocal, the clinician may wish to give a 3 to 5 day trial on an outpatient basis. If symptoms do not remit, hospitalization then would be necessary for medication stabilization.

2. Paranoid schizophrenics are extremely difficult to manage on medication especially when they are acutely psychotic. Taking medication may be seen as an attempt to control or to poison them In reality, of course, the medication does

represent an attempt to control patients' symptoms; however, if this is mentioned by patients, it may be explained that the clinician is trying to help them control the symptoms so they have freedom to act without psychotic thoughts dominating their existence. If medication is refused, intramuscular medication may need to be given to prevent violent assaultive behavior. In addition, paranoid patients, if left unmedicated, may also kill themselves in an attempt to escape their persecutors. If they feel trapped in a room, and fearful of assault, they may jump out of a window. Long-term psychotropic management of an unreliable patient necessitates use of long-acting fluphenazine (e.g., Prolixin decanoate or enanthate) or depot haloperidol (Haldol).

3. In dealing with such patients, it is necessary to be as flexible as possible. A psychiatrist should be prepared for a show of force. Once the diagnosis becomes apparent, patients' families, security guards, or other available hospital or clinical staff should be alerted if there is a need. The door of the clinician's office should be kept open. If patients appear particularly fearful, it may be better to interview them in the lobby or waiting room.

4. External stimulation should be minimized. Beepers and other paging systems may be seen as modes of control, and the voices or other electronic stimuli misconstrued. The clinician should talk calmly. If a clinician is given due cause to be angry, he or she should attempt to control it as any direct expression of it may provoke patients to assault.

5. Patients should not be touched. Be genuine and real. Long silences should be avoided as well as questions about sex, and, in particular, homosexual experiences and thoughts.

6. Medication should first be offered orally, preferably in a liquid form so patients can't "cheek" it and so that absorption is quicker. If patients refuse oral medication, then the intramuscular route should be used. Sufficient help should be summoned if there is any hesitation on the part of patients to accept medication.

7. If patients have command hallucinations (i.e., voices telling them what to do), or if they are very fearful of harm coming to them by an external agency, they should be hospitalized because of the high homicidal and suicidal risk in such cases.

8. Management of paranoid patients with medical problems is exceptionally difficult (Sparr et al, 1986) and entails a combination of use of neuroleptics to reduce the paranoia, establishment of a consistent trustful relationship, and careful and consistent explanation of all procedures and anticipated changes that are part of the medical/surgical treatment plan.

Quality Assurance Issues

1. Have all patients suspected of paranoid schizophrenia been evaluated for other medical/psychiatric/surgical disorders that may indicate paranoia as a presenting symptom?

2. Are all patients who are paranoid schizophrenic provided long-term neuroleptics as an option if compliance has been a problem?

3. Are all paranoid schizophrenic patients evaluated for abuse of substances such as cocaine, which may be contributing to their paranoia?

Ethical/Legal Issues

1. Have all paranoid schizophrenic patients been evaluated for risk of danger to self or others?
2. If a paranoid schizophrenic patient is at risk for harm to self or others, have appropriate precautions been provided?
3. Have significant others been advised of the risk of harm if a patient is paranoid?

PARENTHOOD CRISES

A number of crises emerge that are normal to parenthood. The reason the crisis exists usually is lack of understanding of how a child (and subsequently parents) responds to various developmental milestones. For instance, it is common for a child to temporarily regress just prior to mastering a new task such as recognition of strangers or walking. In other instances, crises emerge because one parent is not willing to share with the other parent responsibilities of parenthood. Much can be read about the parenting ideal, but most is learned through experience. When one parent consistently neglects a coparenting or supportive role of child and spouse, parenthood crises can then lead to marital crises and sometimes divorce, requiring not only parenting courses but also marital therapy (Rasking et al, 1990).

PARKINSON'S DISEASE

Individuals with Parkinson's disease may appear in the psychiatric emergency room or have a psychiatric consultation requested in the hospital because of depression associated with the morbidity of the illness (e.g., resting tremor, hypersalivation, immobile faces), because of the common occurrence of concomitant depression felt due to the underlying changes in dopamine or serotonin metabolism, or because of a side effect (e.g., psychosis, mania, or depression) of the antiparkinson medication. Forty to fifty percent of Parkinson's patients are reported to suffer concomitant depression (Mayeux et al, 1986; Sano et al, 1990). Major depression and, less commonly, dysthymic disorder are reported, sometimes of suicidal proportions.

Dementia incidence in Parkinson's disease is variously reported at between 20 to 80% of sufferers (Harvey, 1986). Patients may be referred because of dementia or due to a sudden change in the degree of dementia due to a toxic effect of the medication they are on or to the development of depression contributing an element of pseudodementia.

Management

1. The management of psychiatric disorders, dementia, and delirium is discussed under the specific sections of this book. The signs and symptoms are the same.

However, the etiology is frequently the primary illness or an antiparkinson drug used to treat it.

Quality Assurance Issues

1. Are all patients with Parkinson's disease evaluated for concurrent medication-responsive depression that may be contributing to their masked facies and psychomotor problems?
2. Are all patients with extrapyramidal disorders evaluated for pharmacologic causes of their disorder?

PATHOLOGIC GAMBLING

Pathologic gamblers generally present after either a loss precipitating a marital or business crises or after their losses have entailed legal action or threat of retribution from an underworld agent who advanced money for debts, which now cannot be paid. The estimates of problem gamblers and pathologic gamblers are approximately 2.8% and 1.4%, respectively (Volberg and Steadman, 1989). Some gamblers clearly are manic or hypomanic and require mood-stabilizing agents. Others are depressed and hope to resolve a career or family problem by ill-advised risk taking. Many, however, tend to be sensation seeking. These gamblers may have a functional disturbance of the noradrenergic metabolism (Roy et al, 1988).

Quality Assurance Issues

1. Have all patients with pathologic gambling been evaluated for a bipolar or cyclothymic disorder as the basis of their pathologic gambling?

Ethical/Legal Issues

1. Are patients and their families advised of the legal problems that may ensue from debts incurred from pathologic gambling?

PEDOPHILIA

Pedophiliacs are a heterogeneous group that includes people with profound sexual problems to individuals who primarily have a mood or thought disturbance or cognitive impairment including mental subnormality that impairs judgement. The task of the emergency psychiatric clinician is often to identify as accurately as possible those with a primary major psychiatric disorder requiring immediate referral to a psychiatric facility so that they are not exposed to the shame and humiliation of a legal proceeding that they do not fully comprehend (as in the instance of Alzheimer's disease or mental subnormality). Pedophiles are divided by their erotic preference (heterosexual or homosexual) and age at presentation (adolescent, middle-aged, or senescent) (Bradford et al, 1988).

Quality Assurance Issues
1. Is support provided to children who have been abused by a pedophiliac and their parents?
2. Are children who have been sexually abused evaluated for a post-traumatic stress disorder as a consequence?

Ethical/Legal Issues
1. Are all pedophiliacs evaluated for a psychiatric/medical disorder and provided diagnostic-specific treatment?

PEMOLINE ABUSE

Pemoline (Cylert) has been reported to cause a paranoid delusional disorder comparable to that seen with other stimulant drugs such as dextroamphetamine (Dexedrine) and methylphenidate (Ritalin) (Polchert and Morse, 1985).

History
1. Pemoline is a stimulant drug commonly used in the management of attention deficit hyperactivity disorder.
2. In addition to a paranoid disorder, pemoline can produce mania.

Management
1. The delusional disorder remits on discontinuation of the drug.
2. Recommencement of use of pemoline may result in another episode of the psychosis.

PEPTIC ULCER

Generally, patients with peptic ulcer are successfully managed with H_2 receptor blockers. In some instances these agents cause psychiatric disturbances necessitating psychiatric consultation. The psychiatric changes seen are not necessarily due to a side effect of the drug. They are at times due to comorbid psychiatric illness (Haggerty and Drossman, 1985).

PERGOLIDE WITHDRAWAL

Acute cessation of pergolide alone in patients treated for Parkinson's disease has been reported to lead to a subacute worsening of confusion, hallucinations, and paranoid ideation as well as to a Parkinson's-like reaction in patients who have received chronic levodopa and pergolide treatment (McHale and Sage, 1988).

Management
1. Reassumption of the prior dose of pergolide would be expected to be associated with restoration of symptoms of the prewithdrawal level.

PERIODIC CATATONIA

Periodic catatonia is characterized by the rapid onset and subsequent disappearance of catatonic excitement or stupor.

History
1. Sudden onset of catatonic symptoms in an individual who is otherwise without manifest psychopathology is felt to be due to a shift from a predominantly cholinergic state to an adrenergic state characterized by salivation, pallor, mydriasis, inhibited peristalsis, tachycardia, increased blood pressure, and sleep disturbance.

Management
1. Lithium carbonate is the recommended mode of treatment.

Quality Assurance Issues
1. Are all patients presenting with catatonia evaluated for medical and surgical causes of the disorder in addition to psychogenic ones?

PERNICIOUS ANEMIA

The clinical manifestation of vitamin B_{12} deficiency (pernicious anemia) includes, in addition to subacute combined degeneration of the spinal cord and anemia, a number of psychiatric symptoms. Alterations of mood, thought, and behavior (including mania) may antedate the anemia and cord disease and may respond only to vitamin B_{12} replacement (Goggans, 1984).

History
1. Psychiatric symptoms that have been reported with vitamin B_{12} deficiency include dementia, delirium, depression, mania, schizophreniform psychoses, and personality disorders.

Clinical Studies
1. Electroencephalographic studies have demonstrated abnormalities in patients with pernicious anemia which are reversible with vitamin B_{12} replacement. Improvement of the EEG changes correlates with clinical improvement in the mental status examination (Evans et al, 1983b).
2. Diagnosis is made by serum B_{12} assay.

Management
1. Psychiatric symptoms generally resolve with B_{12} injections if identified early and aggressively treated.
2. The longer the illness remains untreated, the greater the likelihood of permanent neurologic dysfunction.

PERSONALITY DISORDERS

Personality disorders may occur concomitantly with Axis I disorders complicating management and precipitating a crisis or, as in the instance of borderline personality disorder, be the major reason for presentation in a drug crisis, suicidal crisis, micropsychotic episode, or panic state (Widiger and Rogers, 1989; Zimmerman M et al, 1988b). The management of crises specific to the various personality disorders is provided in the sections on the disorders.

PHENCYCLIDINE INTOXICATION, DELUSIONAL STATE, AND DELIRIUM

Phencyclidine is a potent hallucinogen. It was originally marketed as Sernylan, a veterinary anesthetic with sympathomimetic properties. In 1978, all legal manufacture was discontinued after it was classified as a class II drug under the criteria of the Comprehensive Drug Abuse Prevention and Control Act of 1970. Evidence suggested that phencyclidine has specific dopaminergic, cholinergic, and opiate-like properties (Giannini et al, 1984b).

History
1. Phencyclidine is sold and taken under a number of names including PCP, angel dust, Kay Jay, Hog, Pill, Peace, Crystal, and Rocket Fuel.
2. Ketamine, a structurally comparable anesthetic is still sold. Some individuals have reported adverse reactions to this drug comparable to that reported with phencyclidine.
3. Phencyclidine is a white crystalline solid that may be taken by mouth, snorted, smoked, or taken intravenously. Chronic users prefer to smoke it. Oral ingestion is rare among sophisticated users save as a suicide attempt.
4. It is quite easily manufactured in a kitchen laboratory.
5. Phencyclidine may be misrepresented as cocaine, tetrahydrocannabinol (THC), psilocybin, mescaline, and LSD, or may contaminate any of the above.
6. Phencyclidine's presence in the body can be documented by serum assay.
7. The onset of symptoms is rapid with a bizarre clinical picture that is sometimes confused with schizophrenia. Symptoms can be quite incapacitating and the patients may be at risk of injury to themselves or others.
8. The clinical picture following phencyclidine use seems less dependent on the

user's personality structure than do the clinical presentations of other hallucinogenic drugs.

9. Aggressive behavior of patients hospitalized for PCP detoxification has not been found to be greater than that of patients admitted for heroin detoxification (Khajarwall et al, 1982).

10. A study of the umbilical cord blood of 200 women randomly selected from the labor and delivery unit of the Los Angeles County University of Southern California Women's Hospital during a 7-week period revealed that 24 (12%) of the samples were positive for PCP (Kautman et al, 1983). No obvious defects were found in the population studied, but there exists the possibility of later developmental abnormalities.

Symptoms

1. Thought disorders.
2. Hostility and combativeness.
3. Tangentiality.
4. Ideas of reference.
5. Agitation.
6. Grandiosity.
7. Disorientation.
8. Euphoria.
9. Depression.
10. Body image distortion.
11. Paranoia.
12. Irritability.
13. Suspiciousness.
14. Tactile, auditory, and visual hallucinations.
15. Suicide ideation.
16. Negativism.
17. Anxiety.
18. Paresthesias or analgesias.
19. Circumstantiality.
20. Disassociation of somatic sensation.

Signs

1. Clouded sensorium.
2. Constricted or normal-sized pupils.
3. Elevated blood pressure.
4. Hypersalivation.
5. Diaphoresis.
6. Hyperpyrexia.
7. Tachycardia.
8. Increased deep tendon reflexes.
9. Ataxia.
10. Rigidity.

11. Myoclonus.
12. Psychomotor excitement.
13. Mutism.
14. Decreased peripheral sensation to pain and touch.
15. Decreased position sense.
16. Stereotypies.
17. Loss of motor control.
18. Vomiting.
19. Nystagmus (at first horizontal then vertical).
20. Hiccoughs.
21. Muscle spasticity.
23. Hyperacusis.
24. Tachypnea.

Differential Diagnosis
1. Phencyclidine intoxication.
2. Other hallucinogenic intoxication.
3. Amphetamine or other sympathomimetic intoxication.
4. Schizophrenia.
5. Mania.
6. Encephalitis.

Clinical Studies
1. Blood, urine, and hair analyses provide evidence of PCP use (Sramek et al, 1985).

Management
1. Phencyclidine intoxication is always considered serious until proven otherwise. Medical consultation should be sought if there is any question of a medical complication or a change in status for the worse and transfer to a medical service considered.
2. Haloperidol (Haldol) is more effective than chlorpromazine (Thorazine) in the management of PCP psychoses (Giannini et al, 1984b).
3. Individuals with mild intoxication can be expected to clear in a short while. In these instances, diazepam (Valium) and minimal stimulation may be all that is required for treatment.
4. In some cases, the psychosis may persist for weeks or be attended by severe medical complications. In these instances, life support measures may be necessary with transfer to an intensive care unit and protection of patients from harming themselves or others. Haloperidol or thiothixene (Navane) 5 mg IM every hour as indicated, is usually sufficient to handle these patients.
5. Patients who have intentionally or unintentionally taken large doses of the drug may develop status epilepticus and adrenergic crises. Respiratory failure is a late sequelae.
6. External stimuli are reduced and vital signs monitored. Voice contact is estab-

lished and some attempt made to talk down the patient. Instrumentation is avoided where possible. Muscles are massaged and diazepam 10–30 mg is given. Cranberry juice and ascorbic acid are given to acidify the urine and enhance excretion of PCP. If adequate facilities are not available for prolonged observation, the patient will need to be hospitalized. Serum half-life in overdoses is 1 to 3 days. Samples of blood, urine, and gastric contents are sent for analysis. Patients must be protected from harming themselves or others.

7. If a patient's condition worsens, there is serious risk of respiratory or cardiovascular complication and the patient will require transfer to a medical service.
8. Individuals who do not support use of neuroleptics for the management of acute phencyclidine intoxication argue that phenothiazines may induce dangerous orthostatic hypotensive crises.
9. Those who oppose use of diazepam in the management of PCP intoxication argue that it impairs recovery by retarding PCP excretion.
10. While intramuscular physostigmine (12 mg) has been found to significantly improve several symptoms of acute PCP intoxication as measured by the Brief Psychiatric Rating Scale (Castellani et al, 1982a), it is not recommended because it can produce dangerous cholinergic side effects such as bronchial constriction, brachycardia, hypersecretion, and seizures. In addition, there are several relative contraindications to physostigmine use including diabetes, heart disease, bronchitis, peptic ulcer, and asthma.
11. Schizophreniform symptoms have been reported to improve with 5 mg of intramuscular haloperidol (Castellani et al, 1982b). Use of haloperidol is limited by its potentially serious side effects and interaction with concurrent disease.
12. Quantitative urine PCP levels do not provide clinically useful data beyond that which could be obtained by qualitative measures (Walker et al, 1981). Urinary PCP levels do not predict hypotensive episodes or drug interactions and do not correlate with any parameter relating to violent behavior (Walker et al, 1981).

Quality Assurance Issues

1. Are all patients with phencyclidine-induced disorders evaluated for other substance abuse disorders?
2. Are all patients with PCP-induced disorders evaluated for an underlying nonsubstance abuse psychiatric disorder?
3. Are all patients with PCP-induced psychiatric disorders evaluated for medical, cardiovascular, and respiratory complications?
4. Are all patients with PCP-induced disorders evaluated for risk of harm to self and others?

Ethical/Legal Issues

1. Are appropriate safeguards provided for patients with a PCP-induced disorder to prevent harm to self and others?
2. Are patients and families warned of the danger to self and others when PCP is used?

PHENELZINE-INDUCED DISORDERS

Monoamine oxidase inhibitors are increasingly being used for clearly defined affective illness, for heterogeneous groups of disorders in which depression does not appear with neurovegetative signs as part of the clinical picture, and for panic disorder.

History
1. Phenelzine has been reported to induce a psychosis in some patients.
2. The mechanism may be similar to the psychoses precipitated in borderline patients treated with tricyclic antidepressants and lie at a central catecholamine level.
3. Patients who received tryptophan in addition to phenelzine have been reputed to exhibit both behavioral changes and neurotoxicity (Thomas and Rubin, 1984).
4. In addition to behavioral and cardiovascular disturbance with phenelzine, leukopenia has been reported as a potential side effect (Tiperman et al, 1984).

Management
1. The behavioral disturbances generally abate with cessation of phenelzine.

Quality Assurance Issues
1. Are all patients on phenelzine advised of the side effects of the drug?

PHENYLKETONURIA

Phenylketonuria is a rare (Willet et al, 1980) and sometimes unrecognized cause of behavioral disorders in adults and included in the differential diagnosis of a thought disorder. Even individuals who have been provided the appropriate diet from birth may show poor motor coordination, limits in the amount of information that can be processed simultaneously, and limits in the complexity of spatial problem solving (Faust et al, 1986). Misdiagnosis of such individuals as schizophrenic when seen briefly in an emergency setting would have dire consequences for the individual and possibly result in exposure to risks of neuroleptic medication that is not needed.

PHENYLPROPANOLAMINE-INDUCED DISORDERS

Psychosis has been reported as a result of self-medication with over-the-counter oral diet aids containing phenylpropanolamine (Schaffer and Pearl, 1980) as well as from use of the same agent as an oral and a nasal decongestant.

History
1. Phenylpropanolamine is a decongestant for sinusitis, colds, and hay fever

Symptoms
1. Psychosis.
2. Paranoia.
3. Insomnia.
4. Restlessness.
5. Nervousness.
6. Headache.

Management
1. Symptoms abate with cessation of use of the drug.

PHOBIAS

Phobias are characterized by persistent avoidance of a specific object, activity, or situation based on an irrational fear. Phobias are frequently a symptom of another anxiety disorder such as panic disorder.

History
1. Patients with simple phobias report a higher incidence of phobias among first-degree relatives than do controls (Fyer AJ et al, 1990).
2. While a significant increase in heart rate is reported with most phobias, a significant decrease is seen when the phobia is related to blood and injury situations (Hugdahl, 1988).
3. Individuals with phobias are more frequently seen in outpatient clinics or in private consultation than on an emergency psychiatric service. When seen in crisis, they are usually flooded with anxiety or panic at a near actual encounter with the phobic object.

Management
1. Management of the crisis entails ventilation, support, and use of a benzodiazepine such as alprazolam (Xanax) or lorazepam (Ativan).
2. Longer-term management involves use of one or more of a number of therapeutic modalities including behavioral techniques, tricyclic antidepressants, monoamine oxidase inhibitors, serotonin agonists, and supportive psychodynamic psychotherapy.
3. In placebo-controlled studies, the effect of imipramine hydrochloride (Tofranil) is clearly superior to that of placebo for patients with spontaneous attacks. Individuals with simple phobia without spontaneous attacks do not appear to benefit from imipramine (Zitrin et al, 1978).
4. Systematic hierarchical desensitization and supportive psychotherapy appear largely efficacious for patients with agoraphobia, mixed phobia, and simple phobia, with patients reporting benefit from both (Klein DF et al, 1983). The critical component of the psychotherapeutic endeavor, regardless of whether it entails

formal behavioral modification techniques or not, appears to be that the psycho-therapy session serves as an instigator with the specific corrective activity occurring outside of the formal session when the patient experiences exposure to the phobic stimulus in vivo.

5. The most frequent error in the management of phobias is inadequate diagnostic investigation. The clinician must delineate the pattern of avoidance behavior; the development of secondary psychiatric disorders (e.g., depression); suicidal ideation or actual attempts; impact on social, economic, and work life; and the degree to which self-medication with alcohol or other substances has occurred (Levin and Liebowitz, 1987). Fear of driving, for instance, can lead to a severely constricted lifestyle.

4. Pharmacologic treatment of phobias (e.g., tricyclic antidepressants, MAOIs, or benzodiazepines) coupled with behavior therapies has proven effective but long-term results are limited due to a high dropout rate with a tendency to relapse (Noyes et al, 1986) hence precipitating an emergency psychiatric visit in some cases.

Quality Assurance Issues
1. Are all patients with a phobia evaluated for psychiatric disorders other than anxiety disorders of which the phobia may be a symptom?
2. Are patients with phobias provided knowledge of the risks and benefits of behavioral and psychopharmacologic approaches to treatment?
3. Have all patients with phobias been evaluated for a concurrent substance abuse disorder developed in an effort to self-medicate?
4. Are all phobic patients evaluated for concurrent depression?

Ethical/Legal Issues
1. Are all patients who are provided benzodiazepines for phobias advised of the potential for addiction?

PODOPHYLLIN-INDUCED DISORDERS

Podophyllin resin is an extract of the rhitone roots of *Podophyllum peltatum* (the mandrake plant) used, because of its antimitotic properties, to treat veneral warts.

History
1. Medical and psychiatric complications have been reported from both oral and cutaneous absorption including delirium after topical absorption (Stoudemire et al, 1981).
2. The resin, when applied topically, is given in a diluted benzoin tincture.
3. Systemic toxicity occurs when the resin is not removed in the recommended time (3 hours), is applied excessively, or is taken orally.
4. Death may result from excessive ingestion without treatment
5. The drug is teratogenetic (Stoudemire et al, 1981).

Symptoms
1. Visual hallucinations.
2. Hypersomnia.
3. Paranoia.
4. Nausea.
5. Lethargy.

Signs
1. Confusion.
2. Dysmnesia.
3. Dysattention.
4. Bizarre behavior.
5. Rambling speech.
6. Easy distractibility.
7. Vomiting.
8. Respiratory stimulation.
9. Fever.
10. Tachycardia.
11. Adynamic ileus.
12. Renal failure.
13. Hepatic failure.
14. Pancytopenia.
15. Peripheral renopathy.
16. Paralysis.
17. Obturation.
18. Stupor.
19. Coma.

Differential Diagnosis
1. Schizophrenia.
2. Encephalitis.
3. Podophyllin-induced organic mental disorder.
4. Other drug-induced organic mental disorders.

Management
1. Management entails supportive measures in mild cases to charcoal hemoperfusion in extreme cases.

POLYCYSTIC OVARY DISEASE

Patients with polycystic ovary disease report more physical and psychological symptoms than infertile women with tubal disease or normal controls (Orenstein et al, 1986). In many instances, these women meet the criteria for Briquet's syndrome and may require concomitant psychiatric management to reduce discomfort and psychiatric crises.

PORTAL–SYSTEMIC ENCEPHALOPATHY

A number of psychiatric symptoms are reported with portal–systemic encephalopathy resulting from cirrhosis of the liver. These frequently result in need for emergency consultation on a medical service or in the emergency room. These problems are complicated by need to tailor dose and type of the psychopharmacologic agents to the capacity of a patient with impaired liver functioning to metabolize them as well as made worse by associated acute alcohol-induced disorders such as intoxication or withdrawal (Tarter et al, 1986).

Management
1. The discussion of the management of attendant complications is in the section on the specific emergencies (e.g., delirium, alcohol withdrawal).

POSTCARDIOTOMY DELIRIUM

Delirium may follow cardiac surgery. The usual sequence is a lucid interval followed by a period of illusions or disorientation and at times progression to hallucinations or delusions. A number of factors have been posted for these changes including: impact of the heart surgery recovery room in patients made vulnerable by cardiac disease and surgery, change in the postoperative cardiac index, postoperative infections, atelectasis, blood loss, concurrent medication, pain, effect of anesthetic agents used, electrolyte imbalance, and pre-existent psychiatric disorders. Confusion appears to peak during the first 2 preoperative days (Harrell and Othmer, 1987). Insomnia appears to be a consequence of the confusion and not a cause of it suggesting delirium rather than insomnia should be treated in the postcardiotomy patient (Harrel and Othmer, 1987).

Quality Assurance Issues
1. Are patients and patients' families advised of the potential for delirium pursuant to cardiac surgery?
2. Are all postcardiotomy intensive care units' staff provided instructions in the recognition and management of postcardiotomy delirium?

POSTCATARACTECTOMY SYNDROME

The postcataractectomy syndrome refers to the acute changes in mental status seen following cataract surgery. Anticholinergic intoxication is posited as one explanation for the changes (Summers and Reich, 1979). Mydriatic agents have access to the vitreous humor because of the disruption in the usual occular physiology. There-fore, the anticholinergic drug can be taken up by the neurons and transported by an-terograde axonal transport into the CNS and give rise to a CNS anticholinergic psy-chosis.

Symptoms

1. Disorientation.
2. Disturbance of recent and remote memory.
3. Delusions.
4. Hallucinations.
5. Illusions.
6. Depersonalization.
7. Anxiety.
8. Fear.
9. Depression.
10. Euphoria.

Signs

1. Increased psychomotor activity.

Management

1. The delirium tends to abate as the mydriatic agents are metabolized

POST-CONCUSSION SYMPTOMS

Confusion, headaches, and memory disturbance are common consequences of head injury complicating diagnoses and treatment.

Management

1. Patients, their significant others, and caregivers should be made aware of the cognitive limitations in the post-concussion recovery period so that environmen-tal demands are maintained at a level commensurate with a patient's ability to handle them to avoid the catastrophic reaction experienced when patients are confronted with tasks they assume they should be able to handle but cannot (Wood et al, 1984).

Quality Assurance Issues

1. Are all patients who sustained concussions evaluated neuropsychologically for sequelae?
2. Are efforts made to minimize secondary gain from psychological sequelae of a concussion to reduce long-term morbidity?
3. Are patients with neuropsychological sequelae provided training to maximize post-morbid functioning?

POST-TRAUMATIC STRESS DISORDER

Post-traumatic stress disorder (PTSD) has been reported to occur months to years after a number of traumatic events and is believed to have both psychological and neurobiologic etiologic factors (Davidson and Nemeroff, 1989). These include stress-induced sensitization, possible microstructural alterations, inescapable shock/learned helplessness, conditioned hyperarousal to stimuli, and endogenous opioid dysregulation.

History

1. Patients with PTSD show an induced analgesia assumed due to endogenous opioid release when exposed to situations reminiscent of the original trauma (Van der Kolk et al, 1989; Pitman et al, 1990; Pitman et al, 1987b). The autonomic hyperactivity seen with PTSD after exposure to a traumatic stimulus (such as gunfire to a Vietnam war veteran) resembles opiate withdrawal (Salloway et al, 1990).

2. A number of studies (Pitman et al, 1987b; Pitman et al, 1990; Orr et al, 1990) indicate muscular, skin conductance, and heart rate changes when individuals with PTSD imagine the details of the event that provided the disorder.

3. Fundamental changes in CNS processes generating REM sleep may play a role in the pathogenesis of dream disturbance and startle response, which are cardinal features of the disorder (Ross et al, 1989).

4. Factors contributing to the development of PTSD in veterans of war include threat to life, exposure to grotesque death, prewar functioning (Green et al, 1990), participation in atrocities at a young age, and cumulative exposure to combat stressors (Breslaw and Davis, 1987).

5. It is estimated that approximately 15% of Vietnam veterans experienced PTSD at some time during the service or in the ensuing months after (CDC Vietnam Exposure Study, 1988), with as great as 40% of wounded veterans experiencing the disorder (Pitman et al, 1989a).

6. Symptoms of PTSD have been reported following natural disasters (McFarlane, 1988b) including floods (Donal et al, 1985), fires (McFarlane, 1988b), and earthquakes as well as after airplane crashes (Smith EM et al, 1990; Shuchter and Zisoot, 1984), suicides (McNiel et al, 1988a), mass murders (North et al, 1989), torture (Goldfeld et al, 1988), forced emigration (e.g., in Southeast Asian refugees) (Kroll et al, 1987; Kinzie et al, 1990), volcanic eruptions (Shore et al, 1986), concentration camp experience (Boehnlein et al, 1985), car accidents (Rubinstein, unpublished mimeo), exposure to toxic substances at work (Schottenfeld and Cullen, 1985) and, of course, war (Penk and Rabinowitz, 1989; Solomon Z et al, 1987b; Lerer et al, 1987).

7. Greater observed rates of PTSD among black veterans are attributed to more conflicted feelings about their wartime experiences with limited opportunities for blacks in the postwar period and greater difficulty rationalizing brutality against the Vietnamese (Allen IM, 1986).

8. Individuals who observe a disaster, as well as those directly impacted upon by it, may show long-term signs of PTSD such as flashbacks, anxiety, startle, and frightening nightmares (Wilkinson, 1985; Horowitz, 1985).
9. Psychometric scales have been designed to monitor the severity of long-term response to a traumatic event and the impact of treatment (McFarlane et al, 1990).
10. Firefighters, policemen, rescue workers, emergency medical technicians, and those in the military who have experienced combat are at particular risk.
11. A past personal history and family history of psychiatric disorders, introversion, and neuroticism have been found to enhance risk of development of PTSD (McFarlane, 1988a).
12. Patients with PTSD are significantly more able to be hypnotized than individuals without the disorder (Spiegel et al, 1988). Dissociative phenomena, fugue states, and even emergence of a multiple personality disorder have been reported as sequelae to trauma giving rise to PTSD (McDougle and Southwick, 1990).
13. Not all enduring responses to traumatic life events comport with current or proposed criteria for the diagnosis of PTSD (Brett et al, 1988; Husband and Platt, 1987).
14. The diagnosis of delayed PTSD is made when symptoms emerge for the first time after a period of at least 6 months without any antecedent warning (Solomon Z et al, 1987a).
15. Intrusive auditory hallucinations have been reported in combat-related PTSD in instances of more intense PTSD symptoms and greater combat exposure and forebode a poorer prognosis for treatment (Mueser and Butler, 1987).
16. Paranoid ideation may evolve and complicate treatment (Woolfolk and Grady, 1988).
17. Factitious PTSD has been seen in individuals without military experience seeking veteran-related benefits (Sparr and Pankratz, 1983; Perconte and Goreczny, 1990).
18. Anorexia nervosa has been reported as a sequela to car accidents that caused physical injuries and suggest a response to real or perceived figure distortion (Damlouji and Ferguson, 1985).
19. Suicide is always a risk in individuals with PTSD (Solursh, 1988).
20. Chronic pain syndromes, major depression, anxiety disorders, and substance abuse disorders may coexist with PTSD (Benedikt and Kolb, 1986).
21. Sleep is lighter and more disrupted than normal in many combat veterans without PTSD (Kramer and Kinney, 1988).
22. Symptoms of PTSD have been reported to first appear as long as 30 years after the initial traumatic event (Van Dyke et al, 1985).

Symptoms
1. Recurrent frightening nightmares of the traumatic event.
2. Intrusive memories of the traumatic event.
3. Anxiety.
4. Depression.
5. Impulsive behavior including self-destructive and assaultive behavior.

6. Insomnia.
7. Startle.
8. Agitation.
9. Internal loss of control.
10. Dissociation.
11. Alcohol and drug abuse.
12. Panic attacks.
13. Irritability.
14. Headaches.
15. Hyperventilation.
16. Phobias.
17. Obsessions.
18. Gastrointestinal disturbances.
19. Depersonalization.
20. Fugues.
21. Paranoia.
22. Anger.

Signs
1. Tachycardia.
2. Tremulousness.
3. Diaphoresis.
4. Elevated blood pressure.
5. Galvanic skin response changes.
6. Explosive violent behavior

Management
1. Group support of others who have experienced the same or similar trauma appears to be a critical component of the treatment plan. Nothing helps one to understand as much as to be understood.
2. Phenelzine sulfate (Nardil) and other MAOIs and tricyclics have been reported effective in treatment of the flashbacks and recurrent frightening nightmares as well as of the depressive symptoms (Hogben and Cornfeld, 1981; Davidson and Nemeroff, 1989; Lerer RP, 1986; Davidson J et al, 1990).
3. Carbamazepine (Tegretol) has been reported effective in reducing intensity and frequency of the nightmares, intrusive recollections and flashbacks, poor impulse control, violent behavior, and angry outbursts suggesting that PTSD may be a paroxysmal disorder or have a kindling effect (Lipper et al, 1986; Wolf ME et al, 1988).
4. Crisis-oriented therapy with ventilation, support, psychoeducation, clarification, and interpretation facilitates both compliance with psychopharmacotherapy and enhances functioning (Shuchter and Zisook, 1984; Wilkinson and Vera, 1985; Epstein, 1989).
5. Duration of treatment required varies tremendously from 3 months to years (Burstein, 1986).

Quality Assurance Issues
1. Are patients suffering PTSD provided the group support of others who have suffered a similar tragedy when available?
2. Are PTSD patients evaluated for risk to self and others and for substance abuse disorders?
3. Are PTSD patients provided antidepressants for the recurrent nightmares and intrusive memories?

Ethical/Legal Issues
1. Is the PTSD sufficiently documented for any medico-legal action that may occur pursuant to the trauma?
2. Was treatment offered early after the trauma to minimize occurrence?

PREGNANCY AND THE PUERPERIUM

Pregnancy is sometimes remarkably protective against major psychiatric disturbances. Most problems tend to occur at the time of birth or in the months of the puerperium. When problems occur during pregnancy, both psychopharmacologic and psychotherapeutic interventions present problems.

History
1. Schizophrenic women may develop delusions regarding the change of body image during pregnancy and regarding the putative father (Spielvogel and Wile, 1986).
2. Bipolar patients are prone to development of depression at the time of birth and in the postpartum period (Spielvogel and Wile, 1986).
3. Women experiencing postpartum depression report more life events during pregnancy and less spouse support during the pregnancy and after delivery (O'Hara, 1986). Women who get depressed during their pregnancy report somewhat less support from spouses and more support from confidants than do nondepressed pregnant women (O'Hara, 1986).
4. Mild to moderate depression is common among women during the first 3 months postpartum and seldom requires psychiatric intervention (Saks et al, 1985).
5. Acute psychoses during labor are rare with an incidence of postpartum psychosis between one and two cases per 1000 births (Ticknor and Vogtsberger, 1987).

Management
1. There is no effective psychopharmacologic treatment for a pregnant woman without some risk (Nurnberg, 1989). The risks and benefits of treatment should be explained to the patient and her significant others and appropriate gynecologic consultation sought to minimize risk to patient and fetus and enhance informed consent.
2. Diagnostic-specific interventions for depression and psychosis are the same as in the nonpregnant state save for the need for awareness of the risk to mother and

child of treatment, the need for informed consent to the greatest degree possible, and appropriate consultation.

Quality Assurance Issues
1. When a mother suffers a postpartum disorder, are efforts made to facilitate normal mother–child bonding to the degree it is possible?
2. Are parents-to-be advised of the potential psychiatric complications of pregnancy and delivery?

PREMENSTRUAL AFFECTIVE SYNDROME

Affective and behavioral changes in women have been reported to increase premenstrually and include irritability, heightened sensitivity, depression, anxiety, and suicidal ideation. Women with psychiatric disorders are more likely to suffer premenstrual syndrome (PMS) (Ascher-Svanum and Miller, 1990).

History
1. A menstrually related mood is one that is cyclic, occurs in regular relationship to the menses, and is of sufficient intensity to interfere with functioning (Rubinow and Roy-Byrne, 1984).
2. Although black women use PMS clinics less frequently than white women, there appears to be no difference in frequency of occurrence of symptoms (Stout et al, 1986).
3. Affective changes are reported to occur in the week prior to menses that are of sufficient intensity (Rubinow et al, 1984) to merit the use of mood stabilizers in some instances.
4. Patients with rapidly cycling mood disorders are found to have more severe forms of PMS (Price and DiMarzio, 1986).

Management
1. The acute management is generally that of psychoeducation, evaluation of suicidal and violent potential, referral for further evaluation of endocrine and psychiatric changes, and referral for diagnostic-specific treatment.

Quality Assurance Issues
1. Are patients with PMS offered pharmacologic options to alleviate symptoms?
2. Are young women warned of PMS and advised in how to manage it?

PREPUBERTAL MAJOR DEPRESSIVE DISORDER

Major depressive disorder as diagnosed by Research Diagnostic Criteria may be seen in prepubertal children.

History

1. About one-third of children with major depressive disorder may experience psychotic symptoms including auditory, visual, and tactile hallucinations as well as delusional thinking (Chambers et al, 1982).
2. The symptoms reported are similar to those seen in adults, although the pattern of frequency differs.
3. The higher incidence of hallucinations seen in children with major depressive disorder may reflect cognitive immaturity, less social development, or suggestibility (Chambers et al, 1982).

Management

1. The management of major depression in children is the same as for adults including need for recurrent monitoring for presence of and intensity of suicidal ideation. If a child wishes to die by suicide, appropriate referral for inpatient treatment is indicated as children do kill themselves.
3. Psychopharmacologic doses differ for children by weight. Informed consent must be obtained from parents to administer the medication except where laws provide for emergency psychopharmacotherapy.
4. A chronically depressed child may develop low self-esteem and an enduring sense of learned helplessness leading to lower aspirations in school and career and to selection as an adult of lovers and friends who reduce rather than enhance self-esteem.

Quality Assurance Issues

1. Was consent obtained from parents to administer medication?
2. Are depressed children evaluated for suicide potential?
3. Are accident-prone children evaluated for affective illness?

PROCAINE PENICILLIN-INDUCED DISORDERS

Psychosis has been reported following injection of procaine penicillin. Symptoms reported include paranoia, a Capgras-like syndrome, visual and auditory hallucinations, fear, religious delusions, and somatic hallucinations. The symptoms observed are believed to be due to the impact of procaine on the limbic system (Cummings JL et al, 1987).

PROPOXYPHENE-INDUCED DISORDERS

Abstinence-induced withdrawal symptoms have been described following abrupt cessation of propoxyphene use.

Symptoms

1. Vomiting.

2. Nausea.
3. Muscle cramps.
4. Headaches.
5. Agitation.
6. Tremulousness.

Signs
1. Diaphoresis.
2. Seizures.

Management
1. Very gradual reduction of propoxyphene dosage in addicted patients avoids withdrawal symptoms.
2. Methadone, thioridazine (Mellaril), and clonidine have all been used to minimize withdrawal symptoms (Johnson and Bohan, 1983).

PROPRANOLOL-INDUCED DISORDERS

Propranolol (Inderal), introduced in 1964, is used in the treatment of panic disorder, cardiac arrhythmias, hypertension, lithium-induced tremor, angina pectoris, obstructive cardiomyopathies, thyrotoxicosis, essential tremor, septic shock, and migraine headaches.

History
1. When occurring, depressive symptoms tend to be severe and dose dependent (Petrie et al, 1982; Griffin and Friedman, 1986).
2. Propranolol-induced affective changes are believed to be related to central beta blockade.
3. Symptoms even occur at low or therapeutic doses (less than 100 mg).
4. Depressive symptoms are more likely to occur with propranolol in individuals with a positive personal or family history of depression (Griffin and Friedman, 1986).

Symptoms
1. Depression.
2. Psychosis.
3. Fatigue.
4. Hallucinations.
5. Irritability.
6. Giddiness.
7. Restlessness.
8. Agitation.
9. Insomnia.
10. Dizziness.
11. Lassitude.

12. Nightmares.

Signs
1. Confusion.
2. Acute organic mental disorder.
3. Chronic organic mental disorder (Cummings J et al, 1980).

Management
1. The half-life of propranolol is 2 to 4 hours. It is necessary, however, to reduce or discontinue the drug for 24 to 72 hours to confirm the diagnosis.
2. Symptoms remit when propranolol is discontinued.
3. It is important to remember that sudden cessation of propranolol leads to a withdrawal syndrome that includes, in addition to psychiatric changes, medical problems such as malaise, tremulousness, ventricular tachycardia, diaphoresis, unstable angina, myocardial ischemia, and florid psychosis (Golden RN et al, 1989).

Quality Assurance Issues
1. Are all patients on propranolol advised of the risk of depression associated with taking the medication?
2. Are all patients on propranolol monitored for symptoms of depression?
3. Are patients who develop depression on propranolol offered an alternative pharmacologic agent?
4. Are beta-blocker-induced depressions included in the differential diagnosis of depression?

Ethical/Legal Issues
1. Are all patients with propranolol-induced depressions evaluated for suicide risk?

PSEUDOCYESIS

Pseudocyesis is a term used for the development of the psychological and physiologic concomitants of pregnancy in the absence of a true gravid state.

History
1. The incidence of pseudocyesis appears to be decreasing (Cohen LM, 1982).
2. Patients with pseudocyesis have menstrual abnormalities, breast changes, and galactorrhea.
3. It is felt that the majority of individuals with pseudocyesis have the galactorrhea–amenorrhea hypermallactinemia syndrome. A small portion probably represent variants of monosymptomatic hypochondriasis or Munchausen's syndrome (Cohen LM, 1982).

Symptoms
1 Sensation of fetal movement

2. Nausea.
3. Capricious appetite.

Signs
1. Menstrual abnormalities.
2. Enlarged breasts.
3. Changes in abdominal size.
4. Lactation.
5. Vomiting.
6. Weight gain.
7. Uterine enlargement.
8. Cervical changes.

Management
1. The management of pseudocyesis consists of management of the primary disorder. The galactorrhea–amenorrhea hypermallactinemia syndrome and other causes of pseudocyesis have been shown to have a dramatic response to brief psychotherapy in selected cases (Cohen LM, 1982).

Quality Assurance Issues
1. Are all patients suspected of pseudocyesis given a pregnancy test to assure the diagnosis is not in error?
2. Are all patients with pseudocyesis provided diagnostic-specific treatment?

PSEUDODEMENTIA

Pseudodementia is defined as intellectual impairment in individuals with a primary psychiatric disorder in which the intellectual abnormality resembles that of neuropathologically induced cognitive deficit (Caine et al, 1978).

History
1. Pseudodementia is reversed without residual impairment when the primary disorder is treated.
2. The intellectual impairment of pseudodementia resembles that of a subcortical dementia (Caine et al, 1978).
3. Pseudodementia may be seen with a number of psychiatric disorders. Although it is most common in older depressed patients, it is also seen with schizophrenia (Blumenfield and Hartford, 1982) and conversion disorders (Fieldman and Lipowski, 1981) and the Ganser syndrome (Good, 1981).
4 Pseudodementia may coexist with true dementia. Some apparent recovery of cognitive functioning will occur with treatment of the primary psychiatric disorder presenting with pseudodementia, although the deficit that is part of the "true" dementia is irreversible (McAllister and Price, 1982).
5 It is felt by some clinicians (McAllister and Price, 1982) that the subtype of pseu

dodementia in which cognitive impairment is associated with affective disorders should be labeled as depression-induced organic mental disorder.

6. In a study of 289 randomly selected medical inpatients using the Mini Mental State Examination and the Beck Depression Inventory, no relationship was found between severity of depression and cognitive dysfunction for those under 65. A nearly significant relationship was found for those 65 or older (Cavanaugh and Wettstein, 1983).
7. Depression appears to be more frequently found to occur with mild to moderate dementia than with more severe dementia, although a significant number of individuals with all levels of cognitive impairment are found to be depressed (Reifler et al, 1982).
8. Reported rates of depression among the elderly vary from quite low in the Epidemiologic Catchment Area studies to as great as 25% of elderly individuals in other studies (Hendrie and Crossett, 1990); Jeste et al, 1990).
9. Amnestic pseudodementia may occur without depression (Markowitz and Viederman, 1986).

Signs
1. Paucity of verbal production.
2. Slowed mental processing.
3. Inattention.
4. Concrete thinking.

Management
1. The management of patients with pseudodementia is that of the primary psychiatric disorder (e.g., antidepressants and/or electroshock with supportive psychotherapy for patients with a major depression).

Quality Assurance Issues
1. Are all patients who are diagnosed to have cognitive changes evaluated to ascertain if pseudodementia explains all or part of their mental disorder?
2. Are all patients with pseudodementia evaluated for concurrent true dementia?
3. Have families of pseudodementia patients been advised of the etiology of the cognitive changes and the expected response to treatment?

Ethical/Legal Issues
1. Are all patients who appear to be demented evaluated for pseudodementia before any of their rights are terminated?

PSEUDOSEIZURES

Pseudoseizures vary in presentation and may be difficult to distinguish from true epilepsy and amnestic states (Lesser IM, 1987; Theodore, 1989; Ruedrich et al, 1985). In some instances, true seizures and pseudoseizures coexist. In a pseudoseizure, a patient does not become cyanotic, bite their tongue, or soil themselves despite the motor activity. The Babinski sign is negative with a pseudoseizure unlike the case with a true grand mal attack. Electroencephalography is required to document the absence of true epileptogenic discharges and to ascertain the coexistence of true and pseudoseizures.

Management
1. It is sometimes quite difficult to determine in the emergency situation if a seizure observed by a patient's friends or relatives represents the onset of epilepsy or a pseudoseizure at a time of stress. All patients should be evaluated for treatable causes, as a seizure may be due to a medical condition requiring acute intervention such as a cardiac arrhythmia with decreased blood flow to the brain, hypoglycemia, drug withdrawal or intoxication (e.g., seizures associated with cocaine or meperidine toxicity), or a brain tumor.

Quality Assurance Issues
1. Were all patients suspected of having pseudoseizures evaluated for the presence of epilepsy?
2. Conversely, were all patients diagnosed to have epilepsy and prescribed anticonvulsants evaluated to ascertain if they have pseudoseizures?
3. Are patients with both pseudoseizures and epilepsy provided psychotherapy for the pseudoseizure component?

Ethical/Legal Issues
1. Are patients with pseudoseizures advised of the risks when operating mechanical equipment or driving?

PSYCHOGENIC PAIN

Patients with intractable pain sometimes suffer psychogenic pain disorder, which is responsive to antidepressant medication (Valdes et al, 1989). If they are referred to psychiatry in the emergency room or on a consultation liaison service, they often have not been yet provided a trial of antidepressant therapy. Even if there is a structural change (e.g., metastatic cancer) responsible for the pain, antidepressants alone or in combination with other analgesics may provide a modicum of relief.

Quality/Assurance Issues
1. Are all patients suspected of psychogenic pain evaluated for a medical/surgical explanation for their pain syndrome?
2. Were patients with psychogenic pain provided medication for relief of pain that is addicting?
3. Were all patients with psychogenic pain evaluated for concurrent illnesses that may contribute to their pain syndrome and provided diagnostic-specific treatment?

PSYCHOTIC DEPRESSION

Psychotic depression is distinguishable from nonpsychotic depression by the presence of symptoms normally associated with psychosis such as auditory or olfactory hallucinations and delusions. The content of the delusions may be paranoid, nihilistic, somatic, religious, or otherwise.

History

1. While suicidal behavior may be seen with nonpsychotic depressions, it is generally more of a risk in patients who have a history of psychotic thinking that impedes reality testing. Patients who are delusional, have hallucinations that are of a command or imperative nature, alcoholic, physically ill, homosexual, or have a personal history of previous attempts or a family history of suicide are especially at risk.

2. Patients who are psychotically depressed are particularly adept at hiding certain telltale symptoms such as hallucinations, ideas of reference, and paranoid ideation. It sometimes takes exceptional skill to extract a reliable story.

3. Assessment of social supports is the key in the evaluation of patients who are psychotically depressed. In many instances, the presence or absence of a viable social matrix may be the crucial factor in determining whether a patient should be hospitalized.

4. The nosological difference between a psychotically depressed patient from a nonpsychotic patient is qualitative, based on the presence of delusions and hallucinations or other evidence of psychotic thinking. A nonpsychotic patient may be profoundly depressed with marked weight loss and sleep disturbance without hallucinations or delusions but be more of a suicide risk than some psychotic patients.

5. Depression sometimes follows initiation of treatment of a psychosis. When this occurs, the depression is referred to as postpsychotic depression. In some instances, the observed depression may be due to a toxic effect of the antipsychotic medication. Treatment of akinesia with appropriate antiparkinson medication has been found to bring about improvement in depression, anxiety, blunted affect, somatic concern, motor retardation, and emotional withdrawal in several of these instances.

6. The fact that psychotic depressions with or without delusions appear less responsive to tricyclics, tetracyclics, trazadone, and MAOIs and frequently require the addition of neuroleptics or ECT to manage has led some authors to see them as an entity distinct from other major depressive disorders (Frances A et al, 1981).

7. Although delusionally depressed patients have been found to have a relatively poor short-term outcome regardless of whether or not they have received psychiatric treatment, at long-term followup (40 years), no difference is found between groups of patients who have experienced delusional or nondelusional depressions in terms of psychiatric symptoms; occupational, marital or residential status; final diagnosis of bipolar disorder; or suicide (Coryell and Tsuang, 1982).

Symptoms

The symptoms of a nonpsychotic depression are also found in patients who are psychotically depressed. In addition, however, depressed patients who are psychotic may show:

1. Somatic delusions (e.g., brain being eaten by worms).
2. Hallucinations (particularly auditory and olfactory).
3. Illusions.
4. Ideas of reference.
5. Paranoid delusions.
6. Delusions of guilt and self-reproach (e.g., accusing oneself of sins never committed).

Differential Diagnosis

The differential diagnosis of a psychotic depression is the same as that for a nonpsychotic depression.

Management

1. The mere fact that patients are psychotically depressed does not mean that they must automatically be hospitalized. Suicide risk and strength of social supports coupled with previous history and previous response to outpatient antidepressant therapy, psychotherapy, and sociotherapy are important factors in determining need for inpatient treatment.
2. Some patients become psychotically depressed in a matter of days to weeks and this group tends to respond quickly to antidepressants. When there is a history of rapid onset without risk of suicide, the patient should be started on an antidepressant coupled with psychotherapy and sociotherapy. Response to a particular antidepressant may be somewhat predicted by a patient's previous response to a particular medication or by the response of another member of his biologic family.
3. If a patient has been using barbiturates for sleep, he or she should be withdrawn from them. Not only are barbiturates potentially addictive and dangerous for patients who are at risk for suicide to have, but, like alcohol, barbiturates also increase the amount of tricyclic antidepressant needed to achieve a clinical response.
4. If there is a history of a cyclic mood disturbance with either recurrent episodes of depression or of depression and mania or hypomania, lithium carbonate maintenance therapy should be initiated. Like commencement of antidepressants, this is not an emergency room procedure. Before either is begun, the appropriate laboratory tests should be obtained such as an electrocardiogram, BUN, T_3, T_7, creatinine, urinalysis, and serum electrolytes.
5. If the depression is part of bipolar disorder, the patient may respond better on a monoamine oxidase inhibitor such as phenelzine (Nardil) or tranylcypromine (Parnate) in appropriate doses. A number of foods and medications must not be taken by patients on these drugs (e.g., sherry, beer, pickled herring, amphetamines, serotonin agonists, tricyclic antidepressants). The patient will require

careful medical supervision, particularly when phenelzine is used in doses in excess of 75 mg/day or tranylcypromine in doses in excess of 30 mg/day.

6. If there is evidence of paranoid ideation, if the level of anxiety is high, or if hallucinations or agitation are evident, a neuroleptic should be used in conjunction with the antidepressant. Patients with delusional depression have been found to respond better to combined antipsychotic–antidepressant pharmacotherapy than antidepressant therapy alone. In fact, delusional thinking may be worsened by tricyclic medication even in the absence of a schizophrenic or manic process (Nelson et al, 1979).

7. Indications for hospitalization include high suicide risk, lack of viable social supports, previous history of a long illness, and lack of response to antidepressant medication as an outpatient.

8. Some patients who are psychotically depressed, particularly the elderly, are labile and respond to adjustment of social support. In such instances, social engineering may be more important than psychopharmacotherapy or psychotherapy. This may entail something as simple as calling in a depressed widow's children to make them alert to her depression, and/or contacting her clergy person so that other members of the parish who have some free time may engage her in social activities.

9. A number of pharmacologic agents either increase (e.g., methylphenidate (Ritalin) and phenothiazines) or decrease (e.g., barbiturates) plasma levels of tricyclic antidepressants.

10. Patients who appear nonresponsive to tricyclics may be at inadequate levels and require serum tricyclic level assay. A significant relationship has been documented between plasma levels of imipramine (Tofranil) and its metabolite desipramine hydrochloride (desmethylimipramine) and clinical responsiveness. Older depressed patients treated with amitriptyline (Elavil), imipramine, and desipramine (Norpramin) show a decreased rate of elimination of these drugs from the plasma. This in part may explain the heightened susceptibility of older patients to side effects of these drugs. Smaller doses, therefore, are often required in the management of older depressed patients.

11. Electroshock is indicated for acutely suicidal and severely depressed patients not responsive to antidepressant medication. Electroshock is still considered the treatment of choice for severe depression when monoamine oxidase inhibitors and tricyclics are not successful. Right unilateral electroshock is deemed preferable to bilateral electroshock because the risk of anterograde memory loss is less.

12. Lithium augmentation may be helpful in patients with delusional depression who are unresponsive to neuroleptic and tricyclic therapy alone (Price et al, 1983) by augmentation of a pre-existing pharmacologic effect (DeMontigny et al, 1981).

13. Amoxapine (Asendin) has been recommended for the treatment of delusional and other psychotic major depression disorders because its pharmacologic structure has some of the characteristics of an antipsychotic agent.

Quality Assurance Issues

1. Were all patients sufficiently evaluated for suicide and homicidal ideation and intent?

2. If suicidal or homicidal, were measures taken to prevent harm to self and others?
3. Were significant others warned of the risk of suicide and homicide for patients who present with psychotic depression and how to recognize it?
4. Was the patient evaluated for medical/surgical causes of psychotic depression?
5. Were patients with psychotic depression provided neuroleptic medication if required?

Ethical/Legal Issues

1. Were all patients who were diagnosed to suffer psychotic depression evaluated during the illness for the presence of or evolution of suicidal thoughts and interest?
2. Were all patients with psychotic depression evaluated for the presence of a medical/surgical basis for their depression?

PSYCHOTROPIC MEDICATION SIDE EFFECTS
(General)

Every medication can cause side effects of some kind. In some instances (e.g., the extrapyramidal effects or sedative qualities of the phenothiazines) these may diminish with time. In other cases it may be necessary to lower the dose of the medication, to discontinue medication, or to stop the medication and institute immediate treatment (e.g., acute agranulocytosis with clozapine) or to continue the medication but add another medication to counteract the side effects (e.g., benztropine mesylate [Cogentin] with perphenazine [Trilafon]).

In the following sections we will discuss management of some common as well as uncommon side-effects of psychotropic medication.

Postural Hypotension

Postural hypotension is a frequent concomitant of neuroleptic and antidepressant treatment. At times, blood pressure may drop to dangerously low levels, particularly in patients with atherosclerotic disease or peripheral neuropathy. The adverse sequelae of orthostatic hypotension include chronic fatigue, dizziness, myocardial infarction, cerebrovascular occlusion, and injuries sustained from fainting. The latter may have grave consequences, especially in older people prone to fractures of the femoral neck with its attendant risks (e.g., pulmonary embolism from immobility, adverse reaction to anesthesia).

A predictor of orthostatic hypotension secondary to treatment with imipramine (Tofranil) is a significant drop in pressure in the vertical compared to the supine position. This predictor probably also holds true for the neuroleptics. Patients should have their blood pressure measured both after lying at rest for 5 minutes and while standing. A prominent drop in pressure would indicate need for use of a neuroleptic or antidepressant with small hypotensive risk.

Patients on neuroleptics and antidepressants should be warned not to change posture abruptly. When arising in the morning patients should swing both legs over the side of the bed and sit there for a few minutes. Hot baths are to be avoided, and patients should kneel before standing in the bath. Similar precaution is to be exercised when getting out of a car, particularly following a long drive. Taking medication after meals slows its absorption so that pressure does not drop as abruptly. Increasing fluid and salt intake and wearing tight-fitting elastic stockings may be of benefit.

Emergency measures include bed rest with the head positioned below the pelvis and administration of supplementary fluids and salt. Severe hypotension can be treated with norepinephrine, which combats the alpha adrenergic-blocking effects of neuroleptics. Epinephrine should be avoided as it causes vasodilation. Hospitalization may be necessary to stabilize a patient with severe hypotension.

Decreased Visual Acuity and Blindness

Decrease in visual acuity, and in some instances, blindness, may be associated with the maintenance use of some phenothiazines. Therefore, a patient on a drug like thioridazine (Mellaril) should ideally have regular ophthalmological examinations. Improvement in visual acuity after drug discontinuation may occur rapidly in some cases. Subjectively, patients report reduced visual acuity or an amber hue in vision when ocular pathology is present. If continued medication is required, primary prevention of these changes involves:

1. Keeping dosage relatively low.
2. Using drugs holidays.
3. Switching to drugs other than chlorpromazine (Thorazine) or thioridazine.
4. Concurrent use of a relatively low dose of thioridazine with another phenothiazine such as trifluoperazine (Stelazine).
5. Use of dark glasses.
6. Protection from sunlight.

Ventricular Tachycardia

Sudden death due to malignant cardiac arrhythmia has been reported on patients being treated with neuroleptics and tricyclic antidepressants. This is extremely rare. A case of hemodynamically compromising ventricular tachycardia has been reported in a patient taking therapeutic dosages of desipramine (Norpramin) and thioridazine (Wilens and Stern, 1990).

Dry Mouth

The dry mouth that occurs with the use of a number of psychoactive agents may be somewhat relieved by chewing dietetic gum, sucking a dietetic candy, and by frequently rinsing the mouth out with water.

Drowsiness

Most patients become tolerant to the drowsiness that occurs with some drugs early in treatment and do not complain of it after the first few weeks. If they do, the medication should be reduced temporarily or substituted with a less sedating one. Patients should be warned not to drive or to operate heavy machinery if drowsiness occurs.

Constipation

A serious side effect of some medication is constipation. Fecal impaction may occur and necessitate use of an enema or digital disimpaction. Hardening of stools, which may be accompanied by abdominal cramping, is treated by dioctyl sodium sulfosuccinate (Colace). If this is not effective, Milk of Magnesia 30 mL at bedtime or bisacodyl (Dulcolax) should be initiated. If symptoms persist, the patient should be instructed to insert a glycerine or a bisacodyl suppository in the morning.

Excess Appetite

Some drugs may cause an increase in appetite with a weight gain far in excess of that desired by the patient. Some antidepressants cause a craving for candy and chocolates.

Pseudoparkinsonism

This syndrome includes akinesia, muscular rigidity, tremor, mask-like facies, alterations of posture, and hypersalivation. It usually develops within 5 to 20 days after initiation of treatment with neuroleptics, save clozapine (Clozaril). It occurs more frequently in females than males. An antiparkinsonian drug such as benztropine mesylate 0.5–1.0 mg (bid or qid) or trihexyphenidyl 2–5 mg PO (bid or tid) may be helpful.

Akathisia

An inability to sit still, tendency to pace constantly, motor restlessness, and fidgeting sometimes misdiagnosed as psychotic exacerbation may occur. Akathisia generally develops within 5 to 40 days after commencement of neuroleptic medication and occurs more frequently in females than in males. Akathisia has been reported to emerge toward the end of each injection interval in some patients receiving long-term depot antipsychotic treatment (Braude and Barnes, 1983). Treatment consists of use of antiparkinsonian agents in dosages mentioned above or diphenhydramine (Benadryl) 50 mg PO bid or tid.

Dystonia

Particularly distressing, this symptom may occur from 1 hour to 5 days after commencement of neuroleptic treatment. It consists of uncoordinated spasmodic movements of the limbs and body such as torticollis, retrocollis, opisthotonos, and oculogyric crises. Coordinated stereotyped involuntary movements may occur (dyskinesia). Men are more prone to develop these symptoms. Cases have been reported where lowering of neuroleptic dosage precipitated dystonia (Gardos, 1981). Antiparkinsonian agents are quite effective (e.g., 2–4 mg of benztropine mesylate daily). With acute and particularly distressing symptoms, benztropine mesylate or diphenhydramine are given intramuscularly. The intramuscular dose of diphenhydramine is 50–100 mg and the dose of benztropine mesylate is 1–2 mg. These symptoms are somewhat misdiagnosed as catatonia, tetany, or hysteria.

Tardive Dyskinesia

This result of neuroleptic treatment may persist indefinitely. It is very resistant to treatment and sometimes appears after a neuroleptic has been discontinued. It generally occurs late in the course of treatment.

Tardive dyskinesia consists of buccolingual or buccofaciomandibular movements such as sucking or smacking movements of the lips; rhythmical forward, backward, or lateral movements of the tongue; and lateral jaw movements. These may be accompanied by athetoid movements of the ankles, toes, and fingers. These movements interfere with swallowing and the respiratory rate may be disturbed. Symptoms subside during sleep. They are often irreversible and resistant to all known treatment; however, preventive measures may be employed such as drug holidays, discontinuing medication unless it is absolutely necessary, switching to another drug, or combining lorazepam (Ativan) with neuroleptics to minimize dosage of the latter. Tardive dyskinetic symptoms are sometimes deceptively decreased when the dose of neuroleptic is elevated. These symptoms do not respond to antiparkinsonian agents nor to switching to another neuroleptic. Tardive dyskinesia has not been reported as a side effect of the antipsychotic clozapine.

Tremor

A nonparkinsonian tremor may occur at relatively low doses of lithium. Improvement occurs with lowering of lithium dose, discontinuation of the drug where possible, and in some instance when a beta blocker is given concurrently (Gaby et al, 1983).

Withdrawal Hypomania

Tricyclic withdrawal is accompanied by alterations in the turnover rate of neurotransmitters as well as by shifts in equilibrium between various transmitter systems. This may lead to changes in behavior. While relapse to depression is most frequent, mania or hypomania are also seen. Recommencement of the drug (Nelson et al, 1979) or initiation of neuroleptic or benzodiazepine therapy generally is sufficient to manage the mood change (Mirin et al, 1981).

Blurred Vision

Blurred vision is an especially annoying side effect. Medication, where possible, should be reduced. "Trilafon glasses" may be used for close reading. The patient should be instructed to avoid driving if possible, or at least to be very careful when driving, and to avoid operating heavy machinery. In a number of cases blurred vision subsides with time alone.

Agranulocytosis

This rare side effect occurs so suddenly and dramatically that serial complete blood counts, unless measured weekly, do not protect against it. Suggestive symptoms are sore throat and fever. Treatment includes immediate discontinuation of the offending drug, isolation, use of antibiotics, and possibly transfusion of blood.

Jaundice

This rare side effect is treated by immediate discontinuation of the offending drug, bedrest, and initiation of a high-protein, high-carbohydrate diet.

Gastrointestinal Upset

Heartburn and nausea may occur with some phenothiazines, lithium, fluoxetine (Prozac) and sertraline (Zoloft). This is minimized by taking the medication with milk or after meals.

Megaloblastic Anemia

There is some evidence suggesting that lithium therapy may induce a folic acid deficiency megaloblastic anemia (Prakash et al, 1981). The anemia responds to cessation of lithium and to concurrent use of folic acid.

Retarded Ejaculation

Painful and abnormally protracted ejaculation has been reported with amoxapine (Asendin). Symptoms abate with cessation of the drug or commencement of therapy with an alternate medication (Kerlik and Wilbur, 1982; Schwarz, 1982).

Asphyxia

Asphyxia may occur during use of psychotropic medication. In some instances deaths relate to serious medical illness and not to psychotropic drug use. In other cases, asphyxia is associated with seizures or choking. In the former, the question is raised about subtherapeutic use of anticonvulsants in association with psychotropic drugs. Choking has been linked to a combination of strong anticholinergic effects and dopamine blockade leading to impairment of swallowing. A drug monitoring system and the Heimlich maneuver serves to reduce the cases of choking secondary to psychotropic therapy (Craig TJ, 1980).

Rapid Cycling

Rapid cycling of mood change has been reported to be induced by antidepressants. Cessation of thymoleptics leaves patients manic, depressed, euthymic, or in a condition of continued rapid cycling (Appenheim, 1982).

Stuttering

Stuttering is reported as a rare side effect of phenothiazine use (Nurnberg and Greenwald, 1981).

Seizures

Seizures have been reported with use of both neuroleptic and antidepressant medications. Anticonvulsant medication may have to be increased if the patient is epileptic. Generalized motor seizures have been reported with acute loxapine overdose (Gelesson, 1981).

Phototoxicity

Phenothiazines such as chlorpromazine produce a phototoxicity so that painful sunburn occurs after only a few minutes of exposure. Patients should be warned of this hazard and advised to use sunscreens.

Cardiovascular Effects

Tricyclic antidepressants cause tachycardia and changes in cardiac conduction (Rudorfer and Young, 1980). The EKG may show prolonged Q-T intervals, depressed S-T segments, and flattened T waves, which may be the forerunner of ventricular arrhythmias. Tricyclics exhibit a quinidine-like effect manifested on the EKG by signs of first-degree atrioventricular block. Extreme caution is therefore required in administering tricyclics to patients with bundle branch disease.

The propensity of tricyclics to inhibit activity of antihypertensive drugs such as quanethidine and clonidine may complicate treatment of older patients who have both hypertension and depression. Combined use of a tricyclic and a thiazide diuretic may produce profound hypotension.

Concentrations of imipramine routinely obtained in the treatment of severe depression may markedly suppress spontaneously occurring atrial ventricular premature contractions (Rasking et al, 1982).

Trazadone (Desyrel) has been found to increase ventricular ectopic activity in patients with pre-existing ventricular arrhythmias and mitral valve prolapse (Janowsky et al, 1982).

Marked sinus tachycardia has been reported in a patient who smoked marijuana receiving therapeutic doses of nortriptyline (Aventyl) suggesting a synergistic action of the two drugs. Propranolol is recommended as treatment of the condition (Hillard and Vieweg, 1983).

Central Nervous System Effects

A number of CNS reactions have been reported with tricyclics. These include hypomania and mania, insomnia, and toxic psychosis primarily occurring in older patients. A fine tremor is occasionally seen, and tricyclics may induce generalized seizures in patients with predisposition to epilepsy. Untoward aggressiveness has also been attributed to tricyclics.

Hepatitis

Hepatitis is a rare side effect of tricyclic use.

Sweating

Flushing and sweating of the upper face and scalp are occasionally encountered, particularly in women.

Lupus-like Illness

Bilateral pleural effusions, low-grade fever, immunological abnormalities, and dyspnea as a manifestation of lupus-like syndromes have been reported with chlorpromazine. The process is reversible when the drug is discontinued (Goldman et al, 1980).

Quality Assurance Issues

1. Were all patients and their significant others advised of potential side effects and how to recognize them?
2. If a side effect is dangerous to the health of a patient, was the patient advised of the need for immediate treatment and how to get it?
3. Does a hospital have a system for reporting actual or potential adverse drug responses that includes as reporters physicians, nursing staff, and pharmacists? Are these reports reviewed by the medical staff? If trends exist, what measures are taken to minimize the occurrence of side effects?
4. Are continuing medical education activities sponsored that address the psychopharmacologic management of patients, the side effects of the drugs used, and the management of side effects?
5. Is physician use of given drugs monitored to ascertain if the drugs are used appropriately and if side effects are monitored and treated?

PSYCHOTROPIC MEDICINE WITHDRAWAL

Subjective behavioral and physiologic changes follow abrupt cessation of antidepressants, anticonvulsants, stimulants, and antianxiety and antipsychotic medications.

History

1. Delirium can develop as long as 8 days after diazepam (Valium) withdrawal, consistent with the observation that symptoms are generally slower to develop following cessation of benzodiazepines than discontinuation of alcohol or barbiturates.
2. People with histories of chronic sedative or alcohol abuse are particularly prone to develop symptoms on benzodiazepine cessation. Withdrawal from lesser amounts may lead to gastrointestinal upset, dysphoria, weight loss, increase in orthostatic pulse rate, and physical discomfort.
3. Severe depression may follow cessation of stimulant drugs such as methylphenidate (Ritalin).
4. Discontinuation of anticonvulsants have been reported in some instances to lead to psychotic symptoms in the context of a clear sensorium with markedly increased electroencephalographic abnormalities.
5. Gastrointestinal dysfunction may result from abrupt cessation of antidepressants.
6. Covert dyskinesia may appear upon discontinuation or reduction in dosage of antipsychotic medication, which mimics symptoms of a psychotic exacerbation. These generally disappear in 6 to 12 weeks and are thought to reflect cholinergic overactivity and changes in dopamine–acetylcholine balance in the basal ganglia. Dyskinesia uncovered at the time of drug cessation may be an early sign of a developing tardive dyskinesia

7. Central cholinergic overdrive is posted as the mechanism of symptoms of withdrawal from antidepressants (Dilsaver et al, 1983).
8. Ability to manage withdrawal symptoms from antidepressants is particularly important when the drugs must be abruptly discontinued or in the instances of an allergic reaction or a drug-induced mania.
9. Withdrawal symptoms are reported as greater among antipsychotic agents with more potent autonomic properties and when they are discontinued simultaneously with antiparkinson agents.
10. Sinus tachycardia with frequent ventricular extrasystoles associated with bigeminy has been reported following withdrawal from imipramine (Tofranil) suggesting that imipramine withdrawal may result in either a rebound arrhythmia or in unmasking pre-existing cardiac instability (Boisverg and Chouinard, 1981).
11. The duration of withdrawal symptoms for diazepam may last as long as a month (Nagy and Dilman, 1981).
12. Benzodiazepines with a shorter half-life (e.g., alprazolam [Xanax], oxazepam [Serax], lorazepam [Ativan]) should have a more abrupt onset of the symptoms of withdrawal than those with a longer half-life such as diazepam and chlordiazepoxide (Librium) (Stewart et al, 1980).
13. Abrupt discontinuation of antiparkinson drugs may result in abnormal lower-extremity movements, hallucinations, physical complaints, and motor agitation in vulnerable individuals (Jellinek T et al, 1981).

Symptoms
1. Abdominal pain.
2. Insomnia.
3. Drowsiness.
4. Agitation.
5. Anxiety.
6. Withdrawal.
7. Apathy.
8. Recurrence or worsening of depression.
9. Moodiness.
10. Headaches.
11. Dizziness.
12. Coryza.
13. Chills.
14. Weakness.
15. Fatigue.
16. Musculoskeletal pain.
17. Malaise.
18. Akathisia.

Signs
1. Diarrhea.
2. Nausea.

3. Vomiting.
4. Behavioral activation.
5. Gooseflesh.
6. Perspiration.
7. Delirium.

Clinical Studies
1. EEG changes.

Management
1. Symptoms of antidepressant drug withdrawal have been successfully treated with anticholinergic agents (e.g., atropine) (Dilsaver et al, 1983).
2. Gradual withdrawal of psychotropic drugs over 2 to 4 weeks generally prevents symptoms (Santos and McCurdy, 1980).
3. Symptoms following abrupt cessation of benzodiazepines generally disappear if the drug is reinstated. Gradual withdrawal is generally without untoward effect.
4. The depression following discontinuation of stimulants may be so severe that antidepressant medication or electroshock is required. Suicide precautions are a required component of treatment if patients' depression is so severe that they may take their own life.
5. Recommencement of the anticonvulsants will bring about amelioration of psychotic symptoms erupting upon cessation of seizure medication.
6. The gastrointestinal symptoms that appear following withdrawal of antidepressants are generally not of sufficient magnitude to merit recommencing the drug. If severe discomfort occurs, reinstitution of the medication and subsequent gradual withdrawal will handle the problem.

Quality Assurance Issues
1. Were all patients on addicting psychotropic medications gradually withdrawn?
2. Were symptoms of withdrawal treated as they emerged?
3. Were the drugs used for withdrawal appropriate and specific?

Ethical/Legal Issues
1. Were all patients on potentially addicting psychotropic medication warned of the risk of addiction and of withdrawal symptoms?
2. Were patients withdrawn in settings appropriate to the intensity of the withdrawal symptoms and the risks to the patients' health?

PUERPERAL PSYCHOSIS

Puerperal (postpartum) psychosis is not considered a psychiatric illness in its own right. Many different psychiatric illnesses may be precipitated by childbirth.

History

1. Postpartum patients as a group have more manic symptoms and confusion. They lack schizophrenic symptoms, suggesting that postpartum psychoses are more frequently of an affective nature (Brockington et al, 1981).
2. Suicide risk is decreased during pregnancy but increased in the postpartum period.

Management

1. Management of a puerperal psychosis is diagnostic specific.
2. Sensitivity must be paid to the impact of the illness (be it psychiatric or medical) on the mother, her child, those individuals close to her and her child, the grandparents of the child, the father of the child, and any other children she may have.

3. Suicide evaluation (and precautions if a patient is suicidal) is necessary for all postpartum psychotic patients.

Quality Assurance Issues

1. Were medical/surgical illnesses investigated to ascertain if they were primarily or in part responsible for a patient's symptoms?
2. Were family members advised of the risks to the infant if the mother is psychotic?
3. Was education in mothering advised to reduce the stress of parenthood, and was it provided to the mother and her partner?

Ethical/Legal Issues

1. Were appropriate measures taken to prevent harm to self or others (particularly the newborn infant)?
2. Were fathers advised of how to recognize recrudescence of the psychosis?
3. Were measures taken to prevent harm to the child in the months of recovery?

PULMONARY EMBOLISM

Pulmonary embolism is associated with sudden behavioral, mood, and cognitive changes including panic, anxiety, paranoia, confusion, and hallucinosis, especially in people who have been immobilized for a long period of time, who have suffered mitral valve prolapse, or who have septic emboli to the brain resulting from subacute bacterial endocarditis (Frisbie, 1986).

Management

1. Immediate medical or surgical intervention is required in addition to whatever psychiatric support must be offered to calm the frightened patient.

PYRIDOSTIGMINE-INDUCED DISORDERS

Pyridostigmine bromide has been reported to alter mental status in rare instances.

RADIATION

Radiation of the CNS may result in necrosis of the brain and psychiatric symptoms including affective and cognitive symptoms (McMahon and Vahora, 1986).

RAPE

Women and men of all ages may present with a variety of psychiatric symptoms after being raped. Those who are very young, men, and older women are particularly vulnerable to the "silent rape syndrome" because of associated shame and stigma.

History
1. Some women and men who have been raped may present with complaints of appetite loss or sleep disturbance, suffering the silent rape syndrome. Many of these adults have been raped or molested in the past, especially in adolescence or childhood, and the recent trauma has reactivated early feelings that have never really been talked about and worked through. When given the opportunity, they may talk as much about the earlier incident as about the recent rape.
2. A high index of suspicion that a woman has experienced a previous rape should be entertained when she begins to show signs of increasing anxiety, such as minor stuttering, blocking of associations, physical distress, and long periods of silence during the evaluation.
3. It is always important to find out what a woman means when she states she has been raped. A housewife may label a sexual advance by her husband at a time she prefers not to have intercourse as a "rape." In other instances, a "rape" may be the label attached to an aggressive sexual advance by a husband after a trial separation or a boyfriend after heavy petting and drinking ("date rape"). In other cases, "rape" is a clear physical assault in which sexual gratification is not a primary end, but rather a violent act in which sex is a weapon and serious physical harm or death a possibility.
4. Men, as well as women, may have been raped and be embarrassed to talk about it. Both men and women can be homosexually raped. Rapists spare no age group. Young children and women in their eighties have been raped.
5. In instances of male rape (Groth and Burgess, 1980) it has been found that for some, but not all, gender of victim appeared immaterial and rapist's assaults were an effort to deal with unresolved psychological conflict. For male rapists

the sexual assault was an expression of power, an act of retaliation and a futile assertion of manhood and strength.

6. If a victim has been emotionally healthy, the focus of crisis intervention is on the trauma using ventilation and support. If the individual suffered pre-existing psychopathology, psychotherapy is provided to minimize exacerbation or worsening of symptoms given the traumatic sexual assault (Rose DS, 1986).

7. Rape has been divided into blitz rape and confidence rape. In the former instance, there is a surprise attack whereas in the latter the assailant is an individual with whom the victim had a nonviolent interaction and false pretenses were used to allow the attacker accesses and betrayal of trust (Silverman et al, 1988).

8. Impact of rape on men is similar to that of women (Groth and Burgess, 1980). As a group they report more depression, anger, and fear, as well as difficulties in peer relationships and somatic symptoms such as insomnia and appetite change. Sexual problems are reported in as many as half of those raped (Goyer and Eddleman, 1984). The same percentage is also reported for women (Greenspan and Samuel, 1989).

9. On the whole, male rape victims (when compared to female rape victims) sustain more physical trauma, are more likely to have experienced multiple assaults from multiple assailants, and more likely to have been held captive longer (Kaufman et al, 1980).

10. Male rape victims are less likely to reveal the genital component of the assault and are more likely to use denial and to attempt to control their emotions (Kaufman et al, 1980).

11. In a study of 41 female rape victims it was found 1 to $2\frac{1}{2}$ years later that half of the victims continued to fear being alone and three-fourths remained suspicious of others (Madelson et al, 1983). Other symptoms that were reported included sexual dysfunction, episodic depression, and restriction in daily life.

12. AIDS may result from both hetero- and homosexual rape.

13. The symptoms and signs of rape include, in the pursuing months and years, signs and symptoms of a post-traumatic stress disorder.

Symptoms
1. Headache.
2. Depression.
3. Panic and generalized anxiety.
4. Recurrent nightmares.
5. Sleep disturbance.
6. Appetite disturbance.
7. Irritability.
8. Stomach pain.
9. Vaginal itching.
10. Dysphoria.
11. Anal pain.
12. Anger.
13. Recurrent intrusive memories of the assault.

14. Fear of reprisal.
15. Shame.
16. Self-blame.
17. Phobias (of being outdoors, of being alone, of crowds, of sex).

Signs
1. Startle.
2. Bruises on the legs, thighs, breasts, arms, and face immediately after the assault.
3. Injuries to the mouth and throat if forced to have oral sex.
4. Rectal bleeding if sodomized.
5. Vaginal discharge.
6. Increased motor activity.

Management
1. The immediate psychotherapeutic approach to the rape victim is modeled on the crisis intervention techniques of allowing ventilation and encouraging return to the previous level of functioning as soon as possible. Previous problems are not as important as the current difficulties except in those with severe psychopathology.
2. If there appears to be a more fundamental psychiatric problem, such as schizophrenia or alcoholism, which may have led the patient to take the risks that led to his or her rape, he or she should be referred for long-term treatment with appropriate psychopharmacotherapy, psychotherapy, and sociotherapy.
3. Not all patients will want more than the initial opportunity to ventilate their feelings and to receive legal counsel and medical care at the time of their rape. Others, however, may want to return for a few follow-up sessions to talk more about what happened and perhaps to talk about earlier comparable experiences that have been reactivated.
4. To prevent pregnancy, the patient should be offered one of several methods available presently. Methoxyprogesterone or diethylstilbestrol orally for 5 days has been recommended. If menstruation does not commence within 1 week after cessation of the estrogen, all alternatives, including abortion, should be made available to the patient. If the patient has been using either an oral contraceptive or an intrauterine device, no further treatment should be necessary to prevent pregnancy.
5. The rapist may have had a venereal disease, so the physician should, with written consent, provide appropriate antibiotic therapy. If the patient is not allergic to penicillin, benzathine penicillin G should be given. Alternately, probenecid should be given orally (followed in 30 to 60 minutes by intramuscular procaine penicillin) or oral ampicillin may be given simultaneously with probenecid. If the patient is allergic to penicillin or to penicillin-like drugs, treatment with oral tetracycline HCl or streptomycin IM may be given.
6. A swab should be taken from the vaginal pool to be saved for the police laboratory to inspect for acid phosphatase and blood antigen of the semen. In addition, both cervical and rectal cultures should be obtained for gonorrhea and a serology

sent off for syphilis and a baseline HIV test obtained. Six weeks later, these tests should be repeated and compared to baseline. Of all the above recommended treatments, only penicillin is effective for the treatment of simultaneously incubating syphilis and gonorrhea. When an alternate treatment regime is used, there must be a follow-up serology for syphilis as well as for HIV infection.

7. Witnessed written permission should be obtained to protect the physician for examination, for photographs, for collection of specimens, and for the release of information to the proper authorities.

8. The question as to whether or not rape has actually occurred is a legal decision and not a medical diagnosis. Physicians may be subpoenaed to justify their statements. Therefore, for protection of the patient and themselves, they should obtain consent, record the history in the patient's own words, obtain the required laboratory tests, record the results of their examination, save all clothing, make no diagnosis, and provide protection against disease, psychic trauma, and pregnancy.

9. Both men and women should be represented on a rape team. This serves several purposes. Men, as well as women, are raped and may feel more comfortable discussing the rape with a man. Rape is a violent act and many women have a disinterest or aversion to sexual intercourse following rape. A warm supportive relationship with a man in crisis intervention following a rape allows a woman to separate out the male and sexual component from the violent physical assault. This helps to immediately desensitize women from seeing men or sex as bad and place the rape in its proper perspective as a brutal violent assault on a person and not a male sexual involvement as such. Finally, male members of rape teams are valuable in talking to spouses and fathers concerning their feelings about having had their wife or daughter raped. Husbands and fathers may unjustly see their spouse or daughter as having colluded in the act (i.e., "asked for it").

10. Proper management of male rape victims requires high index of suspicion and a sensitivity to an unexpressed history of trauma (Kaufman et al, 1980).

11. Rape and rape-murders may occur while an offender is under psychiatric care. Probationary supervision is indicated for continued surveillance of offenders given the drive in some to continue to assault (Ressler et al, 1983)

Quality Assurance Issues

1. Has an opportunity been afforded for the victim to ventilate regarding the psychic trauma?
2. Are all the steps in rape management discussed in this section provided to all patients?
3. Is a psychiatric assessment provided to ascertain if the patient had a psychiatric illness that made him or her vulnerable as well as to provide a baseline index of the psychological sequelae of the assault?

Ethical/Legal Issues

1. Do records reflect concern for the patient's legal rights, confidentiality, and human dignity?

2. Is legal counsel provided the victims?
3. Does the medical record include documentation necessary for prosecution of the rapist if pursued?

REFILL REQUESTER

Patients unfamiliar to psychiatric clinicians appear in the emergency room seeking renewals of prescriptions. All patients requesting refills for psychotropic medication ordinarily obtained elsewhere should be seen so that the immediate situation can be assessed. Some patients who have discontinued therapy seek a refill at the time of crisis. The hidden agenda is a need for help, not medication or at least not primarily medication. These individuals should be encouraged to return to the original clinic or clinician who knows their complete psychiatric and treatment history. An attempt should be made to contact the clinic or clinician at the time of the request for renewal of medication to alert them to the patient's problem. The emergency psychiatric clinician should resist any desire to take over the patient's care as this undermines the patient's treatment and reinforces sporadic use of emergency services rather than supporting continuity of care and commitment to therapy that is needed to provide more long-lasting resolutions of psychological problems. If medication is given, it should be only a sufficient amount to cover the days until the patient's next clinic visit to his or her clinicians.

Quality Assurance Issues
1. Was the need for the medication verified and diagnostic specific?
2. If the drug could be taken in overdose or abused, was the amount given no greater than what could reasonably be required by the patient until his or her next regular appointment?
3. Was an effort made to call the patient's attending physician to document need?
4. Were all precautions regarding prescription of controlled drugs observed?

Ethical/Legal Issues
1. If a prescription is refilled for a controlled drug or one that may endanger the health of the person, has sufficient data been obtained to verify the diagnostic-specific indication for the medication?

REFUSAL OF MEDICATION

Patients sometimes refuse to take medication despite the fact that the attending psychiatrist feels that psychopharmacotherapy is a necessary part of management. In most instances, it is possible to obtain cooperation of patients, but effort and time is required. An understanding of the reasons for refusal is the first step in obtaining patient cooperation.

Quality Assurance Issues
1. Is there documentation that the patient was encouraged to take the needed medication and was provided the rationale for its use and a choice when applicable?
2. Were significant others involved in an effort to assure medication compliance?

Ethical/Legal Issues
1. Were patients rights to refuse treatment respected?
2. Is there a record that appropriate therapy was proposed but refused if a patient does not require it in an emergency situation?

REPEATERS

Frequent users of psychiatric emergency services tend to fall into three general groups. The first consists of individuals whose illness is such that continuity of care with one clinician is difficult although obviously desired. This group includes severe substance abusers, delusional disorder, and noncompliant schizophrenics. The second group consists of people with limited resources who seek help only when absolutely necessary. To them, the emergency room is their primary care provider. Finally, there are those whose psychopathology impels them to split or dilute ongoing therapy (such as borderline personality disordered patients and others with severe character pathology). Use of emergency services or the primary care provider leads to confusion over diagnosis, impractical treatment planning, and very destructive countertransference issues (Ellison et al, 1989).

History
1. Studies of repeater populations indicate that the modal frequent user is male, never married, and under 40 years of age (Casper and Donaldson, 1990).

Management
1. The thrust of management for repeaters is to attempt to get them into clinics where continuity of care may be provided.
2. Repeater substance abusers do best in outpatient settings that combine AA, NA, CA, partial hospital inpatient groups, and crisis-oriented therapy. When only one or two elements of the menu needed to provide an integrated program of care are present, the patient becomes a repeater by virtue of need for an alternate service.
3. Repeated use by chronic schizophrenics is reduced when less dependence is placed on the need for adherence to an oral medication schedule by provision of a regimen of long-acting intramuscular medication (e.g., fluphenazine (Prolixin) or haloperidol (Haldol) decanoate).
4. The availability of patients' therapists' telephone numbers in the emergency room to call (when a patient attempts to get more medication in order to avoid seeing a therapist and to dilute the transference) undercuts the acting out and may extinguish the repeater behavior.

Quality Assurance Issues
1. Is there documentation that efforts are made to involve repeaters in a continuing care program to reduce unnecessary use of emergency services?

Ethical/Legal Issues
1. Are patients with a pattern of repeated usage of emergency services reviewed to ascertain if the treatment afforded has been diagnostic specific? (Some patients continually return because their primary problem for use of an emergency room is not addressed, such as a depressed alcoholic who is provided detoxification but never treatment for his or her depression.)

RESERPINE-INDUCED DISORDERS

The rauwolfia alkaloids are clinically used for a variety of reasons including treatment of hypertension. Psychiatric uses include treatment of schizophrenia, mania, delirium tremens, and senile agitated states. Reserpine is used experimentally in animals by researchers interested in studying the effect of depletion of catecholamines on behavior.

History
1. In therapeutic doses, reserpine produces sedation, tranquilization, and antihypertensive effects.
2. Small doses of reserpine can produce nightmares and depression accompanied by serious suicidal ideation. The depression may be insidious in onset.
3. Elderly patients are particularly prone to depression with this drug.

Symptoms
1. Depression.
2. Nightmares.
3. Suicidal ideation and attempts.
4. Decreased libido.
5. Lassitude.
6. Increased appetite.
7. Weight gain.
8. Nasal stuffiness.
9. Abdominal cramps.
10. Dyspepsia.
11. Diarrhea.
12. Fluid retention.
13. Lactation.
14. Drowsiness.
15. Dizziness.

Signs
1. Cutaneous flushing.
2. Drooling.
3. Extrapyramidal signs.
4. Hypotension.

Differential Diagnosis
Differential diagnosis includes all causes of depression.

Management
1. Carefully reduce the dose of reserpine and, if possible, discontinue use and begin the patient on a suitable alternate drug.
2. These patients can be quite suicidal and the usual precautions may be necessary to prevent patients from harming themselves.
3. Antidepressant medication or electroshock may be required if the depression is profound and persistent following cessation of reserpine.

Quality Assurance Issues
1. Are patients on reserpine monitored for signs of depression?
2. If depressed, are patients evaluated (and precautions provided for as indicated) for suicide potential?
3. Is a patient provided an alternative antihypertensive (if indicated) if they suffer depression on reserpine?

Ethical/Legal Issues
1. Are all patients on reserpine and other depression-producing antihypertensive medications, and their families warned that they may become depressed, and in some instances, suicidal?

RHEUMATOID ARTHRITIS

Approximately 1 to 3% of the population suffer rheumatoid arthritis (Rogers, 1985). Psychiatric symptoms in these patients may be a product of the disease itself or be a reaction to the illness or a side effect of a drug used to treat it.

History
1. Fatigue, anorexia, and malaise are seen together with fever and morning stiffness as nonspecific symptoms of the illness (Rogers, 1985).
2. Medication used to treat the disease (e.g., nonsteroidal anti-inflammatory agents, corticosteroids, and hydroxychloroquine) have both affective and cognitive side effects that may be construed to be a product of the illness itself.
3. A patient may become depressed due to the pain and physical limitation that accompany both the adult and juvenile forms.

Management

1. Treatment of the psychiatric symptoms is diagnostic specific. Antidepressants, for instance, are used when depression seen comports with affective illness that would respond to medication.
2. If the symptoms are a side effect of medication, the first approach is to reduce medication or seek an alternate drug without behavioral impact. If the medication is needed, a psychopharmacologic agent is provided that is symptom specific (e.g., lithium or tranquilizers such as clonazepam [Klonopin] for the euphoria induced by steroids).
3. Group support by others suffering the same illness is always helpful as an adjunctive or primary therapy (Winkel, 1988). Adaptations to crippling symptoms are shared, enhancing the repertoire of means of coping with the illness.

SCHIZOAFFECTIVE DISORDER

Patients with schizoaffective disorder present with disturbance of both mood and thought. In some cases, it is extremely difficult to differentiate bipolar disorder from schizoaffective disorder. The bizarre character of a patient's thoughts help to identify schizoaffective disorder.

History

1. Family history of affective illness and alcoholism as opposed to a family history of schizophrenia helps to distinguish schizoaffective disorder from affective illness.
2. Patients with primary affective illness are less frequently found to have the severe interpersonal and employment derangements than those with schizoaffective disorder.
3. The premorbid personality of patients with bipolar disorder is often cyclothymic.
4. Lifetime prevalence of major affective disorder (including schizoaffective disorder) was 37% in relatives of probands with schizoaffective disorders (Gershon et al, 1982). Comparable figures for probands with bipolar I disorders, bipolar II disorders, unipolar disorders, and normal controls were 24, 25, 20, and 7%, respectively, suggesting the concept that different affective disorders represent thresholds on a continuum of underlying multifactorial vulnerability.
5. Suicide among patients with schizoaffective disorder is difficult to predict.

Symptoms

1. Depression.
2. Elation or mania.
3. Suicidal preoccupation.
4. Paranoid ideation.
5. Auditory hallucinations.
6. Ideas of reference.

7. Bizarre thoughts.
8. Paralogical thinking.
9. Somatic delusions.
10. Hypochondriasis.

Signs
1. Bizarre behavior.

Differential Diagnosis
Differential diagnosis is the same as for schizophrenia and depression. It should be remembered that the superimposition of a disease such as hypothyroidism or use of a drug such as beta blocker with depression may make a person with a thought disorder appear schizoaffective or primarily affectively ill. Treatment of the hypothyroidism or discontinuation of the beta blocker would result in an accentuation of the thought disorder.

Management
1. Patients with schizoaffective disorder, like some depressed borderline and personality disordered patients, may become psychotic when given an antidepressant medication.
2. Since suicide is unpredictable in schizoaffective disorder, the presence of depression or suicidal ideation, especially in a patient who has attempted suicide previously, warrants immediate hospitalization.
3. If a viable social matrix exists in the form of family, friends, or a psychotherapist who is following the patient, outpatient management may be possible. In fact, if the patient has been followed in therapy for some time, the therapist may be able to suggest those interventions that have been successful in the past.
4. The combination of neuroleptics and an antidepressant or mood stabilizer tends to work better than either drug alone in schizoaffective-disordered patients who are depressed. Lithium carbonate is helpful in modulating the mood swings of these patients, but alone it is inferior to a combination of lithium with neuroleptics and antidepressants as indicated (Biederman et al, 1979).
5. There is some evidence to support use of a single neuroleptic with antidepressant action, as opposed to a combination of an antidepressant and a neuroleptic without antidepressant action, in the management of depressive and anergic symptoms observed in the course of a schizophrenic illness (Becker, 1983).

Quality Assurance Issues
1. Is the patient continuously reviewed for the possibility of bipolar disorder masquerading as schizoaffective disorder?
2. Have both mood-stabilizing and antipsychotic agents been prescribed and monitored if the patient has schizoaffective disorder?
3. Was the patient evaluated for organic causes (e.g., AIDS) either causing schizoaffective symptoms or contributing to them?
4. Has the patient been evaluated for concurrent substance abuse?

Ethical/Legal Issues
1. Has the patient been evaluated for suicide risk and, if at risk, have appropriate measures been taken?
2. Has the patient been advised of the neuroleptic malignant syndrome and tardive dyskinesia as complications of neuroleptic treatment?
3. Are patients re-evaluated for evidence of tardive dyskinesia?

SCHIZOPHRENIA

Early recognition and treatment of a patient undergoing a schizophrenic break can reduce the emotional pain to both patient, family, and friends, as well as reduce or actually obviate need for inpatient psychiatric care.

History
1. Gradual withdrawal from interpersonal relationships is an ominous sign and especially suggestive of an insidious schizophrenic deterioration in adolescence or in the twenties. Patients may give a history of increasing difficulty at school (which can be objectively quantified by progressively poorer grades) after promise of a sterling academic career (Heinrichs and Carpenter, 1985).
2. In many instances, interest in sex diminishes (Keefe et al, 1989). In other instances, there may be evidence of increased libido with more time committed to autoerotic behavior (i.e., masturbation) and promiscuous hetero- and homosexual activity with less sensuous gratifications.
3. Interests may turn from sports and the mundane to a preoccupation with unanswerable philosophical and religious questions. A previously politically or religiously indifferent individual may become heavily involved in extreme religious or political groups that, in some cases, dynamically appear to represent an attempt to organize the external world while the internal one is in chaos.
4. Decreasing functioning at work manifests itself by an inability to hold jobs or by a gradual constriction of the patient's responsibilities by superiors.
5. Symptoms seen with psychoses of a variety of etiologies may be seen. Ideas of reference, paranoid ideation, and hallucinations may be reported historically and the advent of these symptoms may serve to document the time course of the illness. Affective disorders and schizophrenia are commonly confused in the early stages (Glazer et al, 1987; Slaby and Moreines, 1990).
6. Classically, hallucinations, when reported in schizophrenia, are of the auditory variety (although all types can occur).
7. Age of onset of schizophrenia is early, with a peak for admissions to hospitals in range of 25 to 34 years of age.
8. Family history is always important in providing clues. This is especially true when there exists confusion as to whether a patient is schizophrenic or suffering from an affective disorder. A family history of schizophrenia inclines the diagnostician to think of a thought disorder (Shenton et al, 1989). Conversely, one

should be cautious about diagnosing schizophrenia in a person with a family history of affective disorder. Schizotypal and paranoid personality disorders may be related to schizophrenia (Baron et al, 1985).

9. Obtaining a good history from schizophrenics or their families is not always easy. The ability to critically evaluate a patient's history is the hallmark of the skilled interviewer. Many patients, when asked the number of close friends they have, will reply "many," "several," or even quantify them (e.g., "10 to 15"). The diagnostician should then ask the patient to name his or her friends, even though the diagnostician will not usually recognize the names. The diagnostician will be impressed with the hesitation or even the inability of the patient to name any friends at all! In other cases, a person may be named who, when the patient is asked "When is the last time you saw him?" will reply, "Last year," "Several years ago," etc. In other instances, another patient who is incapable of any supportive or close relationships will be named. Sometimes a famous actor, actress, psychiatric aide, or a member of a janitorial staff may be mentioned. This again reflects that patients have few close friends of their own.

10. In the family history, it is important to ask about any member of the family who was "institutionalized," committed suicide, spent long times in a hospital for "nervous reasons," or behaved strangely. When the last mentioned is answered in the affirmative, the patient should be asked what was strange. A mother may have left a family when the patient was 8 years old and become a prostitute by picking up men or women at bars. The abandonment of the family and rapid change from the previous pattern of behavior would suggest that the patient may have had an undiagnosed schizophrenic parent.

11. Schizophrenics are more anhedonic than nonschizophrenics.

12. History bears on diagnosis. An insidious onset, impoverished or absent affective component, inability to hold a job, no friends or intimate relationships, no clear precipitant, and a family history of schizophrenia are all associated with a poor prognosis. Good prognosticators include marriage, strong affective component, acute onset, ability to make and maintain close friends, ability to hold a job, a family history of affective disorders, and a clear precipitating event (Harrow et al, 1985).

13. The degree to which genetic factors play a role in the transmission of schizophrenia is a subject of much debate (Abrams and Taylor, 1983). It currently appears that while a genetic predisposition is necessary, environmental and familial factors play roles in whether or not genetic tendency expresses itself, in the time of expression, in the severity of the illness, and in the nature of the illness expressed.

14. A high concentration of latent, chronic, and uncertain schizophrenia or schizotypical personality disorder is found in the biologic relatives of adoptees who develop chronic schizophrenia (Kety, 1983).

15. Neither a familial/environmental nor genetic link has been demonstrated between schizophrenia and anxiety disorder by a blind independent analysis of interviews from the Danish Adoption Study of Schizophrenia using *DSM-III* criteria indicating that schizophrenia and anxiety disorders are distinct unrelated illnesses (Kendler et al, 1981).

16. Schizophrenia spectrum disorders (i.e., schizophrenia and schizotypical personality disorders) but not paranoid psychosis (i.e., delusional disorder) are found in greater concentration in biologic relatives of schizophrenic adoptees suggesting that from a genetic perspective, delusional disorder is not part of the schizophrenia spectrum (Kendler et al, 1981).

17. The overall ventricular brain ratio for chronic schizophrenics has been reported to be significantly above that found in normal populations and appears to have significant correlates with measures of neuropsychological performance such as the Standardized Luria-Nebraska Neuropsychological Battery (Golden CJ et al, 1980; Boronow et al, 1985; DeLisi et al, 1986; Brown et al, 1986a).

18. Shortened survival (i.e., premature death) is found in schizophrenia, bipolar disorder, and major depression (Tsuang and Woolson, 1978). Causes of excess mortality include suicide, accidents, and circulatory and infectious disease. Schizophrenics have approximately a two-fold increase in mortality in all causes of death (Allebeck and Wistedt, 1986).

19. Parental loss before age 17 appears to be greater in patients with schizophrenia who also exhibit depressive symptoms (Roy, 1981b).

20. Mentally subnormal adolescent girls are reported vulnerable to schizophreniform psychoses following sexual assault (Varley, 1984).

21. Behavioral response to methylphenidate (Ritalin) has been used to predict relapse in schizophrenia (Lieberman JA, et al, 1987).

Symptoms

1. Flat or constricted affect.
2. Autistic thinking.
3. Loose associations.
4. Inappropriate affect.
5. Pathologic ambivalence.
6. Auditory hallucinations of voices commenting, arguing, or laughing.
7. Audible thoughts.
8. Thought insertion or withdrawal.
9. Forced will.
10. Extreme passivity.
11. Lack of rapport.
12. Delusions of grandeur.
13. Somatic delusions.
14. Social withdrawal.
15. Declining school and work performance.
16. Paucity of association.
17. Alogia.
18. Anhedonia.
19. Avolition.
20. Dysattention.
21. Confusion.
22. Bizarre behavior.

23. Derealization.
24. Depersonalization.
25. Jamais vu.

Signs
1. There are no pathognomonic signs of schizophrenia.
2. In all cases of acute psychosis, certain non-specific psychophysiological changes may be observed.
3. Physical examination is useful in identifying symptomatic schizophrenia (i.e., clinical pictures that look like schizophrenia but have a potentially identifiable organic base such as hyperthyroidism and frontal lobe tumors). Hyperthyroid patients appear acutely excited, anxious, and feel they are going crazy, but also have an elevated resting pulse and other stigmata of excess thyroid activity. With frontal lobe tumors, Pick's disease, and hypothyroidism there is a gradual social withdrawal and deterioration of personal habits coupled with an emotional distance or inability to develop rapport often used as a clinical indicant of schizophrenia.
4. Frontal lobe signs such as the grasp reflex, the snout reflex and the palmomental reflex suggest frontal lobe disease, one of the dementias (e.g., Pick's or Alzheimer's disease), or a frontal lobe neoplasm.

Differential Diagnosis
1. Schizophrenia.
2. Mania.
3. Depression.
4. Alcoholic hallucinosis.
5. Pick's disease.
6. Frontal lobe neoplasm.
7. Idiosyncratic alcohol intoxication.
8. AIDS.
9. Adjustment disorders.
10. Hysterical psychosis.
11. Alcoholic paranoia.
12. Drug-induced (e.g., PCP, cocaine, amphetamine) psychoses.
13. Steroid psychoses.
14. Syphilis.
15. Endocrine disease.
16. Pernicious anemia.
17. Huntington's chorea.
18. Alzheimer's disease.
19. Temporal lobe epilepsy.
20. Shilder's disease.
21. Arteriosclerotic brain disease.
22. Senile degeneration of the brain.
23. Migraine headache.
24. Cimetidine intoxication.

The symptomatic schizophrenias, as mentioned earlier, include those illnesses of organic nature that may present with the clinical picture of schizophrenia. Of the toxic states, amphetamine, cocaine, and phencyclidine psychosis are remarkable in their resemblance to schizophrenia. Amphetamine psychosis may arise after as little as a single dose of amphetamine. There is no impairment of orientation, or memory, nor any alteration in the level of consciousness. Visual hallucinations may be absent and a marked delusional system may be manifest. Auditory hallucinations and feelings of thought control or audible thoughts may be part of the picture of chronic intoxication. The presence of amphetamine in the serum or urine supports the suspicion of an amphetamine psychosis, although a patient undergoing an acute schizophrenic break may have also taken amphetamines. Recovery generally occurs rapidly following withdrawal from the drug. Chronic alcoholic hallucinosis resembles chronic amphetamine psychosis. The character of hallucinations in alcoholic paranoia is often auditory.

A variety of cerebral lesions may present like schizophrenia. Temporal lobe tumors, like temporal lobe epilepsy, may be accompanied by symptoms suggestive of schizophrenia such as feelings of impending doom, deja vu, derealization, and depersonalization. Cerebral syphilis may present as a number of schizophrenic symptoms, including acute paranoid episodes and catatonia. Tumors of the frontal lobes as well as of other areas such as the brainstem and diencephalon resemble schizophrenia. Endocrine dysfunction can cause behavioral alterations and for this reason routine thyroid function studies and electrolyte studies should be obtained. Cerebral trauma should also be ruled out and evidence of head injury sought. Degenerative diseases resembling schizophrenia include Huntington's chorea and Schilder's disease. In the early stages of Huntington's chorea, paranoid features may predominate the clinical picture. Deficiency states such as pernicious anemia also mimic schizophrenia. An affective disorder may present with schizophrenic-like symptoms in adolescence, and like adolescent turmoil, is often difficult to distinguish from schizophrenia. A history of affective disorder in first-degree relatives lends support to the diagnosis of bipolar disorder. Severe weltschmerz should make one suspicious of schizophrenia, especially if it lasts for several months without remission.

Management

1. There are a number of treatment approaches to the management of a psychotic patient which are nonspecific in nature and which can be generalized to the management of all psychotic patients. The principle tasks that should be achieved in an emergency situation are:

    a. Ascertain whether there are signs of delirium.
    b. Determine whether a patient is homicidal, suicidal, or severely depressed.
    c. Determine the amount of social support present.
    d. Determine whether a psychosis will substantially clear with neuroleptics and minor tranquilizers.
    e. Ascertain whether the remission of symptoms continues over several days.

2. Admission to an inpatient unit for evaluation and treatment is indicated if there

are signs of a delirium. In addition if a patient is seriously suicidal or homicidal; if no viable social supports are present; if the psychosis does not clear with the use of a high-potency, low-dosage neuroleptics and minor tranquilizers; or if a remission obtained does not persist longer than a few days, the patient should be hospitalized.

3. The clinician should always aim to manage a patient outside the hospital. This reduces stigmatization of hospitalization and counters regressive tendencies so often encountered in patients undergoing a psychotic break. In addition, it reduces cost of treatment to the patient and the pessimism often felt by the patient's family. The ability to choose the proper antipsychotic medication and use of it in the dose and for the duration needed obviates many hospitalizations. In addition, it allows clinicians to work with patients and their families or other social supports in the community in which the patient ultimately must function to survive (Geller JL et al, 1990).

4. History and physical examination supplemented by data from friends and relatives should help exclude delirium.

5. Special care should be given to clues to endocrinopathies, seizure disorders, head injuries, cardiopulmonary disease, nutritional disorders, renal and hepatic disease, electrolyte imbalance, and a history of alcohol, drug, or poison ingestion.

6. Physical examination is usually possible although at times sedation may be needed.

7. High-potency, low-dosage antipsychotic drugs, which produce little sedation and are less likely to confuse the picture (Dubin and Weiss, 1986) than will the more sedating drugs such as barbiturates and chlorpromazine (Thorazine), are used most frequently for severely agitated patients (Muskin et al, 1986; Schulz and Pato, 1989). Perphenazine (Trilafon) with or without lorazepam (Ativan) is recommended. Lorazepam reduces the amount of neuroleptic required and thereby reduces risk of tardive dyskinesia. Vital signs should be routinely obtained on all psychiatric patients seen in emergencies and should force the clinician to explain abnormalities such as an elevated pulse rate or temperature. The diagnosis of hyperthyroidism would be much less frequently missed if the diagnosis was included in the differential of all patients with elevated pulse rates. Evidence of trauma should be sought and the fundi observed for evidence of increased intracranial pressure. Signs of meningeal irritation and of focal neurologic dysfunction must be sought.

8. A psychiatrist should be able to evaluate the cranial nerves; motor, cerebeller, and sensory function; and reflexes. Certain signs have localizing value such as the Babinski, grasp, sucking, glabeller, snout, and palomental reflex. If there is evidence of Wernicke's disease with oculomotor palsies, ataxia, and the amnesic-confabulatory syndrome (Korsakov's psychosis), it would be necessary to give thiamine hydrochloride and large doses of other B vitamins immediately. Evidence of a tremor, asterixis, or aphasia should also be recorded.

9. Identification of an acute or chronic organic mental disorder is usually obtained by careful mental status examination. Orientation to time and place is not usually seen in considerably disturbed manic or schizophrenic patients, while those with

organic mental disorders show deficits. In the latter, recent memory is usually impaired. The character of hallucinations is also helpful. Olfactory and visual hallucinations are more suggestive of organic disease, while auditory hallucinations are more frequent with schizophrenia.

10. All patients should be evaluated for risk of harm to self or others. Suicide risk is significantly greater among schizophrenics and difficult to predict (Colton et al,1984).

11. Tardive dyskinesia frequently develops in schizophrenics with years of exposure to neuroleptic medication (Wegner et al, 1985). Clozapine (Clorazil) is without current known risk for development of tardive dyskinesia and has proven especially efficacious in the management of negative symptoms that are particularly resistant to conventional treatment (e.g., social withdrawal, flat affect, avolution) (Breier et al, 1987). Alternately, not all schizophrenics must be indefinitely maintained on neuroleptics. Some do as well or better off medication than on medication (Fenton and McGlashan, 1987). Others can be managed with brief focal neuroleptization minimizing risk for development of tardive dyskinesia (Jolley et al, 1989).

12. Patients admitted under involuntary status are as a group more prone to violence, more in need of medication, and more frequently require restraints or seclusion (Arcuni and Asaad, 1989).

13. Patients who are noncompliant with pharmacotherapy, who are repeatedly hospitalized, or act out in violent self- or other-destructive ways may be managed with depot long-acting neuroleptics such as haloperidol (Haldol) decanoate and fluphenazine (Prolixin) decanoate and enanthate (Kane JM, 1986a; Brown and Silver, 1985; Comaty and Janicak, 1987). Low initial dose is recommended with gradual dosage adjustment over time. Extrapyramidal side effects are dose related (Marder, 1986). Injectable haloperidol has been proven to be as efficacious in management of schizophrenic symptoms as the oral form (Nair et al, 1986).

14. Patients on neuroleptics must be cautioned against prolonged or intense exposure to the sun, as heat stroke may ensue (Lazarus, 1985).

15. Data indicating Asian patients require less neuroleptic dosage are inconclusive (Sramek et al, 1986).

16. Command hallucinations in schizophrenics are ominous, even if patients do not report feeling destructive to themselves or others. Persecutory delusions always increase risk of suicide and violence. Paranoid patients, becoming fearful, may either attempt to "defend" themselves from the "persecutors" or to escape from them by a potentially self-destructive route (e.g., jumping out of a window).

17. The presence of a family alone does not mean that a patient has a viable social matrix. A family must be willing to recognize the seriousness of a patient's illness, be truly interested in the patient's welfare, and be willing to take some responsibility for them. If medication is needed, the family must be able to guarantee that the patient will take it. If a patient becomes unmanageable or more depressed and less communicative of his or her intents, the family must be willing and able to bring him or her back to the hospital. Even with the best intentions, a family may have an unconscious need to deny the seriousness of a

patient's condition and the extent of the patient's potential for violence. In other instances, there may be an unconscious desire on the part of the family to have the patient commit suicide and so the family may neglect to observe the patient or ensure that he or she takes the medication. The family may, in their ambivalence, fail to insist that the patient follow through on a recommendation for outpatient care. This neglect may unconsciously represent a desire on the part of the family that the patient either end his or her life or become so psychotic that he or she has to be hospitalized.

18. High dose haloperidol, thiothixene (Navane), fluphenazine, or perphenazine may bring about remission in treatment-resistant schizophrenia. Failure to respond, however, to doses of 150 mg/day of haloperidol or plasma concentrations of 20–50 ng/mL augurs for continued lack of response (Hollister and Kim, 1982).

19. The high potency antipsychotic agents such as trifluoperizine (Stelazine), haloperidol, fluphenazine, perphenazine, and thiothixene are preferred in emergency situations. The dosage of thiothixene, perphenazine, or haloperidol, when given intramuscularly, is 5–10 mg. This may be repeated in $\frac{1}{2}$ hour if agitation persists. Fifty milligrams of chlorpromazine may also be given intramuscularly, but it is more sedating than the high-potency antipsychotics and tends to cause more hypotension.

20. Sedation itself is often not as important as the antipsychotic effect and sedation may confuse the picture in some cases. Hypotension is less frequently seen with the piperazine phenothiazines, haloperidol, and thiothixene. If a patient is able to take medication orally, it is the preferred route.

21. The initial oral dosage for a mild to moderate schizophrenic psychosis of commonly used antipsychotics with concurrent use of lorazepam is:

100 mg chlorpromazine qid, or
100 mg thioridazine qid, or
8 mg perphenazine qid, or
5 mg trifluoperazine qid, or
5 mg fluphenazine qid, or
5 mg thiothixene qid, or
2 mg haloperidol qid.

22. Choice of antipsychotic agent is based on how much sedation is desired (chlorpromazine is much more sedating than the piperazine phenothiazines) and how patients responded to drugs in the past (Were they allergic? Did they respond better to a butyrophenone [e.g., haloperidol] than they did to a phenothiazine?), and the extrapyramidal and other side effects. If patients are moderately or severely schizophrenic, much higher dosages may be needed, especially in the acute stages and for sleep. For example:

a. Perphenazine 16 mg PO qid and 8–16 mg every hour until sleep.
b. Chlorpromazine 200 mg PO qid and 100–200 mg PO every hour until sleep.

23. Side effects such as hypotension and extrapyramidal dysfunction should always

be monitored. In addition to severity of illness and the presence of side effects, age and weight consideration should determine the dosage used.

24. If there is some question that the medication is not being swallowed, the liquid form may be given.

25. In the acute stage, it may be necessary to repeat the dosage every hour until improvement occurs. For example, 5–10 mg of haloperidol may be given every hour until a patient's symptoms decrease, or until they fall asleep (up to about a total of 60 mg). If fluphenazine is given intramuscularly, the hydrochloride should be used rather than the ethanthate or decanoate (which are long acting (10 to 14 days) and cannot as easily be titrated in an emergency situation).

26. In all instances of use of the major antipsychotic agents—the phenothiazines, the thioxanthenes, and the butyrophenones—extrapyramidal changes may occur. The question, therefore, is whether or not to give an antiparkinson agent prophylactically. If using the piperazine phenothiazines, the thioxanthenes, and butyrophenones in doses sufficient to keep down a psychotic process, we recommend an agent such as benztropine mesylate (Cogentin), 0.5–1 mg tid or qid as recommended.

27. Even though, in many instances, use of an antiparkinson agent may not be necessary, when extrapyramidal effects do occur, they are quite frightening to someone already terrified of the chaos within. After a few weeks, the antiparkinsonian agent can be withdrawn to see if it is really needed.

28. The antiparkinson agents, like the phenothiazines, have anticholinergic properties; therefore, they increase blurriness of vision, constipation, dry mouth, etc.

29. If a dystonic reaction occurs, 50–100 mg of diphenhydramine (Benadryl) or 1–2 mg of benztropine mesylate can be given intramuscularly. There is no significant increase in onset of action when benztropine mesylate is given intravenously.

30. Clozapine, belonging to the dibenzazepine group, is said to be low on extrapyramidal side effects and have strong anxiolytic and hypnotic properties. Hypotension, hypersalivation and sedation are its more common side effects. Molindone has a central anorexigenic effect with a weight reducing property.

31. A study comparing three regimens of oral administration of haloperidol for schizophrenia (i.e., 20 mg on day 1 and then increasing in increments of 20 mg a day until reaching a maximum of 100 mg on day 5; 10 mg on day 1 and then in increasing increments of 10 mg daily until reaching a maximum of 100 mg on day 10; and a fixed dosage of 10 mg daily for 10 days) indicated that all regimens had similar therapeutic efficacy. The drug was well tolerated by all and there were no serious adverse reactions. This suggests that acutely ill schizophrenics respond to a wide variety of doses of haloperidol and that onset of action and efficacy is not enhanced in most patients by providing high initial doses (Donlon et al, 1980).

32. Plasma prolactin levels appear to increase with increasing dosage of haloperidol up to 100 mg but not further with additional increase in dose above 100 mg (Zarifian et al, 1982).

33. Postpsychotic depressive symptomatology relatively frequently occurs in pa-

tients with schizophrenia diagnosed by stringent criteria. The full syndromal manifestation of depression, however, is less frequent (Siri et al, 1981).

34. Biweekly evaluation of symptoms in schizophrenics during the first 4 weeks of hospitalization reveals that recovery from psychotic symptoms occurs rapidly early in hospitalization supporting the use of brief hospitalization for psychotic relapse. Recovery from anxiety and depression is less complete and generally will require continued active treatment aimed at symptom amelioration after discharge (Szymanski et al, 1983).

Quality Assurance Issues

1. Have organic causes for schizophrenic symptoms been sought?
2. Are patients on neuroleptics monitored for development of the neuroleptic malignant syndrome and tardive dyskinesia?

Ethical/Legal Issues

1. Has the patient been evaluated for suicidal ideation and, if suicidal, provided necessary precautions?
2. Are patients and families advised of signs and symptoms of tardive dyskinesia and neuroleptic malignant syndrome?
3. Is the minimum amount of antipsychotic that is effective being used?
4. Has the patient been evaluated for need of antiparkinsonian agents?
5. Has the diagnosis of atypical affective illness been considered?
6. In the acute stage, have benzadiazepines been used to minimize exposure to neuroleptics when sedation is required?

SCHIZOTYPAL PERSONALTY DISORDER

Schizotypal and paranoid personality disorders appear genetically related to schizophrenia (Siever et al, 1990). These patients may present with some of the same problems in management that schizophrenics present with, and may be confused with schizophrenia in the emergency situation.

SEASONAL AFFECTIVE DISORDER
(SAD)

Some people experience affective changes concomitant with seasonal change. This change appears to be directly related to the number of hours of daylight each day, with depressed mood and irritability greatest in the winter (Bick, 1986).

History

1. Seasonal affective disorder (SAD) may impact as great as 4 to 10% of the population, with younger women most severely impacted (Kasper et al, 1989).

2. While seasonal depression occurs in both the summer and winter with opposite vegetative symptoms, phototherapy is specific to the management of winter depression (Wehr and Rosenthal, 1989).
3. Women constitute the majority of people with SAD (83%), with onset of the illness generally in the third decade of life (Rosenthal and Wehr, 1987).
4. Variants of SAD include fluctuation in craving for cocaine paralleling seasonal dysphoria (Satel and Gawin, 1989) and premenstrual tension (late luteal phase dysphoria disorder) that is season dependent (Parry et al, 1987) and responsive to phototherapy.
5. SAD has been described that entails depression in the summer and euthymia, hypomania, or mania during the other months of the year (Wehr et al, 1987b).
6. Rates of winter SAD and subsyndromal SAD are significantly greater in the northern latitudes, while summer SAD is not correlated with latitude (Rosen et al, 1990). Reports from India indicate violations of patterns seen in the United States with mania in summer and depression in winter, mania in early winter and depression in late winter, and depression in summer and mania in early winter (Gupta, 1988).
7. Studies in the Southern hemisphere (Boyce and Parker, 1988) have found winter/autumn onset SAD characterized by carbohydrate craving and increased appetite and sleep. Spring/summer onset SAD is characterized by decreased appetite and sleep.
8. SAD should be considered in the differential diagnosis of children with school difficulties as childhood and adolescent SAD is characterized by school difficulties, fatigue, irritability, sleep change, and sadness during the winter months (Rosenthal NE et al, 1986).
9. SAD tends to have an earlier onset than major depression and more frequently presents with hypersomnia and carbohydrate craving (Garvey et al, 1988).

Symptoms and Signs
Symptoms and signs of SAD are those of other forms of affective illness.

Differential Diagnosis
The differential diagnosis of SAD is that of other mood disorders.

Management
1. Phototherapy (light therapy with or without concurrent antidepressant psychopharmacotherapy) is the treatment of choice. Bright full spectrum light is characteristically used (Kasper et al, 1990; Wehr et al, 1988; Jacobsen FM et al, 1987; Blehar and Rosenthal, 1989).
2. Greater intensity of endogenous symptoms predict poor response to light therapy (Stinson and Thompson, 1990).
3. The usual approach is to extend daylight for a patient by exposure to bright artificial light (Rosenthal NE et al, 1984; Byerley et al, 1987).
4. Bright environmental light impacts favorably on individuals with subsyndromal SAD but not on normal controls (Kasper et al, 1989).

Quality Assurance Issues

1. Have all depressed patients been evaluated for concomitant presence of bipolar or major depressive illness and vice versa?
2. Have patients been provided light therapy when they suffer SAD?
3. Were patients provided antidepressant medication in addition to light therapy if required?

Ethical/Legal Issues

1. Have patients been advised of safety precautions when using light therapy?
2. Were all patients with SAD evaluated for suicide?

SEIZURE DISORDERS

Psychiatrists may be called upon in the emergency room to determine whether abberations of mood, thought, and behavior are due to a seizure disorder rather than an Axis I disorder. In some cases, the diagnosis may be apparent, as with most instances of grand mal epilepsy. At other times, the diagnosis may be extremely difficult, particularly if the seizures are of temporal lobe origin. In addition, a patient may have a psychiatric disorder such as schizophrenia as well as seizures.

History

1. Grand mal seizures typically last 5 to 30 minutes. They may or may not be preceded by an aura. When an aura occurs, it may be experienced as a feeling that a seizure is imminent, or as weakness, numbness, paresthesias, auditory hallucinations, scintillating scotomata, fear, or pain in the abdomen. A shrill cry often heralds the onset of a seizure, then the patient loses consciousness. The body stiffens tonically, with rigid extension of all four extremities, simultaneous clonic movements of the extremities, trismus, and opisthotonus. This may be followed by bilateral simultaneous clonic movements of the extremities, head, and jaw. During the seizure, the patients may bite their tongues, ejaculate, or have fecal or urinary incontinence. If they fall, there may be evidence of trauma. Because of the temporary paralysis of the respiratory musculature, they appear cyanotic. Afterward there is coma followed by sleep. When they awaken, there is often headache, muscle aches, and vomiting. Clinicians observing a grand mal seizure should record the side to which the head and eye turns. If consistent, it suggests a lesion of the opposite cerebral hemisphere. Post-ictal motor weakness (Todd's paralysis) and sensory, speech, or visual changes also suggest localization. Grand mal seizures may occur as frequently as once or more a day or as far apart as years.
2. Petit mal seizures, while usually considered a disorder of childhood, may continue into adulthood. They do not have any aura or warning and usually are quite brief, frequently less than a minute in duration. They may occur several times daily. They can be broadly subsclassified into three types: myoclonic jerks,

absence (staring episodes), and akinetic. The last mentioned consists of either falling to the floor suddenly, or dropping objects. Electroencephalograms recorded at the time of a seizure will show a characteristic bilaterally synchronous 3 per second spike and wave over the entire brain. In fact, the eyelids may flutter at a rate of 3 per second at the time of a seizure. Patients may be aware that they had a petit mal attack.

3. Jacksonian seizures are a result of discharge in the motor or sensory areas of the cerebral cortex. When motor in nature, convulsive twitchings or clonic movements typically begin at the angle of the mouth, great toe, or thumb. They often progress to involve part of the face or extremity, or go on to include an entire side of the body. In some cases, they may become generalized with a resultant grand mal seizure. Jacksonian sensory seizures follow the same pattern as the motor, with or without an accompanying clonic component. The march of movement follows the train of discharges across the contralateral cerebral cortex.

4. Psychomotor or temporal lobe seizures typically last 3 to 5 minutes and consist of involuntary, purposeful, but irrelevant movements for which the patient has no recall. Any attempt to assist patients in what they seem to be doing during an attack is resisted. These seizures are often confused with psychiatric states such as fugues and psychogenic amnesia. Their aura may resemble symptoms of an anxiety disorder. Patients appear to be chewing or having other abnormal mouth movements, tug at their clothes, walk, drive a car or perform a variety of complex tasks. A sleep EEG may reveal spikes or other dysrhythmias over the temporal lobes. A variety of emotional changes have been reported with these seizures including rage attacks, anxiety, and euphoria. The mental cloudiness that sometimes occurs resembles that of a psychosis. Aggressive behavior may occur, particularly during the interictal period (Devinsky and Bear, 1984). Temporal lobe epilepsy is in the differential diagnosis of schizophrenia (Stevens, 1988; McKenna PJ et al, 1985), mood disorders, anxiety disorders (Weilburg et al, 1987; McNamara and Fogel, 1990), violent behavior, and catatonia (Kirubakaran et al, 1987).

Complex Partial Seizures (CPS)

Complex partial seizures (CPS) may present as a variety of behavioral disturbances simulating psychiatric disorders. Schizophrenic-like, schizoaffective, and affective states have been reported (Barczak et al, 1988). Depressive and hypomanic subtypes of the affective form are seen (Barczak et al, 1988). Complex partial status epilepticus can present as gelastic seizures with bizarre outbursts of laughter (Glassman JN et al, 1986). In other instances, CPS may appear as conversion disorder, paranoid disorders, and reactive psychoses. Cocaine (Merriam et al, 1988) is an epileptogenic agent that induces seizures including complex partial status epilepticus with behavior disturbances that confuse the clinical picture of cocaine intoxication leading to the misdiagnosis of a primary non-drug-induced psychotic disorder. Complex partial epilepsy has a familial component that is only slightly less than with other forms of epilepsy (Ottman, 1989).

Other Seizure Disorders

Uncinate seizures present by momentary episodes of strange odors or tastes— usually of an unpleasant nature. Gelastic epilepsy is a convulsive disorder with laughter as a manifestation of an attack. Auditory hallucinatory seizures consist of vague noises or complex scores of music. Both hyperacusis and hypoacusis can occur with the latter. Well-formed images or flashes of light may be seen with visual hallucinatory seizures. These unusual variants of epilepsy can occur alone or as an aura of one of the major convulsive disorders.

Status Epilepticus

Status epilepticus refers to persistent recurrence of seizures without episodes of unconsciousness between. They are usually grand mal in nature, but may also be petit mal, psychomotor, or complex partial in nature. Status epilepticus is a medical emergency requiring immediate medical intervention.

History

1. Seizures have been reported in 0.5% (Lowry and Dunner, 1980) to 4% of individuals receiving antidepressants. Patients who develop seizures during thymoleptic treatment are felt to be predisposed by alcoholism, prior electroshock, barbiturate withdrawal, cerebrovascular disease, intramuscular administration of amitriptyline (Elavil), or a combination of amitriptyline with chlorpromazine (Thorazine) (Lowry and Dunner, 1980). Lithium carbonate has been reported to both increase and decrease seizure frequency, including frequency of petit mal epilepsy (Moore DP, 1981), and aggressive behavior occurring between seizures. Clozapine is associated with producing more seizures than other neuroleptics (Haller and Binder, 1990) as is buproprion (Wellbutrin) more than other antidepressants.

2. Major life events appear to play a role in increasing and decreasing seizure frequency, particularly that of complex partial seizures (Webster and Mawer, 1989).

3. Seizures cause a response in family members without epilepsy which, if negative, can impact negatively on an epileptic patient's development (Levin et al, 1988).

4. Toxic delirium induced by either psychotropic drug overdose or hypnotic–sedative drug withdrawal may be associated with prominent paroxysmal electroencephalographic activity indicating a generalized symptomatic nonconvulsive epileptic state pursuant to transient transmitter dysfunction (Van Sweden and Mellerio, 1989). The condition is responsive to intravenous benzodiazepines.

5 While depression in epileptic patients is the result of complex interaction of genetic, social, psychological, and pathophysiologic variables, as a group patients receiving phenobarbital report more depression and those on carbamazepine (Tegretol) report both less depression and anxiety (Robertson et al, 1987).

6. Complex partial seizures of the frontal lobes can mimic absences and give the illusion a person is "spacy," daydreaming, or otherwise inattentive (Berkovic et al, 1987).

Differential Diagnosis
1. Idiopathic epilepsy.
2. Alcohol withdrawal.
3. Barbiturate withdrawal.
4. Cerebral neoplasia.
5. Cardiac arrhythmias.
6. Uremia.
7. Asphyxia.
8. Granuloma.
9. Hypocalcemia.
10. Carotid sinus sensitivity.
11. Hypoglycemia.
12. Hepatic coma.
13. Meningitis.
14. Cerebral abscesses.
15. Encephalitis.
16. Recent and old infarcts.
17. Cerebral vascular insufficiency.
18. Atrophic lesions.
19. Traumatic scarring.
20. Degenerative brain diseases.
21. Dissociative disorder.
22. Meperidine (Demerol) intoxication.
23. Cocaine, amphetamine, and other stimulant intoxication.
24. Anticonvulsant and neuroleptic toxicity.

Diagnosis of a seizure disorder may be obfuscated by clinical presentation. Patients with seizures who present with signs generally associated with psychogenic or feigned unconsciousness (Drake and Coffey, 1983), catatonia (particularly in childhood) (Shah and Kaplan, 1980), and psychological symptoms without any evidence of motor dysfunction are particularly at risk for misdiagnosis. The coexistence of pseudoseizures and true epilepsy is not rare. Video-EEG monitoring facilitates diagnosis of psychogenic seizures superimposed on CNS-based seizures. Patients diagnosed to have such combined seizure disorder do not always have hysterial personality traits further making diagnosis difficult (Ramani et al, 1980).

Clinical Studies
1. Routine, sleep-deprived, 24-hour, and spenoidal electroencephalography all serve to confirm the diagnosis. Absence of seizure activity, however, does not exclude the diagnosis. A patient may be monitored in an interictal phase or dis-

charges confined to an area of the brain that surface electrodes are unable to detect.

2. Concurrent videography and electroencephalography allow diagnosis of pseudoseizures alone or together with a true seizure disorder.

3. Positron emission tomography (PET scans), magnetic resonance imaging (MRI), and computed tomography (CT scans) are helpful in selected cases. Neoplasia are uncommon if both MRI and CT scans are normal. Focal interictal temporal hypometabolism may be seen in complex partial seizures of the temporal lobes (Theodore et al, 1990).

Pseudoseizures

Psychogenic seizures (pseudoseizures) like bonified epilepsy may occur in rapid succession simulating status epilepticus. Clinicians should be aware of this so as to avoid administration of large and unnecessary doses of medication to patients with pseudoseizures. Patients with pseudoseizures tend to show the absence of any postconvulsive stupor or sleep (Gross, 1979). In some instances, in fact, they may recall the seizure and describe how they behaved. Postictal confusion and mental cloudiness is common after grand mal seizures and a period of brief coma may follow an episode of status epilepticus. During a pseudoseizure the electroencephalogram is normal. Babinski's sign is absent and the patient is not cyanotic. This is just the opposite of the clinical picture with grand mal seizures. Patients with pseudoseizures often appear bizarre and respond the same to placebo and active medication. Patients' eyes may go up when someone is present (i.e., secondary gain). Psychogenic seizures should be suspected when there is no tongue biting or fecal or urinary incontinence. Bodily injury is rare with pseudoepilepsy (Gross, 1979).

Management

1. Pharmacologic, surgical, and behavioral (as in the instance of some of the sensory epilepsies) management of seizures and the side effects of anticonvulsant is discussed in neurologic textbooks.

2. Patients may have both pseudoseizures and real seizures. In such instances, patients must be treated with anticonvulsants in addition to psychotherapy.

3. Patients with ictal seizure disorders may also have nonictal seizure disorders with such symptoms as well circumscribed episodes of fear, derealization, depersonalization, deja vu, or rage attacks. These are most commonly seen in patients with temporal lobe epilepsy. Sphenoidal electrodes with simultaneous audiovisual monitoring is sometimes helpful in diagnosing these patients.

4. Anticonvulsants are associated with a number of behavioral and psychologic effects that may be misdiagnosed as a superimposed mood, behavior, or thought disorder (especially in children) (Ferrari et al, 1983), or inaccurately characterized as an indicant of an "epileptic personality."

5. Patients with combined seizure–pseudoseizure disorders responded to individualized re-educative psychotherapy to teach them alternative coping styles and anticonvulsants (Ramani et al, 1980).

6. Amitriptyline (Elavil) is effective in attenuating both seizure severity and

after-discharge duration. Behavioral seizures are not reduced by buproprion or trazadone (Prozac) (Clifford et al, 1985).
7. In many instances conjoint management by a neurologist and psychiatrist is indicated in the emergency room given attendant psychosocial problems (Krumholz et al, 1989).

Quality Assurance Issues

1. Has a patient suspected of suffering a seizure disorder been evaluated by neurologists and has an effort been made to document the disorder by electroencephalography?
2. Has a patient been provided diagnostic-specific anticonvulsant therapy if he or she suffers epilepsy?
3. Has a cause for the seizure (e.g., hypoglycemia, tumor, vascular malformation) been explored?

Ethical/Legal Issues

1. Have all patients with pseudoseizures been evaluated for concomitant presence of epilepsy?
2. Have patients and families been advised of risk of harm to self or others if seizure patients drive or work with fine equipment?
3. Have patients been advised of long-term effects of anticonvulsant therapy?

SELF-MUTILATION

Self-mutilation is seen as a symptom of a number of psychiatric and medical illnesses and seen in incarcerated criminals.

History

1. In some instances, self-mutilation may take on the aspect of social contagion (Rader and Jones, 1982).
2. Self-mutilation evokes strong feelings in attending staff. Care must be given to staff needs to successfully manage such patients, especially on medical and surgical units.

Symptoms

1. Wrist cutting.
2. Rubbing.
3. Head banging.
4. Insertion of foreign bodies.
5. Scratching.
6. Biting.
7. Enucleation.
8. Removal of body parts or organs.
9. Hair removal.

Management

1. Management of self-mutilation entails treatment of the psychiatric or medical illness or management of the social problem that is the basis of the act.

Quality Assurance Issues

1. Has the patient been evaluated for suicide potential, and if so, have precautions been provided?
2. Has diagnostic-specific therapy been provided?

Ethical/Legal Issues

1. Have precautions been taken, if required, to prevent severe self-harm?
2. Have families been advised of patients' self-mutilation?

SEROTONIN AGONISTS

Serotonin agonists have been used successfully in the management of depression, panic disorder, eating disorder, obsessive–compulsive disorder, depression associated with personality disorders, and refractory depressions (Montgomery, 1988). Commonly used agents include fluoxetine (Prozac), sertraline (Zoloft), paroxetine (Paxel), and trazadone (Desyrel). There is a popular misconception that serotonin agonists increase suicide. At the time of the writing of this book, there is no evidence this is true. With all antidepressants, risk of suicide may increase early in the course of treatment because energy returns often before depressive ideation with hopelessness and worthlessness remits. Serotonin agonists enhance ability to concentrate. If thoughts were present regarding suicide, these may become more intense, transiently causing anxiety for patient and therapist until the thoughts abate with treatment (despite persistence of heightened ability to concentrate). Some patients do not respond for several weeks or months or in some instances not at all. In these cases patients may feel more hopeless being found to have a depression refractory to serotonin agonists and feel more suicidal.

Quality Assurance Issues

1. Have patients been warned of the danger of concomitant use of other antidepressants?
2. Have patients been warned of the need of a washout period prior to use of other antidepressants?

Ethical/Legal Issues

1. Have patients been advised of side effects such as agitation and increased clarity of thought, which may distress some patients and be perceived as worsening of the illness?

SEXUAL AGGRESSION

Sexual abuse includes rape (including date rape), incest, and various activities that either physically or sexually harm the victims or exploit their compromised positions (e.g., sex with minors). In most instances, the victim rather than the perpetrator is seen in the emergency. Some parents involved in incest or men who have sexually abused a woman will present for help. In some instances a person is unjustly accused. For instance, occasionally a preschool child will falsely accuse a parent but actually believes his accusation is correct. This may occur when a child misinterprets caregiving ministrations, when another adult (such as an angry spouse in a divorce) has persuaded the child that the sexual event has actually occurred, when primary process material confuses a child's thoughts, or when a child is involved secondarily in the projective identification of a dominant caregiver (Yates and Musty, 1988). Phallometric studies have resulted in conflicting data. In some instances, no statistical difference has been found between nonrapists and rapists when presented various rape stimuli (Prouix, 1989).

History
1. Histories of sexual abuse are significantly more commonly found (70% compared to 6% in one study) when specific questions are asked directly about sexual molestation among women seen in psychiatric emergency rooms (Briere and Zaidi, 1989).
2. Men surveyed in a psychiatric outpatient clinic report sexual or physical abuse in up to 48% of cases seen (Swett et al, 1990).
3. Substance abuse, suicidality, sexual dysfunction, a number of psychiatric disorders, and Axis II disorders or traits (especially borderline personality) have been associated with histories of sexual abuse (Briere and Zaidi, 1989).

Management
1. If a sexually abused patient is a minor, most states and institutions have fairly strict protocols regarding reporting.
2. Ventilation and support are key to the management of a sexually abused person in addition to the specifics related to the type of abuse as exemplified in the section on rape.
3. Support groups of individuals who have suffered similar experiences help victims both understand the immediate and long-term impact on behavior and feeling.
4. Perpetrators, whether presenting for help voluntarily or by legal mandate, require both evaluation to ascertain if a substance abuse problem or other psychiatric disorder is at the basis of the behavior as well as assessment of what is necessary to minimize occurrence of the behavior in the future. This may involve psychopharmacotherapy, group therapy (e.g., "buddy to buddy" groups), family therapy, individual therapy, couples therapy, or sexual therapy.
5. It is important to educate perpetrators about the law and consequences of abuse

in much the same manner as one who abuses drugs is educated about the consequences of drug abuse on health and the legal consequences of buying, using,
and selling.
6. The specifics of the management of rape and other forms of abuse are given in
the sections on each subject.

Quality Assurance Issues
1. Have patients and families been advised of sexual abuse when it has occurred
and of guidelines to follow for treatment and reporting?

Ethical/Legal Issues
1. Have statutes regarding reporting sexual abuse been followed (e.g, state child
abuse reporting procedures)?

SLEEP APNEA

Sleep apnea with periodic brief arousals is in the differential diagnosis of insomnia and fatigue when patients present with these symptoms in the emergency room.
Many disorders result in impaired sleep with increased sleepiness but sleep disruption is greatest in patients with periodic leg movements, central sleep apnea, and obstructive sleep apnea (Bonnet et al, 1990). Triazolam (Halcion) has been found to
increase total sleep and decrease the number of brief arousals (Bonnet el al, 1990).

SLEEP DISORDERS

Periodic leg movements; central sleep apnea; obstructive sleep apnea; the sleep
disturbances associated with psychiatric disorders such as mania, substance abuse
disorder, depression, and schizophrenia; and sleep panic; and other disorders that impact sleep frequencies vary by sex and age. Evaluation in the emergency room entails
age-specific consideration in diagnosis and treatment to focus management. For instance it is estimated that nearly half of individuals over 65 have some problem with
sleep (Monjan, 1990). Increasing use of medication, changing circadian rhythms, retirement, and loss of spouse or friends can, alone or together, cause sleep to be disturbed in this age group (in addition to other biologic and psychiatric [especially de-
pression] causes) (Monjan, 1990). In older people, more than in younger age groups,
a number of factors may be impacting on sleep efficiency; consideration of all these
factors is necessary to formulate a treatment plan.

Quality Assurance Issues
1. Has diagnostic-specific treatment been provided patients with a sleep disorder?
2. Have non-addicting hypnotics been prescribed to patients with a history of substance abuse?
3. Are patients warned of the diagnostic significance of sleep disorders?

4. Are patients warned of the danger of addiction to some hypnotics?

Ethical/Legal Issues
1. Has care been provided to prevent addiction to sleep medication?

SOCIAL PHOBIA

Social phobia, like separation anxiety, may relate to affective illness and, therefore, use of antidepressants is effective in management. This impact may be on depression and not necessarily relate to the use of antidepressants on anxiety (Stein MB et al, 1989).

History
1. At least about one-third of patients with social phobia have a past history of major depression. The percentage of patients who suffer panic disorder who also suffer a past history of major depression is about twice this (Stein MB et al, 1989).
2. Children with separation anxiety are more likely to have mothers with affective illness than children with social phobia (Last et al, 1987b).
3. Abnormalities of the hypothalamic–pituitary–thyroid axis are not a requisite neuroendocrine correlate of social phobia (Tancer et al, 1990).
4. The fact that the number of patients with social phobias who experience panic when given lactate infusions is significantly lower than individuals with agoraphobia or panic disorder supports the belief that the pathophysiology of social phobias differ from disorders characterized by spontaneous panic attacks (Liebowitz et al, 1985a).

Management
1. The fear of evaluation and scrutiny by others can be best approached by combined use of cognitive therapy or desensitization and relaxation techniques and social skill training coupled with psychopharmacotherapy (Heimberg and Barlow, 1988).
2. Beta-blockers, tricyclics, and monoamine oxidase inhibitors, and benzodiazepines have all been employed in management of the symptoms of social phobias (Reich and Yates, 1988).

Quality Assurance Issues
1. Are patients, if prescribed addicting agents, evaluated for the potential of substance abuse?
2. Are patients evaluated for disorders such as schizophrenia, depression, and panic disorders, which may appear to be social phobia?

Ethical/Legal Issues
1. Are patients, if prescribed an addicting substance such as benzodiazepine, advised of the potential for dependence?

2. If a benzodiazepine is to be discontinued, is the patient advised of a schedule that will minimize discomfort?

SOCIOECONOMIC EMERGENCIES
(Resourceless Patients)

A difficult problem that all psychiatrists and perhaps most human beings sooner or later confront is a patient who asks nothing more than food and shelter. The response is not simple. Many of these individuals have no serious psychiatric or medical problems that require inpatient care. At times, these individuals are inappropriately admitted to a psychiatric service because the psychiatric clinician can either think of no alternative or does not wish to take the time to explore what possibilities existed.

Management
1. It is important to protect a patient's self-esteem. Despite the fact that these individuals appear as the disinherited of the earth, and some of them to collude in maintaining a dependent posture, the clinician should not express anger at them out of frustration in being confronted with what seems an impossible task to perform. Treat the patient with respect and try to empathize and understand what it means to be in such a situation for either psychological reasons or because of extremely limited economic opportunities to better oneself because of social circumstances, age, illness, etc.
2. Clearly identify exactly what the patient wants. While at first glance it may appear that patients want a place to stay, they may only want someone to talk to for a while to relate how badly life has treated them.
3. If there is a need for a particular service, then the psychiatric clinicians should review in their mind the possible alternatives and present those most realistic and readily available. Long enumeration of multiple agencies available in emergencies to one's colleagues may be impressive, but to people in such circumstances it may just be another reminder of how limited they are in their resourcefulness compared to the clinician. It is good to develop a written list of agencies that provide emergency services. Increasingly, mental health professionals are finding that they must rely on themselves to develop alternatives in such circumstances. As social workers have begun to move away from this area in many centers to spend their time in the practice of psychotherapy and other tasks common to a number of professions, no group has clearly emerged to take over the responsibility of becoming expert in knowledge of community resources and how to use them ("case work").
4. The first choice is to assess which relatives and friends are available to provide the service the patient requests. Sometimes a simple call to an aunt or friend may provide a room and the companionship the patient wants for the night.
5. If friends and relatives are not available, there are number of other agencies that

may provide financial aid, food, or shelter to a patient for a time. There is Traveler's Aid, Fish, The Salvation Army, Covenant House, and Christian Community Action, to name a few. Some church groups maintain hostels to provide shelter for an evening, and knowledge of these sometimes only comes from experience. Grassroot drug drop-in centers exist in some cities and provide a special resources for distraught adolescents, and there generally are a number of less expensive hotels or branches of the YMCA and YWCA (or YMHA) with available resources for those with compromised means. For those who require nursing care (e.g., geriatric patients), nursing home policies vary, and some receive referrals at unexpected hours for reasonable rates.

6. If patients themselves are able to contact the agency and follow through, it is best to allow them to take the needed step. If, however, it seems doubtful that patients can manage for themselves, clinicians should phone to see what is available and provide referring information with patients' permission.

7. If legal or accounting advice is required, the clinician should provide the name of either free services (e.g., Public Defender Service) or of those individuals in town who will provide services on a sliding scale or for a nominal fee.

8. Explorative psychotherapy may be helpful in some instances in aiding patients in obtaining an understanding of how they got themselves in such situations and to determine what psychological blocks may exist in preventing the patient from resolving socioeconomic crises him or herself. Obviously, in some instances, the reality of patients' lives are so overwhelming that if any form of therapy is indicated, it may only be of the crisis intervention supportive variety. Sometimes, however, counseling in how to manage money is more important than psychological maneuvers.

9. Avoid pushing. If what seems to be a minor intervention appears to relieve patients, do not force them into more than they want at the time. An aggressive approach may appear to the patient to be paternalistic or may overwhelm the patient (who never wanted more than support and a possible suggestion).

10. Finally, hospitalization may be a needed step for patients such as chronic schizophrenics, in providing social and economic rehabilitation. Use of hospitalization is always a delicate issue. Patients may regress, making it difficult for them to be discharged to a world they feel, by contrast, to be cold and unfriendly. If it is concluded that there appears to be no alternative to hospitalization, it should be on a crisis-type unit or in a partial hospital program that works with a philosophy to help the patient maximize his own internal resources, is antiregressive, and moves toward a speedy discharge with good follow-up care.

Quality Assurance Issues

1. Are indigent patients evaluated for a psychiatric disorder that may contribute to their resourcelessness?

Ethical/Legal Issues

1. Are indigent patients evaluated for need for medical care and prescription renewal?

SOMATOFORM DISORDER

Somatoform disorders are often discussed together with conversion and dissociative disorders because of the tendency of clinicians to confuse these terms and of the frequent occurrence of patients presenting with two or more of these disorders at various times in their lives.

History

1. The essential feature of somatoform disorder is the occurrence of physical symptoms and signs for which there is no demonstrable organic pathology. These symptoms, unlike those of malingering or factitious illness, are not under voluntary control. The individual does not consciously feign illness. Symptom formation is unconscious and the primary management is psychological. No physical basis can be found by physical examination or clinical studies.
2. Somatization disorder is characterized by recurrent and multiple somatic complaints for which no physical basis is found. The disorder tends to commence prior to age 25. Menstrual difficulties may be one of the earliest signs.
3. Complaints are often vague or presented in a dramatic way. Patients have complaints referable to many systems and have seen many physicians. They tend to use a great number of medications, frequently seek medical consultation, and get hospitalized. Sometimes they are found to have had excessive surgery.
4. The natural history is decades of such complaints, with fluctuations in intensity. Interpersonal difficulty is common. Marital problems, depression, anxiety, and suicide threats or attempts may bring these patients to the attention of a psychiatrist.
5. This disorder is most frequently diagnosed among women. Seldom a year goes by without patients seeking help from a physician.
6. Sexual experiences of women with somatization disorders tend to be comparable to those of women with affective disorders with the exception that more women with somatization disorder report being molested as children (Morrison, 1989).
7. NIMH Epidemiologic Catchment Area data indicate a prevalence of the disorder in about 0.38% of the population, with the modal patient described as female, non-white, unmarried, less educated, and from a rural area (Swartz M et al, 1986).
8. Screening indices are available to facilitate identification of *DSM-III-R* somatization disorder among general medical patients with unexplained somatic complaints (Smith and Braun, 1990; Othmer and DeSouza, 1985). The current definition of somatization disorder requires evaluation for 35 symptoms, of which 13 are scored as not meeting specific criteria. These screens serve clinicians well in reducing time allocated to correctly diagnose the disorder (Manu et al, 1989).
9. Axis II and III comorbidity is common (Snyder and Strain, 1989).
10. Patients with conversion disorder present with a loss or alteration of physical functioning suggesting physical pathology as a direct expression of a psychological conflict or need. A conversion disorder is most likely to involve a single site

during a given episode but may vary in site or nature if there is more than one episode.

11. The predominant feature of psychalgia is the complaint of pain in the absence of any physical findings to explain the symptoms and in the absence of any other mental disorders. Psychological factors are usually present to suggest a psychological etiology.

12. Dissociative disorders are characterized by sudden, temporary alteration in the normally integrated functions of consciousness, identity, or motor behavior so that one or more parts of these functions are lost. An individual may be amnesic for a certain period of time (psychogenic amnesia) or another personality or personalities may be taken on at various times which are distinct and separate (multiple personalities).

13. Malingering must be distinguished from conversion and dissociative disorders. Secondary gain is less apparent with conversion and dissociative disorders. Lawsuits may be found to be pending with malingerers.

14. Just because a patient may have some histrionic characteristics or has a past documented history of conversion symptoms does not mean that his present symptoms are not organic. Real physical illness can occur in patients with somatization disorder and in patients with a past history of conversion disorders.

15. Some studies have demonstrated that a significant number of individuals diagnosed to have conversion disorders will turn out to have documented physical illness that can explain the original symptoms.

16. Conversion symptoms first appearing late in life are often associated with an organic disorder or a psychotic depression.

17. Somatoform disorders and conversion disorders should be distinguished from facititious disorders. The latter includes physical and psychological symptoms that are produced by the individual and under his voluntary control. These include Ganser's syndrome and Munchausen's syndrome. The former is sometimes referred to as pseudostupidity. Patients with a Ganser's syndrome seem to understand a question, but give ridiculous answers (e.g., How many legs does a three-legged stool have? "Four." How many eyes does a man have? "Seven."). Munchausen's syndrome is a label given to those individuals who seem addicted to surgery and medical care. They sustain numerous operations without much pathology ever being found.

Symptoms
1. Amnesia.
2. Deafness.
3. Aphoria.
4. Loss of sensation.
5. Vomiting spells.
6. Abdominal pain.
7. Dysmenorrhea.
8. Menstrual irregularity (e.g., amenorrhea or more severe bleeding).
9. Lack of interest in having sex.

10. Sexual indifference.
11. Lack of pleasure during intercourse.
12. Pain during intercourse.
13. More headaches than most people.
14. Back pain.
15. Joint pain.
16. Pain in extremities.

Differential Diagnosis

1. Somatization syndrome.
2. Conversion disorder.
3. Multiple sclerosis.
4. Schizophrenia.
5. Vitamin deficiencies.
6. Toxic nerve damage.
7. Temporal lobe epilepsy.
8. Anxiety disorders.
9. Other forms of epilepsy.
10. Tabes dorsalis.
11. General paresis.
12. Basal ganglia disease.
13. Cerebral neoplasia.
14. Psychalgia.
15. Dissociative disorder.
16. Collagen diseases (e.g., lupus erythematosus, polyarteritis nodosa).
17. Other organic disorders.

Management

1. Carefully take a medical history. Perform a general physical and neurologic examination and order appropriate diagnostic studies to rule out organic disease.
2. Inquire into any recent life events that may have stressed patients. What is their personal past history? Their family history?
3. Do not focus on symptoms. When interviewing patients, remove them from friends and relatives who may be a source of secondary gain.
4. Allow patients to ventilate in a supportive psychotherapeutic relationship.
5. If a crisis intervention mode of psychotherapy does not work with patients with conversion symptoms, dissociative disorders, or psychalgia, try suggestion, hypnotherapy or an amytal interview using the proper precautions (Swartz and McCracken, 1986).
6. If a patient appears excessively anxious, it may be necessary to use an antianxiety agent such as 1–2 mg of lorazepam (Ativan) PO or 1–2 mg of alprazolam (Xanax).
7. If none of the above succeed in removing the symptom, it may be necessary to hospitalize the patient, but both internist and psychiatrist should work together in the evaluation.

8. Long-term, supportive, limit-setting psychotherapy may be required with various degrees of health education and explorative psychotherapy to get at the underlying psychogenetic roots. For instance, if a patient repeatedly becomes psychogenically paralyzed when dating married men, she should be advised not to do so and to explore reasons why she is attracted to them rather than to unmarried men who offer a more stable relationship.

Quality Assurance Issues

1. Are patients with somatoform disorders continuously reviewed to ascertain if symptoms may be due to a medical illness with intermittent symptoms (e.g., early multiple sclerosis)?
2. Have all patients with somatoform disorders been examined physically with appropriate specialist and laboratory studies ordered to rule out a medical/surgical basis of the symptoms?

Ethical/Legal Issues

1. Have patients been advised of the need for continued re-evaluation for a medical/surgical basis of the symptoms, given the fact that some illnesses (e.g., multiple sclerosis, the collagenoses) may present psychiatrically, but eventually take considerable physical toll?

SOMNAMBULISM

Somnambulism (or sleepwalking) is defined as a state of dissociated consciousness in which phenomena of sleeping and waking states combine.

History

1. The disorder is observed to occur in stages 3 and 4 of sleep and considered an impairment of arousal.
2. The typical episode of somnambulism occurs during the first 3 hours of sleep, and consists of the patient sitting up, arising from bed, and moving about in a poorly coordinated manner.
3. Complex activity such as dressing or eating out of context may occur.
4. The patient awakens slowly when aroused with awareness returning gradually (Kales JD et al, 1980).
5. Individuals are usually amnesic for the somnambulistic episode.
6. There is rarely more than one episode per night (Kales JD et al, 1980).
7. Somnambulism is relatively common in childhood but rare in adulthood.
8. When somnambulism is outgrown, its onset is usually prior to 10 years and terminated before 15 years (Kales JD et al, 1980).
9. Adult sleepwalkers tend to have started sleepwalking at a later age, have a higher frequency of events, have more episodes earlier in the night, have more intense clinical manifestations, and have more psychotherapy (Kales JD et al, 1980).

Adult sleepwalkers in particular appear to have difficulty in the management of aggressive feelings.

Management

1. Onset of sleepwalking after age 10, sleepwalking occurring frequently for 6 months to one year, no family history of sleepwalking, daytime symptoms, suggestion of a functional disorder, and onset of sleep disorder after major life stress all suggest underlying psychopathology that should be identified and appropriately treated (Kales JD et al, 1980).
2. Safety measures may be needed to protect sleepwalkers such as bolts on doors and windows and sleeping on the ground floor.
3. If sleepwalkers do not return to their bed unaided, they should be gently led.
4. Sleepwalking episodes should not be interrupted if it is known to lead to confusion or fright.
5. Parents of children who are sleepwalkers can be informed that their child's behavioral disturbance seldom leads to adult difficulty.

Quality Assurance Issues

1. Are all patients and their families advised of the danger of sleep walking so that appropriate measures may be taken to protect the patient?

SPINAL CORD INJURY

Despondency and, in some instances, depression requiring psychopharmacotherapy are expected consequences of severe spinal cord injury (Lloyd, 1980; Radloff, 1980).

History

1. Post-injury depressive disorders as diagnosed by the Schedule for Affective Disorders and Schizophrenia and the Research Diagnostic Criteria have been reported to occur in nearly one-third of patients with spinal cord injury within 1 month of the trauma (Fullerton et al, 1981).
2. Post-injury affective illness is more common in patients with complete (as opposed to partial) spinal cord injury but appears no more commonly in quadriplegia than in paraplegia (Fullerton et al, 1981).
3. The accident causing the injury may relate to a previously diagnosed or nondiagnosed disorder such as substance abuse, major depression, hypomania, or mania.

Management

1. Most individuals with affective symptoms following spinal cord injury recover without use of antidepressants.

STEROID-INDUCED DISORDERS

Steroids such as prednisone are employed in the management of a number of different medical illnesses including collagen disease, Addison's disease, and a number of neoplastic and allergic disorders. In addition, anabolic steroids are used by men and boys (and rarely women and girls) to build up their muscle mass.

History

1. As great as 6 to 7% of high school male seniors report current use or having used anabolic steroids, with about one-fifth acknowledging a health professional as a source (Buckley et al, 1988).
2. In addition to mania, nonspecific psychoses, depression, delirium and schizophreniform psychoses, and dementiform cognitive changes have been reported from administration of steroids. These persist after a steroid psychoses resolves in patients who suffer both the psychotic and cognitive changes and include deficits in concentration, attention, mental speed, retention, efficiency, and occupational performance. Symptoms remit after discontinuation or reduction of steroid use (Varney et al, 1984).
3. Estimated percent of affective symptoms and psychoses in athletes taking steroids is 22 and 12%, respectively (Pope and Katz, 1988). Those who use steroids to enhance skill as weight lifters are often quite refractory to maintaining abstinence and exhibit psychiatric symptoms, especially depression. They tend to exhibit withdrawal symptoms on cessation of use and continue to use despite known adverse circumstances (Brower et al, 1990).
4. Since steroids such as prednisone (a synthetic glucocorticoid medication) cause both euphoria and dysphoria, depressed patients who discover the mood-elevating effect may use it as a euphoriant (Goldberg and Wise, 1986).
5. Dosage is correlated with risk of developing psychologic changes but neither dosage nor duration of treatment affect time of onset, severity, duration, or type of psychologic symptoms (Ling et al, 1981).
6. Females are more prone to psychological symptoms during steroid use than males (Ling et al, 1981).
7. Patients with a past history of mental illness are not necessarily more predisposed to developing mental symptoms when given steroids (Ling et al, 1981).

Symptoms

1. Euphoria.
2. Dysphoria.
3. Cognitive impairment.

Signs

1. Stigmata of steroid use (e.g., moon faces).

Management

1. It is not necessary to reduce or discontinue the steroid being given if the primary clinician feels that it must be continued.
2. Antipsychotic medication may be prescribed in doses sufficient to control symptoms. Haloperidol (Haldol) or thiothixene (Navane), 2 mg PO tid is usually sufficient to manage a steroid psychosis.
3. Symptoms nearly always abate if the steroid therapy is discontinued.
4. It should be remembered that a psychosis may be developed while a patient's dose is being increased, while it is being decreased, or while at a steady state. If psychosis develops during reduction of dosage, it is possible to return to the original dose and decrease dosage more slowly. If it develops while increasing a patient's dose, decrease the dose and increase it more slowly. If psychosis develops while at a steady dose, either reduction of dose or the addition of antipsychotic medication may be used to manage the patient.

Quality/Assurance Issues

1. Was a patient informed of the potential of psychiatric side-effects?
2. Were chronic users examined for presence of medical complications?
3. Were all anorexics, weight lifters, and drug abusers asked about steroid use?
4. Are all patients on steroids advised of the risk of psychosis when decreasing a dosage in anticipation of surgery?

STROKE

Solitary or multiple strokes, as in the instance of multi-infarct dementia, can cause alterations in mood, thought, and behavior that are either specific to the region effected (e.g., the frontal lobe syndrome with infarcts or bleeds in the frontal lobes) or a response to the illness (e.g., depression). There is some evidence (Robinson and Starkstein, 1990) suggesting that major depressions following right hemispheric lesions are associated with a family history of depression and parietal cortical lesions. Generalized anxiety and depression are seen more with cortical damage and depression alone, with subcortical lesions. Direct or indirect dysfunction of the basotemporal cortex of the right hemisphere is associated with mania. Nonsuppression on the dexamethasone suppression test during the year pursuant to a stroke is associated with the presence of poststroke depression (Lipsey et al, 1985). The incidence of major and minor depression following a stroke has been estimated to be 27 and 20%, respectively (Robinson and Starkstein, 1990). The management of poststroke depression involves antidepressants and individual and family therapy in concert with rehabilitative efforts.

Quality Assurance Issues

1. Have all patients who have suffered stroke been evaluated for depression or another psychiatric disorder contributing to their disability?

SUBDURAL HEMATOMA

Subdural hematomas may present with depression, schizophrenia, violent behavior, catatonia (Woods, 1980), dementia, and conversion-like symptoms (Alarcon and Thweatt, 1983). In some instances they will have the associated symptoms and signs of a space-occupying lesion (Allen AM et al, 1940).

Clinical Investigations
Computed tomography confirms diagnosis.

Management
Patients with subdural hematomas are referred to neurosurgery for evacuation of the clot.

SUDDEN DEATH ASSOCIATED WITH ANTIPSYCHOTIC MEDICATION USE

Sudden death has been reported with patients on neuroleptic medication and attributed to seizures and asphyxiation, cardiovascular causes, postural hypotension, and laryngeal–pharyngeal dystonia.

History
1. Chlorpromazine (Thorazine) acts directly on autonomic centers in the midbrain producing a blocking effect on sympathetic ganglia resulting in hypotension.
2. In elderly people and others with compromised cerebral or cardiovascular status, use of antipsychotic medication may result in strokes or myocardial infarctions.
3. In patients treated with phenothiazines there is a diminution of the gag reflex that may result in aspiration asphyxia secondary to regurgitation due to loss of control of the esophageal sphincters and impairment of swallowing.

Management
1. Cardiovascular status and neurologic condition must be monitored throughout the duration of the neuroleptic treatment together with laboratory studies to minimize the occurrence of these potentially lethal consequences.

Quality Assurance Issues
1. Are all patients on neuroleptics advised of the premonitory symptoms of the neuroleptic malignant syndrome?

Ethical/Legal Issues
1. Are patients with symptoms of neuroleptic malignant syndrome provided the acute medical care required?

SUDDEN DEATH OF PSYCHOGENIC ORIGIN

Emotional factors are sufficient to bring about death in individuals not otherwise predisposed by immediate physical factors.

History

1. Individuals may die of heart attacks after they learn that their entire family has been killed in an airplane crash on the way to meet them.
2. Some people die of "fright" and others "give up" and die. Powerlessness, hopelessness, or other intense emotions usually precede these deaths.
3. The cardiovascular system responds to stress under such conditions to make sudden death more likely from cerebrovascular accidents or arrhythmias. People with coronary heart disease are at particular risk.
4. Voodoo deaths are a particular subtype of sudden death. "Root doctors," "conjure doctors," and "two-headed doctors" exist in both isolated rural communities in the deep South as well as in the large urban areas of the West and Northeast and are believed to be able to cause insanity, sickness, and death. They are also felt able to cure those who have been hexed using a mixture of herbs, stones, powders, insects, charms, roots, and incantations. These items are sometimes purchased at folk medicine stores for use by interested laypeople.
5. In order for a hex to work it is felt that victims must believe in the power of the person who places the curse and must have some knowledge that they have been hexed.
6. Evidence demonstrating that CNS input can modify the electrical activity of the heart and trigger sudden death is mounting. Cardiac ischemia, a major factor in the occurrence of ventricular arrhythmias, has been ascribed in animal models to the sympathetic limb of the autonomic nervous system.
7. The fact that beta-adrenergic blocking drugs alone have proven inadequate in the prevention of malignant ventricular arrhythmias indicates that enhanced sympathomimetic stimulation is not alone sufficient to cause a ventricular arrhythmias and that other central and peripheral variables play a role (Lown et al, 1980).

Management

1. Management of patients who believe they are hexed is often quite difficult without the involvement or support of lay or community healers. Ideally, a clinician seeks out a folk healer (e.g., "root doctor") who is perceived by the patient to possess the power both to hex and remove hexes to undo the curse.

Quality Assurance Issues

1. Are victims of voodoo or hexes referred to natural healers for help if medical intervention fails to reverse the spell or to sustain the patient?

SUICIDE IDEATION, SUICIDE ATTEMPTS,
AND THE DELIBERATE SELF-HARM SYNDROME

The evaluation and management of suicidal patients is one of the most anxietogenic components of emergency psychiatric care. Fortunately there are a number of simple guidelines that serve to guide both evaluation and management (Robbins and Kulbok, 1988).

Incidence

1. It is estimated that approximately 0.5 to 1% of individuals (Farmer, 1988) die by their own hand each year with a two- to three-fold increase among adolescents during the past 3 decades (Slaby, 1986; Farmer, 1988; Rudd, 1989).
2. Suicides may be obfuscated when a person is in a single car accident or a child walks in front of a car, particularly on an interstate or other highway.
3. Suicide is the third leading cause of death in the military with a three-fold increase from 6.2 per 100,000 in the mid-1950s to 21.4 per 100,000 in 1980 for white males in the age group 15 to 24 (Rothberg et al, 1987).
4. About one-quarter of all adolescent deaths are due to suicide, with rates of suicide ideation among youth ranging from 2.3 to 60.0% and rates of attempts from 0.6 to 9% (Friedman RC et al, 1983; Smith and Crawford, 1986). It is the second leading cause of death among American youth (Rudd, 1989).
5. Rates of suicidal behavior have been reported as high as 78.5% among child psychiatric inpatients and found to be associated with preoccupation with death, recent and past depression, and recent general psychopathology (Pfeffer et al, 1986).
6. While suicide rates have decreased over the past several decades among older age groups (Murphy E et al, 1986), rates are still highest among older men.
7. The United States ranks about average in rate of suicide with about 10 to 12 per 100,000 per year. It is the fifth major cause of death. Chile, Ireland, and New Zealand have lower rates. Germany, Japan, Sweden, Australia, Denmark, and Hungary have higher rates.
8. Age-specific cohort analyses of Canadian (Hellon and Solomon, 1980), American (Murphy and Wetzel, 1980), and Australian (Goldney and Katsikitis, 1983) populations indicate a substantial increase in suicide rates among each successively younger age group. Currently (Pfeffer, 1986) it is the third most common cause of death among 15- to 24-year-olds (after accidents and homicides) with more than 5000 adolescents and young adults (18.8% of deaths in this age group) dying each year. A 94% increase is predicted by the year 2000 (Pfeffer, 1986).

History

1. Data indicate that between 32 and 60% of those who attempt suicide see their primary care clinician in the 2 months preceding the act with one-half seeing a physician within 1 week of an attempt or suicide (Diekstra and van Egmond, 1989). In most instances the clinicians were unaware of the elevated risk.

2. Suicide behavior among youth relates to family dysfunction, psychiatric disorder, parental arrest (Joffe et al, 1988a), morbid ideas, loss of interest, and nonsuicidal self-directed aggression (Rosenthal and Rosenthal, 1984).

3. Depression has been found to be greater among those born after World War II, contributing to the increase in suicide rates among the young (Klerman, 1987).

4. Reduction in death by suicide entails educating the community about the early signs of depression and reducing the stigma of suicide so that those needing help get it and get it early (McGinnis, 1987).

5. Individuals right to die creates a particular problem in diagnosis and management (Karlinsky et al, 1988). Obviously an individual with severe medical illness such as terminal AIDS or cancer may wish to die and if the desire to suicide is not a product of a mental illness, a psychiatric clinician cannot restrain the person. In many instances however, a person is delusional and thinks he has a terminal illness but does not and rather is profoundly depressed. The thought that he or she is terminally ill is a false belief due to psychotic depression.

6. A reduction in suicide ideation is reported to occur after near death experiences wherein individuals have a brush with death that entails transcendent or mystical elements despite the romanticization of death (Greyson, 1986).

7. A number of biologic correlates have been reported with suicide. In summary, lethal suicide attempts and successful suicide tends to be associated with a decrease in serotonin in the brain and of its principle metabolite, 5-hydroxyindoleacetic acid in the cerebrospinal fluid (Arora and Meltzer, 1989; Gross-Isseroff et al, 1989; Stanley and Stanley, 1988; Mann JJ, 1987). Low serotonin is not consistently reported among schizophrenics who attempt suicide (Karpi et al, 1986). The ratio of norepinephrine to epinephrine is decreased in the urine of people who have made suicide attempts (Ostroff et al, 1985) and corticotropin-releasing factor (CRF) is hypersecreted, suggesting hyperactivity of the hypothalamic–pituitary–adrenal axis in suicidal patients (Nemeroff et al, 1988). The dexamethasone suppression test shows high rates of nonsuppression among those who commit suicide or make suicide attempts (Narman et al, 1990).

8. It is important to evaluate the "murder risk" as well as the suicidal risk among survivors of a suicide pact. The instigator of such pacts most frequently dies and tends to be a depressed male with a history of a previous suicide attempt. The survivor tends to be a cooperative woman who is not psychiatrically ill and does not have a history of a suicide attempt (Rosenbaum M, 1983). It appears in these instances that a depressed male may have convinced a woman who loves him to die with him and she does so out of devotion.

9. Although a number of scales have been devised to predict suicide, their value has been limited (Porkorny, 1983; Clark, et al, 1987; Levine S et al, 1989). The *DSM-III-R*, on the other hand, is seen as a valid instrument for diagnosing affective disorder in children (Cytryn et al, 1980).

10. Garfinkel (1982) found adolescents tend to attempt more frequently in the winter, after school or in the evening with someone nearby, and by overdose.

11. Assessment of suicide risk among children age 6 to 12 should focus on degree of depression, family communication patterns, state of ego functioning, and a

child's concept of death (Pfeffer, 1988). Children who are assaultive or suicidal tend to exhibit intense aggression and have histories of parental suicidal and assaultive behavior (Pfeffer et al, 1983).

12. There is some evidence suggesting that overdose may have a respite function for low suicidal intent individuals (Parker A, 1981). Risk-taking recreational activities and substance abuse may represent cryptic antecedent behaviors to suicide.

13. Suicidal ideation is common among children and young adults. Over 10% of high school and 6% of college students in one study (Wright, 1985) reported suicidal thoughts. Factors correlated with suicidal thoughts include perception that parents have many conflicts and that one or both were chronically depressed and angry, drug or alcohol abuse, identification with depressed parent, depression, hopelessness, and lack of social support (Rudd, 1989; Wright, 1985; Pfeffer, 1985).

14. Suicide rates either are inversely related or not related to state spending for hospitals (Zimmerman SL, 1990).

15. Individuals who repeat suicide attempts tend to have histories of more frequent episodes beginning at an earlier age, feel more powerless and normlessness, and experience more feeling of externally directed hostility (Sakinofsky and Roberts, 1990).

Risk Factors for Suicide

1. **Severe psychiatric illness:** Risk of suicide among the psychiatrically ill is 6 to 11 times that for those without illness (Hirschfeld and Davidson, 1988; Garfinkel BD et al, 1982).

2. **Dementia:** While only 11% of the population is over 65 years of age, 25% of completed suicides occur in this age group with dementia being a factor increasing risk (Margo and Finkel, 1990).

3. **Hopelessness:** Hopelessness, more than depression, predicts suicide. People do not want to die, they just want to end the pain and cannot visualize another way of assuaging it (Prezant and Neimeyer, 1988; Beck AT et al, 1985; Schlebusch and Wessels, 1988; Beck AT et al, 1990; Hendin, 1986).

4. **Personality disorder:** Individuals with personality disorder, particularly borderline, have increased risk of suicide (Casey PR, 1989; Friedman RC et al, 1983). Antisocial, depressed, and histrionic features, and concurrent substance abuse enhance risk with borderline patients (Shearer et al, 1988; Fyer MR et al, 1988a; Paris, 1990).

5. **Lethality of attempt:** Using a method that would result in death increases risk. Wrist cuttings and small overdoses are less lethal than defenestration, gunshot wounds, hanging, and throat cutting. The more violent and painful the attempt, the greater the risk. Use of drugs that cause cardiac arrhythmias to overdose enhances risk. The attempter, if overdosing, must be aware a drug is not lethal to see the attempt as lower risk (Rich et al, 1990). Alcohol and drugs are frequently used prior to an impulsive lethal attempt (Peterson LG et al, 1985).

6. **Depression:** Depression is a major risk factor for all age groups (Goldberg EL,

1981). Approximately 15% of patients with untreated major depression commit suicide (Murphy GE, 1983) with 10 to 20 as many suicide attempts (Asnis et al, 1990). Rates are greatest when neurovegetative signs, marital isolation, suicidal ideation, feelings of failure and comorbid alcoholism and drug abuse, male sex, and a number of previous hospitalizations (particularly with suicidal behavior) are present (e.g., sleep and appetite disturbance). Risk may increase early in the course of treatment as energy returns before depression and feelings of hopelessness abate (Wells et al, 1990; van Praag and Plutchik, 1988; Roy-Byrne et al, 1988; Bulik et al, 1990; Robbins and Alessi, 1985; Modestin and Kopp, 1988; Achte 1986; Roy et al, 1989).

7. **Repression:** Individuals who use repression as a primary defense mechanism tend to turn aggression inward and attempt suicide; those who tend to project and deny are more aggressive (Goldberg and Sakinofsky, 1988; Fernandez-Pol, 1986; Apter et al, 1989).

8. **Secondary gain:** Lack of obvious "message" (i.e., a cry for help) increases risk.

9. **Early separation:** Early loss or separation from parents increases risk (Wasserman and Cullberg, 1989).

10. **Anxiety disorders:** Anxiety disorders, particularly panic disorder, increase risk. Risk is greatest when panic disorder is comorbid with substance abuse or depression (Weissman MM et al, 1989).

11. **Akathisia:** Suicide ideation has been found to occur with akathisia and disappear when the akathisia abates (Drake and Ehrlich, 1985).

12. **Accident proneness:** Increase of accidents may indicate covert depression or personality disorder and enhance suicide risk (Black et al, 1985a).

13. **Homicide:** Homicide is associated with increase in suicide risk, probably indicating a general increase in impulsive violent behavior (Virkkunen et al, 1989a; Griffith and Bell, 1989; Holinger, 1980; Rosenbaum M, 1990).

14. **Criminal behavior:** Rates are greater among adult and juvenile offenders (Alessi et al, 1984). Hanging is a common mode of exodus with substance abuse a contributing cause (Keitner et al, 1990).

15. **Signals:** Individuals who do not give off signals that they had planned to attempt suicide are at greater risk than those who do.

16. **Stopping medication:** Cessation of medication for bipolar illness increases risk (Schou and Weeke, 1988).

17. **Stress:** Increasing life stress is correlated with increased risk of suicide (Kosky, 1983; Cohen-Sandler et al, 1982).

18. **Epidemics:** Risk is increased, particularly among adolescents, after others in the community have suicided (Kessler RC et al, 1988; Rosen and Walsh, 1989; Robbins and Kulbock, 1988).

19. **Setting:** Likelihood of suicide is increased if an attempt was made in a setting where there was little likelihood of being found.

20. **Family pathology:** Risk is greater among children and adolescents who come from disturbed families (Hawton et al, 1982).

21. **Self-esteem:** Those who attempt suicide have low self-esteem (Tischler and Mc-

Kenry, 1983). A feeling of worthlessness is a symptom of major depressive disorder.

22. **Child abuse:** Child abuse and a history of incest increase risk (Deykin et al, 1985).

23. **Time of year:** Suicide rates tend to be highest in spring and fall. December, despite the occurrence of Christmas, tends to be associated with low rates (Hillard et al, 1981).

24. **Marital status:** Rates are highest among the widowed, divorced, and separated. Single persons have twice the rate of suicide as do married persons, and married persons with children have the lowest rate (Roy, 1983). An exception is the married adolescent girl, who is at greater risk.

25. **Sex:** Women attempt more but men succeed more. Women tend to overdose while men use more lethal means (McIntosh and Jewell, 1986; Hassan and Tan, 1989; Sudak et al, 1984; Rich et al, 1988b; Stafford and Weisheit, 1988). Professional women differ. Female medical students have rates three to four times higher than age peers (Pepitone-Arreola-Rockwell et al, 1981). Girls attempt suicide as great as three times more than boys (Garfinkel BD et al, 1982).

26. **Age:** Rates increase with age for men, with men over 65 having the highest rates of any sex-age groups. Rates among women increase until age 65 and then drop off. An exception is rates among adolescents that are not again reached until midlife (Garfinkel and Golombek, 1974; Eisenberg, 1980; Solomon and Hellon, 1980; Husain SA, 1990; Hawton, 1982; Spurlock, 1990; Rich et al, 1986b; Holinger and Offer, 1982; American Academy of Pediatrics Committee on Adolescence, 1980; Angle et al, 1983; Holinger and Offer, 1982; Goldberg EL, 1981; Garfinkel BD et al, 1979; Pfeffer, 1990; Lipsitt, 1986; Brent et al, 1988; Kosky, 1983; Sturner, 1986; Asarnow and Carlson, 1988; Achte, 1988; Maris, 1985).

27. **Religion:** Rates are lower among Jews and Catholics and highest among Protestants.

28. **Creativity:** The perception that the creative sensitive person is more prone to suicide has some data to support it (Clayton, 1985; Slaby, 1991).

29. **Socioeconomic status:** Suicide rates tend to be highest among both the lowest and highest socioeconomic classes. The peak suicide rates (i.e., 117.4 per 100,000) were after the Great Depression (Frederick, 1977).

30. **Race:** Rates for non-whites have characteristically been lower than whites, save in urban centers where rates for blacks and whites are similar. Rates for Native Americans vary from higher to lower than the general population (Thompson and Walker, 1990). Asian and Hispanic Americans have rates similar to those of Caucasians (Heacoch, 1990).

31. **Insomnia:** Severe insomnia, even in the absence of depression, is associated with increased risk.

32. **Substance abuse:** Risk is increased in those who abuse alcohol and drugs, which decrease inhibition and impair judgment. Pedestrian and vehicular accidents may represent covert or overt suicide attempts. Alcohol and drugs may be used to self-medicate depression, schizophrenia, or anxiety disorder (i.e., dual diagnosis) complicating diagnoses and treatment (Fernandez-Pol, 1986; Murphy

GE, 1988; Marzuk and Mann, 1988; Stiffman, 1989; Fowler et al, 1986). Alcoholics who attempt suicide are more likely to be female, younger, to have begun heavy drinking and experienced alcohol-related problems at an early age, and to have a lifetime diagnosis of major depression, panic disorder, antisocial personality disorder, phobic disorder, generalized anxiety disorder, or substance abuse (Roy et al, 1989; Berglund, 1984).

33. **Schizophrenia:** Risk is increased in schizophrenia and difficult to predict (Roy, 1983; Hillard et al, 1983; Reich P, 1989; Weiden and Roy, 1990). Risk is also increased for self-mutilation (Sweeny and Zamechik, 1981). Thought disorder, depressed mood, and suicidal ideation are particularly ominous signs of suicide risk (Tsuang, 1978). Schizophrenics who die by suicide tend to be depressed, male, younger, never married, and fail to communicate their desire to die after a stressful life event (Breier and Astrachan, 1984; Cohen LJ et al, 1990; Prasad and Kumar, 1988).

34. **Ethnic Origin:** Rates among foreign born individuals tend to be higher than those assimilated and reflect the rates of country of origin.

35. **Command hallucinations:** Auditory hallucinations commanding a person to commit suicide or to join someone in the beyond increases risk (Hellerstein et al, 1987) when associated with other risk factors.

36. **Delusions:** Delusionally depressed patients are reported to have as great as five times the suicide rates of nondelusional patients (Roose et al, 1983).

37. **Homosexuality:** Risk is increased, especially among gay youth without social support and among those who are aging, depressed, or substance abusing (Rich et al, 1986a; Schneider et al, 1989).

38. **Physical illness:** Illness increases risk especially if the illness holds a stigma (e.g., AIDS, cancer) or if a previously robust and independent person is afflicted with a painful or disabling disease. Depression is often present in those with terminal illness who are suicidal (Leibenluft and Goldberg, 1988).

39. **Family history:** Risk is increased if suicide is in the family and especially in the same-sex parent. Nearly half of patients in one study (Roy, 1983) who had a family history attempted suicide. More than half of these patients had affective illness. Family history increases risk regardless of diagnoses (e.g., major depression, bipolar disorder, dysthymic disorder, schizoaffective disorder) (Roy, 1983; Egeland and Sussex, 1985; Scheftner et al, 1988; Hutchinson and Draguns, 1987).

40. **Disposing of personal property:** Giving away possessions, especially if cherished, increases risk.

41. **Previous attempts:** Previous attempt increases risk particularly if the previous attempt involved lethal means and the patient gave no warning (Goldacre and Hawton, 1985; Shafi et al, 1985; Steer et al, 1988). As the rates of attempted suicide are quite high, use of other risk factors in addition to attempts are needed to ascertain those at greatest risk for a subsequent fatal attempt (Hawton et al, 1982; Hawton, 1982; Pablo and Lamarre, 1986; Brooksband, 1985; Harkavy and Asnis, 1985; Kienhorst et al, 1990; Gespert et al, 1985; DeVanna et al, 1990).

42. **Lack of future plans:** Absence of future plans increases risk, especially if a

person speaks of how they will be viewed at their funeral and what people will say.

43. **Living alone:** Living alone increases risk. Social contacts and contacts with health care providers reduces risk (Wolk-Wasserman, 1987; Lyons MJ, 1985).

44. **Loss:** Recent loss, especially of a loved one through death or separation, increases risk (Rich et al, 1988a).

45. **Hypochondriasis:** Hypochondrial preoccupation increases risk and may indicate occult depression.

46. **Recent childbirth and surgery:** Recent surgery and childbirth increases risk.

47. **Unemployment:** Financial reverses and unemployment increase risk (Hawton et al, 1988). Suicide rates among whites are more sensitive to fluctuations in the economy than are rates among blacks, with the exception of black women. Rates in high rent districts show increases with economic difficulty while low rent districts do not reflect the vicissitudes of fortune to the same degree. Rates in the age group 15 to 65 increase with financial woe more than those of people over 65. Rates decreased at times of war with the exception of the Vietnam War.

48. **Education:** Rates tend to be higher among the educated, particularly those at the most competitive schools (Iskii, 1985).

49. **Tension:** Lack of decrease of tension during an evaluation with elaboration of a treatment plan and options increases risk.

50. **Occupation:** Rates are highest among professional men and women and least among artisans and farm workers, although notable exceptions (e.g., Kentucky farmers) exist (Stallines, 1990). Vietnam veterans are a group at especial risk (Pollock et al, 1990).

Differential Diagnosis

1. Adjustment disorder.
2. Antisocial personality disorder.
3. Anxiety disorder.
4. Bipolar illness.
5. Borderline personality disorder.
6. Delusional (paranoid) disorder.
7. Drug withdrawal.
8. Dysthymic disorder.
9. Existential angst.
10. Hopelessness without psychiatric disorder.
11. Imitative suicide.
12. Impulse control disorder.
13. Learning disability.
14. Major depression.
15. Narcissistic personality disorder.
16. Organic mental disorder.
17. Panic disorder.
18. Personal choice.
19. Politico-cultural factors

20. Post-traumatic stress disorder.
21. Psychoactive drug use.
22. Reactive psychosis.
23. Schizoaffective disorder.
24. Schizophrenia.

Deliberate Self Harm

1. Patients with a number of psychiatric disorders (but particularly schizophrenia and borderline personality disorder) will mutilate their bodies in painful and bizarre ways without suicidal intent; nevertheless, they require observation, restraints (chemical or physical), and diagnostic-specific treatment.
2. Patients have castrated and enucleated themselves as well as cut off their breasts, hands, or ears. Women have put knives and razor blades in their vaginas and not told their husbands or lovers (Coons PM et al, 1986; Soulios and Firth, 1986; Eisenhauer, 1985).
3. The usual self-mutilation is less dramatic and involves burning, scratching, self-hitting, or biting (Coons PM et al, 1986; Favazza and Conterio, 1989).
4. In some instances self-mutilation occurs in patients who feel unreal or depersonalized and is an attempt to make themselves feel that they exist.
5. The incidence of self-mutilation has been reported to range from rare to 40% of patients in different populations (Coons PM et al, 1986).
6. Typically self-harm commences in late adolescence with multiple episodes of low lethality that continues for years (Pattison and Kahan, 1983).
7. Patients who cut may wrist slash but not always in an attempt to die (House and Thompson, 1985).
8. While most self-harm patients report considerable distress, not all are depressed (Ennis et al, 1989; Darhe, 1989).
9. Self-mutilation, particularly skin cutting and burning, is found in patients with eating disorders (Favazza et al, 1989).
10. Self-harm repeaters are at greater short-term risk for suicide than first cases (Barnes R, 1986).

Management

1. The first step in management of the suicidal patient, even in the emergency room, is to determine the need for observation and restraint. If a person is lethally suicidal, he or she may seek a way to execute the act in the emergency room or crisis unit or regret coming in for help and attempt to flee and kill him- or herself (Goldberg RJ, 1987).
2. Observation ranges from arms' length constraint to within eye range in an open area. If there is fear of eminent harm or escape, restraints may be required.
3. An evaluation is made from risk factors as to whether a patient may be managed outside of the hospital or require confinement for a brief or continued stay (Yu-Chin and Arcuni, 1990). Obviously, if risk of significant self-harm is great, a person must be hospitalized even if this necessitates certification or commitment. Families or patients may resist, but ultimately the clinician's actions will

be evaluated by the prevailing standards of quality care. A family may elect to provide constant surveillance under a physician's supervision but for a family to have the time, resources, and sophistication to provide what is demanded is rare.

4. Clinicians should be aware that spouses and family may be quite ambivalent over patients because of years of pain caused by suicidal threats or attempts or other aspects of their illness. In such instances they may militate against a decision to hospitalize harboring a covert unconscious desire for the patient to die. If, however, a suicide occurred the guilt may lead the family to blame the clinician and pursue legal action contending that as a distraught family they had no recourse but to rely on a clinician's decision and deny or minimize their opposition to it because of the pain of the moment.

4. If a person is to be managed outside of the hospital, a person's family, lover, or friends should be alerted to the risk and treatment plan and informed of signs of deepening depression such as return or worsening of hopelessness.

5. It is good policy to give patients and their significant others the clinician's work and home phone number, the number of a back-up clinician, and instructions how to find an emergency room or crisis center if neither are available and immediate assistance is required.

6. Social supports are always rallied and the patient given opportunity for ventilation. This allows bonding to mollify the pain of depression and opens lines of communication to help develop options and resources and to learn alternative ways to cope with stress.

7. Suicidal ideation, like fever and headache, have a differential diagnosis. After the cause of the desire to suicide is determined, diagnostic-specific treatment is initiated.

8. If a person is profoundly depressed, it will not be possible to instill hope until the depression has been adequately treated. If a person, however, is suicidal due to social factors such as rejection by family for being gay, enhancing awareness that being homosexual is not rare and helping establish connections with a supportive gay community should engender hope and reduce risk.

9. "Murder risk," as well as suicide risk, should be assessed in depressed individuals as they may persuade another person who loves them but is not depressed to die by suicide with them (Rosenbaum M, 1983).

10. Since hopelessness more than depression per se is a risk factor in suicide, elaboration of options and rallying social support with the intention of enhancing hope should be an integral part of the treatment plan (Slaby, 1986).

11. Management of the suicidal child and adolescent poses particular problems. Adolescents are more prone to peer pressure and exposed widely to substances to be abused. In addition, suicidal thoughts and behavior may relate to problems of the parents over which the therapist has little control even if the parents consent to be involved in family or individual therapy (Marks A, 1979; Pfeffer, 1984; Robinson, 1984, Tishler, et al, 1981; McKenry et al, 1982). Outcome is best when family and individual therapy is used in combination with psychopharmacotherapy and hospitalization when indicated.

12. Primary care clinicians should be taught to identify potentially suicidal patients

and means of reducing risks. Approximately 75% of individuals who kill themselves see a family physician within 3 months of killing themselves.

13. If suicidal ideation and depression is secondary to an organic process that is treatable, consultation should be sought and appropriate therapy initiated. For instance, if depression is a side effect of an antihypertensive medication, the medication should be, after consultation with an internist, discontinued, reduced, or substituted for by another drug with less likelihood of depression.

14. If the patient is to be managed as an outpatient:

   a. Social support should be rallied.
   b. Appropriate psychopharmacotherapy, psychotherapy, or sociotherapy should be initiated.
   c. The patient and his family and friends should be given the psychiatric clinician's telephone number as well as that of a backup clinician or emergency room where they can go if the clinician is unavailable.
   d. A return visit (even the next day if it is felt the decision to not hospitalize may need to be reconsidered) should be scheduled.
   e. Friends and families should be alerted to ominous signs such as increasing withdrawal, preoccupation, silence, and moroseness.
   f. Careful records should be kept in all instances documenting why a patient was or was not hospitalized.

15. The thrust of crisis work with a suicidal patient is opening lines of communication, identifying and exploring resources and options, establishing social supports, and initiating therapeutic interventions. Frequency of visits, if the patient is treated as an outpatient, depends on how much the psychiatric clinician can depend on others in the community such as friends, family, lovers, and clergy to provide social support; an opportunity for ventilation and exploring options; and to call the clinician if the patient's condition worsens.

16. Post-discharge risk of suicide is greatest within the first month (Roy, 1989) necessitating more frequent visits for therapy during this time if feasible as part of the treatment plan.

17. Predictors of resolution of parasuicidality include improvement in depression, less internally and externally directed hostility, enhanced self-esteem and perceived ability to control one's environment or fate, less sensitivity to criticism, and better social adjustment (Sakinofsky and Roberts, 1990) including need for problem-solving-oriented therapy and sociotherapy to improve bonding with supportive others as part of the treatment plan.

18. In chronic care facilities the most common suicidal behaviors are refusal of food, drink, and medication. These behaviors are associated with depth of depression, feeling rejected by the family, loneliness, and loss (Osgood and Brant, 1990).

19. Schizophrenics have been reported the most likely to suicide as inpatients and drugs and alcohol abusers as outpatients.

20. When suicide occurs, those who survive must be supportive. Such loss is incomprehensible to many and the pain best understood by others who have experienced the sting. The loss is always painful, never fully forgotten, and unique for

everyone (Boldt, 1982–1983; Rudestam and Imbroll, 1983; Kovarsky, 1989). Referral to a survivor group should be provided to all who have suffered such a loss. They may not wish to exercise the option, but should have it available for when and if the need emerges.

Quality Assurance Issues

1. Is there documentation of patient's suicidal ideation with risk factors (e.g., previous attempts, no plans for future, a plan for the suicide, lethal means for suicide)?
2. Does the treatment plan include the appropriate precautions to prevent suicide?
3. Has the patient been provided diagnostic-specific treatment for the illness presenting with suicide ideation?
4. Have medical/surgical causes been evaluated as contributing to or responsible for the suicide ideation (e.g., antihypertensive medication)?

Ethical/Legal Issues

1. Is there documentation of reassessment of a patient's suicide risk?
2. Have appropriate precautions been taken to protect a patient from self-harm?
3. If prescribed an antidepressant, is it one with low-risk for death by overdose or of an amount not sufficient for the person to kill him or herself?
4. Have family and friends been advised of the risk of suicide and what to do if risk increases?
5. Has the patient been provided resources (e.g., therapist's telephone number, therapist's backup telephone number, emergency room) if desire to kill self increases?
6. Has the patient been scheduled as an outpatient at intervals sufficient to pick up increased risk?

SULFAMETHOXAZOLE

Sulfonamides can produce acute psychoses characterized by delusions, psychomotor agitation, hallucinations, and disorientation. In some instances these psychiatric symptoms are accompanied by agoraphobia and aphasia. Acute psychosis coupled with pseudoseizures have been reported with intravenous use of trimethoprim-sulfamethoxazole.

Management

1. Symptoms tend to remit within 24 hours of discontinuation of the drug.

SURGICAL CRISES WITH DEATH-MINDED PATIENTS

While anecdotal evidence suggested that patients with high anxiety entering surgery may be at greater risk for dying, there is some data reported that fearful or "death-minded" patients do not do more poorly than others not so concerned at surgery.

SURVIVORS OF SUICIDE

When a person dies by suicide there are many who knew the person as family, friends, lovers, colleagues, or therapists that survive who feel the impact for months to decades. Never is a suicide entirely forgotten. Grief, anger, shame, disbelief, and a number of somatic and psychic symptoms may ensue. While empathetic therapists and friends help, nothing helps as much as being understood. This is best provided by someone who has experienced a similar loss and specifically by those whose lost most parallels that of the individual who has experienced a suicide. Some whose father suicided will find another individual whose father has died by suicide also. A mother who has lost a daughter, by another mother whose daughter has suicided.

History
1. Suicide, especially to some people who haven't experienced it, still holds considerable stigma. Some survivors are victims of gossip, others to negative reactions by officials and newspapers. Survivors have been found to show increased suicide attempts themselves, moving to new locations to live, difficulty discussing the event or even denying it, and experiencing a feeling (to some degree true) that no one understands them (Somonon, 1982–83).
2. When compared to survivors of victims of accidents and of unanticipated and expected natural causes, survivors of suicide show more unique grief reactions and rejection (Barrett and Scott, 1990).
3. Obsession over the reasons for suicide and how it may have been prevented (playing the "game of ifs") is a common sequela for both adult and child survivors (Ness and Pfeffer, 1990).
4. In one study, 51% of 259 psychiatrists surveyed experienced a death of a patient by suicide. Both personal and professional lives were impacted with effect the greatest on less-experienced younger clinicians and the least on those who were older and more experienced (Chemtol et al, 1988).

Management
1. Nothing helps us to understand a suicide as to be understood. All survivors should be provided the option of a survivor group.
2. Some survivors may not immediately feel comfortable in a survivor group and, therefore, it sometimes takes months to years before they join.
3. Having a survivor call a person who has recently lost someone to suicide may facilitate healing by allowing access to someone who especially understands the pain of the loss.
4. As survivors are at greater risk for suicide both psychologically as well as often genetically as they may have a genetic proclivity to the same illness (e.g., major depression, bipolar illness), they should always be observed for indications of a

tendency toward self-destructive behavior particularly if mourning becomes melancholia.

5. Therapists, primary clinicians, and others who have cared for the suicide just prior to death are also survivors and need support and in some instances participation in survivor groups themselves.

Quality Assurance Issues
1. Were survivors offered a survivor group to participate in?
2. Were survivors observed for indicia of depressive illness or enhanced risk of self-destructive behavior?

Ethical/Legal Issues
1. Are survivors of suicide evaluated for suicide risk themselves and for the disorders contributing to the death of their family member?

SYDENHAM'S CHOREA

Children and adolescents with Sydenham's chorea, when compared to those who have rheumatic fever without chorea, had more obsessive thoughts and compulsive behaviors and greater interference from these behaviors, suggesting that, at least in some instances, obsessive–compulsive disorder may be related to basal ganglia dysfunction (Swedo et al, 1989).

Management
1. Management of the obsessive–compulsive disorder associated with Sydenham's chorea is the same as that with other obsessive–compulsive disorders: clomipramine (Anafranil) or a serotonin agonist such as fluoxetine (Prozac) or sertraline (Zoloft).

SYSTEMIC LUPUS ERYTHEMATOSIS

Lupus erythematosis may initially present with depression. Consideration of a collagen disorder is part of a comprehensive evaluation of anyone with psychiatric symptoms suggestive of depression, mania, or schizophrenia.

History

1. In a study of 400 admissions to a neuropsychiatric unit using antinuclear antibody tests, 14 patients were found to fulfill criteria of systemic lupus erythematosis (Koranyi and Dewar, 1986). This is approximately 70 to 90 times the prevalence in the general population.
2. Drugs such as phenytoin (Dilantin) and barbiturates may induce systemic lupus erythematosis (Koranyi and Dewar, 1986).
3. Lupus can masquerade as a number of psychiatric disorders.
4. CNS changes including seizure disorders have been reported as a sequela of drug-induced lupus (Koranyi and Dewar, 1986).

Management

1. Depression associated with lupus is often extremely difficult to treat (Koranyi and Dewar, 1986).
2. Clonazepam, the anticonvulsant, has been proven effective in the management of depression and anxiety in lupus patients being managed with steroids (Jones and Chouinard, 1985).

TARDIVE DYSKINESIA

Widespread use of neuroleptic drugs has lead to rising awareness of their potential for adverse side effects. One such side effect is the bucco-lingual-masticatory dyskinesia referred to as tardive dyskinesia.

History

1. Patients presenting with tardive dyskinesia usually have a history of prolonged use of antipsychotic medications. Phenothiazines, butyrophenones, and thioxanthenes are reported to play a role in the genesis of this disorder in predisposed individuals although risk is said to be greater when the high-potency, lower-dosage neuroleptics are used.
2. Symptoms first appear after prolonged use of a drug or when drug dosage is lowered or is discontinued. Increasing the dose of a drug may make the dyskinesia disappear but contributes further to the problem.
3. A higher incidence of the disorder is reported for older people, women, those with brain damage and those with long records of hospitalization.
4. The longer patients are on an antipsychotic drug, the more likely they are to develop the disorder.
5. Frequent eye-blinking has been found by some to be the most frequent prodromal sign of tardive dyskinesia (Gardos et al, 1987).
6. The most frequent subtypes of tardive dyskinesia are tardive dystonia, blepharospasm, tardive akathisia, and choreoathetosis.
7. While some patients with tardive dyskinesia may show changes on CT scan such

as altered ventricle–brain ratio, negative results do not rule out more subtle neuropathologic abnormalities (Swayze et al, 1988).

8. While dopamine receptor supersensitivity is purportedly responsible for the abnormal movements, the neurotransmitters norepinephrine, GABA (gamma-aminobutyric acid), and serotonin all probably play a role in the complex neurophysiology of the disorder (Glazer, 1988).

9. Youth is not a protection against development of a tardive dyskinesia. Children and adolescents are at risk.

10. Prompt detection of early signs of the disorder and neuroleptic withdrawal may result in amelioration of symptoms.

11. Duration of symptoms prior to drug withdrawal appears to be a more important factor than age of onset in determining reversibility of symptoms.

12. The incidence of tardive dyskinesia has been reported to be as high as 25% of those exposed to neuroleptics in the past 5 years. The prevalence of *persistent* tardive dyskinesia that may be attributed to neuroleptics is estimated to be about 13% (Jeste and Wyatt, 1981; Task Force of APA, 1980; Klawans HC et al, 1980).

13. Clozapine (Clozaril) has not been reported to give genesis to tardive dyskinesia (Simpson et al, 1986).

14. Greater steady-state serum levels of thiothixene (Navane) have been associated with tardive dyskinesia (Yesavage et al, 1987).

15. Tardive dyskinesia has been reported in as great as one-third of young mentally retarded individuals treated for prolonged periods with neuroleptics (Gualtieri et al, 1986).

16. Prevalence of tardive dyskinesia symptoms as measured by the AIMS (Abnormal Involuntary Movement Scale) increases with duration of treatment with neuroleptics of older people (Joenniessen et al, 1985).

17. Meige's syndrome, first described by Henri Meige in 1910, is an idiopathic movement disorder consisting of oromandibular dystonia and blepharospasm that may be confused with tardive dyskinesia. It is probably a variant of adult onset idiopathic tension dystonia (Glazer et al, 1983). It affects women more than men and is more prevalent in those over 40. A number of individuals who present with it have been found to have an associated neuropsychiatric disorder (Jankovic, 1981).

18. There is some evidence that there may be a familial genetic predisposition to the development of tardive dyskinesia (Yassa and Ananth, 1981).

19. The severity of tardive dyskinesia as assessed by AIMS correlates significantly with the average daily dose and of total dose of fluphenazine (Prolixin) decanoate (Csernansky et al, 1981).

20. In addition to correlations with age, use of high potency low dosage neuroleptics and depot fluphenazine, the occurrence of tardive dyskinesia is correlated with Parkinsonism, teeth or denture problems, incoherence, and grandiose delusions (Mukerjhee et al, 1982).

21. A belief that all abnormal movements in patients using neuroleptics are due to tardive dyskinesia will lead to a failure to recognize treatable entities (Granacher, 1981) (See Differential Diagnosis, below)

22. Spontaneous involuntary movement disorders as measured by AIMS and the Rockland Scale are seen in as great as 50% of schizophrenics using the former scale and 66% using the latter scale, regardless of whether or not they have been exposed to neuroleptics (Owens et al, 1982), suggesting that spontaneous movement disorders are a part of the natural history of untreated severe chronic schizophrenia.

23. In a review of 56 prevalence surveys of tardive dyskinesia in neuroleptic-treated patients and 19 samples of untreated individuals by Kane and Smith (1982) it was found that 20% of the former and 5% of the latter had "spontaneous" dyskinesia. Prevalence during the last 2 decades has increased. Middle age and, to a certain degree, female sex were observed to be risk factors. It was uncertain whether CNS dysfunction or exposure to antiparkinsonism agents are risk factors in its development.

24. In addition to the strong linear correlation of prevalence and severity of tardive dyskinesia with age there is also a strong inverse correlation between rates of spontaneous remission and age with tardive dyskinesia with those younger than 60 years improving over three times as often as in older persons. These findings are not believed to relate solely to duration of previous exposure to neuroleptics but also to increased sensitivity to the drugs with advancing age (Smith and Baldessarini, 1980).

25. Tardive dyskinesia has been reported in children as young as 10 years following neuroleptic use. In some instances, the movement disorder persisted after discontinuation of the medication (Petty and Spar, 1980).

26. Oculogyric dystonia has been reported to emerge in a chronically medicated patient with severe tardive dyskinesia and attributed to a sudden decrease in dopaminergic activity and the relative increase in cholinergic activity following the dopamine-blocking effects of a neuroleptic (Wasrallan et al, 1980).

Signs
1. Frequent eye-blinking.
2. Lip-smacking.
3. Chewing movements.
4. Choreoathetoid movements of the tongue.
5. Puckering of the lips.
6. Choreoathetoid movements of the limbs and trunk (less frequent).

In addition to the above, potentially life-threatening ventilatory and gastrointestinal disturbances may develop that require rapid reinstitution of neuroleptic therapy (Casey and Rabins, 1978).

Differential Diagnosis
1. Tardive dyskinesia.
2. Meige's syndrome.
3. Hepatolenticular degeneration (Wilson's disease).

4. Drug-induced tremor (e.g., lithium-, neuroleptic-, and tricyclic-induced tremors).
5. Tourette's syndrome.
6. Parkinson's disease.
7. Parkinsonism—dementia complex.
8. Hypoparathyroidism.
9. Creutzfeldt–Jacob disease.
10. Sydenham's chorea.
11. Huntington's disease.
12. Simple or multiple tics.
13. Amphetamine-like substance induced stereotypes.
14. Senile or oral-facial dyskinesia.
15. L-Dopa-induced dyskinesia.
16. Dental conditions.
17. Reserpine-induced Parkinsonism.
18. Systemic lupus erythematosus.
19. Hypernatremia.
20. Methyldopa-induced dyskinesia.
21. Anticholinergic-induced dyskinesia.
22. Antimalarial-induced dyskinesia.
23. Psychosis.
24. Hyperthyroidism.
25. Chorea of pregnancy.
26. Kernicterus.
27. Phenytoin-induced dyskinesia.
28. Oral contraceptive-induced dyskinesia.
29. Familial paroxysmal choreoathetosis.
30. Carbon disulfide-induced dyskinesia.
31. Postencephalitic Parkinsonism.

Treatment

1. Focus of treatment is primary, secondary, and tertiary prevention of impairment. Primary prevention entails reduction of patient exposure to high doses of neuroleptics for prolonged periods of time. Secondary prevention requires early diagnosis and cessation of medication where possible to prevent permanent symptoms. Tertiary prevention involves treatment of severe cases to minimize disability (Gardos and Cole, 1977).
2. Cessation of neuroleptic drugs at the first sign of the development of a tardive dyskinesia is recommended if the patient's condition allows. Early cessation leads to total disappearance of symptoms in about 37% of patients (Jeste and Wyatt, 1982).
3. If a patients' conditions are such that psychotic symptoms that prevent functioning of the individuals in their environment will re-emerge on cessation of medication, another antipsychotic (preferably from a different class) or clozapine should be substituted at equivalent doses. For instance, if the patient develops a

tardive dyskinesia on 24 mg a day of perphenazine (Trilafon) substitute 6 mg a day of Navane.

4. Deanol in doses of 1600–2000 mg/day has been considered helpful in some cases.

5. There is no satisfactory current treatment for persistent tardive dyskinesia.

6. The value of cholinergic agents in the treatment of tardive dyskinesia is uncertain (Jeste and Wyatt, 1982).

7. It is generally recommended not to use anticholinergic drugs in the treatment of dyskinetic patients (Jeste and Wyatt, 1982).

8. Drug-free periods have not been found to prevent tardive dyskinesia (Jeste and Wyatt, 1982).

9. Bromocriptine (a dopamine agonist) may have some impact in managing the dystonic symptoms associated with tardive dyskinesia (Lieberman JA et al, 1989).

10. Clonazepam is somewhat effective in treatment of tardive dyskinesia. Its impact is greatest, like bromocriptine, in patients with predominantly dystonic symptoms (Thaker et al, 1990).

11. Vitamin E treatment has been found to lower AIMS scores (Elkashef et al, 1990).

12. GABA agonists have been proposed as treatment of tardive dyskinesia. Their use has been limited by their side effects and toxicity. One of the lesser toxic GABA analogs and GABA receptor agonists, tetrahydroisoxazalopyridinol (THIP) has not been found to have therapeutic efficacy. Side effects of THIP include confusion, vomiting, dizziness, sedation, and myoclonic jerks (Korssgaard et al, 1982).

13. In some instances of tardive dyskinesia, low-dose propranolol (Inderal) has a markedly inhibitory effect (Bacher and Lewis, 1980).

14. Antiparkinsonian agents tend to produce reversible increases in the severity of dyskinetic movements (Gardos and Cole, 1983).

15. Resumption of treatment with the neuroleptic that is assumed to be the pathogenic agent should be avoided where possible (Klawans HC et al, 1980).

16. Attempts must be made to continue to develop antipsychotic drugs that do not entail the risk of development of tardive dyskinesia such as clozapine.

Prevention

1. The best approach to tardive dyskinesia is to minimize occurrence by judicious use of neuroleptic medication. Only use antipsychotic medication when absolutely necessary and then only at the minimum doses required.

2. Risk is minimized by systematically monitoring side effects and reducing drug doses as soon as a patient's condition permits.

3. Information regarding tardive dyskinesia appears to be retained best when written information is supplemented by informal discussion with patients in therapy (Munetz and Roth, 1985).

4. Patient and family should be apprised of the risk and the ethical necessity to always balance continuation of patient functioning in the community and alleviation of psychic pain against the development of permanent neurologic

dysfunction, which makes both the patient and those around him feel uncomfortable.

5. Drug holidays should be given. Neuroleptic medication can usually be discontinued during weekends with a well-managed, chronically psychotic patient without return of psychotic or aggressive symptoms. Sometimes it is possible to take patients off medication 1 week each month without difficulty. The efficacy of drug holidays to avoid tardive dyskinesia at best appears minimal.

6. Switching from drugs in one class to another (e.g., butyrophenone to a thioxanthene) or from one subgroup of a class of drugs to another subgroup (e.g., aliphatic phenothiazine to a piperazine phenothiazine) is felt to decrease risk if done at relatively frequent intervals (e.g., 6 months to 1 year) in patients who are chronically psychotic.

7. There is some evidence to suggest that use of higher-dosage, lower-potency neuroleptics is associated with less risk than use of the higher-potency, lower-dosage drugs.

8. Risk of development of tardive dyskinesia with clozapine appears minimal or absent.

9. The patient and the patient's family's education regarding risk and involvement in decision making should be part of any treatment plan employing neuroleptic or any psychopharmacotherapy (Munetz, 1985).

Quality Assurance Issues

1. Is the minimal amount of neuroleptic used and for the minimal amount of time?
2. Are neuroleptics and other drugs that have the potential of producing tardive dyskinesia (e.g., amoxapine [Ascendin]) only been used for diagnostic-specific indications?
3. Is a patient evaluated for signs of tardive dyskinesia?
4. If signs of tardive dyskinesia are identified, are steps taken to reduce or reverse tardive dyskinetic changes?

Ethical/Legal Issues

1. Are patients warned of the use of tardive dyskinesia when present?
2. Are cost/benefits of neuroleptic medication discussed with patients and their families?
3. Is treatment provided for tardive dyskinesia?
4. Are illnesses that may mimic tardive dyskinesia sought out?
5. Are patients and their significant others advised of how to recognize signs of tardive dyskinesia if they emerge?

THIAZIDE DIURETIC-INDUCED DISORDERS

Thiazide diuretics may cause anergy and depression by electrolyte imbalance and, in particular, through potassium depletion. When administered together with antihypertensives known to cause depression such as bethanidine, clonidine, reserpine, methyldopa, guanethidine, and propranolol (Inderal), the cause of affective change may be mistakenly attributed to the antihypertensive (Okada, 1985).

THYROID-INDUCED DISORDERS

A number of conditions can alter thyroid metabolism resulting in a number of psychiatric symptoms due to hyper- or hypo-function.

1. Increased thyroid function is known to be associated with a panoply of psychiatric changes including depression, mania, anxiety, dementia, and psychosis.
2. Depression associated with thyrotoxicosis does not appear to be associated with an abnormal dexamethasone depression test although the sleep electroencephalogram may suggest the diagnosis of primary endogenous depression (Kronfol et al, 1982).
3. Especially severe extrapyramidal reactions have been reported in patients with thyrotoxicosis treated with haloperidol (Haldol) and fluphenazine (Prolixin) decanoate (Witschy and Redmond, 1981), suggesting that thyrotoxicosis potentializes the adverse reactions to the drugs.
4. Stress and infection can give rise to thyroid storm characterized by marked tachycardia, gastrointestinal dysfunction, hyperthermia, and a variety of neurologic and psychiatric symptoms such as overwhelming anxiety and psychomotor agitation.
5. Depressed patients who have significantly increased delta thyroid-stimulating hormone on the TRH (Thyroid Releasing Hormone) test may respond to treatment with thyroid hormone without antidepressants (Goodnick et al, 1989).
6. Triiodothyronine (T_3) enhances tricyclic antidepressant action in women and potentiates tricyclic response in some females and males found to be tricyclic resistant. T_3 potentiation may be due to the facilitory role of thyroid hormones in beta-adrenergic receptor activity (Extein and Gold, 1988).
7. In addition to mood change, hypothyroid patients may exhibit cognitive dysfunction (Haggerty et al, 1986).
8. Depressed patients with panic attacks have a greater prevalence of diminished TSH response than depressed patients without panic (Gillette et al, 1989).
9. A controlled study (Stewart DE et al, 1988) of patients with post-partum psychosis failed to identify any significant difference in thyroid functioning.
10. Patients receiving thyroid replacement therapy after thyroidectomy who experience psychiatric symptoms such as increased sadness and anxiety off medication are more likely to have histories of mood lability or affective illness (Denicoff et al, 1990).
11. Patients with a lifetime history of either agoraphobia with panic attacks or panic disorder are more likely than other patients to report histories of goiter or hyperthyroidism in themselves or their first degree relatives (Orenstein et al, 1988).

Management

1. There is a complex interaction between genetic predisposition to psychiatric disorders and alterations in thyroid functioning. Individuals with a history of psychiatric illness who have been rendered hypothyroid surgically or by illness (e.g., autoimmune thyroiditis) should be alerted to their exceptional susceptibility to development of psychiatric symptoms if they fail to take replacement therapy.
2. Routine monitoring of thyroid functioning is not indicated in otherwise healthy individuals being treated for depression with monoamine oxidase inhibitors or tricyclics or receiving neuroleptics for psychosis (Wilson and Jefferson, 1985).
3. Thyroid functioning must be carefully followed in patients on lithium. This is especially true where there is a history of thyroid disease (Wilson and Jefferson, 1985).
4. Psychiatric symptoms associated with hyperthyroidism tend to remit when excess thyroid production is treated. Hypothyroid patients tend to respond more variably but most show considerable improvement when euthyroid (Wilson and Jefferson, 1985).
5. Organic anxiety and affective disorders associated with hyperthyroidism tend to respond to antithyroid therapy without addition of psychopharmacotherapy (Kathol et al, 1986).

Quality Assurance Issues

1. Are patients with thyroid disorders or on thyroid therapy advised of the psychiatric side effects?
2. Are all patients who present psychiatrically evaluated for thyroid disorders?

Ethical/Legal Issues

1. Are patients with a history of thyroid disease or of using thyroid medication evaluated clinically, including serum levels for hypo- or hyperthyroidism?
2. Are patients with thyroid disease or on thyroid medication advised of the serum T_3 or T_4's interaction with some medications?

TRANSPLANTATION

While transplant failure in end-stage renal disease has not been found to always compromise quality of life (Binik and Devins, 1986), failure of any organ transplant does create a crisis for a patient and his or her family that may require crisis-oriented therapy or even very cautious psychopharmacotherapy if a patient is predisposed to psychiatric illness.

TRAZADONE-INDUCED DISORDERS

Trazadone (Desyrel) is a triazolepyridine compound that differs structurally from tricyclic antidepressants. Its mechanism of action is that of a serotonin agonist.

History

1. Trazadone is a drug that is considerably sedating for some people and therefore used to facilitate sleep. Otherwise, on the whole it has far fewer side effects than tricyclic antidepressants.
2. Some patients have been reported to develop delirium on the drug. The risk may be greater in bulimics (Damlouji and Ferguson, 1984).
3. At least one case of complex partial seizures has been assumed to have been induced by trazadone (Tasini, 1986).
4. Abrupt cessation of trazadone and commencement of treatment with imipramine (Tofranil) may result in mania (Haggerty and Jackson, 1985).
5. Trazadone gives rise to priapism in some men, albeit rarely, which in exceptional instances may require surgery (Scher et al, 1983).
6. A few women have been reported to experience increased libido above pre-morbid levels on the drug (Gartrell, 1986).
7. A case report was published describing complete heart block following a single dose of trazadone (Rausch et al, 1984). Single case reports are always somewhat suspect as major physical problems occur independent of a drug taken and may not relate to the psychiatric drug (in this case trazadone) but to other pathologic processes operating independently.
8. Peripheral edema with weight gain has been reported to occur without other outstanding medical illness with trazadone use which remits when the trazadone is discontinued (Barrett et al, 1988).

Management

1. Most side effects abate when trazadone is discontinued.
2. Priapism is a serious concern and the drug should be stopped rapidly if a man finds himself to be partially or fully erect on the drug without external stimulation or erotic fantasies. In extreme cases, surgical intervention is required for this problem.
3. Patients who are rapidly switched from trazadone to another drug should be carefully monitored for emergence of psychiatric symptoms such as mania.
4. Patients prescribed trazadone for bulimia should be observed to ascertain if there is any indication of an organic brain disorder and dosage lower or another drug substituted if symptoms of an acute organic mental disorder do not abate.

Quality/Assurance Issues

1. Have all men on trazadone been advised of the risk of priapism and how to recognize it?
2. Have patients on trazadone been advised of risks of driving or operating fine machinery if lethargic?
3. Has an appropriate wash-out period occurred before trazadone is provided after another antidepressant is used or before another is prescribed if necessary?

Ethical/Legal Issues

1. Is appropriate medical/surgical care provided if necessary when priapism occurs?

TRICYCLIC AND TETRACYCLINE-INDUCED DISORDERS

Tricyclics and tetracyclic antidepressants are used in the management of major depression and depression associated with bipolar disorder. In addition, they are used in selected cases for the management of panic disorder and other disorders such as anorexia nervosa and PTSD.

History

1. It is generally advisable *not* to administer tricyclic or tetracyclic antidepressants (TCAs) within 2 weeks of cessation or commencement of use of monoamine oxidase inhibitors (MAOIs). In selected cases, a tri- or tetracyclic may be given with an MAOI to patients refractory to more conventional antidepressant therapies. In one study patients with major depression given amitriptyline hydrochloride (Elavil) together with tranylcypromine (Parnate) were not found to experience a higher frequency of side-effects. No instances of hypertensive or hyperthermic crises were reported (Razani et al, 1983).
2. Tricyclic and tetracyclic antidepressants cause more anticholinergic side-effects than MAOIs.
3. Epidemiologic studies suggest that amitriptyline is associated with more sudden deaths in patients with cardiac disease than other antidepressants (Moir et al, 1972).
4. Nortriptyline at a standard dose of 150 mg/day has been found to produce serum levels within or slightly above the therapeutic window and was safe in regard to cardiovascular toxicity even in patients with pre-existing heart disease (Reed K et al, 1980).
5. All TCAs and some of the non-tricyclics such as amoxapine and maprotiline can be fatal in overdose (Glassman and Davis, 1987). The selective serotonin uptake inhibitors trazadone (Desyrel), sertraline (Zoloft), and fluoxetine (Prozac) have considerably greater margin of safety making them more desirable for use in patients who may overdose.
6. Delirium may occur in patients on TCAs particularly if they are quite young, old, or medically infirm. Disorientation, altered level of consciousness, memory impairment, confusion, dysattention, poor concentration, agitation, hallucinations, sleep disturbance and memory impairment are seen (Meador-Woodruff, 1990).
7. Myoclonus is sometimes seen in patients on TCAs (Garvey and Tollefson, 1987), which remits on discontinuation of the medication.
8. Tricyclic-induced delirium is, in some instances, an idiosyncratic phenomenon and unrelated to serum drug levels (Goodwin FW et al, 1982).
9. Tolerance has been reported to occur in some instances to the therapeutic effect of TCAs (Cohen and Baldessarini, 1985).
10. Withdrawal symptoms may occur with TCAs and tetracyclics and be mistaken for an exacerbation of the primary disorder (Lawrence, 1985).
11. Serum levels of TCAs may be increased above expected levels when neuroleptic compounds are given concomitantly (Nelson and Jatlow, 1980; Linnoila et al,

1982). Toxic or even lethal levels can result. Slowed conduction in the His–Purkinje system and ventricle due to quinidine-like effects of drugs such as imipramine (Tofranil) or desipramine (Norpramin) is a primary concern (Siris et al, 1982).

12. TCAs can be used safely in patients with cardiac pacemakers if a clinician is aware of the type of cardiac disease and the type, properties and proper functioning of the patient's pacemaker. Pulse should be monitored frequently and serial electrocardiograms obtained. Older patients should be commenced on smaller doses than younger patients and high plasma levels avoided (Alexopalos and Shamoian, 1982).

13. Tricyclic antidepressants are probably passed from serum to breast milk in a passive manner (Bader and Newman, 1980).

14. The wide range of plasma levels and toxicity of TCAs indicates that standardized measurement of plasma levels may be appropriate in routine management (Nutter and Brunswick, 1981).

15. The most common side effects reported with TCAs include orthostatic hypotension, constipation, difficulty passing urine possibly culminating in urine retention, increased appetite, weight gain, dry mouth, and sedation. Dysphoria, insomnia, agitation, and an organic mental disorder are occasional side effects.

16. While TCAs at high concentrations are undisputably associated with serious cardiac effects, patients with ventricular arrhythmias at lower serum levels may show improvement of their arrhythmias. The most common cardiac effect of TCAs is orthostatic hypotension. In patients with pre-existing bundle-branch disease, there is risk of heart block. TCAs at normal therapeutic levels have little adverse effect on left ventricular performance (Glassman and Bigger, 1981).

17. Smoking has been associated with lower plasma amitriptyline and nortriptyline levels (Linnoila et al, 1981).

18. Tinnitus (ringing in the ears), a rare side-effect of TCA use, is usually controlled by reducing drug dosage (Racy and Ward-Racy, 1980).

19. Withdrawal symptoms from TCAs include nausea, vomiting, headache, fatigue, nightmares, and, rarely, akathisia.

20. Withdrawal symptoms from TCAs have been reported that meet *DSM-III* criteria for panic anxiety (Gawin and Markoff, 1981).

21. The most frequently encountered manifestations of TCA and tetracyclic antidepressant overdose are due to the anticholinergic actions: dry mouth, retention of urine, absence of bowel sounds, mydriasis, blurring of vision, and sinus tachycardia. Toxic doses affect the CNS and produce agitation, restlessness, pressure of speech, loss of consciousness, increased tendon reflexes, and extensive plantar reflexes, twitching, and convulsions. In extreme cases of toxicity, prolonged flaccid coma is seen.

22. With a major TCA overdose the plasma levels may be elevated for several days, particularly when the poisoning has been with a tertiary amine TCA such as amitriptyline. In such instances, patients should have continuous cardiac monitoring for 5 to 6 days, particularly because death up to 6 days after TCA overdose has been attributed to arrhythmias.

Management
1. Side effects of TCAs and indica of toxicity remit with discontinuation of the drug or lower dosage.
2. If withdrawal symptoms occur, the drug should be recommenced and more gradually reduced in dosage.
3. If serious heart problems occur, consultation with a cardiologist should be provided in the emergency situation.

TOLUENE ABUSE

Chronic toluene inhalation may lead to cerebellar degeneration.

History
1. Toluene is the main ingredient in a number of glues and related volatile compounds.
2. Glue-sniffing among pre-adolescents and adolescents tends to be faddish and intermittent (Lewis JD et al, 1981).
3. Peak prevalence appears to be in 11 and 12 year-olds (Barnes GE, 1979).
4. The usual duration of use is 1 or 2 years. Rarely is use extensive enough to lead to brain damage (Lewis JD et al, 1981).

Management
1. Neurologic degeneration is non-progressive if toluene use is discontinued and reversible if use is stopped early (Lewis JD et al, 1981).

TYPEWRITER CORRECTION FLUID-INDUCED DISORDERS

Typewriter correction fluid includes the active solvents trichloroethane and trichloroethylene. Inhalation of these can provide a high within minutes. Symptoms include euphoria, incoordination, depression, and auditory and visual hallucinations. If brain damage has not already occurred, symptoms will abate upon discontinuation of the practice (Levy AB, 1986). Prolonged use or inhalation of great amounts can result in permanent cognitive impairment.

ULCERATIVE COLITIS

While the exact role of psychosocial factors in the genesis of ulcerative colitis remains uncertain (Morth et al, 1990), it is clear that like any other illness that has the potential for morbid consequences (e.g., severe blood loss, colostomy). It is a stressor for patients, their friends and families, and lovers. Mollification of illness impact on all helps to maximize the patient's ability to comply with a treatment plan and develop what may be required to live with the illness. It also allows family and friends to provide as much support as possible. Self-help groups comprised of others who suffer the illness allows patients to better learn to live with the illness and to antici- pate with solutions in mind expected problems.

VOLATILE NITRATE-INDUCED DISORDERS

Volatile nitrites such as amyl nitrite have been used for relief of angina pectoris for over a century. Alteration of mood and behavior are not unusual if sufficient amounts have been inhaled. These drugs are sometimes used recreationally, particu- larly in the gay subculture.

History
1. Amyl nitrite is sold in small thin glass capsules covered by webbing so that it can be crushed between the fingers and the fumes inhaled when a patient suffers anginal pain.
2. Volatile nitrites are sold in various "head shops," pornographic stores, novelty shops, and through mail order houses under a number of names including Poppers, Heart-On, Toilet Water, Gas Bullet, Rush, Aroma of Men, and Locker Room.
3. Sometimes nitrous oxide is taken directly from the bottle through a single or double nasal inhaler.
4. Volatile nitrites have been used extensively to expand creativity, promote aban- donment in dancing and art, and to intensify both hetero- and homosexual expe- riences.
5. As with all drug intoxication states, the clinical picture represents an interaction of the amount of drug taken, the setting, the effect of concurrent physical illness, the personality structure of the user, the expectations of the user, and the pharma- cology of the drug

Symptoms
1. Light-headedness.
2. Nausea.
3. Weakness.
4. Fluctuating levels of consciousness.
5. Disorientation.
6. Dysattention.
7. Pulsatile headaches and short-lived nitrite headaches.
8. Syncope.
9. Cutaneous flushing.

Signs
1. Ataxia.
2. Hypotension.
3. Tachycardia.

4. Transient changes on the electrocardiogram (e.g., inverted T waves and depressed S-T segments).

Management
1. Symptoms generally pass with cessation of use of volatile nitrites.

WALDENSTROM'S MACROGLOBULINEMIA

The hyperviscosity disorder associated with Waldenstrom's macroglobulinemia is associated with a number of neuropsychiatric symptoms in addition to congestive heart failure, retinopathy, and bleeding from mucosal membranes. Dementia, complex partial seizures, ataxia, vertigo, nystagmus, diplopia, abnormal gait, paresthesia, impaired hearing, and postural hypotension have been reported (Stern et al, 1985). Complex partial seizures, when they occur, respond to anticonvulsants such as carbamazepine (Tegretol). Management of the macroglobulinemia itself is medical.

WATER-INDUCED DISORDERS

Aberrations of mood, thought, and behavior can result from both excessive hydration as well as from dehydration. Dehydration can result from poor nutrition, chronic illness, and psychiatric states such as severe depression where intake is limited. Overhydration can be due to polydipsia associated with severe psychosis further enhancing severity of symptoms. Self-induced water intoxication is almost exclusively seen in psychiatric patients (Jos et al, 1986).

Symptoms seen with water intoxication include muscle tremor, ataxia, twitching, diarrhea, restlessness, convulsions with frothing at the mouth, vomiting, asthenia, polyuria, salivation, frequent urination, retching, helplessness, stupor, and coma (Jos et al, 1986). In order for individuals to become water intoxicated, their intake must exceed their ability to excrete it (Berl, 1988).

Management
1. Management of psychogenic polydipsia is that of the primary psychiatric disorder.

WERNICKE'S ENCEPHALOPATHY

Wernicke's encephalopathy, regardless of etiology, presents with paralysis of the extraocular muscles, disturbances of consciousness, and ataxia.

History
1. While usually associated with chronic heavy alcoholic use, Wernicke's encephalopathy is also seen with nutritional deficiencies, intestinal carcinomas with vomiting, pernicious anemia, and with pernicious vomiting of pregnancy.

2. It is usually seen in young or middle-aged females but has been reported in adolescent women (Turner et al, 1989).
3. It is due to a deficiency of thiamine.

Symptoms
1. Loss of appetite.
2. Nausea.
3. Vomiting.
4. Delirium.
5. Excitement.
6. Insomnia.
7. Giddiness.
8. Confabulation.
9. Apathy.
10. Apprehension.
11. Diplopia.
12. Photophobia.
13. Tremor.
14. Memory loss for recent events.
15. Intellectual deterioration.
16. Mild confusion.
17. Disorientation.
18. Hallucinations.

Signs
1. Ophthalmoplegia.
2. Clouding of consciousness.
3. Nystagmus.
4. Ataxia.
5. External rectus palsy.
6. Loss of visual acuity.
7. Coma.
8. Ptosis.
9. Spasticity.
10. Pupillary abnormalities.
11. Polyneuritis.
12. Papilledema.
13. Seizures.
14. Hypotension.
15. Other signs of chronic heavy alcohol use, such as evidence of liver damage and anemia.

Management
1. The cerebral changes seen with thiamine deficiency rapidly become irreversible.

Therefore, 100 mg of thiamine should be given intramuscularly in the emergency room to all alcoholic patients.

2. Patients should be placed at bed rest and withdrawn from alcohol.

3. High caloric diet with vitamin supplements is prescribed.

4. A rehabilitation program should be started to maximize remaining muscular potential.

WILSON'S DISEASE

Ten to fifty percent of patients with Wilson's disease (hepatolenticular degeneration) present with psychiatric symptoms prior to the onset of other clinical manifestations such as hepatic insufficiency and hemolytic anemia (Dening and Berrios, 1989; Chung et al, 1986). The changes seen are due to progressive accumulation of copper in the brain and other body tissues. This uncommon familial disease is inherited as an autosomal recessive trait most frequently by children of consanguineous marriages. Behavioral changes reported include anxiety, depression, bizarre behavior, hysterical-like symptoms, adjustment problems, personality changes, and cognitive impairment (Dening and Berrios, 1989). The psychiatric symptoms appear to have a neurologic rather than hepatic basis. Management consists of treatment of the primary deficiency in copper metabolism and symptom-specific psychopharmacotherapy of behavior changes (e.g., antidepressants for depression).

Burn Out | 6

When excessive demands are placed on individuals' energy, strength, or resources, they wear out or become exhausted (Sluyter, 1985). This situation is called burn-out (Beemsterboer and Baum, 1984). It is the occupational hazard of crisis psychiatric clinicians and other health professionals who must work with all pores open picking up and responding to nuances of patients' feelings and to the cruel realities of some peoples' lives. Unless mental health professionals learn early in their careers how to counter this, therapists of potentially great talent are lost as they become inured to the great, sometimes magnificent and at other times painful, varieties of the human experience. The impact of stress, and therefore risk of burn-out, is greatest when many deaths are seen such as in the work of those caring for AIDS and cancer patients and in other critical care areas (Price and Murphy, 1985).

SYMPTOMS

1. Loss of charisma.
2. Doubting ability to lead and to heal.
3. Irritability.
4. Dread of going to "work."
5. Exhaustion.
6. Depression.
7. Cynicism.
8. Self-disgust.
9. Disillusionment.
10. Anger.
11. Paranoia (e.g., fear someone will take your territory away if you are not careful).
12. Sense of isolation.
13. Hyperexcitability (everything appears to be a crisis).
14. Headache.
15. Indigestion.
16. Dread of organization.
17. Free-floating anxiety.
18. Undirected energy.
19. Apathy.
20. Emptiness.
21. Confusion.
22. Loss of innovativeness and creativity.

23. Difficulty prioritizing activities.
24. Negative job attitude.
25. Negative self-image.
26. Loss of concern and feeling for clients.

SIGNS

1. Tearfulness.
2. Ridicule of patients and other professionals.
3. Defensiveness (to keep people away from seeing how burnt out one is).
4. Absenteeism (increased number of sick-leave days taken).
5. Sleeplessness.
6. Diarrhea.
7. Increase in patient drop-out rate.
8. Canceling conferences capriciously.
9. Declining appearance of self and work area.
10. Inability to express oneself in writing and words.
11. Not keeping up with paperwork or reading in one's field.
12. Histrionic responses to relatively minor stresses.
13. More time spent talking with other employees than in patient care directed activity.
14. Decreasing effectiveness at job.
15. Inability to make decisions.
16. Impairment of judgement.
17. Fault-finding in others and self.
18. Detached concern.
19. Intellectualization.
20. Withdrawal.
21. Compartmentalization.

CAUSES

A number of researchers (Pines and Maslach, 1978); Sluyter 1985; Price and Murphy, 1985) have identified specific factors that contribute to burn-out in individuals working in health care and specifically in critical care specialities. These include the following:

Unresolved Grief

The more caregivers must work with suicidal individuals, the terminally ill, and those who suffer sexual, physical, and psychological abuse, the greater the burnout. It takes a toll on people to empathize with the pain of victims and feel the hurt of seeing many people suffer whom they wish they could provide more than is humanly possible.

Working With the Chronically Mentally Ill

The greater the time spent working with the chronically mentally ill, the greater the burn-out.

Lack of Opportunity to Ventilate

If an abscess is not lanced, it may eat away at muscle and bone and a person may die of blood poisoning. So too, if a person does not talk about the painful realities he or she must confront daily, that person will burn-out. Emotion becomes blunted and a person irritable in an attempt, albeit unconsciously, to defend against constant trauma to their psychic integrity.

Lack of Continuing Education

Lack of continuing education with opportunities to share approaches to problems encountered and to network with others who may serve both as consultants and as mentors or facilitators to one's professional growth leads to burn-out.

Lack of Social Support

Crisis workers need social support both at work and in their personal life to prevent burnout. If both their personal world and their professional life is constant confrontation with crises, they burn out.

The Need to Not Fail

Crisis clinicians are not gods. Sometimes even the best treatment plan fails and, in the extreme, a patient may commit suicide if a depression proves refractory to treatment. Having the "Jehovah complex" (feeling one will never fail in treatment) contributes to burn-out.

Time Spent in Administrative Tasks

While good record keeping is essential to good patient care, when time spent in paper work approaches or exceeds time spent in patient care, a clinician becomes cynical. Cynicism is an indicant of burn-out.

Lack of Sense of Humor

Oscar Wilde once said that life is far too important to take seriously. Crisis clinicians without a sense of humor find no relief from the stresses of their work crises or home difficulties. We must be able to find humor in life to assuage some of the pain that leads to burn-out.

Lack of Response of Leadership to Crisis Workers' Needs

A lack of those in charge of providing resources including staff appropriate to demands and reasonable working conditions and praise for work well done leads to burn-out.

Staff–Patient Ratio

The greater the number of staff to provide clinical service and the greater the variety of services offered, the less the burden on any one person to be all things to everyone and the less burn-out.

Patient Mix

Staff burn-out is reduced by seeing higher-functioning patients with personal growth issues involving marital and career choices in addition to patients who are chronically psychiatrically ill or in crisis.

Recreational Time

Individuals who schedule relaxation into their work schedules (e.g., meditation time or time to jog, to visit art museums, or to read) or plan time reserved to be with their best of friends, experience less burn-out.

Limiting Staff Meetings

The more crisis clinicians feel other time is intruded upon by redundant or irrelevant staff meetings (as opposed to clinical case conferences, continuing educational activities, or treatment planning meetings), the greater the staff burn-out.

Time in Service

Those who have spent more years in the field without change in responsibilities or location tend to show more burn-out.

Affiliation with Educational or Research Institutions

Individuals working in institutions where there is active research or dynamic educational programs burn out less.

Position in Institution

Those individuals who have more control over obtaining their resources including space, travel opportunities for continuing education, and staff burn out less. If, however, advance in rank entails more time in administration meetings, burn-out increases.

Work Hours

The longer the work hours, the greater the burn-out.

Education

The greater the professional preparation for the task assigned, the less the anxiety attendant to performance of the task and the less burn-out.

MANAGEMENT

1. The most effective way to prevent burn-out is to cultivate the texture of both the

peoplescape and landscape. Too little attention is paid in training to how important it is for those who must daily face the vicissitudes of physical and mental health and illness to surround themselves with people who provide "soft landings" and a physical environment that challenges their sensitivity to art, literature, nature, and music. We, just like our patients, need to ventilate, to lance psychological abscesses so that work stressors do not eat away at the essential core of our being. Each day must be fresh and each patient, like each new person we meet, must be seen as and made to feel special. Art, music, nature, and literature challenge us to be that which we all could be were it not for the layering of defenses against the realities of our molecular experiences. Art and nature have ways of getting at the core of our being in ways more intellectualized approaches do not. We relax, we laugh, and we cry as we savor texture and form and feel real substance. Our defenses come down as we are polite to others and they, in turn, are courteous to us.

2. Psychiatric clinicians should see a variety of patients. Clinicians become particularly burnt out when they see only one type of patient, especially if patients are chronic or in need of critical care. Patient loads should be mixed to prevent burn-out and to help clinicians maintain a fresh approach to each patient. Those who see terminally ill or demented patients should also see some who have better prognoses.

3. Staff should be hired carefully. Individuals may come well credentialed but show, before commencing their new job, the insidious signs of burn-out such as apathy, overinvolvement with administrative minutia, by history, and by lack of innovativeness and creativity in their previous work.

4. Supervisors should get to know their staff as individuals and help each one develop a sense of specialness. It is good that staff members who have special interests such as alcoholism, work with gay and bisexual populations, ethnic groups with special needs, spouse abuse, or work with adolescents be identified. These individuals should be encouraged to read, spend clinical time, and attend conferences and other teaching exercises in their area of interest. In addition, particularly talented clinicians should provide other staff members with case conferences and seminars in their area of expertise and if possible write on their specialities for the popular press as well as scholarly journals.

5. Social support assauges stresses at work and at home. Research (Etzion, 1984) indicates that those with greater social support to mollify the inevitable stresses of crisis care or home life do better and experience less burn-out and disaffection with work. Men and women show an interesting difference in what particular social support impacts most. For men social support at work is critical; for women, support in their personal nonwork life is critical.

6. Changing the function of staff meetings reduces burn-out (Pines and Maslach, 1978). Change challenges. Paradigms that have proven effective in the past are not always relevant to present needs. If changing priorities dictate that forums are required for discussion of new needs and that old topics or format are either irrelevant or redundant, meetings that are no longer required should be discontinued, and new ones evolve that have firm and limited time frames for new issues.

7. Clinicians do better who periodically have a break from patient care. Universities and some businesses have instituted sabbaticals for this purpose. Opportunities for temporary withdrawal from patient care reduces burn-out, irritability, cynicism about work, and negative views of psychiatric illness and patients (Pines and Maslach, 1978).

8. Responsibilities should be rotated. Dealing with crisis patients is exhausting and must be a shared responsibility of all staff. The artificial separation between staff treating emergency patients and those working with inpatients and outpatients leads to burn-out and decreased creativity in both groups. Responsibility for all types of patients should be shared and rotated both to prevent burn-out as well as fatigue due to overwork. Staff members working with the more seriously ill patients tend to burn-out more rapidly.

9. People should not continue to work too long in areas that they have mastered. The lack of challenge leads to a stereotyping of both other staff and patients that is destructive to an organization and to staff. Individuals need to be challenged to grow and must sometimes move out of a high-ranking position of leadership to allow someone newer with fresh enthusiasm and innovative ideas to take an organization through its next phase of growth.

10. Minimize administrative meetings. Staff burn-out is related to the number of administrative meetings attended. Administrative meetings should be short in duration and goal-directed. They should not exceed 1 hour. Group psychotherapy is not a function of a staff meeting and long discussions over anger can lead to greater frustration and a greater sense of helplessness. One cannot get at core individual staff problems in a group and flirtation at the edge creates a sense of unfilled expectancy rather than therapeutic ventilation.

11. Patient–staff ratio should be low enough so that the staff may approach each patient with renewed optimism and individualized care. The greater the number of patients a staff member sees, the greater the sensory overload, and the more rapidly burn-out develops.

12. Work hours, especially in emergency psychiatry and crisis intervention, should be kept sufficiently low to prevent sleep deprivation and the attendant irritability, anger, and lack of enthusiasm that comes from overwork.

13. Periodic staff retreats should be undertaken to review goals and increase the feeling of support and purpose among staff. Humanistic goals can become obfuscated when we do not step back to see the toll taken on even the most sensitive and idealistic clinician when repeatedly confronted with the realities of human pain and the limitations of the human experience. It is imperative for successful crisis work that the clinician's eyes be set on finding strengths and bringing out human potential rather than focusing in on "psychopathology" and "illness."

14. Both staff and an institution must build in programs of continuing education to keep staff abreast of changes in the field and to review basic principles of evaluation and treatment.

15. Staff must be adequately supervised. This allows both a monitoring of quality of care as well as an opportunity to ventilate anxiety over carrying suicidal and homicidal patients, psychotic patients, patients with diagnostic problems, and

chronic patients who frustrate clinicians' desire to see evidence of great change over time. Supervision should be a time of support, education, and quality control.

16. The best approach to burn-out is primarily prevention using such techniques as continuing education, supervision, rotation of duties, and minimizing administrative meetings. When, despite these approaches, the early symptoms of burn-out (such as irritability, increased absenteeism, and discourtesy to staff and patients) occur, the staff members should be called aside by a supervisor and placed elsewhere in the institutional setting, either temporarily or permanently, to allow some renewal and re-evaluation of where they are going and of their goals as mental health professionals.

QUALITY ASSURANCE ISSUES

1. Are a certain number of continuing education credits required of staff members annually for reprivileging?
2. Is a staff member's formal education and previous training commensurate with that required for their specific tasks (e.g., substance abuse training for those who work with chemically dependent patients, training in minority or gay issues to work with minority or gay groups)?
3. Do staff members take vacation time?
4. Are staff members' work schedules consistent with that which allows best patient care?
5. Are staff members' performance reviewed for early indices of burn-out?
6. Are staff members' patient loads and other tasks varied?
7. Are staff members with specific skills rewarded and acknowledged?
8. Are meetings limited in time to that which is needed and are they relevant to current needs and priorities?
9. Is the work environment attractive?

Disaster Planning | 7

A disaster is defined by the Disaster Relief Act of 1974 as a hurricane, tornado, storm flood, high-water, wind-driven water, tidal wave, tsunami, earthquake, volcanic eruption, landslide, snowstorm, fire, or other catastrophic occurrence that causes damage of sufficient severity and magnitude to warrant disaster assistance. In summary, a disaster appears, by the definition, to be any situation that creates such widespread suffering and needs that victims cannot alleviate without assistance beyond personal resources.

MANAGEMENT

1. Planning for a disaster is an especially difficult task. Expertise in crisis intervention comes from training under those skilled in the field supplemented by practical experiences. The patient is always the best teacher. Comparably, expertise in management of disasters comes from both training under those who have been involved in disaster themselves and by field experience in a disaster. Unfortunately (or perhaps fortunately) there are few who have such training in actual disasters because disasters are rare events. A disaster is simply not a multi-car accident or a house burning with three families in it. It may involve whole communities, townships, or even countries as in a hurricane in the Caribbean Isle of Dominica where nearly 90% of the property may be destroyed in a single storm or the riots in Los Angeles following the Rodney King decision. In instances where a disaster is more circumscribed, it may involve unfathomable human carnage such as in the famous Coconut Grove Nightclub fire in Boston in the early 1940s, the Kentucky supper club fire outside of Cincinnati, or the aircrash over San Diego in 1978. In the latter instance, the problem is not the lack of skills in physical or psychological medicine, but rather that the task has elements that counter all we are taught in the management of more specific individual crises.
2. In the management of a simple crisis such as sudden death of a loved one or a rape, we are called upon to be empathetic, sensitive, and supportive. We ride the tide of feeling and listen with all our pores open to hear nuances of words and subtle distinctions of feeling. In a large disaster mental health clinicians are called upon to undertake tasks for which they have had no preparation and which they have never even imagined themselves doing. Following a large fire involving the death of over 100 people, they may be called upon to guide relatives and friends seeking someone who did not return home the night before who was reported to have been in the building that burned. The psychiatric clinician may

have to view over 100 charred bodies with the relative before a ring on a charred hand or a scar or tattoo on a part of the chest not burned provides a clue to the identity of the victim. Caregivers as well as friends and relatives of victims need support and time for ventilation in disaster work. Burn-out may occur over months or years in crisis work. In disaster work, it can occur over hours.

3. Disasters provide, even for those accustomed to seeing mutilated bodies and human violence, unprecedented tests to our fears of unexpected destruction and helplessness against the forces of nature or man (as in the explosion of a nuclear bomb, a nuclear reactor accident, or terrorist attack).

4. In disasters with great loss of life and mutilation of bodies, sensitive-feeling psychotherapists may become a psychological casualty as will many sensitive firemen, policemen, clergy, and other health professionals who empathize with the pain of the survivors and feel their own vulnerability and helplessness anew again and again as each new victim is found. The task of collecting fragmented body parts on a hot humid afternoon after an airplane crash over a city tests human limits. Those who handle it best are often those who do not think about the nuances and do not empathize with the horror of victim and survivor. This is just the opposite of who serves best in most other crisis intervention work.

5. There are a number of studies of disasters of varying epidemiologic sophistication that have contributed to our understanding of what must be included in the psychosocial component of specific disaster plans if they are to meet the needs of those affected and prevent or minimize long-term impairment. These studies have included research on the reactions of psychiatric patients to the Three Mile Island Nuclear Accident (Bromet et al, 1978), on the response of children to a severe winter snowstorm (Burke JD et al, 1982), the impact of the collapse of a dam holding coal wastes in Buffalo Creek, West Virginia, on the inhabitants of the area (Newman, 1976; Erikson KT, 1976), the effect of the Belfast riots (Lyons HA, 1971), the response of a Kibbutz civilian population under war stress (Kaffman, 1977; Ziv and Israeli, 1973; Milgram and Milgram, 1976), and the response of caregivers to recovering and identifying human remains of a religious cult in Jamestown, Guyana in 1978 (Jones DR, 1985). In the study of the reaction of psychiatric patients to the Three Mile Island Nuclear Accident by Bromet et al (1978), patients who were least distressed were those with the greatest network of social support and those who did not continue to view Three Mile Island as dangerous. Disaster did not significantly increase the abnormalities of the psychiatric patient population. The subgroups of children who were at higher risk for behavioral problems following the severe snowstorm studied by Burke et al (1982) included more boys (whose anxiety scores increased from prestorm levels) and children accepted for Head Start because their parents felt they had special needs (whose aggressive conduct scores increased). Burke's study indicated that parents tend to deny their childrens' problems, a finding corroborated by other studies of parents and children after natural disaster (Penick et al, 1976). The Airforce personnel (Jones, 1985) involved in identifying the nearly 1000 people in the mass murder/suicide in Guyana showed more dysphoria especially if they were under 25, enlisted men, black, or had great exposure to the bodies

STEPS IN DEVELOPMENT OF THE PSYCHOSOCIAL
COMPONENT OF A DISASTER PLAN

The steps in the development of the psychosocial component of a disaster plan include:

Enumeration of all the Possible Disasters That May Occur in the Area

Snowstorms are usual in New England, but rare or unheard of in parts of California, while tidal waves and earthquakes are less unusual. Plane crashes and large fires could occur in both places. Explosion of nuclear reactors is limited to those areas where nuclear energy sources have been constructed. Each disaster has its own characteristics and requires specific planning for both the psychosocial and medical component of a disaster assistance program. Floods entail great property loss in a given community. Crisis intervention work focuses around unexpected loss, usually of property, rarely of life, and recruitment of physical, psychological, social, and spiritual strength to go on and begin anew from what little may remain. Disaster work for a large airplane crash may entail working with caregivers, rather than relatives of victims, as victims may be from a number of cities both here and abroad and, other than during the brief period entailed in claiming a body, the victim's relatives will need support at home in their own communities. Caregivers may, however, be overcome by the horror of human carnage and the feeling of the transience of life and man's helplessness. Psychiatric clinicians can play critical roles in structuring time schedules allowing adequate rest and nutrition and ventilation for caregivers. An important part of a disaster assistance program is the secondary prevention of psychiatric illness by early recognition of those who may become psychiatric casualties and their prompt removal from the scene of action.

Individuals Should be Screened for Work on Disaster Teams

In the time of a major disaster, casualties due to an oversensitivity to the horror of the reality compound the work of disaster assistance teams. Well meaning individuals may volunteer but will not be able to be used in the task because they would decompensate. There are a number of films available that are used to train people in disaster assistance that are helpful in making the choice of who may best serve. In addition, some work in a large city riding shift with a police officer takes an individual into contact with serious injury and death in automobile accidents. This will, in a small degree, prepare the individual for the reality of death and bodily mutilation seen in large airplane crashes and chemical explosions.

An Individual Should Be Identified to Coordinate the Psychosocial
Aspect of a Disaster Assistance Program

It is important to have several people identified so that if one or more leadership people are not available at the time of an unexpected disaster, or lost as a victim, another may take leadership. On-call lists with all telephone numbers included (both listed and unlisted) must be in the hands of all leadership people. A clear administrative chain of command and alertness is essential for success of a disaster assistance program.

Mock Disaster Assistance Programs Should Be Held to Test Out Flaws in the Organization and Delivery of Medical and Psychosocial Services

A plan may look good on paper, but delays in arrival of staff or unavailability may be unanticipated. A mock disaster allows one to work out logistic problems. Unfortunately, the exercise usually does not sufficiently engender emotion to test the strength of team members to function in a disaster when flooded with unexpected emotion.

Assistance to Disaster Victims and to Casualties Among the Caregivers Should Be of a Crisis-Oriented Nature

There are certain sample crisis principles that are essential for effective delivery of the psychosocial component of a disaster assistance plan:

1. Individual strengths rather than liability should be brought into focus.
2. Treatment should be given as near to the front lines as possible to reduce the potential for regression, dependency, and guilt.
3. False assurances about loss of life or property or about extent of injuries should not be given.
4. Victims and families should be reunited as soon as possible.
5. Ventilation about the horror of the experience should be encouraged in a warm supportive atmosphere, either with the psychiatric clinician alone or in groups with other victims.
6. Use drugs sparingly as they may delay working through of pent-up emotion.
7. Help victims realistically face the extent of the disaster and its effect on their life.
8. Help individuals plan, given resources present, for what they must do over the ensuing days. This may include burying loved ones and finding shelter, food, and medical assistance (e.g., diabetics needing insulin).
9. Information should be disseminated regarding the extent and severity of the disaster. This information should be updated as needed.
10. Victims who can still function should be encouraged to join in the task of reconstruction.
11. Shelter and food should be found for victims, if needed, with families, neighbors, or with available social agencies in their own or neighboring community.
12. Patients should be provided with the expectation of recovery from the psychological crisis. Even though they may be flooded with anxiety, guilt, depression, anger, panic, and shame for having survived, they should be helped to see it as but a moment in time. It, as other great sorrows and stresses, will pass (even though at the moment the impact may be so predominant that they can see no tomorrow).
13. Community resources should be used rather than creating new ones. Crisis is a time for allowing individuals to find ways of coping within themselves that they

may have had no idea existed before. So too, communities should be encouraged to find undiscovered resources as well as to discover new ways of using extant resources to manage crisis on a community level.

14. Records of individual contacts should be developed to coordinate and document services so that individuals may be referred for continued treatment if needed.

15. Physical facilities should be identified if hospitalization is needed as well as other shelters for the care of victims and their relatives.

16. Psychiatric clinicians and other caregivers should be appropriately identified by badges, armbands, or other means.

17. Care should be provided for caregivers. We do not need to compound tragedy with tragedy. Food, shelter, and sleep are needed, as is careful evaluation and re-evaluation to assure that the caregiver does not become part of the toll. The coordinator of the psychosocial component of the disaster assistance program should set clear time boundaries on all staff to prevent burnout and to maintain high-quality assistance.

18. Always, a crisis is a time for value reassessment. Even in the worst of disasters it is possible to come out of the experience richer for the stress. Individuals who can find a "why" to live will be able to find a "how" to survive. We should help individuals at a time of disaster to find the "why," either in terms of human relationships or in terms of longer altruistic or spiritual goals.

Bibliography

A Treatment Manual for Acute Drug Abuse Emergencies, PG Bourne, ed. Rockville, Md., National Clearinghouse for Drug Abuse Information, National Institute in Drug Abuse, NCDAI Publication, November 16, 1974.

Aagaard, J; Vestergaard, P: Predictors of outcome in prophylactic lithium treatment: A 2-year prospective study. *J Affective Disord,* 18:259–266, 1990.

Abel, GG; Barlow, DH; Blanchard, EB; et al: The components of rapists' sexual arousal. *Arch Gen Psychiatry,* 34:895–903, 1977.

Abernethy, DR; Greenblatt, DJ; Divoll, M; et al: Impairment of diazepam metabolism by low-dose estrogen-containing oral-contraceptive steroids. *N Engl J Med,* 306:791–792, 1982.

Abou-Saleh, MT; Coppen, AJ: Acute treatment, long-term management, and prophylaxis of affective disorders. *Psychiatric Annals,* 17:301–308, 1987.

Abraham, HD: L-5 Hydroxytryptophan for LSD-induced psychosis. Am J Psychiatry, 140:456–458, 1983

Abram, HS; Moore, GL; Westervelt, FB: Suicidal behavior in chronic dialysis patients. *Am J Psychiatry,* 172:1199–1204, 1971.

Abrams, R; Taylor, MA: The genetics of schizophrenia: A reassessment using modern criteria. *Am J Psychiatry,* 140:171–175, 1983.

Abrams, R; Taylor, MA; Faber, R: Bilateral versus unilateral electroconvulsive therapy: Efficacy in melancholia. *Am J Psychiatry,* 140:463–465, 1983.

Achenheil, M; Clozapine-pharmacokinetic investigations and biochemical effects in men. *Psychopharmacology,* 99:S32–S37, 1989.

Achte, K: Depression and suicide. *Psychopathology,* 19:210–214, 1986.

Achte, K: Suicidal tendencies in the elderly. *Suicide and Life-Threatening Behavior,* 18:55–64, 1988.

Adams, F; Fernandez, F; Andersson, B: Emergency pharmacotherapy of delirium in the critically ill cancer patient. *Psychosomatics,* 27:33–37, 1986.

Addington v. Texas, U.S., 47 *L.W.* 4473 (April 30, 1979).

Addonizio, G; Susman, VL; Roth, SD; Neuroleptic malignant syndrome: Review and analysis of 115 cases. *Biol Psychiatry,* 22:1004–1020, 1987.

Addonizio, G; Susman, VL; Roth, SD: Symptoms of neuroleptic malignant syndrome in 82 consecutive inpatients. *Am J Psychiatry,* 143:1587–1590, 1986.

Aden v. Younger, 57 Cal. App. 3d 662, 129 *Cal Rptr* 535 (1976).

Adler LE; Angrist, B; Peselow, E; Corwin, J; et al: Efficacy of propranolol in neuroleptic-induced akathisia. *J Clin Psychopharmacol,* 5:164–166, 1985.

Adler, LE; Bell, J; Kirch, D; et al: Psychosis associated with clonidine withdrawal. *Am J Psychiatry,* 139:110–112, 1982.

Adler, Le; Sadja, L; Wilets, G: Cimetidine toxicity manifested as paranoia and hallucinations. *Am J Psychiatry,* 1367:1112–1113, 1980.

Agle, D; Gluck, H; Pierce, G: The risk of AIDS: Psychologic impact on the hemophilic population. *Gen Hosp Psychiatry,* 9:11–17, 1987.

ALI Model Penal Case, (1955) Section 4.01 (1) (Tent. Draft No. 4).

Alarcon, RD; Thweatt, RW: A case of subdural hematoma mimicking severe depression with conversion-like symptoms. *Am J Psychiatry,* 140:1360–1361, 1983.

Albert, RE; Shore, RE; Sayers, AJ; et al: Follow-up of children over-exposed to lead. *Environ Health Perspect,* 7:33–39, 1974.

Alessi, NE; Magen, J: Panic disorder in psychiatrically hospitalized children. *Am J Psychiatry,* 145:1450–1452, 1988.

Alessi, NE; McManus, M; Brickman, A; Grapetine, L: Suicidal behavior among serious juvenile offenders. *Am J Psychiatry*, 141:286–287, 1984.

Alexander, DA: Bereavement and the management of grief. *Br J Psychiatry*, 153:860–864, 1988.

Alexander, PE; Alexander, DD: Alprazolam treatment for panic disorders. *J Clin Psychiatry*, 47:301–304, 1986.

Alexopoulos, GS; Frances, RJ: ECT and cardiac patients with pacemakers. *Am J Psychiatry*, 137:1111–1112, 1980.

Allebeck P; Wistedt, B: Mortality in schizophrenia: A ten-year follow-up based on the Stockholm County inpatient register. *Arch Gen Psychiatry*, 43:650–653, 1986.

Allen, AM; Moore, M; Daly, BB: Subdural hemorrhage in patients with mental disease. *N Engl J Med* 223:324–329, 1940.

Allen, IM: Posttraumatic stress disorder among black Vietnam Veterans. *Hospital and Community Psychiatry*, 37:55–61, 1986.

Allen, JC: Rosen, G: Transient cerebral dysfunction following chemotherapy for osteogenic sarcoma. *Am Neurol*, 3:441–444, 1978.

Allen, MD; Greenblatt, DJ; Noel, BJ: Overdosage with antipsychotic agents. *Am J Psychiatry*, 137:234–236, 1980.

Allen, RM; Young, SJ: Phencyclidine-induced psychosis. *Am J Psychiatry*, 135:1081–1084, 1978.

Altshuler, LL; Cummings, JL; Mills, MJ: Mutism: Review, differential diagnosis, and report of 22 cases. *Am J Psychiatry*, 143:1409–1414, 1986.

American Bar Association, Commission of the Mentally Disabled: Mental Disability. *Law Reporter*, 2:337–354, September–December, 1977.

Amsterdam, JD; Henle, W; Winokur, A; Wolkowitz, OM; et al: Serum antibodies to Epstein-Barr virus in patients with major depressive disorder. *Am J Psychiatry*, 143:1593–1596, 1986.

Amsterdam, JD; Winokur, A; Lucki, I; et al: A neuroendocrine test battery in bipolar patients and healthy subjects. *Arch Gen Psychiatry*, 40:515–521, 1983.

Ananth, J: Antiasthmatic effect of amitriptyline. *CMA Journal*, 110:1131, 1974.

Ananth, J; Edelmuth, E; Dargan, B: Meige's syndrome associated with neuroleptic treatment. *Am J Psychiatry*, 145:513–515, 1988.

Ananth, J; Kaur, A; Djenederdjian, AH: Simultaneous folie a deux and Capgras syndrome. *Psychiatr J Univ Ottawa*, 15:41–43, 1990.

Ananth, J; Solyom, L; Bryntwick, S; Krishnappa, U: Chlorimipramine therapy for obsessive-compulsive neurosis. *Am J Psychiatry*, 136:700–701, 1979.

Anderson, DJ; Noyes, R; Crowe, RR: A comparison of panic disorder and generalized anxiety disorder. *Am J Psychiatry*, 141:572–575, 1984.

Andersen, H; Kristiansen, ES: Tofranil treatment of endogenous depression. *Acta Psychiatric Neurol Scand*, 34:387–397, 1959.

Andersen, SM; Horthorn, BH: Changing the psychiatric knowledge of primary care physicians: The effects of a brief intervention on clinical diagnosis and treatment. *Gen Hosp Psychiatry*, 12:177–190, 1990.

Andersen, WH; Kuehnle, JC: Strategies for the treatment of acute psychosis. *JAMA*, 229:1884, 1974.

Anderson, A; Ghali, AY; Bansil, RK: Weapon carrying among patients in a psychiatric emergency room. *Hospital and Community Psychiatry*, 40:845–847, 1989.

Andreasen, NC: The American concept of schizophrenia. *Schizophrenia Bulletin*, 16:519–831, 1989.

Andreasen, NC: Negative symptoms in schizophrenia: Definition and reliability. *Arch Gen Psychiatry*, 39:789–794, 1982.

Andreasen, NC; Rice, J; Endicott, J; Reich, T; et al: The family history approach to diagnosis: How useful is it? *Arch Gen Psychiatry*, 43:421–429, 1986.

Andreasen, NC; Swayze, V; Haun, M; et al: Ventricular abnormalities in affective disorder: clinical and demographic correlates. *Am J Psychiatry*, 147:893–900, 1990.

Andreasen, NC; Wasek, P: Adjustment disorders in adolescents and adults. *Arch Gen Psychiatry*, 37:1166–1170, 1980.

Andreasen, NC; Winokur, G: Secondary depression: Familial, clinical, and research perspectives. *Am J Psychiatry*, 136:62–66, 1979.

Andrulonis, PA; Donnelly, J; Glueck, BC; et al: Preliminary data on ethosuximide and the episodic dyscontrol syndrome. *Am J Psychiatry,* 137:1455–1456, 1980.

Angle, C; O'Brien, T; McIntire, M: Adolescent self-poisoning: A nine-year follow-up. *J Develop Behav Ped,* 4:83–87, 1983.

Angold, A: Childhood and adolescent depression: I. Epidemiological and aetiological aspects. *Br J Psychiatry,* 152:601–617, 1988.

Appelbaum, PS: The right to refuse treatment with antipsychotic medications: Retrospect and prospect. *Am J Psychiatry,* 145:413–419, 1988.

Appelbaum, PS; Jackson, AJ; Shoder, RI: Psychiatrists' responses to violence: pharmacologic management of psychiatric inpatients. *Am J Psychiatry,* 140:301–304, 1983.

Appels, A: Mental precursors of myocardial infarction. *Br J Psychiatry,* 156:465–471, 1990.

Appenheim, G: Drug-induced rapid cycling: Possible outcomes and management. *Am J Psychiatry,* 139:939–941, 1982.

Apter, A; Plutchik, R; Sevy, S; Korn, M; et al: Defense mechanisms in risk of suicide and risk of violence. *Am J Psychiatry,* 146:1027–1031, 1989.

Aquilera, DC; Messick, JM; Farrell, MS: *Crisis Intervention: Theory and Methodology.* St. Louis, CV Mosby, 1970.

Arana, JD: Characteristics of homeless mentally ill inpatients. *Hospital and Community Psychiatry,* 41:674–676, 1990.

Arana, GW; Goff, DC; Baldessarini, RJ; Keepers, GA: Efficacy of anticholinergic prophylaxis for neuroleptic-induced acute dystonia. *Am J Psychiatry,* 145:993–996, 1988.

Arana, GW; Barreira, PJ; Cohen, BM; Lipinski, JF; et al: The dexamethasone suppresssion test in psychotic disorders. *Am J Psychiatry,* 140:1521–1523, 1983.

Arcuni, OJ; Asaad, G: Voluntary and involuntary schizophrenic patient admissions on the same general hospital psychiatric unit. *Gen Hosp Psychiatry,* 11:393–396, 1989.

Arnold, LE; Christopher, J; Huestis, R; et al: Methylphenidate vs. dextroamphetamine vs. caffeine in minimal brain dysfunction: Controlled comparison for placebo workout design with Bayes' Analysis. *Arch Gen Psychiatry,* 35:463–473, 1978.

Arnold, WH: *The Techniques of Withdrawal of Opiates and Barbiturate-Sedatives.* Mimeo; Lexington, Kentucky, 1961.

Aronowitz, R: Civil commitment of narcotics addicts. *Columbia L Rev,* 67:405, 1967.

Aronson, TA; Shukla, S: Life events and relapse in bipolar disorder: The impact of a catastrophic event. *Acta Psychiatr Scand,* 75:571–576, 1987.

Arora, RC; Meltzer, HY: Serotonergic measures in the brains of suicide victims: 5-HT2 binding sites in the frontal cortex of suicide victims and control subjects. *Am J Psychiatry,* 146:730–736, 1989.

Asarnow, JR; Carlson, G: Suicide attempts in preadolescent child psychiatry inpatients. *Suicide and Life-Threatening Behavior,* 18:129–136, 1988.

Ascher-Svanum, H; Miller, MJ: Premenstrual changes and psychopathology among psychiatric inpatients. *Hospital and Community Psychiatry,* 41:86–88, 1990.

Asernansky, JG; Grabowski, K; Cervantes, O; et al: Fluphenazine decanoate and tardive dyskinesia: A possible association. *Am J Psychiatry,* 138:1362–1365, 1981.

Ashtroy, MA; Vijayam, N: Clorazepam treatment of insomnia due to sleep myoclonus. *Arch Neurol,* 37:119–120, 1980.

Asnis, GM: Harkavy Friedman, JM; Iqbal, N; et al: The drug-free period: A methodological issue. *Biol Psychiatry* 15;27(6):657–660, 1990.

Astrada, CA; Licamele, WL; Walsh, TL; et al: Recurrent abdominal pain in children and associated DSM-III diagnoses. *Am J Psychiatry,* 138:687–688, 1981.

Astroff, R; Gillen, E; Bonese, K; et al: Neuroendocrine risk factors of suicidal behavior. *Am J Psychiatry,* 139:1323–1325, 1982.

Atkinson, JH; Grant, I; Kennedy, CJ; Richman, DD; et al: Prevalence of psychiatric disorders among men infected with human immunodeficiency virus. *Arch Gen Psychiatry,* 45:859–864, 1988.

Augaard, J; Vestergaard, P: Predictors of outcoming prophylactic lithium treatment: A 2-year prospective study. *J Affective Disord,* 18:259–266, 1990.

Avery, D; Winokur, G: Suicide, attempted suicide, and relapse rates in depression. Occurrence after ECT and antidepressant therapy. *Arch Gen Psychiatry*, 35:749–753, 1978.

Azar, J; Turndorf, H: Paroxysmal left bundle branch block during nitrous oxide anesthesia in a patient on lithium carbonate. A case report. *Anesth Anal*, 56:868–870, 1977.

Bacher, NM; Lewis, HA: Addition of reserpine to antipsychotic medication in refractory chronic schizophrenic outpatients. *Am J Psychiatry*, 135:488–489, 1978.

Bacher, NM; Lewis, HA: Low-dose propranolol in tardive dyskinesia. *Am J Psychiatry*, 137–495,497, 1980.

Bachman, DS: Pemoline-induced Tourette's disorder: A case report. *Am J Psychiatry*, 138:1116–1117, 1981.

Bach-Y-Rita, G: Habitual violence and self-mutilation. *Am J Psychiatry*, 131:1018, 1974.

Bach-Y-Rita, G; Veno, A: Habitual violence: A profile of 62 men. *Am J Psychiatry*, 131:1015, 1974.

Bach-Y-Rita, G; Lion, JR; et al: Episodic dyscontrol: A study of 130 violent patients. *Am J Psychiatry*, 127:1473–1478, 1971.

Bader, TF; Newman, K: Amitriptyline in human breast milk and the nursing infant's serum. *Am J Psychiatry*, 137:855–856, 1980.

Baer, JW: Case Report: Munchausen's/AIDS. *Gen Hosp Psychiatry*, 9:75–76, 1987.

Bailine, SH; Lesser, MS; Krubit, G; Ravasz, TJ; et al: Comparison of IM haloperidol and IM chlorpromazine in the treatment of acutely psychotic patients. *The Psychiatric Hospital*, 18:127–129, 1990.

Bailos, DS: Adverse marijuana reactions: A critical examination of literature with selected case material. *Am J Psychiatry*, 40:569–573, 1983.

Bakish, D; LaPierre, YD: Disulfiram and bipolar affective disorder: A case report. *J Clin Psychopharmacol*, 6:178–180, 1986.

Ball, PG; Wyman, E: Battered wives and powerlessness: What can counselors do? *Victimology: An International Journal*, 2:545–552, 1977–1978.

Ballenger, JC: Pharmacotherapy of the panic disorders. *J Clin Psychiatry*, 47:27–32, 1986.

Ballenger, JC; Burrows, GD; DuPont, RL; Lesser, IM; et al: Alprazolam in panic disorder and agoraphobia: Results from a multicenter trial. *Arch Gen Psychiatry*, 45:413–422, 1988.

Ballenger, JC; Carek, DJ; Steele, JJ; Cornish-McTighe, D: Three cases of panic disorder with agoraphobia in children. *Am J Psychiatry*, 146:922–924, 1989.

Ballenger, JC; Post, RM: Carbamazepine in manic-depressive illness: A new treatment. *Am J Psychiatry*, 137:782–790, 1980.

Ballenger, JC; Rues, VI; Post, RM: "The "atypical" clinical picture of adolescent mania. *Am J Psychiatry*, 139:602–605, 1982.

Balster, GA; Bienenfeld, D; Marvel, NT; et al: Cognitive impairment among geropsychiatric outpatients. *Hospital and Community Psychiatry*, 41:556–558, 1990.

Band, TC: Recognition of acute delirious mania. *Arch Gen Psychiatry*, 37:553–554, 1980.

Barczak, P; Edmunds, E; Betts, T: Hypomania following complex partial seizures: A report of three cases. *Br J Psychiatry*, 152:137–139, 1988.

Barker, JD; Barns, JF; Barns, BJ; et al: Changes in children's behavior after a natural disaster. *Am J Psychiatry*, 139:1010–1014, 1982.

Barkley, RA; Cunningham, CE: The effects of methylphenidate on the mother-child interactions of hyperactive children. *Arch Gen Psychiatry*, 36:201–208, 1979.

Barnes, GE: Solvent abuse: A review. *Int J Addict*, 14:1–36, 1979.

Barnes, GE; Volcano, BA: Bibliography of the solvent abuse literature. Int J Addict, d14:401–421, 1979.

Barnes, R: The recurrent self-harm patient. *Suicide and Life-Threatening Behavior*, 16:399–408, 1986.

Barnes, R; Veith, R; Okimoto, J; et al: Efficacy of antipsychotic medications in behaviorally disturbed dementia patients. *Am J Psychiatry*, 139:1170–1174, 1982.

Barnes, RF; Raskind, MA: DSM-III criteria and the clinical diagnosis of dementia: a nursing home study. *J Gerontol*, 36:20–27, 1981.

Baron, M; Gruen, R; Rainer, JD; Kane, J; et al: A family study of schizophrenic and normal control probands: Implications for the spectrum concept of schizophrenia. *Am J Psychiatry*, 142:447–455, 1985.

Baron, M; Klotz, J; Medlewicz, J; et al: Multiple-threshold transmission of affective disorders. *Arch Gen Psychiatry,* 130:753, 1973.

Barrett, DH; Boyle, CA; Decoufle, P; DeStefano, F; et al: Health status of Vietnam Veterans: 1. Psychosocial characteristics. *JAMA,* 259:2701–2707, 1988.

Barrett, TW; Scott, TB: Suicide bereavement and recovery patterns compared with non-suicide bereavement patterns. *Suicide and Life-Threatening Behavior,* 20:1–14, 1990.

Barrnett, J; Frances, A; Kocsis, J; Brown, R; et al: Peripheral edema associated with trazodone: A report of ten cases. *J Clin Psychopharmacol,* 5:161–164, 1985.

Bass, C; Chambers, JB; Kiff, P; et al: Panic anxiety and hyperventilation in patients with chest pain: A controlled study. *Quarterly Journal of Medicine,* 69:949–959, 1988.

Bassuk, EL; Apsler, R: Are there sex biases in rape counseling? *Am J Psychiatry,* 140:305–308, 1983.

Bassuk, EL; Gerson, S: Chronic crisis patients: A discrete clinical group. *Am J Psychiatry,* 137:1513–1517, 1980.

Bassuk, EL; Minden, S; Apsler, R: Geriatric emergencies: Psychiatric or medical? *Am J Psychiatry,* 140:539–542, 1983a.

Bassuk, EL; Winter, R; Apsler, R: Cross-cultural comparison of British-American psychiatric emergencies. *Am J Psychiatry,* 140:1180–1184, 1983b.

Basto, U; Kaplan, HL; Sellers, EM: Benzodiazepine-associated emergencies in Toronto. *Am J Psychiatry,* 137:224–227, 1980.

Bates, WJ; Smeltzer, DJ: Electroconvulsive treatment of psychotic self-injurious behavior in a patient with severe mental retardation. *Am J Psychiatry,* 139:1355–1356, 1982.

Battaglia, J; Coverdale, JH; Bushing, CP: Evaluation of a mental illness awareness week program in public schools. *Am J Psychiatry,* 147:324–339, 1990.

Battaglia, J; Spector, J: Utility of the CAT scan in a first psychotic episode. *Gen Hosp Psychiatry,* 10:398–401, 1988.

Bauer, MS; Whybrow, PC: Rapid cycling bipolar affective disorder. Treatment of refractory rapid cycling with high dose levothyroxine: A preliminary study. *Arch Gen Psychiatry,* 47:427–432, 1990.

Bauer, MS; Whybrow, PC; Winokur, A: Rapid cycling bipolar affective disorder: I. Association with grade I hypothyroidism. *Arch Gen Psychiatry,* 47:427–432, 1990.

Bauer, S; Balter, L: Emergency psychiatric patients in a municipal hospital. *Psychiat Q,* 45:382–393, 1971.

Baxter, LR: Desipramine in the treatment of hypersomnolence following abrupt cessation of cocaine use. *Am J Psychiatry,* 140:1525–1526, 1983.

Bazelon, DL: Psychiatrists and the adversary process. *Sci Am,* 230:18, 1974.

Bear, D: Fedio, P: Quantitative analysis of interictal behavior in temporal lobe epilepsy. *Arch Neurol,* 34:454–467, 1977.

Beck, AT: *Depression: Clinical, Experimental and Theoretical Aspects.* New York, Harper and Row, 1967.

Beck AT; Beck, R; Kovacs, M: Classification of suicidal behaviors: I. Quantifying intent and medical lethality. *Am J Psychiatry,* 135:285–287, 1975.

Beck, AT; Brown, G; Berchick, RJ; et al: Relationship between hopelessness and ultimate suicide: A reparation with psychiatric outpatients. *Am J Psychiatry,* 147:190–195, 1990.

Beck, AT; Steer, RA; Kovacs, M; Garrison, B: Hopelessness and eventual suicide: A 10-year prospective study of patients hospitalized with suicidal ideation. *Am J Psychiatry,* 142:559–563, 1985.

Beck, JC; Staffin, RD; Patients' competency to give informed consent to medication. *Hospital and Community Psychiatry,* 37:400–402, 1986.

Becker, R: The historical background. *Psychiatr Ann,* 3:8, 1973.

Becker, RE: Implications of the efficacy of thiothixene and a chlorpromazine-lmipramine combination for depression in schizophrenia. *Am J Psychiatry,* 140:208–211, 1983.

Beckett, A; Summergrad, P; Manschreck, T; Vitagliano, H; et al: Symptomatic HIV infection of the CNS in a patient without clinical evidence of immune deficiency. *Am J Psychiatry,* 144:1342–1344, 1987.

Beech, HR; Vaughan, M: *Behavioral Treatment of Obsessional States.* New York, John Wiley & Sons, 1978.

Beecher, HK: *Research and the Individual Human Studies.* Boston, Little, Brown & Co., 1970.

Beemsterboer, J; Baum, BH: "Burnout": Definitions and health care management. *Social Work in Health Care,* 10:97–109, 1984.

Beitman, BD; Carlin, AS: Night terrors treated with imipramine. *Am J Psychiatry,* 136:8, 1979.

Bellak, L; Siegel, H: *Handbook of Intensive, Brief, and Emergency Psychotherapy.* Larchmont, NY, CRS, 1983.

Bellak, L; Small, L: *Emergency Psychotherapy and Brief Psychotherapy.* New York, Grune & Stratton, 1965.

Belmaker, RH; Lehrer, R; Epstein, RP; et al: A possible cardiovascular effect of lithium. *Am J Psychiatry,* 136:577–579, 1979.

Benedek, ED: Children and disaster: Emerging issues. *Psychiatric Annals,* 15:168–172, 1985.

Benedikt, RA; Kolb, LC: Preliminary findings on chronic pain and posttraumatic stress disorder. *Am J Psychiatry,* 143:908–910, 1986.

Beresford, TP; Blow, FC; Hall, RCW; Nichols, LO; et al: CT scanning in psychiatric inpatients: Clinical yield. *Psychosomatics,* 27:105–135, 1986.

Berglund, M: Suicide in alcoholism. *Arch Gen Psychiatry,* 41:888–891, 1984.

Bergman, D; Futterweit, W; Segal, R; et al: Increased estradiol in diazepam related gynecomastia. *Lancet,* i:1225, 1981.

Berkovic, SF; Andermann, F; Andermann, E; Gloor, P: Concepts of absence epilepsies: Discrete syndromes or biological continuum? *Neurology,* 37:993–1000, 1987.

Berl, T: Psychosis and water balance. *N Engl J Med,* 318:441–442, 1988.

Berlin, RM; Conell, LJ: Withdrawal symptoms after long-term treatment with therapeutic doses of flurazepam: A case report. *Am J Psychiatry,* 140:488–490, 1983.

Bernhart, CC; Bowden, CL: Toxic psychosis with cimetidine. *Am J Psychiatry,* 136:725–726, 1979.

Berrios, GE; Samuel, C: Affective disorder in the neurological patient. *J Nerv Ment Dis,* 175:173–175, 1987.

Berson, RJ: Capgras' Syndrome. *Am J Psychiatry,* 140:969–978, 1983.

Bick, PA: Seasonal major affective disorder. *Am J Psychiatry,* 143:90–91, 1986.

Biederman, J; Lerner, Y; Belmaker, RH: Combination of lithium carbonate and haloperidol in schizoaffective disorders: A controlled study. *Arch Gen Psychiatry,* 36:327–333, 1979.

Bien, RD: Cogwheel rigidity early in lithium therapy. *Am J Psychiatry,* 133:1093–1094, 1976.

Bienenfield, D; Hartford, JT: Pseudodementia in an elderly woman with schizophrenia. *Am J Psychiatry,* 139:114–115, 1982.

Bigelow, LB; Weinberger, DR; Wyatt, RJ: Synergism of combined lithium neuroleptic therapy: A double-blind, placebo-controlled case study. *Am J Psychiatry,* 138:81–83, 1981.

Biggs, JT; Spiker, DG; Petit, JM; et al: Tricyclic antidepressant overdose: Incidence of symptoms. *JAMA,* 238:135–138, 1977.

Bille-Brahe, U; Juel-Nielsen, N: Trends in attempted suicide in Denmark, 1976–1980. *Suicide and Life-Threatening Behavior,* 16:46–55, 1986.

Binder, RL: Three case reports of behavioral disinhibition with clonazepam. *Gen Hosp Psychiatry,* 9:151–153, 1987.

Binder, RL: AIDS antibody tests on inpatient psychiatric units. *Am J Psychiatry,* 144:176–181, 1987.

Binder, RL; Levy, R: Extrapyramidal reactions in Asians. *Am J Psychiatry,* 138:1243–1244, 1981.

Binder, RL; McNiel, DE: Effects of diagnosis and context on dangerousness. *Am J Psychiatry,* 145:728–732, 1988.

Bingham, RL; Plante, DA; Bronson, DL; Tufo, HM; McKnight, K: Establishing a "quality" improvement process for identification of psychosocial problems in a primary care practice. *J Gen Intern Med,* 5(4):342–346, 1990.

Binik, YM; Devins, GM: Transplant failure does not compromise quality of life in end-stage renal disease. *Int J Psychiatry Med,* 16:281–292, 1986–87.

Birch, NJ: A note of animal and human studies of possible kidney damage caused by lithium. in *Lithium in Medical Practice,* FN Johnson & S Johnson, Baltimore University, *Lancet,* i:468–472, 1979.

Bishop, LC; Riley, WT: The psychiatric management of the Globus syndrome. *Gen Hosp Psychiatry,* 9:214–219, 1988.

Bixler, EO: Kales, A; Soldatos, CR; et al: Prevalence of sleep disorders in the Los Angeles metropolitan area. *Am J Psychiatry,* 136:1257–1262, 1979.

Blachly, P; Disher, D; Roduner, G: Suicide by physicians. *Bulletin of Suicidology.* Washington, D.C., U.S. Government Printing Office, December 1968.

Black, DW; Winokur, G; Bell, S; Nasrallah, A; et al: Complicated mania: Comorbidity and immediate outcome in the treatment of mania. *Arch Gen Psychiatry,* 45:232–236, 1988.

Black, DW; Warrack, G; Winokur, G: The Iowa record-linkage study: 1. Suicides and accidental deaths among psychiatric patients. *Arch Gen Psychiatry,* 42:71–75, 1985a.

Black, DW; Warrack G; Winokur, G: The Iowa record-linkage study: II. Excess mortality among patients with organic mental disorders. *Arch Gen Psychiatry,* 42:78–81, 1985b.

Blackwell, B; Marley, E; Price, J; et al: Hypertensive interactions between MAOIs and foodstuffs. *Br J Psychiatry,* 113:349–365, 1967.

Blackwell, B; Stepopoulos, A; Endess, P; et al: Anticholinergic activity of two tricyclic antidepressants. *Am J Psychiatry,* 135:722–724, 1978.

Blattner, WA; Blair, A; Masin, TJ: Multiple myeloma in the United States, 1950–1974. *Cancer,* 48:2547–2554, 1981.

Blehar, MC; Rosenthal, NE: Seasonal affective disorders and phototherapy. *Arch Gen Psychiatry,* 46:469–474, 1989.

Blazer, DG: Impact of late-life depression on the social network. *Am J Psychiatry,* 140:162–166, 1983.

Bliss, EL: Multiple personalities: A report of 14 cases with implications for schizophrenia and hysteria. *Arch Gen Psychiatry,* 140:162–166, 1983.

Bloch, DA; Silber, E; Perry, SE: Some factors in the emotional reaction of children to disaster. *Am J Psychiatry,* 140:162–166, 1983.

Bloch, M; Simmott, J: *The Battered Elder Syndrome.* College Park, University of Maryland Center on Aging, 1979.

Block, SH: The grocery store high. *Am J Psychiatry,* 135:126–127, 1978.

Blomhoff, S; Seim, S; Friis, S: Can prediction of violence among psychiatric inpatients be improved? *Hospital and Community Psychiatry,* 41:771–775, 1990.

Blouin, J; Minoletti, A; Blouin, A; Nahon, D: Effects of patient characteristics and therapeutic techniques on crisis intervention outcome. *Psychiatr J Univ Ottawa,* 10:153–157, 1985.

Blum, A: Patients at risk of developing severe side effects from depot fluphenazine treatment. *Am J Psychiatry,* 137:254–255, 1980.

Blumenfield, M; Milazzo, J;Wormser, GP: Noncompliance in hospitalized patients with AIDS. *Gen Hosp Psychiatry,* 12:166–169, 1990.

Blumenfield, M; Smith, PJ; Milazzo, J; Seropian, S; et al: Survey of attitudes of nurses working with AIDS patients. *Gen Hosp Psychiatry,* 9:58–63, 1987.

Blumenthal, MD; Davie, JW: Dizziness and falling in elderly psychiatric outpatients. *Am J Psychiatry,* 137:203–206, 1980.

Bock, JL; Cummings, KC; Jatlow, PI: Amoxapine overdose: A case report. *Am J Psychiatry,* 139:1619–1620, 1982.

Boehnert, CE: Surgical outcome in "death-minded" patients. *Psychosomatics,* 27:638–642, 1986.

Boehnlein, JK; Kinzie, JD; Ben, R; Fleck, J: One-year follow-up study of posttraumatic stress disorder among survivors of Cambodian concentration camps. *Am J Psychiatry,* 142:956–959, 1985.

Boelhouwer, C; Henry, CE; Glueck, BD: Positive spiking: A double-blind control study of its significance in behavior disorders both diagnostically and therapeutically *Am J Psychiatry,* 1225:473–481, 1968.

Bohman, M; Cloninger, CR; Sigvardsson, S; et al: Predisposition to petty criminality in Swedish adoptees: I. Genetic and environmental heterogeneity. *Arch Gen Psychiatry* 39:1233–1241, 1982.

Bohman, M; Sigvardsson, S; Cloninger, R: Maternal inheritance of alcohol abuse: Cross-fostering analysis of adopted women. *Arch Gen Psychiatry,* 38:965–969, 1981.

Boisverg, D; Chouinard, G: Rebound cardiac arrhythmia after withdrawal from imipramine: A case report. *Am J Psychiatry,* 138:985–986, 1981.

Bokstrom, K; Balldin, J; Langstrom, G: Alcohol withdrawal and mood. *Acta Psychiatr Scand,* 80:505–513, 1989.

Boldt, J: Normative evaluations of suicide and death: A cross-generational study. *Omega,* 13:145–155, 1982–1983.

Bond, TC: Recognition of acute delirious mania. *Arch Gen Psychiatry,* 37:553–554, 1980.

Bond, WS; Mandos, LA; Kurtz, MB: Midazolam for agressivity and violence in three mentally retarded patients. *Am J Psychiatry,* 146:925–926, 1989.

Bondareff, W; Baldy, R; Levy, R: Quantitative computed tomography in senile dementia. *Arch Gen Psychiatry,* 38:1365–1368, 1981.

Bonnet, MH; Dexter, Jr; Arand, DL: The effect of triazolam on arousal and respiration in central sleep apnea patients. *Sleep,* 13:31–41, 1990.

Boronow, J; Pickar, D; Ninan, PT; Roy, A; et al: Atrophy limited to the third ventricle in chronic schizophrenic patients. *Arch Gen Psychiatry,* 42:266–271, 1985.

Borson, S: Behcet's disease as psychiatric disorder: A case report. Am J Psychiatry, 139:1348–1349, 1982.

Boulenger, JP; Uhde, TW; Wolff, EA III; Post, RM: Increased sensitivity to caffeine in patients with panic disorders: Preliminary evidence. *Arch Gen Psychiatry,* 41:1067–1071, 1984.

Bowen, RC; Kobout, J: The relationship between agoraphobia and primary affective disorders. *Can J Psychiatry,* 24, 317–321, 1979.

Bowen, RC; Orchard, RC; Keegan, DL; D'Arcy, C: Mitral valve prolapse and psychiatric disorders. *Psychosomatics,* 26:926–929, 1985.

Bowers, MB: Psychoses precipitated by psychotomimetic drugs. A follow-up study. *Arch Gen Psychiatry,* 34:882–885, 1977.

Bowers, MB; Mazure, CM; Nelson, JC; et al: Psychotogenic drug use and neuroleptic response. *Schizophrenia Bulletin,* 16:81–85, 1990.

Bows, JF; Anostasi, M; Casoni, R; et al: Psychotherapy in the goldfish bowl: The role of the indigenous therapist. *Arch Gen Psychiatry,* 36:187–190, 1979.

Boyce, P; Parker, G: Seasonal affective disorder in the southern hemisphere. *Am J Psychiatry,* 145:96–99, 1988.

Boyd, JH; Weissman, MM: Epidemiology of affective disorders: A re-examination Braden, W: Response to lithium in a case of L-dopa-induced psychosis. *Am J Psychiatry,* 134:808–809, 1981.

Bradford, J: Dimock, J: A comparative study of adolescents and adults who willfully set fires. *Psychiatr J Univ Ottawa,* 11:228–234, 1986.

Bradford, JMW; Gloomberg, D; Bourget, D: The heterogeneity/homogeneity of pedophilia. *Psychiatr J Univ Ottawa,* 14:217–226, 1988.

Branchey, MH; Charles, J; Simpson, EM: Extrapyramidal side-effects in lithium maintenance therapy. *Am J Psychiatry,* 133:4444–4451, 1976.

Braude, WM; Barnes, TRE: Late-onset akathisia—an indicant of covert dyskinesia: Two case reports. *Am J Psychiatry,* 140:611–612, 1983.

Breed, W: Suicide, migration and race: A study of cases in New Orleans. *J Soc Issues,* 22:30–43, 1966.

Breier, A; Astrachan, BM: Characterization of schizophrenic patients who commit suicide. *Am J Psychiatry,* 141:206–209, 1984.

Breier, A; Charney, DS; Heninger, GR: Agoraphobia with panic attacks. *Arch Gen Psychiatry,* 43:1029–1036, 1986.

Breier, A; Charney, DS; Nelson, JC: Seizures induced by abrupt discontinuation of alprazolam. *Am J Psychiatry,* 141:1606–1607, 1984.

Breier, A; Wolkowitz, OM; Doran, AR; Roy, A; et al: Neuroleptic responsivity of negative and positive symptoms in schizophrenia. *Am J Psychiatry,* 144:1549–1555, 1987.

Brenner, F: Bromism: Alive and well. *Am J Psychiatry,* 135:857–858, 1978.

Brenner, I; Rheubon, WJ: The catatonic dilemma. *Am J Psychiatry,* 135:1242–1243, 1978.

Brent, DA; Perper, JA; Goldstein, CE; Kolko, DL; et al: Risk factors for adolescent suicide. *Arch Gen Psychiatry,* 45:581–588, 1988.

Breslau, N; Davis, GC: Posttraumatic stress disorder: The etiologic specificity of wartime stressors. *Am J Psychiatry,* 144:578–583, 1987.

Brett, EA; Spitzer, RL; Williams, JBW: DSM-III-R criteria for posttraumatic stress disorder. *Am J Psychiatry,* 145:1232–1236, 1988.

Brewster, JM: Prevalence of alcohol and other drug problems among physicians. *JAMA,* 255:1913–1920, 1986.

Briere, J; Zaidi, LY: Sexual abuse histories and sequelae in female psychiatric emergency room patients. *Am J Psychiatry,* 146:1602–1606, 1989.

Briggs Law (The), Mass. Gen. Laws c 123, Sec 100A, (Ter Ed) (1932).

Brill, H; Malzberg, B: *Statistical report based on the arrest record of 5354 male ex-patients released from New York State Mental Hospitals during the period 1946–48.* Mimeo, New York, 1950.

Brill, NQ; Storrow, HA: Social class and psychiatric treatment. *Arch Gen Psychiatry,* 3:340, 1960.

Brinkley, JR; Beitman, BD; Friedel, RO: Low-dose neuroleptic regimens in the treatment of the borderline patient. *Arch Gen Psychiatry,* 36:319–326, 1979.

Brinton, WT; Vastbinder, EE; Greene, JW; Marz, JJ; et al: An outbreak of organic dust toxic syndrome in a college fraternity. *JAMA,* 258:1210–1212, 1987.

Bristol, JH; Giller, E; Docherty, JP: Trends in emergency psychiatry in the last two decades. *Am J Psychiatry,* 138:623–628, 1981.

Brizer, DA; Manning, DW: Delirium induced by poisoning with anticholinergic agents. *Am J Psychiatry,* 139:1343–1344, 1982.

Brockington, IF; Cernick, KF; Schofield, EM; et al: Puerperal psychosis: Phenomena and diagnosis. *Arch Gen Psychiatry,* 38:829–833, 1981.

Brockington, IF; Hillier, VF; Francis, AF; et al: Definitions of mania: Concordance and prediction of outcome. *Am J Psychiatry,* 140:435–439, 1983.

Brockington, IF; Margison, FR; Schofield, E; Knight, RJE: The clinical picture of the depressed form of puerperal psychosis. *J Affective Disord,* 15:29–37, 1988.

Bromet, E; Schuberg, HC; Dunn, L: Reaction of psychiatric patients to the Three Mile Island nuclear accident. *Arch Gen Psychiatry,* 35:1261–1264, 1978.

Brooksband, DJ: Suicide and parasuicide in childhood and early adolescence. *Br J Psychiatry,* 146:459–463, 1985.

Brothman, AW; Forstein, M: AIDS obsessions in depressed heterosexuals. *Psychosomatics,* 29:428–430, 1988.

Brower, KJ; Eliopulos, GA; Blau, FC; et al: Evidence for physical and psychological dependence on anabolic androgenic steroids in eight weight lifters. *Am J Psychiatry,* 142:570–572, 1990.

Brown, GR; Rundell, JR: Prospective study of psychiatric morbidity in HIV-seropositive women without AIDS. *Gen Hosp Psychiatry,* 12:30–35, 1990.

Brown, R; Colter, N; Gorsellis, JAN; Crow, TJ; et al: Postmortem evidence of structural brain changes in schizophrenia: Differences in brain weight, temporal horn area, and parahippocampal gyrus compared with affective disorder. *Arch Gen Psychiatry,* 43:36–42, 1986a.

Brown, SR; Schwartz, JM; Summergrad, P; Jenike, MA: Globus hystericus syndrome responsive to antidepressants. *Am J Psychiatry,* 143:917–918, 1986b.

Brown, WA; Bamen, M; D'Agostino, C; et al: Cortisol level response to 1- and 2-mg doses of dexamethasone. *Am J Psychiatry,* 140:609–611, 1983.

Brown, WA; Shuey, I: Response to dexamethasone and subtype of depression. *Arch Gen Psychiatry,* 37:747–751, 1980.

Brown, WA; Silver, MA: Serum neuroleptic levels and clinical outcome in schizophrenic patients treated with fluphenazine decanoate. *J Clin Psychopharmacol,* 5:143–147, 1985.

Brownell, LG; West, P; Sweatman, P; et al: Protriptyline in obstructive sleep apnea. A double-blind trial. *N Engl J Med,* 307(17):1037–1042, 1982.

Browning, DH; Boatman, B: Incest: Children at risk. *Am J Psychiatry,* 134:69–72, 1977.

Bruce, ML; Kim, K; Leaf, PJ; et al: Depressive episodes and dysphoria resulting from conjugal bereavement in a prospective community sample. *Am J Psychiatry,* 147:608–611, 1990.

Bruch, H: Anorexia nervosa: Therapy and theory. *Am J Psychiatry,* 139:1531–1538, 1982.

Brune v. Belinkoff, (1978) 354 Mass 102, 235 NE 2d 793 (1978).

Brunton, J; Hawthorne, H: The acute non-hospital: A California model. *The Psychiatric Hospital,* 20:95–99, 1990.

Buchanan, DC: Group therapy for kidney transplant patients. *Int J Psychiat Med,* 6:523–532, 1975.

Buchanan, RW; Kirkpatrick, B; Heinrichs, DW; et al: Clinical correlates of the deficit syndrome of schizophrenia. *Am J Psychiatry,* 147:290–294, 1990.

Buchsbaum, MS; Ingvar, DH; Kessler, R; et al: Cerebral glucography with position tomography: Use in normal subjects and in patients with schizophrenia. *Arch Gen Psychiatry,* 39:251–259, 1982.

Buckley, WE; Yesalis, CE; Friedl, KE; Anderson, WA; et al: Estimated prevalence of anabolic steroid use among male high school seniors. *JAMA,* 260:3441–3445, 1988.

Bulik, CM: Drug and alcohol abuse by bulimic women and their families. *Am J Psychiatry,* 144:1604–1606, 1987.

Bulik, CM; Carpenter, LL; Kupfer, DV; et al: Features associated with suicide attempts in recurrent major depression. *J Affective Disord,* 18:29–37, 1990.

Burd, L; Kerbeshian, J; Wilkenbergerk, M; et al: Prevalence of Gilles de la Tourette's syndrome in North Dakota adults. *Am J Psychiatry,* 143:787–788, 1986.

Burgess, AW; Holmstrom, L: Rape trauma syndrome. *Am J Psychiatry,* 131:981, 1974.

Burgess, AW; Holmstrom, L: *Rape: Victims of Crisis.* Bowie, Maryland, Robert J. Brady. 1974.

Burke, JD; Boruw, JF; Burns, BJ; et al: Changes in children's behavior after a natural disaster. *Am J Psychiatry,* 139:1010–1014, 1982.

Burke, KC; Burke, JD, Regier, DA; Rae, DS: Age at onset of selected mental disorders in five community populations. *Arch Gen Psychiatry,* 47:511–518, 1990.

Burks, JS; Walker, JE; Rumack, BH; et al: Tricyclic antidepressant poisoning: Reversal of coma, choreoathetosis, and myoclonus by physostigmine. *JAMA,* 230(10):1402–1407, 1974.

Burns, RS; Lerner, SE; Corrado, R: Phencyclidine states of acute intoxication and fatalities. *West J Med,* 123:345–349, 1975.

Burstein, A: Treatment length in posttraumatic stress disorder. *Psychosomatics,* 27:632–637, 1986.

Burten, W; Ballard, BL: Hypomania as a stable state: Lithium prophylaxis in two patients. *Am J Psychiatry,* 138:523–524, 1981.

Busto, U; Kaplan, HL; Sellers, EM: Benzodiazepine-associated emergencies in Toronto. *Am J Psychiatry,* 138:523–524, 1981.

Butler, RN: Psychiatry and the elderly: An overview. *Am J Psychiatry,* 132:893–900, September, 1975.

Butters, N; Sax, D; Montgomery, K; et al: Comparison of neuropsychological deficits associated with early and advanced Huntington's disease. *Arch Neurol,* 35:535–589, 1978.

Butzer, JF; Silber, DE; Sahs, AC: Amantadine in Parkinson's disease. *Neurology,* 25:603–606, 1975.

Buydens-Branchey, L; Branchey, MH; Noumair, D: Age of alcoholism onset: I. Relationship to psychopathology. *Arch Gen Psychiatry,* 46:225–230, 1989a.

Buydens-Branchey, L; Branchey, MH; Noumair, D; Lieber, CS: Age of alcoholism onset: II. Relationship to susceptibility to serotonin precursor availability. *Arch Gen Psychiatry,* 46:231–236, 1989b.

Byerley, WF; Brown, J; Lebegue, B: Treatment of seasonal affective disorder with morning light. *J Clin Psychiatry,* 48:447–448, 1987.

Cadoret, RJ; Cain, C: Sex differences in predictors of antisocial behavior in adoptees. *Arch Gen Psychiatry,* 37:1171–1175, 1980.

Cadoret, RJ; Cain, CA; Grove, WM: Development of alcoholism in adoptees raised apart from alcoholic biologic relatives. *Arch Gen Psychiatry,* 37:561–563, 1980.

Caffeinism. *Pharmacy Newsletter of the Connecticut Mental Health Center,* Department of Pharmacy Services, 1:22, 1974.

Caine, ED; Hunt, RD; Weingartner, H; et al: Huntington's dementia: Clinical and neuropsychological features. *Arch Gen Psychiatry,* 35:377–384, 1978.

Caine, ED; Shoulson, I: Psychiatric syndromes in Huntington's disease. *Am J Psychiatry,* 140:728–733, 1983.

Cal. Welf. & Inst'ns Code Section, 5325(f) (W. Supp. 1973) Statute that gives the patient the right to refuse electroshock treatment. Calif. Welf. & Inst'ns Code (West 1966) (Supp. 1968) Section 5276.

Calabrese, JR; Delucchi, GA: Spectrum of efficacy of valproate in 55 patients with rapid-cycling bipolar disorder. *Am J Psychiatry,* 147:431–434, 1990.

Caldwell, JM: Military psychiatry. In: *Comprehensive Textbook of Psychiatry.* AM Freedman; HI Kaplan; HS Kaplan, eds. Baltimore, Williams and Wilkins, 1967.

Calif. Wel. & Inst. Code Sec. 600.

Cameron, OG; Hudson, CJ: Influence of exercise on anxiety level in patients with anxiety disorders. *Psychosomatics,* 27:720–723, 1986.

Campbell, DR: Sinha, BK: Brief group psychotherapy with chronic hemodialysis patients. *Am J Psychiatry,* 137:1234–1237, 1980.

Campbell, R; Simpson, GM: Alternative approaches in the treatment of psychotic agitation. *Psychosomatics,* 27:23–27, 1986.

Campion, JF; Cravens, JM; Covan, F: A study of filicidal men. *Am J Psychiatry,* 145:1141–1144, 1988.

Camron, TD; Mednick, SA; Parnas, V: Antecedents of predominantly negative—and predominantly positive—symptom schizophrenia in a high-risk population. *Arch Gen Psychiatry,* 47:522–532, 1990.

Canton, CLM; Mayers, L; Gralnick, A: The long-term hospital treatment of the young chronic patient: Follow-up findings. *The Psychiatric Hospital,* 21:25–30, 1988.

Cantopher, T; Oliveri, S; Cleave, N; et al: Chronic benzodiazepine dependence: A comparative study of abrupt withdrawal under propranolol cover versus gradual withdrawal. *Br J Psychiatry,* 156:406–411, 1990.

Cantwell, DP; Sturzenberger, S; Burroughs, J; et al: Anorexia nervosa: an affective disorder? *Arch Gen Psychiatry,* 34:1087–1093, 1977.

Caplan, G: *An Approach to Community Health.* New York, Grune and Stratton, 1961.

Caplan, G: *Concepts of Mental Health and Consultation.* Washington, U.S. Dept of Health, Education and Welfare, Children's Bureau, 1959.

Caplan, G: *Manual for Psychiatrists Participating in the Peace Corps Program.* Washington, Medical Program Division, Peace Corps. 1962.

Caplan, G: Mastery of stress: Psychosocial aspects. *Am J Psychiatry,* 138:413–420, 1981.

Caplan, G: *Principles of Preventive Psychiatry.* New York, Basic Books, 1964.

Caplan, RA; Posner, KL; Cheney, FW: Effect of outcome on physician judgments of appropriateness of care. *JAMA,* 265:1957–1960, 1991.

Carlson, GA; Cantwell, DP: A survey of depressive symptoms, syndrome and disorder in a child psychiatric population. *J Clin Psychol Psychiatry,* 21:10–25, 1980.

Carlson, GA; Davenport, YB; Jamison, K: A comparison of outcome in adolescent and late-onset bipolar manic-depressive disease. *Am J Psychiatry,* 134:919–922, 1977.

Carlson, GA; Miller, DC: Suicide, affective disorder, and women physicians. *Am J Psychiatry,* 138:1330–1335, 1981.

Carmel, H; Hunter, M: Compliance with training in managing assaultive behavior and injuries from inpatient violence. *Hospital and Community Psychiatry,* 41:558–560, 1990.

Carmen, E; Brady, SM: AIDS risk and prevention for the chronic mentally ill. *Hospital and Community Psychiatry,* 41:652–653, 1990.

Carpenter, WT; Bartko, JJ; Strauss, JS; et al: Signs and symptoms as predictors of outcome: A report from the international pilot study of schizophrenia. *Am J Psychiatry,* 135:940–945, 1978.

Carpiniello, B; Carta, MG; Rudas, N: Depression among elderly people: A psychosocial study of urban and rural populations. *Acta Psychiatr Scand,* 80:445–450, 1989.

Carroll, BJ; Feinberg, M; Greden, JF; et al: A specific laboratory test for the diagnosis of melancholia. *Arch Gen Psychiatry,* 38:15–22, 1981.

Carter v. United States, 252 F.2d 608 (D.C. Cir. 1957).

Casey, DE: Clozapine: Neuroleptic induced EPS and tardive dyskinesia. *Psychopharmacology,* 99:S47–S53, 1989.

Casey, DE; Rabins, P: Tardive dyskinesia or a life-threatening illness. *Am J Psychiatry,* 135:486–488, 1978.

Casey, PR: Personality disorder and suicide intent. *Acta Psychiatr Scand,* 79:290–295, 1989.

Casper, ES; Donaldson, B: Subgroups in a population of frequent users of inpatient services. *Hospital and Community Psychiatry,* 41:189–191, 1990.

Casper, RC; Davis, JM: On the course of anorexia nervosa. *Am J Psychiatry,* 134:974–978, 1977.

Casper, RC; Eckert, ED; Halmi, KA; et al: Bulimia: Its incidence and clinical significance in patients with anorexia nervosa. *Arch Gen Psychiatry,* 37:1030–1035, 1980.

Cassens, G; Wolfe, L; Zola, M: The neuropsychology of depressions. *J Neuropsychiatry,* 2:202–213, 1990.

Castellani, S; Adams, PM; Giannini, AJ: Physostigmine treatment of acute phencyclidine intoxication. *J Clin Psychiatry,* 43:10–11, 1982a.

Castellani, S; Giannini, AJ; Adams, PM: Physostigmine and haloperidol treatment of acute phencyclidine intoxication. *Am J Psychiatry,* 139:508–510, 1982b.

Castro, KG; Lifson, AR; White, CR; Bush, TJ; et al: Investigations of AIDS patients with no previously identified risk factors. *JAMA,* 259:1388–1342, 1988.

Caton, CLM: Effect of length of inpatient treatment for chronic schizophrenia. *Am J Psychiatry,* 139:856–861, 1982.

Cavanaugh, SA; Wettstein, RM: The relationship between severity of depression, cognitive dysfunction, and age in medical inpatients. *Am J Psychiatry,* 140:495–496, 1983.

Cavenar, JO; Sullivan, JL; Maltbie, AA: A clinical note on hysterical psychosis. *Am J Psychiatry,* 136:830–832, 1979.

Chalmers, TC; Aster, RH; Bloom, JR; Collins, JJ; et al: The impact of routine HTLV-111 antibody testing of blood and plasma donors on public health. *JAMA,* 256:1778–1783, 1986.

Chamberlain, MJ; Reynolds, AC; Yeoman, WB: Toxic effect of podophyllum application in pregnancy. *Br Med J,* 3:319–392, 1972.

Chamberlain, S; Hahn, PM; Casson, P; et al: Effect of menstrual cycle phase and oral contraceptive use on serum lithium levels after a loading dose of lithium in normal women. *Am J Psychiatry,* 147:907–909, 1990.

Charness, ME; Simon, RP; Greenberg, DA: Ethanol and the nervous system. *N Engl J Med,* 321:442–454, 1989.

Charney, DS; Heninger, GR; Jatlow, PI: Increased anxiogenic effects of caffeine in panic disorders. *Arch Gen Psychiatry,* 42:233–243, 1985.

Charney, DS; Heninger, GR; Kleber, HD: The combined use of clonidine and naltrexone as a rapid, safe, and effective treatment of abrupt withdrawal from methadone. *Am J Psychiatry,* 143:831–837, 1986a.

Charney, DS; Nelson, JC: Delusional and non-delusional unipolar depression: Further evidence for distinct subtypes. *Am J Psychiatry,* 138:328–333, 1981.

Charney, DS; Riordan, CE; Kleber, HD; et al: Clonidine and naltrexone: A safe, effective, and rapid treatment of abrupt withdrawal from methadone therapy. *Arch Gen Psychiatry,* 39:1327–1332, 1982.

Charney, DS; Woods, SW; Goodman, WK; Rifkin, B; et al: Drug treatment of panic disorder: The comparative efficacy of imipramine, alprazolam, and trazodone. *J Clin Psychiatry,* 47:580–586, 1986b.

Chemtol, CM; Hamada, RS; Bauer, G: Patients' suicides: Frequency and impact on psychiatrists. *Am J Psychiatry,* 145:224–228, 1988.

Chiles, JA; Miller, ML; Cox, GB: Depression in an adolescent delinquent population. *Arch Gen Psychiatry,* 37:1179–1184, 1980.

Chopra, HD; Beatson, JA: Psychotic symptoms in borderline personality disorder. *Am J Psychiatry,* 143:1605–1607, 1986.

Chouinard, G: Antimanic effects of clonazepam. *Psychosomatics,* 26:7–12, 1985.

Chouinard, G; Annable, L; Ross-Chouinard, A; et al: Factors related to tardive dyskinesia. *Am J Psychiatry,* 136:79–83, 1979.

Christie, KA; Burke, JD; Reigier, DA; Rae, DS; et al: Epidemiologic evidence for early onset of mental disorders and higher risk of drug abuse in young adults. *Am J Psychiatry,* 145:971–975, 1988.

Christodoulou, GN: The syndrome of Capgras. *Br J Psychiatry,* 130:556–564, 1977.

Christodoulou, GN; Kokevi, A; Lykouras, EP; et al: Effects of lithium on memory. *Am J Psychiatry,* 138:847–848, 1981.

Christy v. Saliterman, 288 Minn 144, 179 NW 2d 288 (1970).

Chronholm, B; Ottosson, JO: The experience of memory function after electroconvulsive therapy. *Br J Psychiatry,* 109:251–258, 1963.

Chu, JA; Dill, DL: Dissociative symptoms in relation to childhood physical and sexual abuse. *Am J Psychiatry,* 147:887–892, 1990.

Chuang, HT; Devins, GM; Hunsley, J; Gill, MJ: Psychosocial distress and well-being among gay and bisexual men with human immunodeficiency virus infection. *Am J Psychiatry,* 146:876–880, 1989.

Chung, YS; Ravi, SD; Borge, GF: Psychosis in Wilson's Disease. *Psychosomatics,* 27:65–66, 1986.

Civil Commitment of the Mentally Ill. De Paul L Rev, 23:1276–97 (Spring, 1974).

Clark v. State, 12 Ohio Rep 483 (1843).

Clark, DC; Clayton, PJ; Andreasen, NC; Lewis, C; Fawcett, J; Scheftner, WA: Intellectual functioning and abstraction ability in major affective disorders. *Comprehensive Psychiatry,* 26:313–325, 1985.

Clark, DC; Taylor, CB; Roth, WT; et al: Surreptitious drug rise by patients in a panic disorder study. *Am J Psychiatry*, 147:507–509, 1990.

Clark, DC; Young, MA; Schefner, WA; et al: A field test of Matto's risk estimator for suicide. *Am J Psychiatry*, 144:923–926, 1987.

Clarkin, JF; Glick, ID; Haas, GL; et al: A randomized clinical trial of inpatient family intervention: V. Results for affective disorders. *J Affective Disord*, 18:17–28, 1990.

Cleary, PD; Goldberg, ID; Kessler, LG; et al: Screening for mental disorder among primary care patients: Usefulness of the general health questionnaire. *Arch Gen Psychiatry*, 39:837–840, 1982.

Clifford, DB; Rutherford, JL; Hicks, FG; Zorumski, CF: Acute effects of antidepressants on hippocampal seizures. *Ann Neurol*, 18:692–697, 1985.

Climo, LH: Treatment-resistant catatonic stupor and combined lithium-neuroleptic therapy: A case report. *J Clin Psychopharmacol*, 5:166–170, 1985.

Cloninger, CR; Sigvardsson, S; Bohman, M; et al: Predisposition to petty criminality in Swedish adoptees: II. Cross-fathering analysis of gene-environment interaction. *Arch Gen Psychiatry*, 39:1242–1247, 1982.

Cloninger, CR; Bohman, M; Sigvardsson, S: Inheritance of alcohol abuse: Cross-fostering analysis of adopted men. *Arch Gen Psychiatry*, 38:861–868, 1982.

Cochrane, N: The role of aggression in the psychogenesis of depressive illness. *Am J Med Psychol*, 48:113–130, 1975.

Cocozza, JJ; Steadman, HJ: Some refinements in the measurement and prediction of dangerous behavior. *Am J Psychiatry*, 131:1012, 1974.

Coffey, CE; Figiel, GS; Weiner, RD, et al: Caffeine augmentation of ECT. *Am J Psychiatry*, 147:579–585, 1990a.

Coffey, CE; Figiel, GS; Djang, WT; Weiner, RD: Subcortical hyperintensity on magnetic resonance imaging: A comparison on normal and depressed elderly subjects. *Am J Psychiatry*, 147:187–189, 1990b.

Coffey, CE; Weiner, RD: Electroconvulsive therapy: An update. *Hospital and Community Psychiatry*, 41:515–521, 1990.

Cohen, BM; Baldessarini, RJ: Tolerance to therapeutic effects of antidepressants. *Am J Psychiatry*, 142:489–490, 1985.

Cohen, BM; Lipinski, JF: Treatment of acute psychosis with non-neuroleptic agents. *Psychosomatics*, 27:7–16, 1986.

Cohen, DJ; Detlor, J; Young, GF; et al: Clonidine ameliorates Gilles de la Tourette Syndrome. *Arch Gen Psychiatry*, 37:1350–1357, 1980.

Cohen, LH; Freeman, H: How dangerous to the community are state hospital patients? *Connecticut State Medical Journal*, 9:E97, 1945.

Cohen, LJ; Test, MA; Brown, RL: Suicide and schizophrenia: data from a prospective community treatment study. *Am J Psychiatry*, 147:602–607, 1990.

Cohen, LM: A current perspective of pseudocyesis. *Am J Psychiatry*, 139:1140–1144, 1982.

Cohen, M; Kern, JC; Hassett, C: Identifying alcoholism in medical patients. *Hospital and Community Psychiatry*, 37:398–400, 1986.

Cohen, MAA: Biopsychosocial approach to the human immunodeficiency virus epidemic: A clincian's primer. *General Hospital Psychiatry*, 12:98–123, 1990.

Cohen, MAA; Weisman, HW: A biopsychosocial approach to AIDS. *Psychosomatics*, 27:245–249, 1986.

Cohen, S; Chiles, J; MacNaughton, A: Weight gain associated with clozapine. *Am J Psychiatry*, 147:503–504, 1990.

Cohen S; Khan, A: Antipsychotic effect of milieu in the acute treatment of schizophrenia. *General Hospital Psychiatry*, 12:178–186, 1982.

Cohen v. New York State, 282 New York Supplement 2d 128 (1976).

Cohen-Sandler, R; Berman, AL; King, RA: Life stress and symptomatology: Determinants of suicidal behavior in children. *J Am Acad Child Psychiatry* 21:178–186, 1982.

Cohn, JB; Wilcox, CS: Low-sedation potential of buspirone compared with alprazolam and lorazepam in the treatment of anxious patients: A double-blind study. *J Clin Psychiatry*, 47:409–412, 1986.

Cohn, JV: The psychiatric emergency. *South Med J*, 52:547–553, 1989.

Colt, EWD; Kimbrell, D; Fieve, RR: Renal impairment, hypercalcemia, and lithium therapy. *Am J Psychiatry,* 138:106–108, 1981.

Comaty, JE; Janicak, PG: Depot neuroleptics. *Psychiatric Annals,* 17:491–496, 1987.

Committee on Adolescents of the American Academy of Pediatrics: Teenage suicide. *Pediatrics,* 66:144–146, 1980.

Committee on Trauma—American College of Surgeons: *Emergency Care.* Philadelphia, WB Saunders, 1966.

Comroe, BI: Follow-up study of 100 diagnosed as neurosis. *J Nerv Ment Dis,* 83:679–684, 1936.

Conn Gen Stat Sec 17–183 (1975).

Conn Gen Stat Sec 17–206d (1974).

Conn, LM; Rudnick, BF; Lion, JR: Psychiatric care for patients with self-inflicted gunshot wounds. *Am J Psychiatry,* 141:261–263, 1984.

Connelly, CE; Davenport, YB; Nurnberger, JI: Adherence to treatment regimen in a lithium carbonate clinic. *Arch Gen Psychiatry,* 39:585–588, 1982.

Conners, CK; Taylor, E: Pemoline, methylphenidate, and placebo in children with minimal brain dysfunction. *Arch Gen Psychiatry,* 37:922–930, 1980.

Cookson, HM: A survey of self-injury in a closed prison for women. *Br J Criminol,* 17:332–347, 1977.

Coons, DJ; Hillman, FJ; Marshall, RW: Treatment of neuroleptic malignant syndrome with dantrolene sodium: A case report. *Am J Psychiatry,* 139:944–945, 1982.

Coons, PM; Ascher-Svanum, H; Bellis, K: Self-amputation of the female breast. *Psychosomatics,* 27:667–668, 1986.

Cooper, AJ: Tyramine and irreversible monoamine oxidase inhibitors in clinical practice. *Br J Psychiatry,* 155(Suppl 6):38–45, 1989.

Cooperstock, R: A review of women's psychotropic drug use. *Can J Psychiatry,* 24:29–34, 1979.

Coppen, A: The prevalence of menstrual disorders in psychiatric patients. *Br J Psychiatry,* 111:155–167, 1965.

Cornelius, JR; Soloff, PH; Reynolds, CF: Paranoia, homicidal behavior, and seizures associated with phenylpropanolamine. *Am J Psychiatry,* 141:120–121, 1984.

Coryell, W; Andreasen, NC; Endicott, J; Keller, M: The significance of past mania or hypomania in the course and outcome of major depression. *Am J Psychiatry,* 144:309–315, 1987.

Coryell, W; Keller, M; Lavori, P; et al: Affective syndromes, psychotic features, and prognosis in depression. *Arch Gen Psychiatry,* 47:651–657, 1990.

Coryell, W; Noyes, R; Clancy, J: Excess mortality in panic disorder: A comparison with primary unipolar depression. *Arch Gen Psychiatry,* 39:701–703, 1982.

Coryell, W; Sherman, A: Slow tricyclic antidepressant metabolism polypharmacy, and cardiac arrest. *Am J Psychiatry,* 137:108–109, 1982.

Cotton, PG; Drake, RE; Gates, C: Critical treatment issues in suicide among schizophrenics. *Hospital and Community Psychiatry,* 36:534–536, 1985.

Cowley, DS; Arana, GW: The diagnostic utility of lactate sensitivity in panic disorder. *Arch Gen Psychiatry,* 47:277–284, 1990.

Cox, WH: An indication for use of imipramine in attention deficit disorder. *Am J Psychiatry,* 139:1059–1060, 1982.

Coyle, PK; Sterman, AB: Focal neurologic symptoms in panic attacks. *Am J Psychiatry,* 143:648–649, 1986.

Craig, AG; Pitts, FN: Suicide by physicians. *Dis Nerv Syst,* 29:763–772, 1968.

Craig, J; Abu-Saleh, M; Smith B; Evans, I: Diabetes mellitus in patients on lithium. *Lancet,* ii:1028, 1977.

Craig, RJ; Olson, R; Shalton, G: Improvement in psychological functioning among drug abusers: Inpatient treatment compared to outpatient methadone maintenance. *J Substance Abuse,* 7:11–19, 1990.

Craig, TJ: An epidemiologic study of problems associated with violence among psychiatric inpatients. *Am J Psychiatry,* 139:1266, 1982.

Craig, TJ: Medication use and deaths attributed to asphyxia among psychiatric patients. *Am J Psychiatry,* 137:1366–1371, 1980.

Craig, TJ; Abeloff, MD: Psychiatric symptomatology among hospitalized patients. *Am J Psychiatry,* 131:1323–1327, 1974.

Craig, TJ; Lin, SP: Mortality among psychiatric inpatients: Age-adjusted comparison of populations before and after psychotropic drug era. *Arch Gen Psychiatry,* 38:935–938, 1981.

Craig, TJ; Van Nattan, PA: Disability and depressive symptoms in two communities. *Am J Psychiatry,* 140:598–601, 1983.

Craig, TJ; Van Natta, PA: Influence of demographic characteristics on two measures of depressive symptoms: The relation of prevalence and persistence of symptoms with sex, age, education and marital status. *Arch Gen Psychiatry,* 35:149–154, 1979.

Crane, GE: The prevention of tardive dyskinesia. *Am J Psychiatry,* 134:756–758, 1977.

Crawshaw, R: Reactions to a disaster. *Arch Gen Psychiatry,* 9:157–162, 1963.

Cravens, JM; Campion, J; Rotholc, A; Covan, F; et al: A study of 10 men charged with patricide. *Am J Psychiatry,* 142:1089–1092, 1985.

Croughan, JL; Woodruff, RA; Reich, T: The management of patients with undiagnosed psychiatric illness. *Arch Gen Psychiatry,* 36:341–346, 1979.

Crowder, MK; Pate, JK: A case report of cimetidine-induced depressive syndrome. *Am J Psychiatry,* 137:1451, 1980.

Crowe, MJ; Lloyd, GG; Bloch, S; et al: Hypothyroidism in patients treated with lithium: a review and two case reports. *Psychol Med,* 3:337–342, 1973.

Crowe, RR; Noyes, R; Pauls, DL; Slymen, D: A family study of panic disorder. *Arch Gen Psychiatry,* 40:1065–1069, 1983.

Crowe, RR; Pauls, DL; Slymen, DJ; et al: A family study of anxiety neurosis. *Arch Gen Psychiatry,* 37:77–99, 1981.

Crowley, DS; Roy-Byrne, PP: Hyperventilation and panic disorder. *Am J Med,* 83:929–937, 1987.

Crowley, TJ; Wagner, JE; Zerbe, G: Macdonald, M: Naltrexone-induced dysphoria in former opioid addicts. *Am J Psychiatry,* 142:1081–1084, 1985.

Crumley, FE: Substance abuse and adolescent suicidal behavior. *JAMA,* 263:3051–3060, 1990.

Csernansky, JG; Grabowski, K; Cervantes, J; et al: Fluphenazine decanoate and tardive dyskinesia: A possible association. *Am J Psychiatry,* 138:1362–1365, 1981.

Cumming, RG: *Casebook of Psychiatric Emergencies: The "On Call" Dilemma.* Baltimore, University Park Press, 1983.

Cummings, J; Benson, F; Loverme, S: Reversible dementia: Illustrative cases, definition, and review. *JAMA,* 243:2434–2439, 1980.

Cummings, JL: Multi-infarct dementia: Diagnosis and management. *Psychosomatics,* 28:117–126, 1987.

Cummings, JL; Barritt, CF; Horan, M: Delusions induced by procaine penicillin: Case report and review of the syndrome. *Int J Psychiatry Med,* 16:163–168, 1986–1987.

Cummings, MA; Cummings, KL; Rapaport, MH; Atkinson, JH; et al: Acquired immunodeficiency syndrome presenting as schizophrenia. *West J Med,* 146:615–618, 1987.

Curtis, GC; Cameron, OG; Nesse, RM: The dexamethasone suppression test in panic disorder and agoraphobia. *Am J Psychiatry,* 139:1043–1046, 1982.

Curtis, GC; Thyer, B: Fainting on exposure to phobic stimuli. *Am J Psychiatry,* 140:771–774, 1983.

Cutler, NR; Anderson, DJ: Proven as asymptomatic eosinophilia with imipramine. *Am J Psychiatry,* 134:1296–1297, 1977.

Cutler, NR; Zavadil, AP; Eisdorfer, C; et al: Concentrations of desipramine in elderly women. *Am J Psychiatry,* 138:1235–1237, 1981.

Cytryn, L; McKnew, DH, Bunney, WE: Diagnosis of depression in children: A reassessment. *Am J Psychiatry,* 137, 22–25, 1980.

Dackis, CA; Bailey, J; Pottash, ALC; Stuckey, RF; et al: Specificity of the DST and the TRH Test for major depression in alcoholics. *Am J Psychiatry,* 141:680–683, 1984.

Dackis, CA; Estroff, TW; Sweeney, DR; Pottash, ALC; et al: Specificity of the TRH test for major depression in patients with serious cocaine abuse. *Am J Psychiatry,* 142:1097–1099, 1985.

Dackis, CA; Gold, MS; Sweeney, DR; Byron, JP; et al: Single-dose bromocriptine reverses cocaine craving. *Psychiatry Research,* 20:261–264, 1987.

Daggett, LR; Rolde, EJ: Decriminalization of public drunkenness: The response of suburban police. *Arch Gen Psychiatry,* 34:937–941, 1977.

Damlouji, NF; Ferguson, JM: Trazodone-induced delirium in bulimic patients *Am J Psychiatry,* 141:434–435, 1984.

Damlouji, NF; Ferguson, JM: Three cases of posttraumatic anorexia nervosa. *Am J Psychiatry,* 142:362–363, 1985.

Daniel, AE; Harris, PW; Husain, SA: Differences between midlife female offenders and those younger than 40. *Am J Psychiatry,* 138:1225–1228, 1981.

Daniel, WF; Weiner, RD; Crovitz, HF; Strong, GB; et al: ECT-induced delirium and further ECT: A case report. *Am J Psychiatry,* 140:922–924, 1983.

Darbonne, A: Crisis: A review of theory, practice and research. *Int J Psychiatry,* 6:371, 1968.

Darhe, MA: Psychological factors differentiating self-mutilating and non-self-mutilating adolescent inpatient females. *The Psychiatric Hospital,* 21:31–35, 1989.

Darling v. Charleston Memorial Hospital, 33 III 2nd 326, NE 2d 253 (1965); cert. denied 383 U.S 946 (1966).

DasGupta, K; Jefferson, JW: The use of lithium in the medically ill. *General Hospital Psychiatry,* 12:83–97, 1990.

David, OJ; Grad, G; McGann, B; et al: Mental retardation and "nontoxic" lead levels. *Am J Psychiatry,* 139:806–809, 1982.

Davidson, HA: *Forensic Psychiatry,* 2nd ed. New York, The Ronald Press, 1965.

Davidson, J; Kudler, H; Smith, R; et al: Treatment of post-traumatic stress disorder with amitriptyline and placebo. *Arch Gen Psychiatry,* 47:259–266, 1990.

Davidson, JRT: Post-traumatic stress disorder: Recent advances in basic science and clinical research. *Psychopharmacology Bulletin,* 25:(3)415, 1989.

Davidson, JRT; Nemeroff, CB: Pharmacotherapy in posttraumatic stress disorder: Historical and clinical considerations and future directions. *Psychopharmacology Bulletin,* 25:422–425, 1989.

Davis, BD; Fernandez, F; Adams, F; Holmes, V; et al: Diagnosis of dementia in cancer patients. *Psychosomatics,* 28:175–179, 1987.

Davis, MH; Casey, DA: Utilizing cognitive therapy on the short-term psychiatric unit. *General Hospital Psychiatry,* 12:170–176, 1990.

Deaton, AV; Craft, S; Skenazy, J: Enduring psychiatric and neuropsychologic sequelae in the postencephalitis patient. *Int J Psychiatry Med,* 16:275–280, 1986.

DeBard, ML: Diazepam withdrawal syndrome: A case with psychosis, seizure, and coma. *Am J Psychiatry,* 136:104–105, 1979.

Decker, S; Fins, J; Frances, R: Cocaine and chest pain. *Hospital and Community Psychiatry,* 38:464–466, 1987.

de Figueiredo, JM; Boerstler, H: The relationship of presenting complaints to the use of psychiatric services in a low-income group. *Am J Psychiatry,* 145:1145–1148, 1988.

Dekret, JJ; Maany, I; Ramsey, TA; et al: A case of oral dyskinesia associated with imipramine treatment. *Am J Psychiatry,* 134:1297–1298, 1977.

Delga, I; Heinssen, RK; Fritsch, RC; et al: Psychosis, aggression and self-destructive behavior in hospitalized adolescents. *Am J Psychiatry,* 146:521–525, 1989.

DeLisi, LE; Goldin, LR; Hamovit, JR; Maxwell, ME; et al: A family study of the association of increased ventricular size with schizophrenia. *Arch Gen Psychiatry,* 43:148–153, 1986.

Delworth, V; Rudow, EH; Taub, J: *Crisis Center/Hotline.* Springfield, Illinois, Charles C. Thomas, 1972.

Demitivek, MA; Lesem, MD; Brandt, HA; et al: Neurohypophysical dysfunction implications for the pathophysiology of eating disorders. *Psychopharmacology Bulletin,* 25:439–443, 1989.

DeMontigny, C; Grunberg, F; Mayer, A; et al: Lithium-induced rapid relief of depression in tricyclic antidepressant drug nonresponders. *Br J Psychiatry,* 138:252–256, 1981.

Demers, R; Lukesh, R; Prichard, J: Convulsion during lithium therapy. *Lancet,* ii:315–316, 1970.

Demers-Desrosiers, LA; Nestoros, JN; Vaillancourt, P: Acute psychosis precipitated by withdrawal of anticonvulsant medication. *Am J Psychiatry,* 135:981–982, 1978.

Demuth, GW; Rand, BS: Atypical major depression in a patient with severe primary degenerative dementia. *Am J Psychiatry,* 137:1609–1610, 1980.

DeMyer, MK; Hendrie, HC; Gilmor, RL; DeMyer, WE: Magnetic resonance imaging in psychiatry. *Psychiatric Annals,* 15:262–267, 1985.

Denicoff, KD; Joffe, RT; Lakshmanan, MC; Robbins, J; et al: Neuropsychiatric manifestations of altered thyroid state. *Am J Psychiatry*, 147:94–99, 1990.

Dening, TR; Berrios, GE: Wilson's Disease: Psychiatric symptoms in 195 cases. *Arch Gen Psychiatry*, 46:1126–1134, 1989.

Dennehy, CM: Childhood bereavement and psychiatric illness. *Br J Psychiatry*, 112:1049–1069, 1966.

Der, G; Gupta, S; Murray, RM: Is schizophrenia disappearing? *Lancet*, 335:513–516, 1990.

Dershowitz, AN: Dangerousness as a criterion for confinement. *Bulletin of the American Academy of Psychiatry and the Law*, 2:172–179 (September), 1974.

Detre, TP; Jarecki, HG: *Modern Psychiatric Treatment*. Philadelphia, JP Lippincott Co., 1971.

Deutsch, H: Some forms of emotional disturbance and their relationship to schizophrenia. *Psychoanal Q*, 11:301, 1942.

DeVanna, M; Paterniti, S; Mitievich, C; et al: Recent life events and attempted suicide. *J Affective Disord*, 18:57–58, 1990.

Deveaugh-Geiss, J; Bandurangi, A: Confusional paranoid psychosis after withdrawal from sympathomimetic amines: Two case reports. *Am J Psychiatry*, 139:1190–1191, 1982.

Developments in the Law—Civil commitment of the mentally ill. *Harvard L Rev*, 87:1190, April, 1974.

Devins, GM; Seland, TP: Emotional impact of multiple sclerosis: Recent findings and suggestions for future research. *Psychological Bulletin*, 101:363–375, 1987.

Devinsky, O; Bear, D: Varieties of aggressive behavior in temporal lobe epilepsy. *Am J Psychiatry*, 141:651–656, 1984.

Dewan, MJ; Pandurangi, AK; Boucher, MI; et al: Abnormal dexamethasone suppression test results in chronic schizophrenic patients. *Am J Psychiatry*, 139:1501–1503, 1982.

Dewhurst, K; Oliver, J; Trick, KLK; et al: Neuropsychiatric aspects of Huntington's disease. *Confin Neurol*, 31:258–268, 1969.

Deykin, EY; Alpert, JJ; McNamarra, JJ: A pilot study of the effect of exposure to child abuse or neglect on adolescent suicidal behavior. *Am J Psychiatry*, 142:1299–1303, 1985.

Dhib-Jalbut, S; Hesselbrock, R; Mouradian, MM; Means, ED: Bromocriptine treatment of neuroleptic malignant syndrome. *J Clin Psychiatry*, 48:69–73, 1987.

Diagnostic and Statistical Manual of Mental Disorders, 3rd ed., Revised. Washington, D.C., American Psychiatric.

Dickson, LR; Ranseen, JD: An update on selected organic mental syndromes. *Hospital and Community Psychiatry*, 41:290–300, 1990.

Diekstra, RFW; van Egmond, M: Suicide and attempted suicide in general practice, 1979–1986. *Acta Psychiatr Scand*, 79:268–275, 1989.

Dilley, JW; Ochitill, HN; Perl, M; Volberding, PA: Findings in psychiatric consultations with patients with acquired immune deficiency syndrome. *Am J Psychiatry*, 142:82–86, 1985.

Dilsaver, SC; Coffman, JA: Antipsychotic withdrawal phenomena in the medical-surgical setting. *Gen Hosp Psychiatry*, 10:438–446, 1988.

Dilsaver, SC; Feinberg, M; Greden, JF: Antidepressant withdrawal symptoms treated with anticholinergic agents. *Am J Psychiatry*, 140:249–151, 1983.

Dimsdale, JE: Emotional causes of sudden death. *Am J Psychiatry*, 134:1361–1366, 1977.

Dimsdale, JE; Hackett, TP: Effect of denial on cardiac health and psychological assessment. *Am J Psychiatry*, 139:1477–1480, 1982.

Disclosure of confidential information. *JAMA*, 216:385, April 12, 1971.

District of Columbia Alcoholic Rehabilitation Act (1968): P.L. 90-452, 82 Stat 618.

Dixon, KN; Arnold, LE; Calestro, K: Father-son incest: Underreported psychiatric problem? *Am J Psychiatry*, 135:835–838, 1978.

Dixon, L; Haas, G; Weiden, P; et al: Acute effects of drug abuse in schizophrenic patients: Clinical observations and patients' self-reports. *Schizophrenia Bulletin*, 16:69–79, 1990.

Donaldson, JA; Hale, MS; Klau, M: A case of reversible pure-word deafness during lithium toxicity. *Am J Psychiatry*, 138:242–243, 1981.

Donaldson, SR: Sialorrhea as a side effect of lithium: A case report. *Am J Psychiatry*, 139:1350–1351, 1982.

Donlon, PT; Hopkin, JT; Tupin, JP; et al: Haloperidol for acute schizophrenia patients: an evaluation of three oral regimens. *Arch Gen Psychiatry*, 37:691–695, 1980.

Donlon, PT; Hopkin, JT; Tupin, JP: Overview: Efficacy and safety of the rapid neuroleptization method with injectable haloperidol. *Am J Psychiatry,* 136:273–278, 1979.

Donlon, PT; Tupin, JP: Successful suicides with thioridazine and mesoridazine. *Arch Gen Psychiatry,* 34:955–957, 1977.

Dorpat, T; Anderson, WF; Ripley, HS: "The relationship of physical illness to suicide" in *Suicidal Behaviors.* HLP Resnick, ed. Boston, Little, Brown, & Co., 1968.

Dorus, W; Kennedy, J; Gibbons, RD; Ravi, SD: Symptoms and diagnosis of depression in alcoholics. *Alcoholism: Clinical and Experimental Research,* 11:150–156, 1987.

Douglas, CJ; Schwartz, HI: ECT for depression caused by lupus cerebritis: A case report. *Am J Psychiatry,* 140:800–801, 1983.

Douyon, R; Angrist, B; Peselow, E; Cooper, T; et al: Neuroleptic augmentation with alprazolam: Clinical effects and pharmacokinetic correlates. *Am J Psychiatry,* 146:231–234, 1989.

Drake, RE; Ehrilich, J: Suicide attempts associated with akathisia. *Am J Psychiatry,* 142:499–501, 1985.

Drake, RE; Osher, FC; Noordsy, DL; et al: Diagnosis of alcohol use disorders in schizophrenia. *Schizophrenia Bulletin,* 16:57–67, 1990.

Drake, ME: Cotard's syndrome and temporal lobe epilepsy. *Psychiatr J Univ Ottawa,* 13:36–40, 1988.

Drimmer, EJ; Gitlen, MJ; Gwirtsman, HE: Desipramine and methylphenidate combination treatment for depression: Case report. *Am J Psychiatry,* 140:241–242, 1983.

Driver v. Hinnant, 356 F. 2d 761 (4th Cir. 1966).

Drossman, DA: Patients with psychogenic abdominal pain: Six years' observation in the medical setting. *Am J Psychiatry,* 139:1549–1557, 1982.

Drug Interactions—a review. *Pharmacy Newsletter of the Connecticut Mental Health Center.* Department of Pharmacy Services, 1:21, 1974.

Drummond, LM; Gravestock, S: Delayed emergence of obsessive-compulsive neurosis following head injury: Case report and review of its theoretical implications. *Br J Psychiatry,* 153:839–842, 1988.

Dubey, J: Confidentiality as a requirement of the therapist: Technical necessities for absolute privilege in psychotherapy. *Am J Psychiatry,* 131:1093–1096, 1974.

Dubin, WR: The role of fantasies, countertransference, and psychological defenses in patient violence. *Hospital and Community Psychiatry,* 40:1280–1283, 1989.

Dubin, WR: Evaluating and managing the violent patient. *Ann Emerg Med,* 10:481–484, 1981.

Dubin, WR; Stalberg, R: *Emergency Psychiatry for the House Officer.* New York, SP Medical and Scientific Books, 1981.

Dubin, WR; Weiss, KJ: Rapid tranquilization: A comparison of thiothixene with Loxapine. *J Clin Psychiatry,* 47, 294–297, 1986.

Dubin, WR; Weiss, KJ; Doran, JM: Pharmacotherapy of psychiatric emergencies. *J Clin Psychopharmacol,* 6:210–222, 1986.

Dublin, L: Suicide: A public health problem. In: *Essays in Self-Destruction,* ES Schneidman, ed. New York, Science House, 1967.

Dubner, NP; Durant, Dl; Creech, FR: Epstein-Barr antibodies in three psychiatric syndromes. *The Psychiatric Hospital,* 20:167–170, 1987.

Duffy, DL; Hamerman, D; Cohen, MA: Communications skills of house officers: A study in medical clinic. *Ann Intern Med,* 93:354–357, 1980.

Dulit, RA; Fyer, MR; Haas, GL; Sullivan, T; et al: Substance use in borderline personality disorder. *Am J Psychiatry,* 147:1002–1007, 1990.

Dune, AK: The toxic emergency: Phencyclidine. *Emergency Medicine,* 12:129–182, 1978.

Dunn, CG; Gross, D: Treatment of depression in the medically ill geriatric patient: A case report. *Am J Psychiatry,* 134:448–450, 1977.

Dunner, DL: Anxiety and panic: Relationship to depression and cardiac disorders. *Psychosomatics,* 26:18–22, 1985.

Dunner, DL; Fieve, RR: Clinical factors in lithium carbonate prophylaxis failure. *Arch Gen Psychiatry,* 30:229–233, 1974.

Dunner, DL; Fleiss, JL; Fieve, RR: Lithium carbonate prophylaxis failure. *Br J Psychiatry,* 129:40–44, 1976.

Durham v United States, 214 F. 2d 862 (D.C. Cir. 1954).

Durkheim, E: *Le Suicide: Etude de Sociologic.* Paris, Alcan, 1897.

Durnal, C; Gaviria, M; Flaherty, J; Birz, S: Perceived disruption and psychological distress among flood victims. *J Operational Psychiatry,* 16:9–16, 1985.

Dworkin, RH: Patterns of sex differences in negative symptoms and social functioning consistent with separate dimensions of schizophrenic psychopathology. *Am J Psychiatry,* 147:347–349, 1990.

Dworkin, SF; Van Korff, M; Leresche, L: Multiple pains and psychiatric disturbance: An epidemiologic investigation. *Arch Gen Psychiatry,* 47:239–244, 1990.

Dysken, MW; Chan, CH: Diazepam withdrawal psychosis: A case report. *Am J Psychiatry,* 134:573, 1977.

Eagles, JM; Wilson, AM; Hunter, D, et al: A comparison of anorexia nervosa and affective psychosis in young females. *Psychological Medicine,* 20:119–123, 1990.

Easter v. District of Columbia, 361 F. 2d 50 (D.C. Cir. 1966).

Eastwood, MR; Rifat, SL; Nobbs, H; Ruderman, J: Mood disorder following cerebrovascular accident. *Br J Psychiatry,* 154:195–200, 1989.

Eaton, LF; Menolascino, FJ: Psychiatric disorders in the mentally retarded: Types, problems, and challenges. *Am J Psychiatry,* 139:1297–1303, 1982.

Edelstein, CK; Roy-Byrne, P; Fawzy, FI; et al: Effects of weight loss on the dexamethasone suppression test. *Am J Psychiatry,* 140:338–341, 1983.

Egeland, JA; Sussex, JN: Suicide and family loading for affective disorders. *JAMA,* 254:915–918, 1985.

Eisenberg, L: Adolescent suicide: On taking arms against a sea of troubles. *Pediatrics,* 66:315–320, 1980.

Eisendrath, SJ; Goldman, B; Douglas, J; Dimatteo, L; et al: Meperidine-induced delirium. *Am J Psychiatry,* 144:1062–1065, 1987.

Eisendrath, SJ; Sweeney, MA: Toxic neuropsychiatric effects of digoxin at therapeutic serum concentrations. *Am J Psychiatry,* 144:506–507, 1987.

Eisendrath, SJ; Way, LW; Ostroff, JW; Johanson, CA: Identification of psychogenic abdominal pain. *Psychosomatics,* 27:705–712, 1986.

Eisenhauer, GL: Self-inflicted ocular removal by two psychiatric inpatients. *Hospital and Community Psychiatry,* 36:189–191, 1985.

Elkashef, AM; Ruskin, PE; Bacher, N; et al: Vitamin E in the treatment of tardive dyskinesia. *Am J Psychiatry,* 147:505–506, 1990.

Elliott, RL; Thomas, BJ: A case report of alprazolam-induced stuttering. *J Clin Psychopharmacol,* 5:159–160, 1985.

Ellison, JM; Blum, N; Barsky, AJ: Repeat visitors in the psychiatric emergency service: A critical review of the data. *Hospital and Community Psychiatry,* 37:37–41, 1986.

Ellison, JM; Blum, NR; Barsky, AJ: Frequent repeaters in a psychiatric emergency service. *Hospital and Community Psychiatry,* 40:958–960, 1989.

Ellison, JM; Wharff, EA: More than a gateway: The role of the emergency psychiatry service in the community mental health network. *Hospital and Community Psychiatry,* 38:180–185, 1985.

Emergency Psychiatric Care: The Management of Mental Health Crises, H.L.P. Resnik and H.L. Ruben, eds. Bowie, Maryland, Charles Press, 1975.

Emmerson, JP; Burvill, PW; Finlay-Jones, R; et al: Life events, life difficulties and confiding relationships in the depressed elderly. *Br J Psychiatry,* 155:787–792, 1989.

Emslie, GJ; Rosenfield, A: Incest reported by children and adolescents hospitalized for severe psychiatric problems. *Am J Psychiatry,* 140:708–711, 1983.

Endicott, J; Cohen, J; Nee, J; et al: Brief vs. standard hospitalization. For Whom? *Arch Gen Psychiatry,* 36:706–712, 1979.

Engel, G: *Fainting: Physiological and Psychological Considerations,* 2nd ed. Springfield, Illinois, Charles C. Thomas. 1962.

Engel, GL; Ramano, J: Delirium: A syndrome of cerebral insufficiency. *J Chron Dis,* 9:260–277, 1959.

Ennis, BJ; Barnis, RA; Kennedy, S; et al: Depression in self-harm patients. *Br J Psychiatry,* 154:41–47, 1989.

Ennis, BJ: Emerging legal rights for the mentally handicapped. *The Bulletin of the American Academy of Psychiatry and the Law,* 2:185, 1974.

Ennis, BJ; Litwack, TR: Psychiatry and the presumption of expertise: Flipping coins in the courtroom. *California L Rev,* 62:693–754, May, 1974.

Epstein, RS: Posttraumatic stress disorder: A review of diagnostic and treatment issues. *Psychiatric Annals,* 19:556–563, 1989.

Epstein, RS: Withdrawal symptoms from chronic use of low-dose barbiturates. *Am J Psychiatry,* 137:107–108, 1980.

Erikson, KT: *Everything in its Path: Destruction of A Community in the Buffalo Creek Flood.* New York, Simon and Schuster, 1976.

Erikson, E: *Childhood and Society.* New York, WW Norton Co., 1950.

Erwin, CW; Gerber, CJ; Morrison, SD; et al: Lithium carbonate and convulsive disorders. *Arch Gen Psychiatry,* 28:646–648, 1973.

Estroff, TW; Extein, IL; Malaspina, D; Gold, MS: Hepatitis in 101 consecutive suburban cocaine and opiate users. *Int J Psychiatry Med,* 16:237–242, 1986–87.

Estroff, TW; Gold, MS: Psychiatric presentations of marijuana abuse. *Psychiatric Annals,* 16:221–224, 1986a.

Estroff, TW; Gold, MS: Medical and psychiatric complications of cocaine abuse with possible points of pharmacological treatment. *Controversies in Alcoholism and Substance Abuse,* 61–76, 1986b.

Ethics of Health Care. LR Tancredi, ed. Washington, D.C., National Academy of Sciences, 1973.

Etzion, D: Moderating effect of social support on the stress-burnout relationship. *J Appl Psychol,* 69:615–622, 1984.

Evans, DL; Burnett, CB; Nemeroff, CB: The dexamethasone suppression test in the clinical setting. *Am J Psychiatry,* 140:568–586, 1983a.

Evans, DL; Edelsohn, GA; Golden, RN: Organic psychosis without anemia of spinal cord symptoms in patients with vitamin B12 deficiency. *Am J Psychiatry,* 140:218–221, 1983b.

Evans, DL; Nemeroff, CB: The dexamethasone suppression test in mixed bipolar disorder. *Am J Psychiatry,* 140:615–617, 1983.

Extein, IL; Gold, MS: Thyroid hormone potentiation of tricyclics. *Psychosomatics,* 29:166–174, 1988.

Extein, I; Rosenberg, G; Pottash, ALC; et al: The dexamethasone suppression test in depressed adolescents. *Am J Psychiatry,* 139:1617–1619, 1982.

Fairburn, CG; Beglin, SJ: Studies of the epidemiology of bulimia nervosa. *Am J Psychiatry,* 147:401–408, 1990.

Falks, DG; King, LD; Dowdy, SB; et al: Carbamazepine treatment of selected affectively disordered inpatients. *Am J Psychiatry,* 139:115–117, 1982.

Faltus, FJ: The positive effect of alprazolam in the treatment of three patients with borderline personality disorder. *Am J Psychiatry,* 141:802–803, 1984.

Faquet, RA; Rowland, KF: Spice cabinet intoxication. *Am J Psychiatry,* 135:860–861, 1978.

Farberow, NL; Shneidman, ES: *The Cry for Help.* New York, McGraw-Hill, 1965.

Farmer, RDT: Assessing the epidemiology of suicide and parasuicide. *Br J Psychiatry,* 153:16–20, 1988.

Farsy, D; Baldessarini, RJ: The tardive dyskinesia syndrome, in *Clinical Neuropharmacology,* Volume 1. HL Klawans, ed. New York, Raven Press, 1976.

Fauman, MA: Quality assurance monitoring in psychiatry. *Am J Psychiatry,* 146:1121–1130, 1989.

Faust, D; Libon, D; Pueschel, S: Neuropsychological functioning in treated phenylketonuria. *Int J Psychiatry Med,* 16:169–177, 1986–87.

Fava, J; Anderson, K; Rosenbaum, JF: Anger attacks: Possible variants of panic and major depressive disorders. *Am J Psychiatry,* 147:867–870, 1990.

Favazza, AR; Conterio, AR: Female habitual self-mutilators. *Acta Psychiatr Scand,* 79:283–289, 1989.

Favazza, AR; DeRosear, L; Conterro, K: Self-mutilation and eating disorders. *Suicide and Life-Threatening Behavior,* 19:352–361, 1989.

Favazza, AR; Martin, P: Chemotherapy for delirium tremens: A survey of physician's preferences. *Am J Psychiatry,* 131:1031, 1974.

Feibel, JH; Shiffer, RB: Sympathoadrenomedullary hyperactivity in the neuroleptic malignant syndrome: A case report. *Am J Psychiatry,* 138:1115–1116, 1981.

Feighner, JP; Aden, GC; Fabre, LF; et al: Comparison of alprazolam, imipramine, and placebo in the treatment of depression. *JAMA,* 249:3057–3064, 1983.

Feighner, JP; et al: Diagnostic criteria for use in psychiatric research. *Am J Psychiatry,* 26:57, 1972.

Feinglass, EJ; Arnett, FC; Dorsch, CA; et al: Neuropsychiatric manifestations of systemic lupus erythematosis, diagnosis, clinical spectrum and relationship to other features of the disease. *Medicine,* (Baltimore), 55:323–339, 1976.

Feingold, BF: *Why Your Child is Hyperactive.* New York, Random House, 1975.

Feirstein, A; Weisman, G; Kamas, C: A crisis intervention model for inpatient hospitalization. In: *Current Psychiatric Therapies,* Vol. 11, JH Masserman, ed. New York, Grune and Stratton, 1971.

Feldman, S; Goldstein, HH: Community mental health centers in the United States: An overview. *Int J Nursing Studies,* 8:247–257, 1971.

Females Lead Suicide Attempts. *NAMH Reporter,* Winter, 1972–73.

Fenichel, GS; Murphy, JG: Factors that predict psychiatric consultation in the emergency department. *Medical Care,* 23:258–265, 1985.

Fenichel, U: *The Psychoanalytic Theory of Neurosis.* New York, WW Norton Co., 1945.

Fenley, J; Posers, PS; Miller, J; et al: Untreated anorexia nervosa: A case study of the medical consequences. *General Hospital Psychiatry,* 12:264–270, 1990.

Fenn, H: Violence: Probability versus prediction. *Hospital and Community Psychiatry,* 41:117, 1990.

Fenton, WS; McGlashan, TH: Sustained remission in drug-free schizophrenic patients. *Am J Psychiatry,* 144:1306–1309, 1987.

Ferguson, JM: Bulimia: A potentially fatal syndrome. *Psychosomatics,* 26:252–253, 1985.

Fernandez, F; Adams, F; Levy, JK; et al: Cognitive impairment due to AIDS-related complex and its response to psychostimulants. *Psychosomatics,* 29:38–46, 1988a.

Fernandez, F; Levy, JK; Galizzi, H: Response of HIV-related depression to psychostimulants: Case reports. *Hospital and Community Psychiatry,* 39:628–631, 1988b.

Fernandez-Pol, B: Characteristics of 77 Puerto Ricans who attempted suicide. *Am J Psychiatry,* 143:1460–1463, 1986.

Ferrari, M; Barabas, G; Matthews, WS: Psychologic and behavioral disturbance among epileptic children treated with barbiturate anticonvulsants. *Am J Psychiatry,* 140:112–113, 1983.

Fetzer, J; Kader, G; Danahy, S: Lithium encephalopathy: A clinical, psychiatric, and EEG evaluation. *Am J Psychiatry,* 138:1622–1623, 1981.

Fink, M: Missed seizures and the bilateral-unilateral electroconvulsive therapy controversy. *Am J Psychiatry,* 140:198–199, 1983.

Firsch, DO; Hasfield, WB; Change, PN; et al: An adult phenyketonuric with schizophrenia. *Minn Med,* 62:243–46, 1979.

Fishbain, DA; Rosomoff, H: Capgras Syndrome associated with metrizamide myelography. *Int J Psychiatry Med,* 16:131–136, 1986–87.

Flavin, DK; Franklin, JE; Frances, RJ: The acquired immune deficiency syndrome (AIDS) and suicidal behavior in alcohol-dependent homosexual men. *Am J Psychiatry,* 143:1440–1442, 1986.

Flaherty, JA; Lahmeyer, HW: Laryngeal-pharyngeal dystonia as a possible cause of asphyxia with haloperidol treatment. *Am J Psychiatry,* 135:1414–1415, 1978.

Fleishman, M: Board and Care Homes 1984: Return of the house call. *Psychiatric Annals,* 15:654–660, 1985.

Flippin, J; Henn, FA: Modified leukotemy in the treatment of intractable obsessional neurosis. *Am J Psychiatry,* 139:1601–1603, 1982.

Folks, DG; King, LD; Dowdy, SB; et al: Carbamazepine treatment of selected affectively disordered inpatients. *Am J Psychiatry,* 139:115–117, 1982.

Foltin, RW; Fischman, MW; Pedroso, JJ; Pearlson, GD: Marijuana and cocaine interactions in humans: Cardiovascular consequences. *Pharmacology Biochemistry and Behavior,* 28:459–464, 1987.

Fontaine, R: Clonazepam for panic disorders and agitation. *Psychosomatics,* 26:13–18, 1985.

Forrest, NJ; Cohen, JD; Iorretti, J; et al: On the mechanism of lithium induced diabetes insipidus in man and the rat. *J Clin Invest,* 53:115, 1974.

Forster, FM: *Synopsis of Neurology.* St Louis, CV Mosby Co., 1962.

Fowler, RC; Krontol, ZA; Perry, PJ: Water intoxication, psychosis, and inappropriate secretion of antidiuretic hormone. *Arch Gen Psychiatry,* 34:1097–1099, 1977.

Fowler, RC; Rich, CL; Young, D: San Diego Suicide Study: II. Substance abuse in young cases. *Arch Gen Psychiatry,* 43:962–965, 1986.

Frances, A; Brown, RP; Kocsis, JH; et al; Psychotic depression: A separate entity? *Am J Psychiatry,* 138:831–833, 1981.

Frances, A; Susman VL: Managing an acutely manic 17-year-old girl with neuroleptic malignant syndrome. *Hospital and Community Psychiatry,* 37:771–788, 1986.

Frances, RJ; Timm, S; Bucky, S: Studies of familial and nonfamilial alcoholism: I. Demographic Studies. *Arch Gen Psychiatry,* 37:564–566, 1980.

Frankel, M: Narcotic addiction, criminal responsibility and civil commitment. *Utah L Rev,* 581, 1956.

Frank, E; Kupfer, DJ; Jacob, M; Blumenthal, SJ; et al: Pregnancy-related affective episodes among women with recurrent depression. *Am J Psychiatry,* 144:288–293, 1987.

Frankl, VE: *Man's Search for Meaning.* New York, Washington Square Press, 1963.

Frankl, VE: *The Doctor and the Soul.* New York, Knopf, 1955.

Franks, RD; Dubovsky, SL; Lifshitz, M; et al: Long-term lithium carbonate therapy causes hyperparathyroidism. *Arch Gen Psychiatry,* 39:1074–1077, 1982.

Franks, RD; Richter, AJ: Schizophrenia-like psychosis associated with anticonvulsant toxicity. *Am J Psychiatry,* 136:973–974, 1979.

Fras, I; Karlavage, J: The use of methylphenidate and imipramine in Gilles de la Tourette's disease in children. *Am J Psychiatry,* 134:195–197, 1977.

Fraser, AR: Choice of antidepressants based on the dexamethasone suppression test. *Am J Psychiatry,* 140:786–787, 1983.

Fraser, HF; Wikler, A; Essig, EF; et al: Degree of physical dependence induced by secobarbital or pentobarbital. *JAMA,* 166:126–129, 1958.

Frederick, CJ: *Current Trends in Suicidal Behavior in the United States.* Paper presented in abridged form at Thirteenth National Scientific Meeting of the Association for the Advancement of Psychotherapy, Toronto, Canada, May 1, 1977.

Frederick, CJ: *Ecological Aspects of Self-Destruction: Some Legal, Legislative and Behavioral Implications in Health and Human Values.* A Jefcoat, ed. New York, John Wiley and Sons, 1972.

Frederick, CJ; Farberow, NL: Group psychotherapy with suicidal persons: A comparison with standard group methods. *Int J Soc Psychiat,* 16:103–111, 1970.

Frederick, CJ; Lague, L: *Dealing with the Crisis of Suicide.* New York, Public Affairs Pamphlet No. 406A, 1972. Copyright Public Affairs Committee, Inc., Eighth printing revised November, 1978.

Frederick, CJ; Resnik, HLP: How suicidal behaviors are learned. *Am J Psychotherapy,* 25:37–55, 1971.

Frederick, CJ; Resnik, HLP: Interventions with suicidal patients. *J Contemporary Psychotherapy,* 2:103–109, 1970.

Frederick, CJ: The present suicide taboo in the United States. *Mental Hygiene,* 55:178–183, 1971.

Frederick, CJ: The role of the nurse in crisis intervention and suicide prevention. *J Psychiat Nursing,* 11:27–31, 1973.

Frederick, CJ: The school guidance counselor as a preventive agent to self-destructive behavior. *New York State Personnel and Guidance Journal,* 5:1–5, 1970.

Freedman, R; Schwab, PJ: Paranoid symptoms in patients on a general hospital psychiatric unit: Implications for diagnosis and treatment. *Arch Gen Psychiatry,* 35:387–390, 1978.

Freud, S: *Beyond the Pleasure Principle.* London, Hogarth, 1950.

Freud, S: Mourning and melancholia. In: *Collected Papers IV.* London, Hogarth Press, 1925.

Freudenberger, HJ: The staff burn-out syndrome in alternative institutions. *Psychotherapy: Theory, Research and Practice,* 12:73–82, 1975.

Fricchione, GL; Vlay, SC: Psychiatric aspects of patients with malignant ventricular arrhythmias. *Am J Psychiatry,* 143:1518–1526, 1986.

Fried, PH; Rakoff, AE; Schopbach, RR; et al: Pseudocyesis: A psychosomatic study in gynecology. *JAMA,* 145:1329–1335, 1951.

Friedman, E: Death from Ipecac intoxication in a patient with anorexia nervosa. *Am J Psychiatry,* 141:702–703, 1984.

Friedman, I; Von Mering, O; Hinko, EN: Intermittent patienthood. *Arch Gen Psychiatry,* 33:386, 1976.

Friedman, MJ; Lipowski, ZJ: Pseudodementia in a young Ph.D. *Am J Psychiatry,* 138:381–382, 1981.

Friedman, RC; Aronoff, MS; Clarkin, JF; Corn, R; et al: History of suicidal behavior in depressed borderline inpatients. *Am J Psychiatry,* 140:1023–1026, 1983.

Friedman, RC; Hurt, SW; Clarkin, J; et al: Sexual histories and premenstrual affective syndrome in psychiatric inpatients. *Am J Psychiatry,* 139:1484–1486, 1982.

Frierson, RL; Lippmann, SB: Psychiatric consultation for acute amputees. *Psychosomatics,* 28:183–189, 1987.

Frierson, RL; Lippmann, SB; Johnson, J: AIDS: Psychological stresses on the family. *Psychosomatics,* 28:65–68, 1987.

Frisbie, JH: Behavioral disturbance, embolism, and mitral stenosis. *Int J Psychiatry Med,* 16:249–256, 1986–87.

Fudge, JL; Perry, PJ; Garvey, MJ; et al: A comparison of the effect of fluoxetine and trazodone on the cognitive functioning of depressed outpatients. *J Affective Disord,* 18:259–266, 1990.

Fullerton, DT; Harvey, RF; Klein, MH; et al: Psychiatric disorders in patients with spinal cord injuries. *Arch Gen Psychiatry,* 38:1369–1371, 1981.

Fulop, G; Strain, JJ: Psychiatric emergencies in the general hospital. *Gen Hosp Psychiatry,* 8:425–431, 1986.

Fyer, AJ; Liebowitz, MR; Gorman, JM; Campeas, R; et al: Discontinuation of alprazolam treatment in panic patients. *Am J Psychiatry,* 144:303–308, 1987.

Fyer, AJ; Mannuzza, S; Gallops, MS; et al: Familial transmission of simple phobias and fears. A preliminary report. *Arch Gen Psychiatry,* 47:277–284, 1990.

Fyer, MR; Frances, AJ; Sullivan, T; Hurt, SW; et al: Suicide attempts in patients with borderline personality disorder. *Am J Psychiatry,* 145:737–739, 1988a.

Fyer, MR; Frances, AJ; Sulivan, T; Hurt, SW: Comorbidity of borderline personality disorder. *Arch Gen Psychiatry,* 45:348–352, 1988b.

Gaby, NS; Lefkowitz, DS; Israel, JR: Treatment of lithium tremor with metoprolol. *Am J Psychiatry,* 140:593–595, 1983.

Gaff, DC; Brotman, AW; Waites, M; et al: Trial of flouoxetine added to neuroleptus for treatment resistant schizophrenic patients. *Am J Psychiatry,* 147:492–494, 1990.

Gaitz, CM; Varner, RV; Overall, JE: Pharmacotherapy for organic brain syndrome in late life. Evaluation of an Ergot derivative vs. placebo. *Arch Gen Psychiatry,* 34:839–845, 1977.

Galanter M: Cults and zealous self-help movements: A psychiatric perspective. *Am J Psychiatry,* 147:543–551, 1990.

Gallagher, RM; Stewart, FI; Weissbein, T; Weissbein, A: Nonnarcotic analgesic abuse: A common biopsychosocial problem. *Gen Hosp Psychiatry,* 9:102–107, 1988.

Gallner, G; Haldipua, CV: Life events and early and late onset of bipolar illness. *Am J Psychiatry,* 140:215–217, 1983.

Gammon, GD; Hansen, C: A Case of akinesia induced by amoxapine. *Am J Psychiatry,* 141:283–284, 1984.

Gancher, S; Cponant-Norville, D; Anzell, R: Treatment of Tourette's syndrome with transdermal clonidine: A pilot study. *J Neuropsychiatry,* 2:66–69, 1990.

Garber, HJ; Weilburg, JB; Buonanno, FS; Manschreck, TC; et al: Use of magnetic resonance imaging in psychiatry. *Am J Psychiatry,* 145:164–171, 1988.

Garbus, SB; Weber, MP; Priest, RT; et al: The abrupt discontinuation of antihypertensive treament. *J Clin Pharmacol,* 1:476–486, 1979.

Garbutt, J; Malepoar, B; Brunswick, O; et al: Effects of triiodothyromine on drug levels and cardiac function in depressed patients treated with imipramine. *Am J Psychiatry,* 136:980–982, 1979.

Garcia, RI; Gutierrez, JM; Faraone, SV; et al: Use of lorazepam for increased anxiety after neuroleptic dose reduction. *Hospital and Community Psychiatry,* 41:197–198, 1990.

Gardner, DL; Cowdry, RW: Alprazolam-induced dyscontrol in borderline personality disorder. *Am J Psychiatry,* 142:98–100, 1985.

Gardner, HJ; Fischer, E; Hess, J: Side effects of clozapine. *Psychopharmacology,* 99:S97–S100, 1989.

Gardos, G: Dystonic reaction during maintenance antipsychotic therapy. *Am J Psychiatry,* 138:114–115, 1981.

Gardos, G; Cole, JO: Overview: Public health issues in tardive dyskinesia. *Am J Psychiatry,* 140:200–202, 1983.

Gardos, G; Cole, JO: Weight reduction in schizophrenics by molindone. *Am J Psychiatry,* 134:302–304, 1977.

Gardos, G; Cole, JO: Salomon; M; Schniebolk, S: Clinical forms of severe tardive dyskinesia. *Am J Psychiatry,* 144:895–902, 1987.

Gardos, G; Cole, JO; Tarsy, D: Withdrawal syndromes associated with antipsychotic drugs. *Am J Psychiatry,* 135:1321–1324, 1978.

Garfield, P: Nightmares in the sexually abused female teenager. *Psychiatr J Univ Ottawa,* 12:93–97, 1987.

Garfinkel, BD; Golombek, H: Suicide and depression in childhood and adolescence. *Can Med Assoc J,* 110:1278–1281, 1974.

Garfinkel, BD; Froese, A; Hood, J: Parasuicide in children and adolescents. Paper presented at the International Association for Suicide Prevention, Ottawa, June 1979.

Garfunkel, BD; Froese, A; Hood, J: Suicide attempts in children and adolescents. *Am J Psychiatry,* 139:1257–1261, 1982.

Garfinkel, PE; Kaplan, AS; Garner, DM; Darby, P: The differentiation of vomiting/weight loss as a conversion disorder from anorexia nervosa. *Am J Psychiatry,* 140:1019–1022, 1983.

Garfinkel, PE; Moldofsky, H; Garner, DM: Prognosis in anorexia nervosa as influenced by clinical features, treatment and self-perception. *Can Med Assoc J,* 117:1041–1045, 1977.

Garfinkel, PE; Moldofsky, H; Garner, DM: The heterogeneity of anorexia nervosa: bulimia as a distinct subgroup. *Arch Gen Psychiatry,* 37:1036–1040, 1980.

Garkani, H; Zitrin, CM; Klein, DF: Treatment of panic disorder with imipramine alone. *Am J Psychiatry,* 141:446–448, 1984.

Garland, BJ; Ganz, VH; Fleiss, JL; et al: The study of the psychiatric symptoms of systemic lupus erythematosus. *Psychosom Med,* 34:199–206, 1972.

Gartrell, N: Increased libido in women receiving trazodone. *Am J Psychiatry,* 143:781–782, 1986.

Garvey, MJ; Tollefson, GD: Occurrence of myoclonus in patients treated with cyclic antidepressants. *Arch Gen Psychiatry,* 44:269–272, 1987.

Garvey, MJ; Wesner, R; Godes, M: Comparison of seasonal and nonseasonal affective disorders. *Am J Psychiatry,* 145:100–102, 1988.

Gastfriend, DR; Biederman, J; Jellinek, MS: Desipramine in the treatment of adolescents with attention deficit disorder. *Am J Psychiatry,* 141:906–908, 1984.

Gastfriend, DR; Rosenbaum, JF: Adjunctive buspirone in benzodiazepine treatment of four patients with panic disorder. *Am J Psychiatry,* 146:914–916, 1989.

Gastout, J; Broughton, R: A clinical and polygraphic study of episodic phenomena during sleep. *Biol Psychiatry,* 7:197–221, 1965.

Gawin, FH; Ellinwood, EH: Cocaine dependence. *Annu Rev Med,* 40:149–161, 1989.

Gawin, FH; Kleber, HD: Cocaine abuse treatment: Open pilot trial with desipramine and lithium carbonate. *Arch Gen Psychiatry,* 41:903–909, 1984.

Gawin, FH; Kleber, HD: Abstinence symptomatology and psychiatric diagnosis in cocaine abusers. *Arch Gen Psychiatry,* 43:107–113, 1986.

Gawin, FH; Kleber, HD; Byck, R; Rounsaville, BJ; et al: Desipramine facilitation of initial cocaine abstinence. *Arch Gen Psychiatry,* 46:117–121, 1989.

Gawin, FH; Markoff, RA: Panic anxiety after abrupt discontinuation of amitriptyline. *Am J Psychiatry,* 138:117–118, 1981.

Gelenberg, AJ: Single case study: Amoxapine, a new antidepressant appears in human milk. *J Nerv Ment Dis,* 167:635–636, 1979.

Gelenberg, AJ: The catatonic syndrome. *Lancet,* 1:1339–1341, 1976.

Gelenberg, AJ; Mandel, MR: Catatonic reactions to high-potency neuroleptic drugs. *Arch Gen Psychiatry,* 34:947–950, 1977.

Gelenberg, AJ; Bellinghausen, B; Wojcik, JD; Falk, WE; et al: A prospective survey of neuroleptic malignant syndrome in a short-term psychiatric hospital. *Am J Psychiatry,* 145:517–518, 1988.

Geller, B; Cooper, TB; Faroohi, ZO; et al: Dose and plasma levels of nortriptyline and chlorpromazine in delusionally depressed adolescents and of nortriptyline in nondelusionally depressed adolescents. *Am J Psychiatry,* 142:336–338, 1989.

Geller, B; Rogol, AD; Knitter, EF: Preliminary data on the dexamethasone suppression test in children with major depressive disorder. *Am J Psychiatry,* 140:620–622, 1983.

Geller, JL: Firesetting in the adult psychiatric population. *Hospital and Community Psychiatry,* 38:501–506, 1987.

Geller, JL; Fisher, WH; Wirth-Cauchon, JL; Simon, LJ: Second-generation deinstitutionalization, I: The impact of *Brewster v. Dukakis* on state hospital case mix. *Am J Psychiatry,* 147:982–987, 1990.

George, DT; Ladenheim, JA; Nutt, DJ: Effect of pregnancy on panic attacks. *Am J Psychiatry,* 144:1078–1079, 1987.

Gerbert; Badner; Maquire; Altman; et al: Why fear persists: health care professionals and AIDS. *JAMA,* 260:3481, 1988.

Gerle, B: Clinical observations on the side-effects of haloperidol. *Acta Psychiat Scand,* 40:65, 1964.

Gerner, RH; Gwirtsman, HE: Abnormalities of dexamethasone suppression test and urinary MHPG in anorexia nervosa. *Am J Psychiatry,* 138:650–653, 1981.

Gershon, ES; Hamovit, J; Guroff, JJ; et al: A family study of schizoaffective bipolar I, bipolar II, unipolar, and normal control probands. *Arch Gen Psychiatry,* 39:1157–1167, 1982.

Gerson, S; Bassuk, E: Psychiatric emergencies: An overview. *Am J Psychiatry,* 137:1–11, 1980.

Gerson, S; Shopsen, B (eds): *Lithium: Its Role in Psychiatric Research and Treatment* 2nd ed. New York, Plenum Press, 1976.

Gespert, M; Wheeler, K; Marsh, L; Davis, MS: Suicidal adolescents: Factors in evaluation. *Adolescence,* 20:753–762, 1985.

Ghadirian, AM; Gauthier, S; Bertrand, S: Anxiety attacks in a patient with a right temporal lobe meningioma. *J Clin Psychiatry,* 47:270–271, 1986.

Ghoneim, MM; Hinrichs, JV; Mewaldt, SP; Petersen, RC: Ketamine: Behavioral effects of subanesthetic doses. *J Clin Psychopharmacol,* 5:70–77, 1985.

Giannini, AJ; Eighan, MS; Loiselle, RH; Giannini, MC: Comparison of haloperidol and chlorpromazine in the treatment of phencyclidine psychosis. *J Clin Pharmacol,* 24:202–204, 1984a.

Giannini, AJ; Giannini, MC; Price, WA: Antidotal strategies in phencyclidine intoxication. *Int J Psychiatry Med,* 14:315–321, 1984b.

Giannini, AJ; Houser, WL; Loiselle, RH; Giannini, M; et al: Antimanic effects of verapamil. *Am J Psychiatry,* 141:1602–1603, 1984c.

Giannini, AJ; Slaby, AE: *Handbook of Overdose and Detoxification Emergencies.* New York, Medical Examination Publishing Company, 1983.

Gift, TE; Strauss, JS; Young, Y: Hysterical psychosis: An empirical approach. *Am J Psychiatry,* 142:345–347, 1985.

Gillette, GM; Garbutt, JC; Quade, DE: TSH response to TRH in depression with and without panic attacks. *Am J Psychiatry,* 146:743–748, 1989.

Gillig, PM; Dumaine, M; Stammer, JW; et al: What do police officers really want from the mental health system? *Hospital and Community Psychiatry,* 41:663–665, 1990.

Gillig, PM; Hillard, JR; Bell, J; et al: The psychiatric emergency service holding area: Effect on utilization of inpatient resources. *Am J Psychiatry,* 146:369–372, 1989.

Gilliland, K; Andress, D: Ad lib caffeine consumption symptoms of caffeinism, and academic performance. *Am J Psychiatry,* 138:512–514, 1981.

Gindolf, EW; Mulvey, EP; Ledz, CW: Characteristics of perpetrators of family and nonfamily assaults. *Hospital and Community Psychiatry,* 41:191–195, 1990.

Ginzburg, HM; MacDonald, MG; The epidemiology of human T-cell lymphotropic virus, type-III (HTLV-III disease). *Psychiatric Annals,* 16:153–157, 1986.

Glass, AJ: Psychotherapy in the combat zone. *Am J Psychiatry,* 110:725, 1954.

Glass, GS; Heninger, GR; Lansky, M; et al: Psychiatric emergencies related to the menstrual cycle. *Am J Psychiatry,* 128:705–711, 1971.

Glassman, A; Davis, JM: Overdose with tricyclic drugs. *Psychiatric Annals,* 17:410–411, 1987.

Glassman, AH; Arana, GW; Baldessarini, RJ; Brown, WA; et al: The dexamethasone suppression test: An overview of its current status in psychiatry. *Am J Psychiatry,* 144:1253–1262, 1987.

Glassman, AH; Bigger, JT: Cardiovascular effects of therapeutic doses of tricyclic antidepressants: A review. *Arch Gen Psychiatry,* 38:815–820, 1981.

Glassman, AH; Bigger, JT; Giardina, EV; et al: Clinical characteristics of imipramine-induced orthostatic hypotension. *Lancet,* i, 468–472, 1979.

Glassman, AH; Perel, JM; Shostak, M; et al: Clinical implications of imipramine plasma levels for depressive illness. *Arch Gen Psychiatry,* 34:197–204, 1977.

Glassman, AH; Roose, SP: Delusional depression: A distinct clinical entity? *Arch Gen Psychiatry*, 38:424–427, 1981.

Glassman, JN; Dryer, D; McCartney, JR: Complex partial status epilepticus presenting as gelastic seizures: A case report. *Gen Hosp Psychiatry*, 8:61–64, 1986.

Glassman, JN; Magulac, M; Darko, DF: Folie a famille: Shared paranoid disorder in a Vietnam veteran and his family. *Am J Psychiatry*, 144:658–660, 1987.

Glassner, B; Haldipur, CV: Life events and early and late onset of bipolar disorder. *Am J Psychiatry*, 140:215–217, 1983.

Glazer, WM: An introduction to tardive dyskinesia. *Psychiatric Annals*, 288, 1988.

Glazer, WM: Moore, DC; Hansen, TC; et al: Meige syndrome and tardive dyskinesia. *Am J Psychiatry*, 140:798–799, 1983.

Glazer, WM; Pino, CD; Quinlan, D: The reassessment of chronic patients previously diagnosed as schizophrenic. *J Clin Psychiatry*, 48:430–434, 1987.

Glick, I; Hargreaves, WA; Drues, J; et al: Short vs. long hospitalization: a prospective controlled study. VII. Two-year follow-up results for nonschizophrenics. *Arch Gen Psychiatry*, 34:314–317, 1977.

Glothlin, WH; Anglin, MD: Shutting off methadone: Costs and benefits. *Arch Gen Psychiatry*, 38:885–892, 1981.

Godwin, CD: Case report of tricyclic-induced delirium at a therapeutic drug concentration. *Am J Psychiatry*, 140:1517–1518, 1983.

Goff, DC: The stimulant challenge test in depression. *J Clin Psychiatry*, 47:538–543, 1986.

Goffman, E: *Asylums*. New York, Anchor, 1961.

Goggans, FC: A case of mania secondary to vitamin B_{12} deficiency. *Am J Psychiatry*, 141:300–301, 1984.

Goggans, FC; Odgers, RP; Luscombe, SM; Foust, R; et al: Chemical dependency and anxiety disorders. *The Psychiatric Hospital*, 20:79–83, 1990.

Goin, MK; Goin, JM: Mid-life reactions to mastectomy and subsequent breast reconstruction. *Arch Gen Psychiatry*, 38:225–227, 1981.

Gold, M: *Psychiatric Emergencies*. Unpublished mimeo. Summit, New Jersey, Fair Oaks Hospital, 1979.

Gold, MS; Herridge, P; Hapworth, WE: Depression and "symptomless" autoimmune thyroiditis. *Psychiatric Annals*, 17:750–757, 1987.

Gold, MS; Pottash, ALC; Extein, I: "Symptomless" autoimmune thyroiditis in depression. *Psychiatry Research*, 6:261–269, 1982.

Gold, MS; Pottash, ALC; Sweeney, DR; et al: Further evidence of hypothalamic–pituitary dysfunction in anorexia nervosa. *Am J Psychiatry*, 137:101–102, 1980.

Goldacre, M; Hawton, K: Repetition of self-poisoning and subsequent death in adolescents who take overdoses. *Br J Psychiatry*, 146:395–398, 1985.

Goldberg, D; Steele, JJ; Johnson, A; et al: Ability of primary care physicians to make accurate ratings of psychiatric symptoms. *Arch Gen Psychiatry*, 39:829–833, 1982.

Goldberg, EL: Depression and suicide ideation in the young adult. *Am J Psychiatry*, 128:35–40, 1981.

Goldberg, J; Sakinofsky, I: Intropunitiveness and parasuicide: Prediction of interview response. *Br J Psychiatry*, 153:801–804, 1988.

Goldberg, MC: Women's friendships—women's groups. *Pychiatric Annals*, 20:398–401, 1990.

Goldberg, RJ; Slaby, AE: *Diagnosing Disorders of Mood, Thought and Behavior*. New York, Medical Examination Publishing Company, 1981.

Goldberg, RJ; Cullen, LO: Use of psychotropics in cancer patients. *Psychosomatics*, 27:687–700, 1986.

Goldberg, RJ; Slaby, AE: Psychosocial aspects of living with cancer. In: *Medical Oncology*. P. Calabresi, PS Shein, SA Rosenberg, eds. New York, MacMillan Co. 1985.

Goldberg, RL; Wise, TN: Corticosteroid abuse revisited. *Int J Psychiatry Med*, 16:145–149, 1986–87.

Goldberg, VJ; Dubin, WR; Fogel BS: Behavioural emergencies: Assessment and psychopharmacologic management. *Clin Neuropharmacol*, 12:233–248, 1989.

Goldberg, RJ: Use of constant observation with potentially suicidal patients in general hospitals. *Hospital and Community Psychiatry*, 38:303–305, 1987.

Golden, RN; Hoffman, J; Falk, D; Provenzale, D; et al: Psychoses associated with propranolol withdrawal. *Biol Psychiatry*, 25:351–354, 1989.

Golden, CJ; Graber, B; Coffman, J; et al: Structural brain deficits in schizophrenia. Identification by computed tomographic scan density measurements. *Arch Gen Psychiatry,* 38:1014–1017, 1981.

Golden, CJ; Moses, JA; Zelazowski, R; et al: Cerebral ventricular size and neuropsychological impairment in young chronic schizophrenics: Measurement by the standardized Luria-Medroska Neuropsychological Battery. *Arch Gen Psychiatry,* 37:619–623, 1980.

Golden, KM: Voodoo in Africa and the United States. *Am J Psychiatry,* 134:1425–1427, 1977.

Golden, RN; James, SP; Sherer, MA; Rudorfer, MV; et al: Psychoses associated with bupropion treatment. *Am J Psychiatry,* 142:1459–1462, 1985.

Goldfeld, AE; Mollica, RF; Pesavento, BH; Faraone, SV: The physical and psychological sequelae of torture. *JAMA,* 259:2725–2729, 1988.

Golding, JM; Karno, M; Rutter, CM: Symptoms of major depression among Mexican-Americans and non-Hispanic whites. *Am J Psychiatry,* 147:861–866, 1990.

Goldman, LS; Hudson, JI; Weddington, WW: Lupus-like illness associated with chlorpromazine. *Am J Psychiatry,* 137:1613–1614, 1980.

Goldman, LS; Tiller, JA: Hypomania related to phenelzine and isoetharine interaction in one patient. *J Clin Psychiatry,* 48:170, 1987.

Goldney, RD; Katsikitis, M: Cohort analysis of suicide rates in Australia. *Arch Gen Psychiatry,* 40:71–74, 1983.

Goldstein, DM; Goldberg, RL: Monoamine oxidase inhibitor-induced speech blockage. *J Clin Psychiatry,* 47:604, 1986.

Goldstein, J; Windle, C: *Ideas for Improving Telephone Emergency Services.* Unpublished mimeo available from C. Windle, Room 11-C-03, NIMH, 5600 Fishers Lane, Rockville, Maryland, 20857.

Goldstein, MJ; Rodnick, EH; Evan, JR; et al: Drug and family therapy in the aftercare of acute schizophrenics. *Arch Gen Psychiatry,* 35:1169–1177, 1978.

Gonsalves-Ebrahim, L; Sternin, G; Gulledge, AD; Gipson, WT; et al: Noncompliance in younger adults on hemodialysis. *Psychosomatics,* 28:34–41, 1987.

Good, MI: Pseudodementia and physical findings masking significant psychopathology. *Am J Psychiatry,* 138:811–814, 1981.

Good, MI: Primary affective disorders, aggression, and criminality. A review and clinical study. *Arch Gen Psychiatry,* 35:954–960, 1978.

Good, MI; Shoder, RI: Behavioral toxicity and equivocal suicide associated with chloroquine and its derivatives. *Arch J Psychiatry,* 134:798–801, 1977.

Goodman, LS; Gilman, A: *The Pharmacological Basis of Therapeutics.* 5th ed. New York, MacMillan Publishing Co., 1975.

Goodman, LS; Gilman, A: *The Pharmacological Basis of Theapeutics,* 4th ed. New York, MacMillan, 1970.

Goodman, WK; Charney, DS; Price, LH; Woods, SW; et al: Ineffectiveness of clonidine in the treatment of the benzodiazepine withdrawal syndrome: Report of three cases. *Am J Psychiatry,* 143:900–903, 1986.

Goodman, WK; Price, LH; Charney, DS: Fluvoxamine in obsessive–compulsive disorder. *Psychiatric Annals,* 19:92–96, 1989.

Goodnick, PJ; Fieve, RR; Schlegel, A; Kaufman, K: Lithium level and inter-episode symptoms in affective disorder. *Acta Psychiatr Scand,* 75:601–603, 1987.

Goodnick, PJ; Extein, IL; Gold, MS: TRH test identification of thyroid-responsive depression. *Ann Clin Psychiatry,* 1:175–178, 1989.

Goodstein, RK: Overview: Cerebrovascular accident and the hospitalized elderly—a multidimensional clinical problem. *Am J Psychiatry,* 140, 141–147, 1983.

Goodstein, RK; Page, AW: Battered wife syndrome: Overview of dynamics and treatment. *Am J Psychiatry,* 138:1036–1044, 1981.

Goodwin, D: *Is Alcoholism Hereditary?* New York, Oxford University Press, 1976.

Goodwin, DW; Guze, SB: *Psychiatric Diagnosis.* New York, Oxford University Press, 1979.

Goodwin, FW; Prange, AF; Post, RM; et al: Potentiation of antidepressant effects by L-triiodothyromine in tricyclic nonresponders. *Am J Psychiatry,* 139:34–38, 1982.

Goodwin, JM; Cheever, K; Connell, V: Borderline and other severe symptoms in adult survivors of incestuous abuse. *Psychiatric Annals,* 20:22–32, 1990.

Gordon, JS: The runaway center as community mental health center. *Am J Psychiatry,* 135:932–935, 1978.

Gorman, JM; Fyer, AF; Glicklich, J; et al: Effect of imipramine in prolapsed mitral valves of patients with panic disorder. *Am J Psychiatry,* 138:977–978, 1981a.

Gorman, JM; Fyer, AF; Glicklich, J; et al: Effect of sodium lactate on patients with panic disorder and mitral valve prolapse. *Am J Psychiatry,* 138:247–249, 1981b.

Gorman, JM; Liebowitz, MR; Fyer, AJ; Stein, J: A neuroanatomical hypothesis for panic disorder. *Am J Psychiatry,* 146:148–161, 1989.

Gorman, JM; Martinez, JM; Liebowitz, MR; Fyer, AJ; et al: Hypoglycemia and panic attacks. *Am J Psychiatry,* 141:101–102, 1984.

Gostin, L: Confusion from pyridostigmine bromide: Was there bromide intoxication? *JAMA* 264:454–456, 1990.

Gottlieb, GL: Sleep disorders and their management: Special considerations in the elderly. *Am J Med,* 88 (suppl 3A):295–300, 1990.

Goyer, PF; Eddleman, HC: Same-sex rape of nonincarcerated men. *Am J Psychiatry,* 141:576–579, 1984.

Graber, HJ; Weilburg, JB; Daffy, FH; et al: Clinical use of typographic brain electrical activity mapping in psychiatry. *J Clin Psychiatry,* 50:205–211, 1989.

Graham, D; Kabler, J; Lunsford, L: Vasovagal fainting: A diphasic response. *Psychosom Med,* 23:493–507, 1961.

Grahmann, R; Ruther, E; Sanin, W; et al: Adverse effects of clozapine. *Psychopharmacology,* 99:S101–S104, 1989.

Grakash, R; Sethi, N; Agrarval, S; et al: A case report of megatoblastic anemia secondary to lithium. *Am J Psychiatry,* 138:849, 1981.

Gram, LF; Overo, KF: Drug interaction: Inhibitory effect of neuroleptics on metabolism of tricyclic antidepressants in man. *Br Med J,* I:463–465, 1972.

Granacher, RP: Differential diagnosis of tardive dyskinesia: An overview. *Am J Psychiatry,* 138:1288–1297, 1981.

Grant, BL; Lindsay, PB: Psychosis and water intoxication as presenting symptoms of pulmonary carcinoma. *Psychosomatics,* 27:732–733, 1986.

Grant, I; Reed, R; Adams, KM: Diagnosis of intermediate-duration and subacute organic mental disorders in abstinent alcoholics. *J Clin Psychiatry,* 48:319–323, 1987.

Greaves, G; Ghant, L: Comparison of accomplished suicides with persons contacting a crisis intervention clinic. *Psychol Rep,* 3:390, 1972.

Greden, JF: Anxiety or caffeinism: A diagnostic dilemma. *Am J Psychiatry,* 131:1089, 1974.

Greden, JF; Gardner, R; King, D; et al: Dexamethasone suppression tests in antidepressant treatment of melancholia: The process of normalization of test-retest reproductability. *Arch Gen Psychiatry,* 40:493–500, 1983.

Green, AI; Salzman, C: Clozapine: Benefits and risks. *Hospital and Community Psychiatry,* 41:379–380, 1990.

Green, BL; Grace, MC; Lindy, JD, et al: Risk factors for PTSD and other diagnoses in a general sample of Vietnam veterans. *Am J Psychiatry,* 142:729–733, 1990.

Greenberg, L; Fink, M: Electroconvulsive therapy in the elderly. *Psychiatric Annals,* 20:99–101, 1990.

Greenblatt, DJ; Kock-Wesner, J: Adverse reactions to propranolol in hospitalized medical patients: A report from the Boston Collaborative Drug Surveillance Program. *Am Heart J,* 86:478–484, 1973.

Greenblatt, DJ; Shader, RI; Abernethy, DR: Current status of benzodiazepines. *N Engl J Med,* 309:354–358, 1983.

Greenblatt, DJ; Shader, RI; Abernethy, DR: Current status of benzodiazepines. *N Engl J Med,* 309:410–415, 1983.

Greenblatt, DJ; Shader, RI: *Benzodiazepines in Clinical Practice.* New York, Raven Press, 1974.

Greenblatt, M: Efficacy of ECT in affective and schizophrenic illness. *Am J Psychiatry,* 134:1001–1005, 1977.

Greenfeld, D: Feigned psychosis in a 14-year-old girl. *Hospital and Community Psychiatry,* 38:73–75, 1987.

Greenfield, TK; McNiel, DE; Binder, RL: Violent behavior and length of psychiatric hospitalization. *Hospital and Community Psychiatry,* 40:809–814, 1989.

Greenspan, GS; Samuel, SE: Self-cutting after rape. *Am J Psychiatry,* 146:789–790, 1989.

Greilsheimer, H; Groves, JE: Male genital self-mutilation. *Arch Gen Psychiatry,* 36:441–446, 1979.

Greyson, B: Incidence of near-death experiences following attempted suicide. *Suicide and Life-Threatening Behavior,* 16:40–45, 1986.

Griffin, ML; Weiss, RD; Mirin, SM; Lange, U: A comparison of male and female cocaine abusers. *Arch Gen Psychiatry,* 46:122–126, 1989.

Griffin, SJ; Friedman, JM; Depressive symptoms in propranolol users. *J Clin Psychiatry,* 47:453–457, 1986.

Griffith, EEH; Bell, CC: Recent trends in suicide and homicide among blacks. *JAMA,* 262:2265–2289, 1989.

Grinker, RR; Werble, B; Urye, R: *The Borderline Syndrome: A Behavioral Study of Ego Function.* New York, Basic Books, 1968.

Gross, M: Pseudoepilepsy: A study in adolescent hysteria. *Am J Psychiatry,* 136:210–213, 1979.

Gross-Isseroff, R; Israeli, M; Biegon, A: Autoradiographic analysis of tritiated imipramine binding in the human brain post mortem: Effects of suicide. *Arch Gen Psychiatry,* 46:237–241, 1990.

Groth, AN; Burgess, AW: Male rape: Offenders and victims. *Am J Psychiatry,* 157:806–810, 1980.

Groves, JE; Mandel, MR: The long-acting phenothiazines. *Arch Gen Psychiatry,* 32:893–900, 1975.

Gualtieri, CT; Schroeder, SR; Hicks, RE; Quade, D: Tardive dyskinesia in young mentally retarded individuals. *Arch Gen Psychiatry,* 43:335–340, 1986.

Gualtieri, CT; Staze, J: Withdrawal symptoms after abrupt cessation of amitriptyline in an eight-year-old boy. *Am J Psychiatry,* 136:457–459, 1979.

Gukstien, OG; Brent, DA; Kaminer, Y: Comorbidity of substance abuse and other psychiatric disorders in adolescents. *Am J Psychiatry,* 146:1131–1141, 1989.

Guilleminault, C; Raynal, D; Takahashi, S; et al: Evaluation of short-term and long-term treatment of the narcolepsy syndrome with clomipramine hydrochloride. *Acta Neurol Scand,* 54:71–87, 1976.

Gunderson, JG; Elliott, GR: The interface between borderline personality disorder and affective disorder. *Am J Psychiatry,* 142:277–288, 1985.

Gunderson, JG; Singer, MT: Defining borderline patients: An overview. *Am J Psychiatry,* 132:1, 1975.

Gunderson, JG; Zanarini, MC: Current overview of the borderline diagnosis. *J Clin Psychiatry,* 48:5–11, 1987.

Gupta, MA; Gupta, AK; Haberman, HF: The self-inflicted dermatoses: A critical review. *Gen Hosp Psychiatry,* 9:45–52, 1987.

Gupta, R: Alternative patterns of seasonal affective disorder: Three case reports from North India. *Am J Psychiatry,* 145:515–516, 1988.

Gurland, BJ; Ganz, VH; Fleiss, JL; et al: The study of the psychiatric symptoms of systemic lupus erythematosus. *Psychosom Med,* 34:199–206, 1972.

Gutheil, TG: The effect of Rogers on forensic emergency psychiatry. *Am J Psychiatry,* 142:1521–1522, 1985.

Guttmacher, M; Weihofen, H : *Psychiatry and the Law.* New York, WW Norton, 1952.

Guze, SB; Robbins, E: Suicide and primary affective disorders. *Br J Psychiatry,* 117:437–438, 1970.

Guze, SB: The validity and significance of the clinical diagnosis of hysteria (Briquet's syndrome). *Am J Psychiatry,* 140:559–563, 1983.

Hackett, TP: Depression following myocardial infarction. *Psychosomatics,* 26:23–30, 1985.

Hadl, J: *Short Term Therapy: A Personal Exposition and a Historical Perspective.* (Unpublished mimeo). Bethesda, Maryland, 1979.

Haggerty, JJ; Drossman, DA: Use of psychotropic drugs in patients with peptic ulcer. *Psychosomatics,* 26:277–284, 1985.

Haggerty, JJ; Evans, DL; Pringe, AJ: Organic brain syndrome associated with marginal hypothyroidism. *Am J Psychiatry,* 143:785–786, 1986.

Haggerty, JJ; Jackson, R: Mania following change from trazodone to imipramine. *J Clin Psychopharmacol,* 5:342–343, 1985.

Hahn, TJ: Drug-induced disorders of vitamin D and mineral metabolism. *Clin Endocrinol Metab,* 9:107–129, 1980.

Hajal, F; Leach, AM: Familial aspects of Gilles de la Tourette syndrome. *Am J Psychiatry,* 138:90–95, 1981.

Halbreich, V; Endicott, J; Nee, J: Premenstrual depressive changes: Value of differentiation. *Arch Gen Psychiatry,* 40:535–542, 1983.

Hales v. Petit, 75 *Eng. Rep.* 387 (KB) (1562).

Hall, PE; Multiple personality disorder and homicide: Professional and legal issues. Paper presented at the Fourth International Conference on Multiple Personality/Dissociative States, in Chicago, Illinois, November 6, 1987.

Hall, RCW; Gardner, ER; Papkin, MK; et al: Unrecognized physical illness prompting psychiatric admission: A prospective study. *Am J Psychiatry,* 138:629–634, 1981.

Hall, RCW; Gardner, ER; Perl, M; et al: *Psychiatric Opinion,* pp. 12–17, 1979.

Hall, RCW; Gardner, ER; Stickney, SK; et al: Physical illness manifesting as psychiatric illness: II. Analysis of a state hospital inpatient population. *Arch Gen Psychiatry,* 37:989–995, 1980.

Hall, RCW; Popkin, MK; McHenry, LE: Angel's trumpet psychosis: A central nervous system anticholinergic syndrome. *Am J Psychiatry,* 134:312–314, 1977.

Haller, E; Binder, RL: Clozapine and seizures. *Am J Psychiatry,* 147:1069–1071, 1990.

Halliday, JL: Principles of etiology. *Brit J Med Psychol,* 19:367, 1943.

Halmi, KA; Falk, JR; Schwartz, E: Binge eating and vomiting: A survey of a college population. *Psychol Med,* 11:697–706, 1981.

Halperin, DA: Psychiatric perspectives on cult affiliation. *Psychiatric Annals,* 20:206–213, 1990.

Hammer, DW; Matsuo, V; Malkowitz, O; et al: Benzodiazepine sensitivity in normal human subjects. *Arch Gen Psychiatry,* 43:542–551, 1986.

Hammer v. Rosen, 7 NY 2d 376, 165 NE 2d 756, 198 *NYS* 2d 65 (1960).

Harcherik, DF; Cohen, DJ; Ort, S; Paul, R; et al: Computed tomographic brain scanning in four neuropsychiatric disorders of childhood. *Am J Psychiatry,* 142:731–734, 1985.

Hardy, MC; Lecrubier, Y; Widlocher, D: Efficacy of clonidine in 24 patients with acute mania. *Am J Psychiatry,* 143:1450–1453, 1986.

Hargreaves, WA; Glick, ID; Drues, J; et al: Short vs. long hospitalization: A prospective controlled study. VI. Two-year follow-up results for schizophrenics. *Arch Gen Psychiatry,* 34:305–311, 1977.

Harkavy, JM; Asnis, G: Suicide attempts in adolescence: Previolence and implications. *N Engl J Med,* 313:1290–1291, 1985.

Harkavy-Friedman, JM; Asnis, GM: Assessment of suicidal behavior: A new instrument. *Psychiatric Annals,* 19:382–387, 1989.

Harkavy-Friedman, JM; Asnis, GM; Boeck, M; DiFiore, J: Prevalence of specific suicidal behaviors in a high school sample. *Am J Psychiatry,* 144:1203–1206, 1987.

Harkoff, LD: *Emergency Psychiatric Treatment. A Handbook of Secondary Prevention.* Springfield, Charles C. Thomas, 1969.

Harper, RW; Knothe, JC: Coloured lilliputian hallucinations with amantadine. *Med J Aust,* 1:444–445, 1973.

Harrell, RG; Othmer, E: Postcardiotomy confusion and sleep loss. *J Clin Psychiatry,* 48:445–446, 1987.

Harrington, R; Fudge, H; Rutter, M; et al: Adult outcomes of childhood and adolescent depression. I. Psychiatric statistics. *Arch Gen Psychiatry,* 47:465–473, 1990.

Harris, EL; Noyes, R; Crowe, RR; Chaudhry, DR: Family study of agoraphobia. *Arch Gen Psychiatry,* 40:1061–1064, 1983.

Harrow, M; Carone, BJ; Westermeyer, JF: The course of psychosis in early phases of schizophrenia. *Am J Psychiatry,* 142:702–707, 1985.

Harrow, M; Goldberg, JF; Grossman, LS; et al: Outcome in manic disorders: A naturalistic follow-up study. *Arch Gen Psychiatry,* 47:665–671, 1990.

Harrow, M; Grinker, RR; Holzman, PS; Kayton, L: Anhedonia and schizophrenia. *Am J Psychiatry,* 134:794–797, 1977.

Harrow, M; Grossman, LS; Silverstein, ML; Meltzer, HY; et al: A longitudinal study of thought disorder in manic patients. *Arch Gen Psychiatry,* 43:781–785, 1986.

Hartman, N; Kramer, R; Brown, WT; et al: Panic disorder in patients with mitral valve prolapse. *Am J Psychiatry,* 139:1563–1566, 1982.

Hartmann, E; Russ, D; Oldfield, M; Sivan, I: Who has nightmares? The personality of the lifelong nightmare sufferer. *Arch Gen Psychiatry,* 44:49–56, 1987.

Harvey, NS: Psychiatric disorders in parkinsonism: 2. Organic cerebral states and drug reactions. *Psychosomatics*, 27:175–182, 1986.

Haskett, RF: Diagnostic categorization of psychiatric disturbance in Cushing's syndrome. *Am J Psychiatry*, 142:911–916, 1985.

Hassan, R; Tan, G: Suicide trends in Australia, 1901–1985: An analysis of sex differentials. *Suicide and Life-Threatening Behavior*, 19:362–380, 1989.

Hausman, A; Rioch, DM: Military psychiatry. *Arch Gen Psychiatry*, 16:727, 1967.

Hausner, RS: Amantadine-associated recurrence of psychosis. *Am J Psychiatry*, 137:240–242, 1980.

Haverkos, HW, Edelman, R: The epidemiology of acquired immunodeficiency syndrome among heterosexuals. *JAMA*, 260:1922–1929, 1988.

Hawkins, DR; Taub, JM; Van de Castle, RL: Extended sleep (hypersomnia) in young depressed patients. *Am J Psychiatry*, 142:905–910, 1985.

Hawton, K: Attempted suicide in children and adolescents. *Journal of Child Psychology and Psychiatry and Allied Disciplines*, 23:497–503, 1982.

Hawton, K; Cole, D; O'Grady, J; Osborn, M: Motivational aspects of deliberate self-poisoning in adolescents. *Br J Psychiatry*, 141:286–291, 1982.

Hawton, K; Fagg, J; Simkin, S: Female unemployment and attempted suicide. *Br J Psychiatry*, 152:632–637, 1988.

Hawton, K; O'Grady, J; Osborn, M; Cole, D: Adolescents who take overdoses: Their characteristics, problems and contacts with helping agencies. *Br J Psychiatry*, 140:118–123, 1982.

Hay, GG; Jolley, DJ; Jones, RG: A case of Capgras syndrome in association with pseudohypoparathyroidism. *Acta Psychiat Scand*, 50:73–77, 1974.

Heacoch, DR: Suicidal behavior in black and hispanic youth. *Psychiatric Annals*, 20:134–142, 1990.

Hechtman, L: Attention-deficit hyperactivity disorder in adolescence and adulthood: A updated follow-up. *Psychiatric Annals*, 19:597–603, 1989.

Hegedus, AM; Tarter, RE; VanThiel, DH; Schade, RR; et al: Neuropsychiatric characteristics associated with primary biliary cirrhosis. *Int J Psychiatry Med*, 14:303–314, 1984.

Heh, CWC; Smith, R; Wu, J; Hazlett, E; et al: Positron emission tomography of the cerebellum in autism. *Am J Psychiatry*, 146:242–245, 1989.

Heimberg, RG; Barlow, DH: Psychosocial treatments for social phobia. *Psychosomatics*, 29:27–32, 1988.

Heinrichs, DW; Carpenter, WT: Prospective study of prodromal symptoms in schizophrenic relapse. *Am J Psychiatry*, 142:371–373, 1985.

Heiser, JF; Wilbert, DE: Reversal of delirium induced by tricyclic antidepressant drugs with physostigmine. *Am J Psychiatry*, 131:1275, 1974.

Helfer, R; Kempe, C: *The Battered Child*. Chicago, University of Chicago Press, 1968.

Heller, SS; Kornfeld, DS; Frank, KA; et al: Postcardiotomy delirium and cardiac output. *Am J Psychiatry*, 136:337–339, 1979.

Hellerstein, D; Frosch, W; Koenigsberg, HW: The clinical significance of command hallucinations. *Am J Psychiatry*, 144:219–221, 1987.

Hellon, CP; Solomon, MI: Suicide age in Alberta, Canada, 1951 to 1977. The changing profile. *Arch Gen Psychiatry*, 37:505–510, 1980.

Helson, L; Duque, L: Acute brain syndrome after propranolol. *Lancet*, 1:98, 1978.

Helzer, JE; Canino, GJ; Eng-Kung, Y; et al: Alcoholism—North America and Asia: A comparison of population surveys with the diagnostic internal schedule. *Arch Gen Psychiatry*, 47:313–319, 1990.

Henderson, J: *Emergency Medical Guide*. New York, McGraw-Hill, 1963.

Henderson, VW; Wooten, GF: Neuroleptic malignant syndrome: A pathogenetic role for dopamine receptor blockage. *Neurology*, 31:132–137, 1981.

Hendin, H: Suicide: A review of new directions in research. *Hospital and Community Psychiatry*, 37:148–154, 1986.

Hendin, H: *Suicide and Scandinavia*. New York, Grune and Stratton, 1964.

Hendin, H: Suicide. In: *Comprehensive Textbook of Psychiatry*. AM Freedman, HI Kaplan, eds. Baltimore, Williams and Wilkins, 1967.

Hendrie, HC; Crossett, JHW: An overview of depression in the elderly. *Psychiatric Annals*, 20:64–70, 1990.

Henn, FA; Bardwell, R; Jenkins, RL: Juvenile delinquents revisited: Adult criminal activity. *Arch Gen Psychiatry,* 37:1160–1163, 1980.

Henry, AF; Short, JF: *Suicide and Homicide: Some Economic, Sociological and Psychological Aspects of Aggression.* New York, Free Press, 1954.

Henslin, JM: Problems and prospects in studying significant others of suicides. *Bull Suicidology,* No. 8, Fall, pp. 81–84, 1971.

Heritch, AJ; Capwell, R; Roy-Byrne, PP: A case of psychosis and delirium following withdrawal from triazolam. *J Clin Psychiatry,* 48:168–169, 1987.

Herman, J; Hirschman, L: Families at risk for father-daughter incest. *Am J Psychiatry,* 138:967–970, 1981.

Herman, J; Russell, D; Trocki, K: Long-term effects of incestuous abuse in childhood. *Am J Psychiatry,* 143:1293–1296, 1986.

Hermesh, H; Aizenberg, D; Lapidot, M; Munitz, H: Risk of malignant hyperthermia among patients with neuroleptic malignant syndrome and their families. *Am J Psychiatry,* 145:1431–1434, 1988.

Herrero, FA: Lithium carbonate toxicity. *JAMA,* 226:1109–1110, 1973.

Herridge, CF: Physical disorders in psychiatric illness: A study of 209 consecutive admissions. *Lancet,* 2:949–951, 1960.

Herridge, PL; Pope, HG: Treatment of bulimia and rapid-cycling bipolar disorder with sodium valproate: A case report. *J Clin Psychopharmacol,* 5:229–235, 1985.

Herz, MI; Endicott, J; Gibbon, M: Brief hospitalization. Two-year follow-up. *Arch Gen Psychiatry,* 36:701–705, 1979.

Herzberg, JL; Fenwick, PBC: The aetiology of aggression in temporal-lobe epilepsy. *Br J Psychiatry,* 153:50–55, 1988.

Hestbech, J; Mansen, HE; Amdisen, A; et al: Chronic renal lesions following long-term treatment with lithium. *Kidney International,* 12:205–213, 1977.

Heston, LL; Hastings, D: Psychosis with withdrawal from ethchlorvynol. *Am J Psychiatry,* 137:249–250, 1980.

Hilberman, E: Overview: The "wife-beater's wife" reconsidered. *Am J Psychiatry,* 137:1336–1347, 1980.

Hill, D: Discussion on surgery of temporal lobe epilepsy. Indications and contraindications to temporal lobectomy. *Proc Roy Soc Med,* 51:610, 1958.

Hillard, JR; Holland, JM; Ramm, D: Christmas and psychopathology: Data from a psychiatric emergency room population. *Arch Gen Psychiatry,* 38:1377–1381, 1981.

Hillard, JR; Ramm, D; Zung, WWK; et al: Suicide in a psychiatric emergency room population. *Am J Psychiatry,* 140:459–462, 1983.

Hillard, JR; Slomowitz, M; Deddens, J: Determinants of emergency psychiatric admission for adolescents and adults. *Am J Psychiatry,* 145:1416–1419, 1988.

Hillard, JR, Slomowitz, M; Levi, LS: A retrospective study of adolescents' visits to a general hospital psychiatric emergency service. *Am J Psychiatry,* 144:432–436, 1987.

Hillard, JR; Vieweg, WVR: Marked sinus tachycardia resulting from the synergistic effects of marijuana and nortriptyline. *Am J Psychiatry,* 140:626–627, 1983.

Hillard, JR; Zung, WW; Ramm, D; Holland, JM; et al: Accidental and homicidal death in a psychiatric emergency room population. *Hospital and Community Psychiatry,* 36:640–643, 1985.

Himmelhoch, JM; Detre, T; Kupfer, DJ; et al: Treatment of previously intractable depressions with tranyl-cypromine and lithium. *J Nerv Ment Dis,* 155:216–220, 1972.

Hirschfeld, RMA; Davidson, L: Clinical risk factors for suicide. *Psychiatric Annals,* 18:628–635, 1988.

Hoch, P; Polatin, P: Pseudoneurotic forms of schizophrenia. *Psychiat Q,* 23:248, 1949.

Hochman, J: Miracle, mystery, and authority: The triangle of cult indoctrination. *Psychiatric Annals,* 20:175–187, 1990.

Hodges, K; Kline, JJ; Barbero, G; Woodruff, C: Anxiety in children with recurrent abdominal pain and their parents. *Psychosomatics,* 26:859–866, 1985.

Hoes, MJAMJ; Colla, P; van Doorn, P; Folgering, H; et al: Hyperventilation and panic attacks. *J Clin Psychiatry,* 48:435–437, 1987.

Hoffman, JA; Forssmann-Falck, R: Emergency psychiatry training: The new old problem. *Gen Hosp Psychiatry,* 6:143–145, 1984.

Hoffman, WH; Chodoroff, G; Piggott, LR: Haloperidol and thyroid storm. *Am J Psychiatry,* 135:485–486, 1979.

Hogben, GL; Cornfield, RB: Treatment of traumatic war neurosis with phenelzine. *Arch Gen Psychiatry,* 38:440–445, 1981.

Hoge, SK; Sachs, G; Appelbaum, PS; Greer, A; et al: Limitations on psychiatrists' discretionary civil commitment authority by the stone and dangerousness criteria. *Arch Gen Psychiatry,* 45:764–769, 1988.

Holinger, PC: Violent deaths as a leading cause of mortality: An epidemiologic study of suicide, homicide, and accidents. *Am J Psychiatry,* 137:472–476, 1980.

Holinger, PC; Offer, D: Prediction of adolescent suicide: A population model. *Am J Psychiatry,* 139:302–307, 1982.

Holinger, PC; Offer, D; Ostrov, E: Suicide and homicide in the United States: An epidemiologic study of violent death, population changes, and the potential for prediction. *Am J Psychiatry,* 144:215–219, 1987.

Holland, J; Fasanello, S; Ohnuma, T: Psychiatric symptoms associated with L-asparaginase administration. *J Psych Res,* 10:105–113, 1974.

Holland, JC; Korzun, AH; Tross, S; Silberfarb, P; et al: Comparative psychological disturbance in patients with pancreatic and gastric cancer. *Am J Psychiatry,* 143:982–986, 1986.

Hollander, E; Liebowitz, MR; Gorman, JM; Cohen, B; et al: Cortisol and sodium lactate-induced panic. *Arch Gen Psychiatry,* 46:135–140, 1989.

Hollingshead, AB; Redlich, FC: *Social Class and Mental Illness.* New York, Wiley, 1958.

Hollister, LE: Tricyclic antidepressants (I). *N Engl J Med,* 299(20):1106–1109, 1978.

Hollister, LE: Tricyclic antidepressants (II). *N Engl J Med,* 299(21):1168–1172, 1978.

Hollister, LE; Davis, KL; Berger, PA: Subtypes of depression based on excretion of MHPG and response to nortriptyline. *Arch Gen Psychiatry,* 37:1107–1110, 1980.

Hollister, LE; Kim, DY: Intensive treatment with haloperidol of treatment-resistant chronic schizophrenic patients. *Am J Psychiatry,* 139:1466–1468, 1982.

Hollister, LE: Monitoring tricyclic antidepressant plasma concentrations. *JAMA,* 241:2530–2533, 1979.

Hollister, LE; Pfefferbaum, A; Davis, KL: Monitoring nortriptyline plasma concentrations. *Am J Psychiatry,* 137:485–486, 1980.

Hollister, LE: Pharmacology and pharmacokinetics of the minor tranquilizers. *Psychiatric Annals,* 11(Nov. Suppl.):26–31, 1981.

Hollister, LE: Psychiatric Disorders, in GS Avery (ed) *Drug Treatment.* Seaforth, Australia, ADN Press, 1976.

Hollon, TH: Modified group therapy in the treatment of patients on chronic hemodialysis. *Am J Psychotherapy,* 26:501–510, 1972.

Holmberg, G: Anxiety disorders: Classification and diagnosis. *Acta Psychiatr Scand,* 76:7–13, 1987.

Holmes, JM: Cerebral manifestations of vitamin B12 deficiency. *Br Med J,* 2:1394–1398, 1956.

Hooper, JF; Minter, G: Droperidol in the management of psychiatric emergencies. *J Clin Psychopharmacol,* 3:362–363, 1983.

Hoover, CF; Fitzgerald, RG: Marital conflict of manic-depressive patients. *Arch Gen Psychiatry,* 38:65–67, 1981.

Horhan, DJ; Guerrini, MD: Developing legal trends in psychiatric malpractice. *J Psych Law,* 9:65–89, 1981.

Horney, K: *Self-Analysis.* New York, WW Norton, 1942.

Horowitz, MJ: Disasters and psychological responses to stress. *Psychiatric Annals,* 15:161–167, 1985.

Horowitz, MJ; Marmar, C; Weiss, DS; DeWitt, KN; et al: Brief psychotherapy of bereavement reactions. *Arch Gen Psychiatry,* 41:438–448, 1984.

Horton, AM; Fiscella, RA; O'Connor, K; Jackson, M: Revised criteria for detecting alcoholic patients with attention deficit disorder, residual type. *J Nerv Ment Dis,* 175:371–372, 1987.

Horwitz, D; Lovenberg, W; Engelman, K; et al: Monoamine oxidase inhibitors, tyramine, and cheese. *JAMA,* 188:1108–1110, 1964.

Hotchkiss, AP; Harvey, PD: Effect of distractive and communicative failures in schizophrenic patients. *Am J Psychiatry,* 147:513–515, 1990.

House, RM; Thompson, TL: Acute psychiatric evaluation of self-injuring patients. *Psychosomatics,* 26:845–851, 1985.

Howath, BG; Grace, MGA: Depression, drugs, and delusions. *Arch Gen Psychiatry,* 42:1145–1147, 1985.

Hsu, LKG: Outcome of anorexia nervosa: A review of the literature (1954 to 1978). *Arch Gen Psychiatry,* 37:1041–1046, 1980.

Hsu, LKG; Starzynski, JM: Mania in adolescence. *J Clin Psychiatry,* 47:596–599, 1986.

Hsu, LKG; Lieberman, S: Paradoxical intention in the treatment of chronic anorexia nervosa. *Am J Psychiatry,* 139:650–653, 1982.

Hubain, PP; Castro, P; Mesters, P; et al: Alprazolam and amitriptyline in the treatment of major depressive disorder: A double-blind clinical and sleep EEG study. *J Affective Disord,* 18:67–73, 1990.

Hudson, JI; Laffer, PS; Pope, HG: Bulimia related to affective disorder by family history and response to the dexamethasone suppression test. *Am J Psychiatry,* 139:685–687, 1982.

Hudson, JI; Pope, HG: Affective spectrum disorder: Does antidepressant response identify a family of disorders with a common pathophysiology? *Am J Psychiatry,* 147:552–564, 1990.

Hugdahl, K: Psychophysiological aspects of phobic fears: An evaluative review. *Neuropsychobiology,* 20:194–204, 1988.

Hughes, JR; Gust, SW; Pechacek, TF: Prevalence of tobacco dependence and withdrawal. *Am J Psychiatry,* 144:205–208, 1987.

Hughes, JR; Hatsukami, D: Signs and symptoms of tobacco withdrawal. *Arch Gen Psychiatry,* 43:289–294, 1986.

Hughes, JR; Hatsukami, DK; Skoog, KP: Physical dependence on nicotine in gum. *JAMA,* 255:3277–3279, 1986.

Hunt, RG: Social class and mental illness: Some implications for clinical theory and practice. *Am J Psychiatry,* 116:1065, 1960.

Husain, A; Chapel, JL: History of incest in girls admitted to a psychiatric hospital. *Am J Psychiatry,* 140:591–593, 1983.

Husain, SA: Current perspective on the role of psychosocial factors in adolescent suicide. *Psychiatric Annals,* 20:122–127, 1990.

Husband, SD; Platt, JJ: Criteria for the diagnosis of PTSD. *Am J Psychiatry,* 144:388, 1987.

Hussain, MZ; Khan, AG; Chandry, ZA: Aplastic anemia associated with lithium therapy. *Can Med Assoc J,* 108:724–728, 1973.

Husserl, E: *Ideas.* New York, Macmillan, 1931.

Hutchinson, MP; Draguns, JG: Chronic, early exposure to suicidal ideation in a parental figure: A pattern of presuicidal characteristics. *Suicide and Life-Threatening Behavior,* 17:288–298, 1987.

Hutt, PB; Merrill, RA: *Criminal responsibility and the right to treatment for intoxication and alcoholism.* Georgetown L J 57:835, 1969.

Inamdar, SC; Lewis, DO; Siomopoulos, G: Violent and suicidal behavior in psychotic adolescents. *Am J Psychiatry,* 139:932–935, 1982.

Infantino, JA; Musingo, SY: Assaults and injuries among staff with and without training in aggression control techniques. *Hospital and Community Psychiatry,* 36:1312–1322, 1985.

Inglese-Bieber, M; Slaby, AE: Serum alcohol levels and the incidence of trauma. *Currents in Alcoholism,* Vol VIII, pp 269–282, 1981.

Ingraham, LF; Bridge, PT; Janssen, R; et al: Neuropsychological effects of early HIV-1 infection: Assessment and methodology. *The Journal of Neuropsychiatry and Clinical Neurosciences,* 2:174–182, 1990.

Ingvar, D: Abnormal distribution of cerebral activity in chronic schizophrenia: A neurophysiological interpretation. In: *Perspectives in Schizophrenia Research,* CF Baxter, T Melnechuch, eds. New York, Raven Press, 1980.

Irwin, M: Diagnosis of anorexia nervosa in children and the validity of DSM-III. *Am J Psychiatry,* 138, 1382–1383, 1981.

Irwin, M; Schuchit, M; Smith, TL: Clinical importance of age at onset in type 1 and type 2 primary alcoholics. *Arch Gen Psychiatry,* 47:320–324, 1990.

Iskii, K: Backgrounds of high suicide rates among "name university" students: A retrospective study of the past 25 years. *Suicide and Life-Threatening Behavior,* 15:56–68, 1985.

Iversen, BM; Willassen, Y; Bakke, O: Charcoal hemoperfusion in nortriptyline poisoning. *Lancet*, i:388–389, 1978.

Jablonski v. USA, No. 81–5786 (9th Cir. June 14, 1983).

Jacobs, S; Kim, K: Psychiatric complications of bereavement. *Psychiatric Annals*, 20:314–317, 1990.

Jacobson, A: Physical and sexual assault histories among psychiatric outpatients. *Am J Psychiatry*, 146:755–758, 1989.

Jacobson, A; Richardson, B: Assault experiences of 100 psychiatric inpatients: Evidence of the need for routine inquiry. *Am J Psychiatry*, 144:908–913, 1987.

Jacobson, G; Strickler, M; Morley, E: Generic and individual approaches to crisis intervention. *Am J Public Health* 58:339, 1968.

Jacobson, GF: Crisis theory and treatment strategy. Some socio-cultural and psychodynamic considerations. *J Nerv Ment Dis*, 141:209, 1965.

Jacobsen, FM; Wehr, TA; Skwerer, RA; Sack, DA; et al: Morning versus midday phototherapy of seasonal affective disorder. *Am J Psychiatry*, 144:1301–1305, 1987.

Jacobziner, H: Lead poisoning in childhood: Epidemiology, manifestation, and prevention. *Clin Pediatr* (Phila), 5:277–286, 1966.

Jaffe, CM: First-degree atrioventricular block during lithium carbonate treatment. *Am J Psychiatry*, 135:88–89, 1977.

Jaffe, K; Barnshaw, HD; Kennedy, ME: The dexamethasone suppression test in depressed outpatients with and without melancholia. *Am J Psychiatry*, 140:492–493, 1983.

James, HR; Siekert, RG; Gervi, JE: Neurological manifestations of bacterial endocarditis. *Ann Intern Med*, 71:21–28, 1969.

Jamison, KR; Wellisch, DK; Pasnau, RO: Psychosocial aspects of mastectomy. I. The woman's perspective. *Am J Psychiatry*, 135:432–436, 1978.

Jampala, VC; Abrams, R: Mania secondary to left and right hemisphere damage. *Am J Psychiatry*, 140:1197–1199, 1983.

Janicak, PG; Boshes, RA: Advances in the treatment of mania and other acute psychotic disorders. *Psychiatric Annals*, 17:145–149, 1987.

Janis, IL: *Psychological Stress: Psychoanalytical and Behavioral Studies of Surgical Patients*. New York, Wiley, 1958.

Jankovic, J: Drug-induced and other orofacial-cervical dyskinesias. *Ann Intern Med*, 84:788–793, 1981.

Jann, MW; Bitar, AH; Rau, A: Lithium prophylaxis of tricyclic antidepressant-induced mania in bipolar patients. *Am J Psychiatry*, 139:683–684, 1982.

Jann, MW; Ereshefsky, L; Saklad, SR; Seidel, DR; et al: Effects of carbamazepine on plasma haloperidol levels. *J Clin Psychopharmacol*, 5:106–109, 1985.

Janowsky, D; Curtis, G; Zisoch, S; et al: Ventricular arrhythmias possibly aggravated by trazodone. *Am J Psychiatry*, 139:683–684, 1982.

Jarrett, DB; Coble, PA; Kupter, DJ: Reduced cortisol latency in depressive illness. *Arch Gen Psychiatry*, 40:506–511, 1983.

Jarvik, LF; Ruth, V; Matsuyama, SS: Organic brain syndrome and aging: A six-year follow-up of surviving twins. *Arch Gen Psychiatry*, 37:280–286, 1980.

Jas, A; Villeneuve, A; Gauter, J; et al: Some remarks on the influence of lithium carbonate in patients with temporal lobe epilepsy. *Int J Clin Pharmacol*, 7:67–79, 1983.

Jefferson, JW: Biologic treatment of depression in cardiac patients. *Psychosomatics*, 26:31–38, 1985.

Jefferson, JW: Beta-adrenergic receptor blocking drugs. *Arch Gen Psychiatry*, 31:681–691, 1974.

Jefferson, JW: Central nervous system toxicity of cimetidine: A case of depression. *Am J Psychiatry*, 136:346, 1979.

Jefferson, JW; Greist, JH: Some hazards of lithium use. *Am J Psychiatry*, 138:93–94, 1981.

Jefferson, JW; Greist, JH; Clagnaz, PJ; et al: Effect of strenous exercise of serum lithium level in man. *Am J Psychiatry*, 139:1593–1595, 1982.

Jefferson, JW; Greist, JH: *Primer of Lithium Therapy*. Baltimore, Williams & Wilkins Co., 1977.

Jellinek, EM: *European Seminar on Alcoholism*. October, 1951. (Unpublished monograph).

Jellinek, T; Gardos, G; Cole, JO: Adverse effects of antiparkinsonian drug withdrawal. *Am J Psychiatry*, 138:1567–1571, 1981.

Jenike, MA; Baer, L; Summergrad, P; et al: Sertraline in obsessive–compulsive disorder: a double-blind comparison with placebo. *Am J Psychiatry,* 147:923–928, 1990.

Jenike, MA; Pato, C: Disabling fear of AIDS responsive to imipramine. *Psychosomatics,* 27:143–144, 1986.

Jenkins, PL; Shaw, G: Psychosis in a patient with hyperkalemic periodic paralysis. *Gen Hosp Psychiatry,* 12:56–61, 1990.

Jenner, FA: Lithium and the question of kidney damage. *Arch Gen Psychiatry,* 36:888–890, 1979.

Jensen, JC; Faiman, MD; Harwitz, A: Elimination characteristics of disulfiram over time in five alcoholic volunteers: A preliminary study. *Am J Psychiatry,* 139:1596–1598, 1982.

Jernigan, TL; Zatz, LM; Moses, JA; et al: Computed tomography in schizophrenics and normal volunteers. I. Fluid volume. *Arch Gen Psychiatry,* 39:765–770, 1982a.

Jernigan, TL; Zatz, LM; Moses, JA; et al: Computed tomography in schizophrenics and normal volunteers. II. Cranial asymmetry. *Arch Gen Psychiatry,* 39:771–773, 1982b.

Jeste, DV; Potkin, SG; Sinha, S; et al: Tardive dyskinesia-reversible and persistent. *Arch Gen Psychiatry,* 36:585–590, 1979.

Jeste, DV; Wyatt, RJ: Changing epidemiology of tardive dyskinesia: An overview. *Am J Psychiatry,* 138:297–309, 1981.

Jeste, DV; Wyatt, RJ: Therapeutic strategies against tardive dyskinesia: Two decades of experience. *Arch Gen Psychiatry,* 39:803–816, 1982.

Jobson, K; Linnoila, M; Gillam, J; et al: Successful treatment of severe anxiety attacks with tricyclic antidepressants: A potential mechanism of action. *Am J Psychiatry,* 135:863–864, 1978.

Joffe, RT; Offord, DR; Boyle, MH: Ontario child health study: Suicidal behavior in youth age 12–16 years. *Am J Psychiatry,* 145:1420–1423, 1988a.

Joffe, RT; Post, RM; Uhde, TW: Effect of carbamazepine on body weight in affectively ill patients. *J Clin Psychiatry,* 47:313–314, 1986.

Joffe, RT; Rubinow, DR; Denicoff, KD; Maher, M; et al: Depression and carcinoma of the pancreas. *Gen Hosp Psychiatry,* 8:241–245, 1986b.

Joffe, RT; Swinson, RP; Regan, JJ: Personality features of obsessive-compulsive disorder. *Am J Psychiatry,* 145:1127–1129, 1988b.

Johannessen, DJ; Crowley, DS; Walker, RD; Jensen, CF; et al: Prevalence, onset, and clinical recognition of panic states in hospitalized male alcoholics. *Am J Psychiatry,* 146:1201–1203, 1989.

Johnson, C; Berndt, DJ: Preliminary investigation of bulimia and life adjustment. *Am J Psychiatry,* 140:774–777, 1983.

Johnson, DA; Bohan, ME: Propoxyphene withdrawal with clonidine. *Am J Psychiatry,* 140:1217–1218, 1983.

Johnson, DAW: The evaluation of routine physical examination in psychiatric cases. *Practitioner,* 200:686–691, 1968.

Johnson, GFS; Leeman, MM: Analysis of familial factors in bipolar affective illness. *Arch Gen Psychiatry,* 34:1074–1083, 1977.

Jolley, AG; Hirsh, SR; McRink, A; Manchanda, R: Trial of brief intermittent neuroleptic prophylaxis for selected schizophrenic outpatients: Clinical outcome at one year. *Br Med J,* 298:985–990, 1989.

Jones, BD; Chouinard, G: Clonazepam in the treatment of recurrent symptoms of depression and anxiety in a patient with systemic lupus erythematosus. *Am J Psychiatry,* 142:354–355, 1985.

Jones, DR: Secondary disaster victims: The emotional effects of recovering and identifying human remains. *Am J Psychiatry,* 142:303–307, 1985.

Jones, HR; Siekert, RG; Geraci, JE: Neurological manifestations of bacterial endocarditis. *Ann Intern Med,* 71:21–28, 1969.

Jos, CJ; Evenson, RC; Mallya, AR: Self-induced water intoxication: A comparison of 34 cases with matched controls. *J Clin Psychiatry,* 47:368–370, 1986.

Joseph, AB: Cotard's syndrome in a patient with coexistent Capgras' syndrome, syndrome of subjective doubles, and palinopsia. *J Clin Psychiatry,* 47:605–606, 1986.

Joubert, PH; Oliver, JA: Fatal suicidal ingestion of thioridazine. *Clin Toxicol,* 7:133–138, 1974.

Juergens, SM; Morse, RM: Alprazolam dependence in seven patients. *Am J Psychiatry,* 145:625–627, 1988.

Junginger, J: Predicting compliance with command hallucinations. *Am J Psychiatry,* 147:245–247, 1990.

Jus, A; Pinean, R; Lachance, R; et al: Epidemiology of tardive dyskinesia. *Dis Nerv Syst,* 37:210–214, 1976.

Jus, A; Villeneuve, A; Gautier, J; et al: Some remarks on the influence of lithium carbonate in patients with temporal epilepsy. *Int J Clin Pharmacol,* 7:67–79, 1973.

Kaffman, M: Kibbutz civilian population under war stress. *Br J Psychiatry,* 130:489–494, 1977.

Kahn, EM; Schulz, C; Perel, JM; et al: Change in haloperidol level due to carbamazepine—a conflicting factor in combined medication for schizophrenia. *J Clin Psychopharmacol,* 10:54–57, 1990.

Kales, A; Bixler, EO; Kales, JD; et al: Comparative effectiveness of nine hypnotic drugs: Sleep laboratory studies. *J Clin Psychopharmacol,* 17:207–213, 1977.

Kales, A; Jacobson, A; Paulson, J; et al: Somnambulism: Psychophysiological correlates: I. All night EEG studies. *Arch Gen Psychiatry,* 14:586–594, 1966.

Kales, A; Soldatos, CR; Bixler, EO; et al: Rebound insomnia and rebound anxiety: A review. *J Pharmacol,* 26:121–137, 1983.

Kales, A; Soldatos, CR; Caldwell, AB; et al: Somnambulism: Clinical characteristics and personality patterns. *Arch Gen Psychiatry,* 37:1406–1410, 1980.

Kales, JD; Kales, A: Evaluation and treatment of insomnia. *Psychiatric Annals,* 17:459–464, 1987.

Kales, JD; Kales, A; Soldatos, CR; et al: Night terrors: Clinical characteristics and personality patterns. *Arch Gen Psychiatry,* 37:1413–1417, 1980.

Kalman, T; Warner, GM: Protracted vomiting following abrupt cessation of psychotropics. A case report. *Can Psychiat Assoc J,* 23:163–165, 1978.

Kandel, DB; Davies, M: Epidemiology of depressive mood in adolescents: An empirical study. *Arch Gen Psychiatry,* 39:1205–1212, 1982.

Kane, FJ; Greene, BQ: Psychotic episodes associated with the use of common proprietary decongestants. *Am J Psychiatry,* 123:484–4878, 1966.

Kane, J; Rifkin, A; Quitkin, F; et al: Extrapyramidal side effects with lithium treatment. *Am J Psychiatry,* 135:851–853, 1978.

Kane, JM: Dosage strategies with long-acting injectable neuroleptics, including haloperidol decanoate. *J Clin Psychopharmacol,* 6:20–23, 1986a.

Kane, JM: Prevention and treatment of neuroleptic noncompliance. *Psychiatric Annals,* 16:576–579, 1986b.

Kane, JM; Honigfeld, G; Singer, J; Meltzer, H: Clozapine in treatment-resistant schizophrenics. *Psychopharmacol Bull* 24(1):62–67, 1988.

Kane, JM; Quitkin, FM; Rifkin, A; et al: Comparison of the incidence and severity of extrapyramidal side-effects with fluphenazine enanthate and fluphenazine decanoate. *Am J Psychiatry,* 135: 1539–1542, 1978.

Kane, JM; Quitkin, FM; Rifkin, A; et al: Lithium carbonate and imipramine in the prophylaxis of unipolar and bipolar II illness. *Arch Gen Psychiatry,* 39:1065–1069, 1982.

Kane, JM; Smith, JM: Tardive dyskinesia: Prevalence and risk factors, 1959 to 1979. *Arch Gen Psychiatry,* 39:473–481, 1982.

Kane, JM; Struve, FA; Weinhold, P; et al: Strategy for the study of patients at high risk for tardive dyskinesia. *Am J Psychiatry,* 137:1265–1267, 1980.

Kaney, JM; Quitkin, FM; Rifkin, A; et al: Lithium carbonate and imipramine in the prophylaxis of unipolar and bipolar II illness: A prospective placebo-controlled comparison. *Arch Gen Psychiatry,* 39:1065–1969, 1982.

Kantor, SJ; Bigger, J; Glassman, AH; et al: Imipramine-induced heart block. A longitudinal case study. *JAMA,* 231:1364–1366, 1975.

Kantor, SJ; Glassman, AH; Bigger, JT; et al: Cardiac effects of therapeutic plasma concentrations of imipramine. *Am J Psychiatry,* 135:534–538, 1978.

Kantor, SJ; Zitrin, CM; Zeldis, SM: Mitral valve prolapse syndrome in agoraphobic patients. *Am J Psychiatry,* 137:467–469, 1980.

Kaplan, JE; Spira, TJ; Fishbein, DB; Boze, LH; et al: A six-year follow-up of HIV-infected homosexual men with lymphadenopathy. *JAMA,* 260:2695–2696, 1988.

Kaplan, DM; Mason, EA: Maternal reactions to premature birth viewed as an acute emotional disorder. *Am J Psychiatry,* 135:534–538, 1978.

Kaplan, DM; Mason, EA: Maternal reactions to premature birth viewed as an acute emotional disorder. *Am J Orthopsychiat,* 30:539, 1960.

Karajgi, B; Rifkin, A; Doddi, S; Kolli, R: The prevalence of anxiety disorders in patients with chronic obstructive pulmonary disease. *Am J Psychiatry,* 147:200–201, 1990.

Kardiner, A: *War Stress and Neurotic Illness.* New York, Paul B. Hoeber, Inc. 1947.

Kardiner, A; *The Traumatic Neurosis of War.* Washington, National Research Council, 1941.

Karki, SD; Holden, JMC: Combined use of haloperidol and lithium. *Psychiatric Annals,* 20:154–161, 1990.

Karlinsky, H; Taerk, G; Schwartz, K; Ennis, J; et al: Suicide attempts and resuscitation dilemmas. *Gen Hosp Psychiatry,* 10:423–427, 1988.

Karpi, ER; Kleinman, JE; Goodman, SI; et al: Serotonin and 5-hydroxyindoleacetic acid in brains of suicide victims. *Arch Gen Psychiatry,* 43:594–600, 1986.

Kars, H; Broehema, W; Gloudemans-van Gelderen, I; et al: Naltrexone attenuates self-injurious behavior on mentally retarded subjects. *Biol Psychiatry,* 27:741–746, 1990.

Kashani, JH; Cantwell, DP: Characteristics of children admitted to inpatient community mental health centers. *Arch Gen Psychiatry,* 40:397–400, 1983.

Kashani, JH; Cantwell, DP; Shekim, WO; et al: Major depressive disorder in children admitted to an inpatient community mental health center. *Am J Psychiatry,* 139:671–672, 1982.

Kashani, JH; Husain, A; Shekim, WO; et al: Current perspective on childhood depression: An overview. *Am J Psychiatry,* 138:143–153, 1981.

Kashani, JH; McGee, RO; Clarkson, SE; Anderson JC; et al: Depression in a sample of 9 year-old children: Prevalence and associated characteristics. *Arch Gen Psychiatry,* 40:1217–1223, 1983.

Kashani, JH; Orvaschel, H: A community study of anxiety in children and adolescents. *Am J Psychiatry,* 147:313–318, 1990.

Kashani, JH; Vardya, AF; Soltys, SM; et al: Correlates of anxiety in psychiatrically hospitalized children and their parents. *Am J Psychiatry,* 147:319–323, 1990.

Kasper, S; Rogers, SLB; Madden, PA; et al: The effects of phototherapy in the general population. *J Affective Disord,* 18:211–219, 1990.

Kasper, S; Rogers, SLB; Yancey, A; Schulz, PM; et al: Phototherapy in individuals with and without subsyndromal seasonal affective disorder. *Arch Gen Psychiatry,* 46:837–844, 1988.

Kasper, S; Wehr, TA; Bortho, JJ; et al: Epidemiological findings of seasonal changes in mood and behavior. *Arch Gen Psychiatry,* 46:823–833, 1989.

Kasset, JA; Gershon, ES; Maxwell, ME; et al: Psychiatric disorders in the first-degree relatives of probands with bulimia nervosa. *Am J Psychiatry,* 146:1468–1471, 1989.

Kathol, RG; Mutgi, A; Williams, J; Clamon, G; et al: Diagnosis of major depression in cancer patients according to four sets of criteria. *Am J Psychiatry,* 147:1021–1024, 1990.

Kathol, RG; Noyes, R; Slymen, DJ; et al: Propranolol in chronic anxiety disorders: A controlled study. *Arch Gen Psychiatry,* 37:1361–1365, 1980.

Kathol, RG; Turner, R; Delahunt, J: Depression and anxiety associated with hyperthryoidism: Response to antithyroid therapy. *Psychosomatics,* 27:501–505, 1986.

Katon, W; Raskind, M: Treatment of depression in the medically ill elderly with methylphenidate. *Am J Psychiatry,* 137:963–965, 1980.

Katz, J: Disclosure and consent in psychiatry practice mission impossible. In: *Law and Ethics in the Practice of Psychiatry,* CK Hofling, ed. New York, Brunner/Mazel, 1980.

Kaufman, A; Divasto, P; Jackson, R; et al: Male rape victims: Noninstitutionalized assault. *Am J Psychiatry,* 137:221–223, 1980.

Kaus, RP; Hux, M; Graf, P: Psychotropic drug withdrawal and the dexamethasone suppression test. *Am J Psychiatry,* 144:82–85, 1987.

Kautman, KR; Petrucha, RA; Pitts, RN; et al: Phencyclidine in umbilical cord blood: Preliminary data. *Am J Psychiatry,* 140:450–452, 1983.

Kay, DWK; Bergmann, K; Foster, EM; et al: Mental illness and hospital usage in the elderly: A random sample followed up. *Comp Psychiatry,* 11:26–35, 1970.

Kazdin, AE; Matson, JL; Senatore, V: Assessment of depression in mentally retarded adults. *Am J Psychiatry,* 140:1040–1043, 1983.

Kazdin, AE: Conduct Disorder. *The Psychiatric Hospital,* 20:153–158, 1990.

Keck, Jr., PE; Pope, HG; Cohen, BM; McElroy, SL; et al: Risk factors for neuroleptic malignant syndrome: A case-control study. *Arch Gen Psychiatry,* 146:914–918, 1989.

Keck, Jr., PE; Pope, HG; McElroy, SL: Frequency and presentation of neuroleptic malignant syndrome: A prospective study. *Am J Psychiatry,* 144:1344–1346, 1987.

Keefe, RS; Mohs, RC; Losonczy, MF; Davidson, M; et al: Premorbid sociosexual functioning and long-term outcome in schizophrenia. *Am J Psychiatry,* 146:206–211, 1989.

Keighley, MRB; Gannon, M; Warlow, J; et al: Evaluation of single-dose hypnotic treatment before elective operation. *Br Med J,* 281:829–931, 1980.

Keisling, R: Under-diagnosis of manic-depressive illness in a hospital unit. *Am J Psychiatry,* 138:672–673, 1981.

Keitner, GI; Ryan, CE; Miller, et al: Family functioning, social adjustment, and recurrence of suicidality. *Psychiatry* 53(1):17–30, 1990.

Keller, MB; Lavori, PW; Endicott, J; et al: "Double depression": Two-year follow-up. *Am J Psychiatry,* 140:689–694, 1983.

Keller, MB; Shapiro, RW; Lavori, PW; et al: Recovery in major depressive disorder: Analysis with the life table. *Arch Gen Psychiatry,* 39:911–915, 1982a.

Keller, MB; Shapiro, RW; Lavori, PW; et al: Recovery in major depressive disorder: analysis with the life table and regression models. *Arch Gen Psychiatry,* 39:905–910, 1982b.

Kelley, JG; Snowden, LR; Munnoz, RF: Social and community interventions in MR Rosenzweig and LW Porter (eds.) *Annual Rev Psychol,* 28:323–361, 1977.

Kelley, TW: Prolonged cerebellar dysfunction associated with paint sniffing. *Pediatrics,* 54:605–606, 1974.

Kelly, WA: Suicide and psychiatric education. *Am J Psychiatry,* 130:463–468, 1973.

Kempe, CH; Helfer, RE: *Helping the Battered Child and His Family.* Philadelphia, JB Lippincott, 1972.

Kemph, JP: Psychotherapy with donors and recipients of kidney transplants. In: *Psychiatric Aspects of Organ Transplantation,* A Catelnuovo-Tedesco, ed. New York, Grune & Stratton, 1971.

Kendler, KS: Demography of paranoid psychosis (delusional disorder): A review and comparison with schizophrenia and affective illness. *Arch Gen Psychiatry,* 39:890–902, 1982.

Kendler, KS; Gruenberg, AM; Strauss, JS: An independent analysis of the Copenhagen sample of the Danish adaptation study of schizophrenia: I. The relationship between anxiety disorder and schizophrenia. *Arch Gen Psychiatry,* 38:973–977, 1981a.

Kendler, KS; Gruenberg, AM; Strauss, JS: An independent analysis of the Copenhagen sample of the Danish adaptation study of schizophrenia: II. The relationship between schizothyroid personality and schizophrenia. *Arch Gen Psychiatry,* 38:982–984, 1981b.

Kendler, KS; Gruenberg, AM; Strauss, JS: An independent analysis of the Copenhagen sample of the Danish adaptation study of schizophrenia: III. The relationship between paranoid psychosis (delusional disorder) and the schizophrenia spectrum disorders. *Arch Gen Psychiatry,* 38:985–987, 1981c.

Kerling, R: Underdiagnosis of manic depressive illness in a hospital unit. *Am J Psychiatry,* 138:672–673, 1981.

Kermani, EJ; Borod, JC; Brown, PH; Tunnell, G: New psychopathologic findings in AIDS: Case report. *J Clin Psychiatry,* 46:240–241, 1985.

Kernberg, O: Borderline personality organization. *J Am Psychoanal Assoc,* 15:641, 1967.

Kessler, LG; Cleary, PD; Burke, JD: Psychiatric disorders in primary care: Results of a follow-up study. *Arch Gen Psychiatry,* 42:583–587, 1985.

Kessler, KA; Waletzky, JP: Clinical use of the antipsychotics. *Am J Psychiatry,* 138:202–491, 1981.

Kessler, RC; Downey, G; Milavsky, JR; Stipp, H: Clustering of teenage suicides after television news stories about suicides: A reconsideration. *Am J Psychiatry,* 145:1379–1383, 1988.

Ketal, R: Psychotropic drugs in the management of psychiatric emergencies. *Postgraduate Medicine,* 58:87–93, 1975.

Kety, SS: Mental illness in the biological and adoptive relatives of schizophrenic adoptees: Findings relevant to genetic and environmental factors in etiology. *Am J Psychiatry,* 140:720–727, 1983.

Khajawall, AM; Erickson, TB; Simpson, GM: Chronic phencyclidine abuse and physical assault. *Am J Psychiatry,* 139:1604–1606, 1982.

Khantzian, EJ: An extreme case of cocaine dependence and marked improvement with methylphenidate treatment. *Am J Psychiatry,* 140:784–785, 1983.

Khantzian, EJ; Treece, C: DSM-III psychiatric diagnosis of narcotic addicts: Recent findings. *Arch Gen Psychiatry,* 42:1067–1071, 1985.

Kidd, KK; Brusoff, BA; Cohen, DJ: Familial pattern of Gilles de la Tourette Syndrome. *Arch Gen Psychiatry,* 37:1336–1339, 1980.

Kiely, T: Addicts with AIDs. *Massachusetts Medicine,* 50–52, Nov/Dec 1986.

Kienhorst, CWM; de Wilde, EJ; van den Bout, J; et al: Self-reported suicidal behavior in Dutch secondary education students. *Suicide and Life-Threatening Behavior,* 20:101–112, 1990.

King, MB: Psychological aspects of HIV infections and AIDS: What have we learned? *Br J Psychiatry,* 156:151–156, 1990.

Kingsbury, SJ; Salzman C: Disulfiram in the treatment of alcoholic patients with schizophrenia. *Hospital and Community Psychiatry,* 41:133–134, 1990.

Kinzie, JD; Bochnlein, JK; Leung, PK; et al: The prevalence of posttraumatic stress disorder and its clinical significance among Southeast Asian refugees. *Am J Psychiatry,* 147:850–854, 1990.

Kiriakos, R; Ananth, J: Review of 13 cases of Capras syndrome. *Am J Psychiatry,* 137:1605–1607, 1980.

Kirk, L; Baastrup, PC; Schou, M: Propranolol treatment of lithium-induced tremor. *Lancet,* ii:1086–1087, 1973.

Kirkpatrick, B; Buchanan, RW: Anhedonia and the deficit syndrome of schizophrenia. *Psychiatry Res,* 31:25–30, 1990.

Kiroy, K: Aggressiveness, anxiety and drugs. *Br J Psychiatry,* 155:846, 1989.

Kirstein, L; Prusoff, B; Weissman, M; et al: Utilization review of treatment for suicide attempters. *Am J Psychiatry,* 132:22–27, 1975.

Kirubakaran, V; Sen, S; Wilkinson, CB: Catatonic stupor: Unusual manifestation of temporal lobe epilepsy. *Psychiatr J Univ Ottawa,* 12:244–246, 1987.

Kittrie, N: *The Right to be Different.* John Hopkins Press, Baltimore, 1971.

Klawans, HC; Goetz, CG; Perlik, S: Tardive dyskinesia: Review and update. *Am J Psychiatry,* 137:900–908, 1980.

Klawans, HL: The pharmacology of tardive dyskinesia. *Am J Psychiatry,* 130:82–85, 1973.

Kleber, HD: *Withdrawal from barbiturates and sedatives.* Mimeo, New Haven, Connecticut, 1974.

Kleber, HD: *Withdrawal from opiates.* Mimeo, New Haven, Connecticut, 1974.

Kleber v. Stevens, 39 Misc 2d 712, 241 NYS 2d 497 (Sup. Ct. Aff'd 20 App. Div. 2d 896, 239 *NYS* 2d 668 (1964).

Klee, SH; Garfinkel, BD; Beauchesne, H: Attention deficits in adults. *Psychiatric Annals,* 16:52–56, 1986.

Klein, DE; Sullivan, G; Wolcott, DL; Landsverk, J; et al: Changes in AIDS risk behaviors among homosexual male physicians and university students. *Am J Psychiatry,* 144:742–747, 1987.

Klein, DF; Davis, JM: *Diagnosis and Drug Treatment of Psychiatric Disorders.* Baltimore, Williams and Wilkins Co., 1969.

Klein, DF; Gittelman, R; Quitkin, F; et al: *Diagnosis and Drug Treatment of Psychiatric Disorders: Adults and Children.* 2nd ed. Baltimore, Williams & Wilkins, Co., 1980.

Klein, DF; Zitrin, CM; Woerner, MG; et al: Treatment of phobias. II: Behavior therapy and supportive psychotherapy: are there any specific ingredients. *Arch Gen Psychiatry,* 40:139–145, 1983.

Klein, DW: Symptom criteria and family history in major depression. *Am J Psychiatry,* 147:850–854, 1990.

Klerman, GL: Clinical Epidemiology of Suicide. *J Clin Psychiatry,* 48:33–38, 1987.

Klerman, GL: The current age of youthful melancholia: Evidence for increase in depression among adolescents and young adults. *Br J Psychiatry,* 152:4–14, 1988.

Knesevich, JW; Martin, RL; Berg, L; et al: Preliminary report on affective symptoms in the early stages of senile dementia of the Alzheimer type. *Am J Psychiatry,* 140:233–235, 1983.

Knight, R: Borderline states. *Bull Menninger Clin,* 17:1, 1953.

Ko, GN; Leckman, JF; Heninger, GR: Induction of rapid mood cycling during l-dopa treatment in a bipolar patient. *Am J Psychiatry,* 138:1623–1625, 1981.

Kobazaski, RM: Drug therapy of tardive dyskinesia. *N Engl J Med,* 296:257–260, 1977.

Kobazaski, RM: Orofacial dyskinesia: Clinical features, mechanisms, and drug therapy. *West J Med,* 125:277–288, 1976.

Kocsis, JH; Croughan, JL; Katz, MM; et al: Response to treatment with antidepressants of patients with severe or moderate nonpsychotic depression and of patients with psychotic depression. *Am J Psychiatry,* 147:621–624, 1990.

Koehler-Troy, C; Strober, M; Malenbaum, R: Methylphenidate-induced mania in a prepubertal child. - *J Clin Psychiatry,* 47:566–567, 1986.

Kolansky, H; Moore, WT: Toxic effects of chronic marijuana use. *JAMA,* 222:35–41, 1972.

Kontaxakis, V; Markianos, M; Markidis, M; Stefanis, C: Clonidine in the treatment of mixed bipolar disorder. *Acta Psychiatr Scand,* 79:108–110, 1989.

Koranyi, EK: Morbidity and rate of undiagnosed physical illness in a psychiatric clinic population. *Arch Gen Psychiatry,* 36:414–419, 1979.

Koranyi, EK; Dewar, A: Neuropsychiatric features of drug-induced and spontaneous systemic lupus erythematosus. *Psychiatr J Univ Ottawa,* 11:52–57, 1986.

Koranyi, EK; Ravindrm, A; Seguin, J: Alcohol withdrawal concealing symptoms of subdural hematoma— A caveat. *Psychiatr J Univ Ottawa,* 15:15–17, 1990.

Korsgaard, S; Casey, DE; Gerlach, J; et al: The effect of tetrahydoisoxazolopyridinol (THIP) in tardive dyskinesia: A new gamma-aminobutyric acid agonist. *Arch Gen Psychiatry,* 39:1017–1021, 1982.

Kosky, R: Childhood suicidal behavior. *J Child Psychol Psychiatry,* 24:457–468, 1983.

Kosten, TR; Schumann, B; Wright, D; Carney MK; et al: A preliminary study of desipramine in the treatment of cocaine abuse in methadone maintenance patients. *J Clin Psychiatry,* 48:442–444, 1987.

Kosten, TR; Forrest, JN: Treatment of severe lithium-induced polyuria with amiloride. *Am J Psychiatry,* 143:1563–1568, 1986.

Kovacs, M; Gastsonis, C; Paulauskas, SL; Richards, C: Depressive disorders in childhood: IV. A longitudinal study of comorbidity with and risk for anxiety disorders. *Arch Gen Psychiatry,* 46:776–782, 1989.

Kovarsky, RS: Loneliness and disturbed grief: A comparison of parents who lost a child to suicide or accidental death. *Arch Psych Nursing,* 3:86–96, 1989.

Kozol, R; Boucher, R; Garofalo, R: The diagnosis and treatment of dangerousness. *Crime and Delinquency,* 19:371–392, 1972.

Krakowski, MI; Convit A; Jaeger, J; Lin, S; et al: Neurological impairment in violent schizophrenic inpatients. *Am J Psychiatry,* 146:849–853, 1989.

Kramer, BA: Sleep disturbance associated with fluphenazine HCL: A case report. *Am J Psychiatry,* 136:977–978, 1979.

Kramer, JC; Klein, DF; Fink, M: Withdrawal symptoms following discontinuation of imipramine therapy. *Am J Psychiatry,* 118:549–550, 1961.

Kramer, M; Kinney, L: Sleep patterns in trauma victims with disturbed dreaming. *Psychiatr J Univ Ottawa,* 13:12–16, 1988.

Kramlinger, KG; Swanson, DW; Maruta, T: Are patients with chronic pain depressed? *Am J Psychiatry,* 140:747–749, 1983.

Kramlinger, KG; Post; RM: Addition of lithium carbonate to carbamazepine: Hematological and thyroid effects. *Am J Psychiatry,* 147:615–620, 1990.

Krauthammer, C; Klerman, GL: Secondary mania. Manic syndromes associated with antecedent physical illness or drugs. *Arch Gen Psychiatry,* 35:1333–1339, 1978; 1565–1566, 1978.

Kreek, MJ: Multiple drug abuse patterns and medical consequences. *Psychopharmacology: The Third Generation of Progress,* 172:1597–1604, 1987.

Kreipe, RE; Churchill, BH; Strauss, J: Long-term outcome of adolescents with anorexia nervosa. *Am J Dis Child,* 143:1322–1327, 1989.

Krishnan, RR; Maltbie, AA: Davidson, JRT: Abnormal cortisol suppression in bipolar patients with simultaneous manic and depressive symtpoms. *Am J Psychiatry,* 140:203–205, 1983.

Kroboth, PD; Juhl, RP: Triazolam. *Drug Intelligence and Clinical Pharmacology,* 17:495–500, 1983.

Kroll, J; Habenicht, M; Mackenzie, T; Yang, M; et al: Depression and posttraumatic stress disorder in Southeast Asian refugees. *Am J Psychiatry,* 146:1592–1597, 1987.

Kroll, J; Sines, L; Martin, K; et al: Borderline personality disorder: Construct validity of the concept. *Arch Gen Psychiatry,* 38:1021–1026, 1981.

Kronfol, Z; Greden, JF; Condon, M; et al: Application of biological markers in depression secondary to thyrotoxicosis. *Am J Psychiatry,* 139:1319–1322, 1982.

Kruesi, MJP; Dale, J; Straus, SE: Psychiatric diagnoses in patients who have chronic fatigue syndrome. *J Clin Psychiatry,* 50:53–55, 1989.

Kruesi, MJP; Rapoport, JL; Hamberger, S; et al: Cerebrospinal fluid monoamine metabolites, aggression, and impulsivity in disruptive behavior disorders of children and adolescents. *Arch Gen Psychiatry,* 47:419–426, 1990.

Krumholz, A; Grufferman, S; Orr, ST; Stern, BJ: Seizures and seizure care in an emergency department. *Epilepsia,* 30:175–181, 1989.

Krystal, A; Krishneen, KRR; Raitiere, M; et al: Differential diagnosis and pathophysiology of Cushing's syndrome and primary affective disorder. *J Neuropsychiatry,* 2:34–43, 1990.

Kuhn, WF; Davis, MH; Lippmann, SB: Emotional adjustment to cardiac transplantation. *Gen Hosp Psychiatry,* 10:108–113, 1988.

Kulick, AR; Ahmed, I: Substance-induced organic mental disorders: A clinical and conceptual approach. *Gen Hosp Psychiatry,* 8:168–172, 1986.

Kulik, FA; Wilbur, R: Case report of painful ejaculation as a side effect of amoxapine. *Am J Psychiatry,* 139:234–235, 1982.

Kunzukrishnan, R; Bradford, OMW: The profile of a major affectual disorder offender. *Psychiatr J Univ Ottawa,* 15:11–14, 1990.

Kuperman, S; Black, DW; Burns, TL: Excess mortality among formerly hospitalized child psychiatric patients. *Arch Gen Psychiatry,* 45:277–282, 1988.

Kupfer, DJ; Berger, PA; Janeway, J; Endicott, J; et al: Mood disorders: Pharmacologic prevention of recurrences. *Am J Psychiatry,* 142:469–476, 1985.

Kupfer, DJ; Coble, PA; Rubenstein, D: Changes in weight during treatment for depression. *Psychosom Med,* 41(7):535–544, 1979.

Kupfer, DJ; Frank, E: Relapse in recurrent unipolar depression. *Am J Psychiatry,* 144:86–88, 1987.

Kupfer, DJ; Frank, E; Perel, JM: The advantage of early treatment intervention in recurrent depression. *Arch Gen Psychiatry,* 47:771–775, 1989.

Kurland, ML: Organic brain syndrome with propranolol. *N Engl J Med,* 300:366, 1979.

Kushner, MG; Sher, KJ; Beitman, BD: The relation between alcohol problems and the anxiety disorders. *Am J Psychiatry,* 147:685–695, 1990.

Kwentus, JA; Hart, RP; Calabrese, V; Hekmati, A: Mania as a symptom of multiple sclerosis. *Psychosomatics,* 27:729–731, 1986.

Kwentus, JA; Silverman, JJ; Sprague, M: Manic syndrome after metrizamide myelography. *Am J Psychiatry,* 141:700–702, 1984.

Lacoursiere, RB; Spohn, HE; Thompson, K: Medical effects of abrupt neuroleptic withdrawal. *Compr Psychiatry,* 17:285–294, 1976.

Lacoursiere, RB; Swatek, R: Adverse interaction between disulfiram and marijuana: A case report. *Am J Psychiatry,* 140:243–244, 1983.

Lake, DR; Stirba, AL; Kinneman, RW; et al: Mania associated with LSD ingestions. *Am J Psychiatry,* 138:1508–1509, 1981.

Lamb, HR: The new asylums in the community. *Arch Gen Psychiatry,* 36:129–134, 1979.

Lammi, UK; Kivela, SL; Nissiren, A; et al: Mental disability among elderly men in Finland: Prevalence of psychiatric disorder. *Acta Psychiatr Scand,* 80:459–468, 1989.

Lane, RD; Merikangas, KR; Schwartz, GE; et al: Inverse relationship between defensiveness and lifetime prevalence of psychiatric disorder. *Am J Psychiatry,* 147:573–578, 1990.

Lapierre, YD: A controlled study of penfluridol in the treatment of chronic schizophrenia. *Am J Psychiatry,* 135:956–959, 1978.

Lapierre, YD; Anderson, K: Dyskinesia associated with amoxapine antidepressant therapy: A case report. *Am J Psychiatry,* 140:493–494, 1983.

Last, CG; Hersen, M; Kazdin, AE; Francis, G; et al: Psychiatric illness in the mothers of anxious children. *Am J Psychiatry,* 144:1580–1583, 1987a.

Last, CG; Francis, G; Hersen, M; Kazdin, AE; et al: Separation anxiety and school phobia: A comparison using DSM-III criteria. *Am J Psychiatry,* 144:653–657, 1987b.

Latimer, PR: External contingency management for chronic pain: Critical review of the evidence. *Am J Psychiatry,* 139:1308–1312, 1982.

Lawrence, JM: Reactions to withdrawal of antidepressants, antiparkinsonian drugs, and lithium. *Psychosomatics,* 26:869–877, 1985.

Lazarus, A: Heatstroke in a chronic schizophrenic patient treated with high-potency neuroleptics. *Gen Hosp Psychiatry,* 7:361–363, 1985.

Lazarus, A: Should neuroleptic malignant syndrome be treated in a private psychiatric hospital or a general hospital? *Gen Hosp Psychiatry,* 12:245–247, 1990.

Lazzara, RR; Stoudemire, A; Manning, D; Prewitt, KC: Metoclopramide-induced tardive dyskinesia: A case report. *Gen Hosp Psychiatry,* 8:107–109, 1986.

Leckman, JF; Ort, S; Caruso, KA; Anderson, GM; et al: Rebound phenomena in Tourette's Syndrome after abrupt withdrawal of clonidine. *Arch Gen Psychiatry,* 43:1168–1176, 1986.

Leckman, JF; Weissman, MM; Merikangas, KR; Pauls, DL; et al: Panic disorder and major depression. *Arch Gen Psychiatry,* 40:1055–1060, 1983.

Lee, MA; Flegel, P; Greden, JF; Cameron, OG: Anxiogenic effects of caffeine on panic and depressed patients. *Am J Psychiatry,* 145:632–635, 1988.

Lehman, AF; Myers, CP; Corty, E: Assessment and classification of patients with psychiatric and substance abuse syndromes. *Hospital and Community Psychiatry,* 40:1019–1025, 1989.

Leibenluft, E; Goldberg, RL: The suicidal, terminally ill patient with depression. *Psychosomatics,* 29:379–386, 1988.

Leighton, A: *My Name is Legion, Vol. 1. The Stirling County Study of Psychiatric Disorder and Sociocultural Environment.* New York, Basic Books, 1963.

Leighton, DC; et al: *The Character of Danger, Vol. III. The Stirling County Study of Psychiatric Disorder and Sociocultural Environment.* New York, Basic Books, 1963.

Leighton, DC; et al: *The Character of Danger, Vol. III. The Stirling County Study of Psychiatric Disorder and Sociocultural Environment.* New York, Basic Books, 1963.

Lelliott, P; Marks, I; McNamee, G; Tobena, A: Onset of panic disorder with agoraphobia. *Arch Gen Psychiatry,* 46:1000–1004, 1989.

Lenox, RH; Modell, JG; Weiner, S: Acute treatment of manic agitation with lorazepam. *Psychosomatics,* 27:28–32, 1986.

Leong, GB; Shaner, AL; Silva JA: Narcolepsy, paranoid psychosis, and analeptic abuse. *Psychiatr J Univ Ottawa,* 14:481–483, 1989.

Leppig, M; Bosch, B; Naber, D; et al: Clozapine in the treatment of 121 outpatients. *Psychopharmacology,* 99:S77–S79, 1989.

Lerer, B; Bleich, A; Kotler, M; Garb, R; et al: Posttraumatic stress disorder in Israeli combat veterans. *Arch Gen Psychiatry,* 44:976–981, 1987.

Lessard v. Schmidt, 349 Supp. 1078 (E.D. Wisc. 1972): Vacated and remanded, 94 S. Ct. 713 (1974).

Lesser, IM: Case report of withdrawal dyskinesia associated with amoxapine. *Am J Psychiatry,* 140:1358–1359, 1983.

Lesser, IM; Rubin, RT: Diagnostic considerations in panic disorders. *J Clin Psychiatry,* 47:4–10, 1986.

Lesser, IM; Rubin, RT; Pecknold, JC; Rifkin, A; et al: Secondary depression in panic disorder and agoraphobia: I. Frequency, severity, and response to treatment. *Arch Gen Psychiatry,* 45:437–443, 1988.

Lesser, RP: Psychogenic seizures. *Psychosomatics,* 27:823–829, 1986.

Lester, D; Brockopp, GW: *Crisis Intervention and Counseling by Telephone.* Springfield, Illinois, Charles C. Thomas, 1973.

Lester, D; *Effects of Suicide Prevention Centers on Suicide Rates in the United States.* Health Services Reports, 89:37–39, 1974.

Lester, D: The myth of suicide prevention. *Comp Psychiat,* 13:555–560, 1972.

Levar, I; Greenfield, H; Baruch, E: Psychiatric combat reactions during the Yom Kippur War. *Am J Psychiatry,* 136:637–641, 1979.

Leventstein, S; Klein, DF; Pollack, M: Follow-up study of formerly voluntary psychiatric patients: The first two years. *Am J Psychiatry,* 122:1102–1966.

Levin, AP; Liebowitz, MR: Drug treatment of phobias: Efficacy and optimum use. *Practical Therapeutics,* 34:504–514, 1987.

Levin, R; Banks, S; Berg, B: Psychosocial dimensions of epilepsy: A review of the literature. *Epilepsia,* 296:805–816, 1988.

Levine, S; Ancill, RJ; Roberts, AP: Assessment of suicide risks by computer-delivered self-rating questionnaire: Preliminary findings. *Acta Psychiatric Scand,* 80:216–220, 1989.

Levine, SR; Washington, JM; Jefferson, MF, Kieran, SN; et al: "Crack" cocaine-associated stroke. *Neurology,* 37:1849–1853, 1987.

Levy, AB; Dixon, KN; Stern, SL: How are depression and bulimia related? *Am J Psychiatry,* 146:162–169, 1989.

Levy, AB: Delirium induced by inhalation of typewriter correction fluid. *Psychosomatics,* 27:665–666, 1986.

Levy, AB; Stern, SL: DST and TRH stimulation test in mood disorder subtypes. *Am J Psychiatry,* 144:472–475, 1987.

Levy, JC; Deykin, EY: Suicidality, depression, and substance abuse in adolescence. *Am J Psychiatry,* 146:1462–1467, 1989.

Levy, JK; Fernandez, F: Neuropsychiatric care for critically ill AIDS patients. *J Crit Illness,* 4:33–42, 1989.

Lewis, DO; Shanok, SS; Grant; et al: Homicidally aggressive young children: Neuropsychiatric and experiential correlates. *Am J Psychiatry,* 140:148–153, 1983.

Lewis, JD; Moritz, D; Mellis, LP: Long-term toluene abuse. *Am J Psychiatry,* 138:368–370, 1981.

Leyberg, JT; Denmark, JC: The treatment of depressive states with imipramine hydrochloride (Tofranil). *J Ment Sci,* 105:1123–1126, 1959.

Lieb, J: Degraded protein-containing food and monoamine oxidase inhibitors. *Am J Psychiatry,* 134:1444–1445, 1977.

Lieb, J; Lipstich, II; Slaby, AE: *The Crisis Team: A Handbook for the Mental Health Professional.* New York, Harper and Row, 1973.

Lieb, J; Slaby, AE: How much do you know about clinical psychiatry? *Mod Med,* pp 81–88, March 1, 1975a.

Lieb, J; Slaby, AE: *Integrated Psychiatric Treatment.* New York, Harper and Row, 1975b.

Lieberman, J; Johns, C; Cooper, T; et al: Clozapine pharmacology and tardive dyskinesia. *Psychopharmacology,* 99:554–559, 1989.

Lieberman, JA; Alvir, J; Mukherjee, S; Kane, JM: Treatment of tardive dyskinesia with bromocriptine. *Arch Gen Psychiatry,* 46:908–913, 1989.

Lieberman, JA; Bowers, MB: Substance abuse comorbidity in schizophrenia. Editors' introduction. *Schizophrenia Bulletin,* 16:97–110, 1990.

Lieberman, JA; Kane, JM; Sarantakos, S; Gadeleta, D; et al: Prediction of relapse in schizophrenia. *Arch Gen Psychiatry,* 44:597–603, 1987.

Lieberman, PB; Baker, FM: The reliability of psychiatric diagnosis in the emergency room. *Hospital and Community Psychiatry,* 36:291–293, 1985.

Lieberman, PB; Strauss, JS: Brief psychiatric hospitalization: What are its effects? *Am J Psychiatry,* 143:1557–1562, 1986.

Lieberman, PB; Strauss, JS: The recurrence of mania: Environmental factors and medical treatment. *Am J Psychiatry,* 141:77–80, 1984.

Liebman, WM: Recurrent abdominal pain in children; lactose and sucrose intolerance: A prospective study. *Pediatrics,* 64:43–45, 1979.

Liebowitz, MR; Fyer, AJ; Gorman, JM; Dillon, D; et al: Lactate provocation of panic attacks: I. Clinical and behavioral findings. *Arch Gen Psychiatry,* 41:764–770, 1984a.

Liebowitz, MR; Fyer, AJ; Gorman, JM; Dillon D; et al: Specificity of lactate infusions in social phobia versus panic disorders. *Am J Psychiatry,* 142:947–950, 1985a.

Liebowitz, MR; Gorman, JM; Fyer, AJ; Dillion, DJ; et al: Effects of naloxone on patients with panic attacks. *Am J Psychiatry,* 141:995–997, 1984b.

Liebowitz, MR; Gorman, JM; Fyer, AJ; Levitt, M; et al: Lactate provocation of panic attacks: II. Biochemical and physiological findings. *Arch Gen Psychiatry,* 42:709–719, 1985b.

Liebowitz, MR; Wuetzel, EJ; Bowser, AE; Klein, DF: Phenelzine and delusions of parasitosis: A case report. *Am J Psychiatry,* 135:998–1002, 1978.

Lief, HI; et al: Low dropout rate in psychiatric clinic. *Arch Gen Psychiatry,* 5:200, 1961.

Lifschutz (In re), 2 *Cal.* 3d 330 (1970).

Lin, KM; Finder, E: Neuroleptic dosage for Asians. *Am J Psychiatry,* 140:490–491, 1983.

Lindemann, E: Symptomatology and management of acute grief. *Am J Psychiatry,* 101–141, 1944.

Lindemann, E: The Wellesley Project for the study of certain problems in community mental health, in *Interrelationships Between Social Environment and Psychiatric Disorders.* New York, Milbank Memorial Fund, 1953.

Linder v. United States, 268 *U. S. 5* (1925).

Linet, LS: Mysterious MAOI hypertensive episodes. *J Clin Psychiatry,* 47:563–565, 1986.

Linet, MS; Stewart, WF; Celentano, DD; Ziegler, D; et al: An epidemiologic study of headache among adolescents and young adults. *JAMA,* 261:2211–2216, 1989.

Ling, MHM; Perry, PJ; Tsuant, MT: Side effects of corticosteroid therapy: Psychiatric aspects. *Arch Gen Psychiatry,* 38:471–477, 1981.

Linnoila, M; DeJong, J; Virkkunen, M: Family history of alcoholism in violent offenders and impulsive fire setters. *Arch Gen Psychiatry,* 46:613–616, 1989.

Linnoila, M; George, L; Guthrie, S: Interaction between antidepressants and perphenazine in psychiatric inpatients. *Am J Psychiatry,* 139:1329–1331, 1982.

Linnoila, M; George, L; Guthrie, S; et al: Effect of alcohol consumption and cigarette smoking on antidepressant level of depressed patients. *Am J Psychiatry,* 138:841–842, 1981.

Linnoila, M; Viukari, M; Vaisanen, K; et al: Effect of anticonvulsants on plasma haloperidol and thioridazine levels. *Am J Psychiatry,* 137:819–821, 1980.

Lipinski, JF; Pope, HG: Possible synergistic action between carbamazepine and lithium carbonate in the treatment of three acutely manic patients. *Am J Psychiatry,* 139:948–949, 1982.

Lipper, S; Davidson, JRT; Grady, TA; Edinger, JD; et al: Preliminary study of carbamazepine in posttraumatic stress disorder. *Psychosomatics,* 27:849–854, 1986.

Lipsitt, LP: The "development" of adolescent suicide. *R I Med J,* 69:475–478, 1986.

Lishman, WA: *Organic Psychiatry.* Oxford, Blackwell Scientific Publications, 1978.

Liss, L; Frandes, A: Court-mandated treatment: Dilemmas for hospital psychiatry. *Am J Psychiatry,* 132:924–927, 1975.

Litwack, TR: The role of counsel in civil commitment proceedings: Emerging problems. *California L Rev,* 62:816–839, May, 1974.

Livingston, R; Reis, CJ; Ringdahl, IC: Abnormal dexamethasone suppression test results in depressed and nondepressed children. *Am J Psychiatry,* 141:106–108, 1984.

Livingstone, JB; Portnoi, T; Sherry, SN; et al: A new multidisciplinary child clinic: Description of a research study and a report of clinical results. *J Am Acad Child Psychiatry,* 9:688–706, 1983.

Lloyd, C: Life events and depressive disorder reviewed: II. Events as precipitating factors. *Arch Gen Psychiatry,* 37:541–548, 1980.

Locke, BZ; Slaby, AE: *Monographs in Psychosocial Epidemiology. Volume 1: Studies of Children.* F Earls, ed. Rutgers University Press, New York, 1980.

Locke, BZ; Slaby, AE: *Monographs in Psychosocial Epidemiology. Volume 2: Stressful Life Events.* BS Dohrenwend, BP Dohrenwend, eds. New York, Rutgers University Press, 1981.

Locke, BZ; Slaby, AE: *Monographs in Psychosocial Epidemiolgy. Volume 3: Symptoms, Illness Behavior and Help Seeking.* D Mechanic, ed. New York, Rutgers University Press, 1982.

Locke, S: *Neurology.* Boston, Little, Brown and Co., 1966.

Loewenstein, RJ; Sharfstein, SS: Neuropsychiatric aspects of acquired immune deficiency syndrome. *Int J Psychiatry Med,* 13:255–260, 1983–84.

Loimer, W; Schmid, RW; Resslick, O; et al: Continuous naloxone administration suppresses opiate withdrawal symptoms in human opiate addicts during detoxification treatment. *J Psychiat Res,* 23:81–86, 1989.

Loosen, PT; Kistler, K; Prange, AJ: Use of TSH response to TRH as an independent variable. *Am J Psychiatry,* 140:700–703, 1983.

Loosen, PT; Prange, AJ: Serum thyrotropin response to the thyrotropin-releasing hormone in psychiatric patients: a review. *Am J Psychiatry,* 139:405–416, 1982.

Loranger, AW; Levin, PM: Age at onset of bipolar affective illness. *Arch Gen Psychiatry,* 35:1345–1348, 1978.

Loranger, AW; Oldham, JM; Tulis, EH: Familial transmission of DSM-III borderline personality disorder. *Arch Gen Psychiatry,* 39:795–799, 1982.

Louis, AK; Lannon, RA, Ketter, TA: Treatment of cocaine-induced panic disorder. *Am J Psychiatry,* 146:40–44, 1989.

Lowenstein, M; Binder, RL; McNiel, DE: The relationship between admission symptoms and hospital assaults. *Hospital and Community Psychiatry,* 41:311–330, 1990.

Lown, B; Desilva, RA; Reich, P; et al: Psychophysiologic factors in sudden cardiac death. *Am J Psychiatry,* 137:1325–1335, 1980.

Lowry, MR; Dunner, FJ: Seizures during tricyclic therapy. *Am J Psychiatry,* 137:1461–1462, 1980.

Lucas, CP; Rigby, JC; Lucas SB: The occurrence of depression following mania: A method of predicting vulnerable cases. *Br J Psychiatry,* 154:705–708, 1989.

Luchins, DJ; Freed, WJ; Wyatt, RJ: The role of cholinergic supersensitivity in the medical symptoms associated with withdrawal of antipsychotic drugs. *Am J Psychiatry,* 137:1395–1398, 1980.

Luchins, DJ; Rose, RP: Late-life onset of panic disorder with agoraphobia in three patients. *Am J Psychiatry,* 146:920–921, 1989.

Ludolph, PS; Westen, D; Misle, B; et al: The borderline diagnosis in adolescents: Symptoms and developmental history. *Am J Psychiatry,* 147:470–476, 1990.

Lugaresi, E; Zucconi, M; Bixler, E: Epidemiology of sleep disorders. *Psychiatric Annals,* 17:446–453, 1987.

Lukianowicz, N: Incest. *Br J Psychiatry,* 120:301–313, 1972.

Lydiard, RB; Gelenberg, AJ: Amoxapine: An antidepressant with some neuroleptic properties? A review of its chemistry, animal pharmacology and toxicology, human pharmacology, and clinical efficacy. *Pharmacotherapy,* 1:163–175, 1981.

Lydiard, RB; Laraia, MT; Ballenger, JC; Howell, EF: Emergence of depressive symptoms in patients receiving alprazolam for panic disorder. *Am J Psychiatry,* 144:664–665, 1987.

Lyman, JL: Student suicide at Oxford University. *Student Medicine,* 10:218, 1961.

Lynsey, JR; Robinson, RG; Pearlson, GD; et al: The dexamethasone suppression test and mood following stroke. *Am J Psychiatry,* 142:318–323, 1985.

Lyons, HA: Psychiatric sequelae of the Belfast riots. *Br J Psychiatry,* 118:265–273, 1971.

Lyons, MJ: Observable and subjective factors associated with attempted suicide in later life. *Suicide and Life Threatening Behavior,* 15:168–183, 1985.

Maany, I: Treatment of depression associated with Briquet's syndrome. *Am J Psychiatry,* 138:373–375, 1981.

Maas, JW: Clinical and biochemical heterogeneity of depressive disorders. *Intern Med,* 88:556–563, 1978.

MacDonald, DI; Czechowicz, D: Marijuana: A pediatric overview. *Psychiatric Annals,* 16:215–218, 1986.

Mackenzie, TB; Popkin, MK: Organic anxiety syndrome. *Am J Psychiatry,* 140:342–344, 1983.

MacMahon, B; Johnson, S; Pugh, TF: Relation of suicide rates to social conditions. *Public Health Rep,* 78:285, 1963.

Madakasira, S; Hall, TB: Capgras syndrome in a patient with myxedema. *Am J Psychiatry,* 138:365–367, 1981.

Maes, M; Jacobs, MP; Soy, E; et al: An augmented escape of beta-endorphins to suppression by dexamethasone in severely depressed patients. *J Affective Disord,* 18:149–156, 1990.

Mageux, R; Stern, Y; Williams, JBW: Clinical and biochemical features of depression in Parkinson's disease. *Am J Psychiatry,* 143:756–759, 1981.

Maguire, GP; Granville-Grossman, KL: Physical illness in psychiatric patients. *Brit J Psychiatry,* 115:1365–1369, 1968.

Maitre, L; Waldeier, PC; Greengrass, PM; et al: Maprotiline—its position as an antidepressant in the light of recent neuropharmacological and neurobiochemical findings. *J Int Med Res,* Supplement 2, 1975.

Maldonado, RR; DeFrancisco, CP; Tamajo, L: Lithium dermatitis. *JAMA,* 224:1534, 1973.

Maletta, GJ; Pirozzolo, FJ; Thompson, G; et al: Organic mental disorders in a geriatric outpatient population. *Am J Psychiatry,* 139:521–523, 1982.

Malmquist, CP: Can the committed patient refuse chemotherapy. *Arch Gen Psychiatry,* 36:351–354, 1979.

Man, PL; Chen, CHP: Rapid tranquilization of acutely psychotic patients with haloperidol and chlorpromazine. *Psychosomatics,* 14:59, 1973.

Mann, JJ: Psychobiologic predictors of suicide. *J Clin Psychiatry,* 48:39–43, 1987.

Mann, LS; Johnson, RW; Levine, DJ: Tobacco dependence: Psychology, biology, and treatment strategies. *Psychosomatics,* 27:713–718, 1986.

Mann, SC; Caroff, SN; Bleier, HR; Welz, WKR; et al: Lethal catatonia. *Am J Psychiatry,* 143:1374–1381, 1986.

Manos, N; Gkiouzepas, J; Logthetis, J: The need for continuous use of antiparkinsonian medication with chronic schizophrenic patients receiving long-term neuroleptic therapy. *Am J Psychiatry,* 138:184–188, 1981.

Manu, P; Lane, TJ; Matthews, DA; Escobar, JI: Screening for somatization disorder in patients with chronic fatigue. *Gen Hosp Psychiatry,* 11:294–297, 1989.

Manual of Medical Therapeutics 20th ed. CMG Rosenfeld, ed. Boston, Little, Brown and Co., 1971.

Maquire, P: The psychologist and social sequelae of mastectomy. In: *Modern Perspectives in the Psychiatric Aspects of Surgery,* JC Howells, ed. New York, Brunner/Mazel, 1976.

Marcus, MD; Wing, RR; Ewing, L; et al: A double-blind, placebo-controlled trial of fluoxetine plus behavior modification in the treatment of obese binge-eaters and non-binge eaters. *Am J Psychiatry,* 147:876–881, 1990.

Marder, SR: Depot neuroleptics: Side effects and safety. *J Clin Psychopharmacol,* 6:24–29, 1986.

Margo, GM; Finkel, JA: Early dementia as a risk factor for suicide. *Hospital and Community Psychiatry,* 41:676–678, 1990.

Maris, R: The adolescent suicide problem. *Suicide and Life-Threatening Behavior,* 15:91–109, 1985.

Mark, VH; Ervin, FR: *Violence and the Brain.* New York, Harper & Row, 1970.

Markovitz, PJ; Stagno, SJ; Calabrese, JR: Buspirone augmentation fluoxetine in obsessive-compulsive disorder. *Am J Psychiatry,* 147:798–800, 1990.

Markowitz, J; Viederman, M: A case report of dissociative pseudodementia. *Gen Hosp Psychiatry,* 8:87–90, 1986.

Markowitz, JS; Weissman, MM; Ouellette, R; Lish, JD; et al: Quality of life in panic disorder. *Arch Gen Psychiatry,* 46:984–992, 1989.

Marks, A: Management of the suicidal adolescent on a nonpsychiatric adolescent unit. *J Pediatr,* 95:305–308, 1979.

Marks, I; Lader, M: Anxiety states (anxiety neurosis): A review. *J Nerv Ment Dis,* 156:3–18, 1973.

Marks, IM: The classification of phobic disorders. *Br J Psychiatry,* 116:377–386, 1970.

Marks, J: *The Benzodiazepines: Use, Overuse, Misuse, Abuse,* 2nd ed. Boston, MTP Press Ltd., 1985.

Markusk, RE; Schwab, JJ; Farris, P; et al: Mortality and community mental health. *Arch Gen Psychiatry,* 34:1393–1401, 1977.

Marneros, A: Adult onset of Tourette's Syndrome: A case report. *Am J Psychiatry,* 140:924–925, 1983.

Marsden, CD; Tarsy, D; Baldessarini, RJ: Spontaneous and drug-induced movement disorders in psychiatric patients. In: *Psychiatric Aspects of Neurological Disease,* DF Benson, D Blumer, eds. New York, Grune and Stratton, 1975.

Marshall, H: Incidence of physical disorders among psychiatric inpatients. *Brit Med J,* 2:468–470, 1949.

Marson, DC; McGovern, MP; Pomp, HC: Psychiatric decision making in the emergency room: A research overview. *Am J Psychiatry,* 145:918–925, 1988.

Martin, J; Reichlin, S; Brown, G: *Clinical Neuroendocrinology,* Philadelphia. F.A. Davis Co., 1977.

Martin, RL; Cloninger, R; Guze, SB: Female criminality and the prediction of recidivism: A prospective six-year follow-up. *Arch Gen Psychiatry,* 35:207–214, 1978.

Martin, RL; Cloninger, R; Guze, SB; Clayton, PJ: Mortality in a follow-up of 500 psychiatric outpatients. *Arch Gen Psychiatry,* 42:47–54, 1985a.

Martin, RL; Cloninger, CR; Guze, SB; Clayton, PJ: Mortality in a follow-up 500 psychiatric outpatients: II. Cause-specific mortality. *Arch Gen Psychiatry,* 42:58–66, 1985b.

Marx, AJ; Test, MS; Stein, LI: Extra-hospital management of severe mental illness. *Arch Gen Psychiatry,* 29:505, 1973.

Marzuk, PM; Mann, JJ: Suicide and substance abuse. *Psychiatric Annals,* 18:639–645, 1988.

Marzuk, PM; Tierney, H; Tardiff, K; Gross, EM; et al: Increased risk of suicide in persons with AIDs. *JAMA,* 259:1333–1337, 1988.

Mass. Gen. Laws Ch. 123 ss 7, 8, 12 (1971).

Massie, MJ; Holland J; Glass, E: Delirium in terminally ill cancer patients. *Am J Psychiatry,* 140:1048–1050, 1983.

Matikainen, M: Spontaneous rupture of the stomach. *Am J Surg,* 138:451–452, 1979.

Mattes, JA: Comparative effectiveness of carbamazepine and propranolol for rage outbursts. *J Neuropsych Clin Neurosci,* 2:159–164, 1990.

Mattes, JA: Metoprolol for intermittent explosive disorder. *Am J Psychiatry,* 142:1108–1109, 1985.

Mattes, JA; Gittelman, R: Effects of artificial food colorings in children with hyperactive symptoms: A critical review and results of a controlled study. *Arch Gen Psychiatry,* 38:714–718, 1981.

Mavissakalian, M; Perel, J: Imipramine in the treatment of agoraphobia: Dose-response relationships. *Am J Psychiatry,* 142:1032–1036, 1985.

Mavissakalian, M; Salerni, R; Thompson, ME; Michelson, L: Mitral valve prolapse and agoraphobia. *Am J Psychiatry,* 140:1612–1614, 1983.

Mavissakalian, M; Turner, SM; Michelson, L; Jacob, R: Tricyclic antidepressants in obsessive-compulsive disorder: Antiobsessional or antidepressant agents? II. *Am J Psychiatry,* 142:572–576, 1985.

May, PRA; Van Putten, T; Jenden, DJ; et al: Chlorpromazine levels and the outcome of treatment in schizophrenic patients. *Arch Gen Psychiatry,* 38:202–207, 1981.

May, PRA; Van Putten, T; Yale, C: Predicting outcome of antipsychotic drug treatment from early response. *Am J Psychiatry,* 137:1088–1089, 1980.

Mayfield, DG; Montgomery, D: Alcoholism, alcohol intoxication, and suicide attempts. *Arch Gen Psychiatry,* 27:349–353, 1972.

Mazeade, M; Caron, C; Cote, R; et al: Extreme temperament and diagnosis: A study in a psychiatric sample of consecutive children. *Arch Gen Psychiatry,* 47:477–484, 1990.

Mazza, DL; Martin, D; Spacavento, L; Jacobsen, J; et al: Prevalence of anxiety disorders in patients with mitral valve prolapse. *Am J Psychiatry,* 143:349–352, 1986.

McAllister, TW; Ferrell, RB; Price; TRP; et al: The dexamethasone suppression test in two patients with severe depressive pseudodementia. *Am J Psychiatry,* 139:479–481, 1982.

McAllister, TW; Price, TRP: Severe depressive pseudodementia with and without dementia. *Am J Psychiatry,* 139:626–629, 1982.

McClelland, RJ: Psychosocial sequelae of head injury—anatomy of a relationship. *Br J Psychiatry,* 153:141–146, 1988.

McCoid, AH: A reappraisal of liability for unauthorized medical treatment. *Minnesota L Rev* 41:381, 1957.

McCulloch, LE: McNiel, DE; Binder, RL; Hatcher, C: Effects of a weapon screening procedure in a psychiatric emergency room. *Hospital and Community Psychiatry,* 37:937–838, 1986.

McCurdy, L: Lorazepam, a new benzodiazepine derivative, in the treatment of anxiety: A double-blind clinical evaluation. *Am J Psychiatry,* 136:187–190, 1979.

McDonald v. United States, 114 U.S. App. D.C. 120, 312 F. 2d 847 (en banc) (1962).

McDougle, CJ; Goodman, WK; Price, LH; et al: Neuroleptic addiction in fluvoxamine—refractory obsessive–compulsive disorder. *Am J Psychiatry,* 147:652–654, 1990.

McDougle, CJ; Southwich, SM: Emergence of an alternate personality in combat-related post-traumatic stress disorder. *Hospital and Community Psychiatry,* 41:554–556, 1990.

McEvoy, JP; Lohr, JB: Diazepam for catatonia. *Am J Psychiatry,* 141:284–285, 1984.

McFall, ME; Smith, DE; Raszell, DK, et al: Comergent validity of measures of PTSD in Vietnam combat veterans. *Am J Psychiatry,* 147:645–648, 1990.

McFarlane, AC: The aetiology of post-traumatic stress disorders following a natural disaster. *Br J Psychiatry,* 152:116–121, 1988a.

McFarlane, AC: The phenomenology of posttraumatic stress disorders following a natural disaster. *J Nerv Ment Dis,* 176:22–29, 1988b.

McGarry, AL; Kaplan, HA: Overview: Current trends in mental health law. *Am J Psychiatry,* 130:621–630, 1973.

McGee, RK: *Crisis Intervention in the Community.* Baltimore, University Park Press, 1974.

McGinnis, JM: Suicide in America-moving up the public health agenda. *Suicide and Life-Threatening Behavior,* 17:18–32, 1987.

McGlashan, TH: Adolescent versus adult onset of mania. *Am J Psychiatry,* 145:221–223, 1988.

McGlothlin, WH; Anglin, M: Long-term follow-up of clients of high- and low-dose methadone programs. *Arch Gen Psychiatry,* 38:1055–1063, 1981.

McGrath, PJ; Quitkin, FM; Stewart, JW; et al: An open clinical trial of mianserin. *Am J Psychiatry,* 138:530–532, 1981.

McHale, DM; Sage, JI: Hallucinations and confusion after pergolide withdrawal. *Clin Neuropharmacology,* 11:545–548, 1988.

McHugh, PR; Folstein, MF: Psychiatric syndromes in Huntington's chorea: A clinical and phenomenologic study. In: *Psychiatric Aspects of Neurological Diseases.* DF Benson, D Blumer, eds. New York, Grune & Stratton, 1975.

McIntosh, JL; Jewell, BL: Sex difference trends in completed suicide. *Suicide and Life-Threatening Behavior,* 16:16–27, 1986.

McKenna, MS: Assessment of the eating disordered patient. *Psychiatric Annals,* 19:467–472, 1989.

McKenna, PJ; Kane, JM; Parrish, K: Psychotic syndromes in epilepsy. *Am J Psychiatry,* 142:895–904, 1985.

McKenry, PC; Tishler, CL; Kelley, C: Adolescent suicide: A comparison of attempters and nonattempters in an emergency room population. *Clin Ped,* 21:266–270, 1982.

McKenry, PC; Tishler, CL; Kelley, C: The role of drugs in adolescent suicide attempts. *Suicide and Life-Threatening Behavior* 13(3):166–175, 1983.

McLean, P; Casey, DE: Tardive dyskinesia in an adolescent. *Am J Psychiatry,* 135:969–971, 1978.

McLellan, AT; Luborsky, L; Woody, GE; et al: Predicting response to alcohol and drug abuse treatment: Role of psychiatric severity. *Arch Gen Psychiatry,* 40:620–625, 1983.

McMahon, T: Dyskinesia associated with amoxapine withdrawal and use of carbamazepine and antihistamines. *Psychosomatics,* 27:145–148, 1986.

McMahon, T; Vahora, S: Radiation damage to the brain: Neuropsychiatric aspects. *Gen Hosp Psychiatry,* 8:437–441, 1986.

McNamara, ME; Fogel, BS: Anticonvulsant-responsive panic attacks with temporal lobe EEG abnormalities. *J Neuropsych Clin Neurosci,* 2:193–196, 1990.

McNeil v. Director, Patuxen Institution, 407 U.S. 245, 1972.

McNeil, DE; Binder, RL: Relationship between preadmission threats and later violent behavior by acute psychiatric inpatients. *Hospital and Community Psychiatry,* 40:605–608, 1989.

McNiel, DE; Binder, RL; Greenfield, TK: Predictors of violence in civilly committed acute psychiatric patients. *Am J Psychiatry,* 145:965–970, 1988a.

McNiel, DE; Hatcher, C; Reubin, R: Family survivors of suicide and accidental death: Consequences for widows. *Suicide and Life-Threatening Behavior,* 18:137–148, 1988b.

McPherson, DE: Teaching and research in emergency psychiatry. *Can J Psychiatry,* 29:50–54, 1984.

Meador-Woodruff, JH: Psychiatric side effects of tricyclic antidepressants. *Hospital and Community Psychiatry,* 41:84–86, 1990.

Melia, PI: Prophylactic lithium in recurrent affective disorders: A four year study. *J Ir Med Assoc,* 63:160–170, 1970.

Mellman, LA; Gorman, JM: Successful treatment of obsessive compulsive disorder with ECT. *Am J Psychiatry,* 141:596–597, 1984.

Mellman, TA; Uhde, TW: Obsessive compulsive symptoms in panic disorder. *Am J Psychiatry,* 144:1573–1576, 1987.

Mellman, TA; Uhde, TW: Withdrawal syndrome with gradual tapering of alprazolam. *Am J Psychiatry,* 143:1464–1466, 1986.

Mellman, TA; Uhde, TW: Sleep panic attacks: New clinical findings and theoretical implications. *Am J Psychiatry,* 146:1204–1207, 1989.

Meltzer, HY; Fang, VS: Cortisol determination and the dexamethasone suppression test: A review. *Arch Gen Psychiatry,* 40:501–509, 1983.

Melzack, R: *The Puzzle of Pain.* New York, Basic Books, 1973.

Mendel, WM; Rapport, S: Determinants of the decision for psychiatric hospitalization. *Arch Gen Psychiatry,* 20:321, 1969.

Mendelson, JH; Teoh, SK; Lange, U; Mello, NK; et al: Anterior pituitary, adrenal, and gonadal hormones during cocaine withdrawal. *Am J Psychiatry,* 145:1094–1098, 1988.

Mendelson, JH; Mello, NK; Lex, BW; Bavli, S: Marijuana withdrawal syndrome in a woman. *Am J Psychiatry*, 141:1289–1290, 1984.

Mendelson, W; Johnson, N; Stewart, MA: Hyperactive children as adolescents: A follow-up study. *J Nerv Ment Dis*, 153:273–279, 1971.

Mendez, MF; Martin, RJ; Smyth, KA; et al: Psychiatric syndromes associated with Alzheimer's disease. *J Neuropsychiatry*, 2:28–33, 1990.

Menninger, K: *Man Against Himself.* New York, Harcourt Brace, 1938.

Menninger, WC: *Psychiatry in a Troubled World.* New York, Macmillan, 1948.

Menza, MA; Murray, GB; Holmes, VF; Rafuls, WA: Decreased extrapyramidal symptoms with intravenous haloperidol. *J Clin Psychiatry*, 48:278–280, 1987.

Mermel, LA; Doro, JM; Kabadi, UM: Acute psychosis in a patient receiving trimethoprim-sulfamethoxazole intravenously. *J Clin Psychiatry*, 47:269–270, 1986.

Merriam, AE; Medalia, A; Levine, B: Partial complex status epilepticus associated with cocaine abuse. *Biol Psychiatry*, 23:515–518, 1988.

Meyer, RE: Anxiolytics and the alcoholic patient. *J Stud Alcohol*, 47:269–273, 1986.

Mierenberg, AA; Price, LH; Channey, DS; et al: After lithium augmentation: A retrospective follow-up of patients with antidepressant-refractory depression. *J Affective Disord*, 18:167–175, 1990.

Milby, JB; Girwitch, RH; Wiebe, DJ; et al: Prevalence and diagnostic reliability of methadone maintenance detoxification fear. *Am J Psychiatry*, 143:739–743, 1986.

Milgram, RM; Milgram, NA: The effect of the Yom Kippur war on anxiety level in Israeli children. *J Psychol*, 94:107–113, 1976.

Miller, AL; Faber, RA; Hatch, JP; Alexander, HE: Factors affecting amnesia, seizure duration, and efficacy in ECT. *Am J Psychiatry*, 142:692–696, 1985.

Miller, D; Walker, MC; Friedman, D: Use of a holding technique to control the violent behavior of seriously disturbed adolescents. *Hospital and Community Psychiatry*, 40:520–524, 1989.

Miller, DD; Macklin, M: Cimetidine-imipramine interaction: A case report. *Am J Psychiatry*, 140:351–352, 1983.

Miller, FT; Mazade, NA: *Crisis Intervention Services in Comprehensive Community Mental Health Centers in the United States.* Unpublished mimeo, 1978, available through Dr. Mazade at The Staff College, National Institute of Mental Health, 5635 Fishers Lane, Rockville, Maryland, 20857.

Miller, NS; Gold, MS: The medical diagnosis and treatment of alcohol dependence. *Medical Times*, 115:109–126, 1987.

Miller, NS; Mirin, SM: Multiple drug use in alcoholics: Practical and theoretical implications. *Psychiatric Annals*, 19:248–255, 1989.

Miller, W: A psychiatric emergency service and some treatment concepts. *Am J Psychiatry*, 124:924–933, 1968.

Mills, MJ: Civil Commitment: The relationship between perceived dangerousness and mental illness. *Arch Gen Psychiatry*, 45:770–772, 1988.

Minkoff, K; Bergman, E; Beck, AT; et al: Hopelessness, depression, and attempted suicide. *Am J Psychiatry*, 130:445–459, 1973.

Minnesota ex rel Pearson v. Probate Court, 309 U.S. 270, 1940.

Mintz, RS: A pilot study of the prevalence of persons in the City of Los Angeles who have attempted suicide. Presented at the 120th Annual Meeting of the American Psychiatric Association, Los Angeles, May 4, 1964.

Mirin, SM; Schatzberg, AF; Creasey, DE: Hypomania and after withdrawal of tricyclic antidepressants. *Am J Psychiatry*, 138(1):87–89, 1981.

Mitchell, E; Matthew, KL: Gilles de la Tourette's disorder associated with pemoline. *Am J Psychiatry*, 137:1618–1619, 1980.

Mitchell, JE; Hatsukami, D; Eckert, ED; Pyle, RL: Characteristics of 275 patients with bulimia. *Am J Psychiatry*, 142:482–485, 1985.

Mitchell, JE; Pyle, RL; Eckert, ED: Frequency and duration of binge-eating episodes in patients with bulimia. *Am J Psychiatry*, 138:835–836, 1981.

M'Naghten Case: House of Lords, 1843, 8 *Eng Rep*, 718 (HL), 1843.

Modell, JG; Lenox, RH; Weiner, S: Inpatient clinical trial of lorazepam for the management of manic agitation. *J Clin Psychopharmacol*, 5:109–113, 1985.

Modestin, J; Hoffman, H: Completed suicide in psychiatric inpatients: A comparative study. *Acta Psychiatr Scand*, 79:229–234, 1989.

Modestin, J; Kopp, W: Study on suicide in depressed inpatients. *J Affective Disord*, 15:157–162, 1988.

Modestin, J; Krapf, R; Boker, W: A fatality during haloperidol treatment: Mechanism of sudden death. *Am J Psychiatry*, 138:1616–1617, 1981.

Modigh, K: Antidepressant drugs in anxiety disorders. *Acta Psychiatr Scand*, 76:57–71, 1987.

Moher, LM; Maurer, SA: Podophyllin toxicity: Case report and literature review. *J Fam Pract*, 9:237–240, 1979.

Moir, DC; Crooks, J; Cornwall, WB; et al: Cardiotoxicity of amitriptyline. *Lancet*, 2:561–564, 1972.

Molnar, G; Cameron, P: Incest syndromes: Observations in a general hospital psychiatric unit. *Can Psychiat Assoc J*, 20:373–377, 1975.

Monahan, J: Prediction research and the emergency commitment of dangerous mentally ill persons: A reconsideration. *Am J Psychiatry*, 135:198–201, 1978.

Monahan, J: The prediction of violent behavior: Toward a second generation of theory and policy. *Am J Psychiatry*, 141:10–15, 1984.

Mondimore, FM; Damlouji, N; Folstein, MF; Tune, L: Post-ECT confusional states associated with elevated serum anticholinergic levels. *Am J Psychiatry*, 140:930–931, 1983.

Monjan, AA: Sleep disorders of older people: Report of a concensus conference. *Hospital and Community Psychiatry*, 41:743–744, 1990.

Monopolis, S; Lion, JR: Problems in the diagnosis of intermittent explosive disorder. *Am J Psychiatry*, 140:1200–1202, 1983.

Monroe, RR: *Episodic Behavioral Disorders*. Cambridge, Mass, Harvard University Press, 1970.

Montgomery, SA: New antidepressants and 5-HT uptake inhibitors. *Acta Psych Scand*, 80(suppl 350):107–116, 1988.

Moore, DC: Amitriptyline therapy in anorexia nervosa. *Am J Psychiatry*, 134:1301–1304, 1977.

Moore, DP: A case of petit mal epilepsy aggravated by lithium. *Am J Psychiatry*, 138:690–691, 1981.

Moore, HE: Some emotional concomitants of disaster. *Mental Hygiene*, 42:45–50, 1958.

Mor, V; McHorney, C; Sherwood, S: Secondary morbidity among the recently bereaved. *Am J Psychiatry*, 143:158–163, 1986.

Moreau, DL; Weissman, M; Warner, V: Panic disorder in children at high risk for depression. *Am J Psychiatry*, 146:1059–1060, 1989.

Morgan, SL: Families' experiences in psychiatric emergencies. *Hospital and Community Psychiatry*, 40:1265–1269, 1989.

Morris, GH: Institutionalizing the rights of mental patients: Committing the legislature. *California L Rev*, 62:816–839, 1974.

Morrison, J: Childhood sexual histories of women with somatization disorder. *Am J Psychiatry*, 146:239–241, 1989.

Morse, HN: The tort liability of the psychiatrist. *Baylor L Rev*, 19208, 1971.

Moskovitz, C; Moses, H; Klawans, HL: Levodopa-induced psychosis: A kindling phenomenon. *Am J Psychiatry*, 135:669–675, 1978.

Moskovitz, R; Springer, P; Urguhart, M: Lithium-induced nephrotic syndrome. *Am J Psychiatry*, 138:382–383, 1981.

Mossman, D; Somoza, E: Maximizing diagnostic information from the dexamethasone suppression test. *Arch Gen Psychiatry*, 46:653–660, 1989.

Motet-Grigoras, CN; Schuckit, MA: Depression and substance abuse in handicapped young men. *J Clin Psychiatry*, 47:234–237, 1986.

Motto, JA: Evaluation of a suicide prevention center by sampling the population risk. *Suicide and Life-Threatening Behavior*, 1:18–22, 1971.

Mueser, KT; Butler, RW: Auditory hallucinations in combat-related chronic posttraumatic stress disorder. *Am J Psychiatry*, 144:299–302, 1987.

Mueser, KT; Yarnold, PR; Levinson, DF, et al: Prevalence of substance abuse in schizophrenia: Demographic and clinical correlates. *Schizophrenia Bulletin*, 16:31–58, 1990.

Mukherjee, S; Rosen, AM; Caracci, G; Shukla, S: Persistent tardive dyskinesia in bipolar patients. *Arch Gen Psychiatry*, 43:342–346, 1986.

Mukherjee, S; Rosen, AM; Cardenas, C; et al: Tardive dyskinesia in psychiatric outpatients: A study of prevalence and association with demographic, clinical, and drug history variables. *Arch Gen Psychiatry,* 39:466–469, 1982.

Muller, OE; Goodman, N; Bellet, S: The hypotensive effect of imipramine hydrochloride in patients with cardiovascular disease. *Clin Pharmacol Ther,* 2:300–307, 1961.

Munetz, MR: Overcoming resistance to talking to patients about tardive dyskinesia. *Hospital and Community Psychiatry,* 36:283–287, 1985.

Munetz, MR; Roth, LH: Informing patients about tardive dyskinesia. *Arch Gen Psychiatry,* 42:86–871, 1985.

Munetz, MR; Slawsky, RC; Neil, JF: Tardive Tourette's syndrome treated with clonidine and mesoridazine. *Psychosomatics,* 26:256–257, 1985.

Mungas, D: Interictal behavior abnormality in temporal lobe epilepsy: A specific syndrome or nonspecific psychopathology? *Arch Gen Psychiatry,* 39:108–111, 1982.

Munjack, DJ: Moss, HB: Affective disorder and alcoholism in families of agoraphobics. *Arch Gen Psychiatry,* 38:869–871, 1981.

Munoz, RA; Amado, H; Hyatt, S: Brief reactive psychosis. *J Clin Psychiatry,* 48:324–327, 1987.

Munoz-Millan, RJ; Casteel, CR: Attention-deficit hyperactivity disorder: Recent literature. *Hospital and Community Psychiatry,* 40:699–707, 1989.

Murphy, E; Lindesay, J; Grundy, E: 60 Years of suicide in England and Wales: A cohort study. *Arch Gen Psychiatry,* 43:969–976, 1986.

Murphy, GE: On suicide prediction and prevention. *Arch Gen Psychiatry,* 40:343–344, 1983.

Murphy, GE: Suicide and substance abuse. *Arch Gen Psychiatry,* 45:593–596, 1988.

Murphy, GE; Armstrong, JW; Hermele, SL; Fischer, JR; Clendenin, WW: Suicide and alcoholism: Interpersonal loss confined as a predictor. *Arch Gen Psychiatry,* 36:65–69, 1979.

Murphy, GE; Wetzel, RD: Suicide risk by birth cohort in the United States, 1949 to 1971. *Arch Gen Psychiatry,* 37:519–523, 1980.

Murphy, GE; Wetzel, RD: The lifetime risk of suicide in alcoholism. *Arch Gen Psychiatry,* 47:383–392, 1990.

Murphy, JG; Fenichel, GS; Jacobson, S: Psychiatry in the emergency department: Factors associated with treatment and disposition. *Am J Emerg Med,* 2:309–314, 1984.

Muskin, PR; Mellman, LA; Kornfeld, DS: Emergency psychiatry. *Gen Hosp Psychiatry,* 8:404–410, 1986.

Myers, JK; Bean, LL: *A Decade Later: A Follow-up of Social Class and Mental Illness.* New York, John Wiley and Sons, 1968.

Myers, MJ: Informed consent in medical malpractice. *California L Rev,* 55:396, 1967.

Naber, D; Leppig, M; Grohmann, R; et al: Efficacy and adverse effects of clozapine in the treatment of schizophrenia and tardive dyskinesia a retrospective study of 387 patients. *Psychopharmacology,* 99:S73–S76, 1989.

Nace, EP: Substance use disorders and personality disorders: Comorbidity. *The Psychiatric Hospital,* 20:65–69, 1989.

Nagy, A: Long-term treatment with benzodiazepines: Theoretical, ideological and practical aspects. *Acta Psychiatr Scand,* 76:47–55, 1987.

Naranjo, CA; Kadlec, KE; Sanhueza, P; Woodley-Remus, D; et al: Fluoxetine differentially alters alcohol intake and other consummatory behaviors in problem drinkers. *Clin Pharmacol Ther,* 47:490–498, 1990.

Narman, WH; Brown, WA; Miller, IW, et al: The dexamethasone suppression test and completed suicide. *Acta Psychiatr Scand,* 81:120–125, 1990.

Nasrallah, HA; Churchill, CM; Hamdan-Allan, GA: Higher frequency of neuroleptic-induced dystonia in mania than in schizophrenia. *Am J Psychiatry,* 145:1455–1456, 1988.

Nasrallah, HA; Jacoby, CG; McCalley-Whitters, M; et al: Cerebral ventricular enlargement in subtypes of chronic schizophrenia. *Arch Gen Psychiatry,* 39:774–777, 1982.

National Research Council Committee in Clinical Evaluation of Narcotic Antagonists: Clinical evaluation of naltrexone treatment of opiate-dependent individuals. *Arch Gen Psychiatry,* 135:335–340, 1978.

Navia, BA; Jordan, DB; Price, RW: The AIDS dementia complex: I. Clinical features. *Am Neurol,* 19:517–524, 1986.

Navia, BA; Price, RW: Dementia complicating AIDS. *Psychiatric Annals,* 16:158–166, 1986.

Neil, JF: Himmelhoch, JM; Licata, SM: Emergency of myasthenia gravis during treatment with lithium carbonate. *Arch Gen Psychiatry,* 33:1090–1092, 1976.

Neilsen, AC; Williams, TA: Depression in ambulatory medical patients. Prevalence of self-report questionnaire and recognition by nonpsychiatric physicians. *Arch Gen Psychiatry,* 37:999–1004, 1980.

Nelson, JC; Bowers, MB: Delusional unipolar depression. Description and drug response. *Arch Gen Psychiatry,* 35:1321–1328, 1978.

Nelson JC; Bowers, MB; Sweeney, DR: Exacerbation of psychosis by tricyclic antidepressants in delusional depression. *Am J Psychiatry,* 136:574–576, 1979.

Nelson, JC; Charney, DS: The symptoms of major depressive illness. *Am J Psychiatry,* 138:1–13, 1981.

Nelson, JC; Conwell, Y; Kim, K; Mazure, C: Age at onset in late-life delusional depression. *Am J Psychiatry,* 146:785–786, 1989.

Nelson, JC; Jatlow, PI: Neuroleptic effect on desipramine steady-state plasma concentrations. *Am J Psychiatry,* 137:1232–1234, 1980.

Nelson, JC; Mazone, CM; Jatlow, PI: Does melancholia predict response in major depression? *J Affective Disord,* 18:157–165, 1990.

Nemeroff, CB; Owens, MJ; Bissette, G; Andorn, AC; et al: Reduced corticotropin releasing factor binding sites in the frontal cortex of suicide victims. *Arch Gen Psychiatry,* 45:577–579, 1988.

Nemeroff, CB: Evans, DL: Correlation between the dexamethasone suppression test in depressed patients and clinical response. *Am J Psychiatry,* 141:247–249, 1984.

Neshkes, RE; Gerner, R; Jarvik, LF; Mintz, J; et al: Orthostatic effect of imipramine and doxepin in depressed geriatric outpatients. *J Clin Psychopharmacol,* 5:102–106, 1985.

Ness, DE; Pfeffer, CR: Syndrome of bereavement resulting from suicide. *Am J Psychiatry,* 147:279–285, 1990.

Nesse, RM; Carli, T; Curtis, GC; et al: Pre-treatment nausea in cancer chemotherapy: A conditional response. *Psychosom Med,* 42:33–36, 1980.

Nesse, RM; Carli, T; Curtis, GC; et al: Pseudohallucinations in cancer chemotherapy patients. *Am J Psychiatry,* 140:483–485, 1983.

Neuringer, C; Lettieri, DJ: Cognition attitude and affect in suicidal individuals. *Suicide and Life-Threatening Behavior,* 1:106–124, 1971.

Neuver, MR: Uses and abuses of brain mapping. *Arch Neurol,* 46:1134–1136, 1989.

Neuver, MR: Quantitative EEG: I. Techniques and problems of frequency analysis and topographic mapping. *J Clin Neurophysiol,* 5:1–45, 1980.

Neuver, MR: Quantitative EEG: II. Frequency analysis and topographic mapping in clinical settings. *J Clin Neurophysiol,* 5:46–85, 1988.

New Hampshire v. Jones, 50 NH 369, 1869.

New Hampshire v. Pike, 49 NH 399, 1869.

New York Civil Rights Law, Act 45, Section 4501, 4507, 4508, 1972.

New York Mental Hygiene Law, McKinney, 1951, Supp. 1970.

New York Mental Hygiene Law Sections 15, 29, 31 (McKinney Supp.1973).

New York State Department of Mental Hygiene: *Application for Admission of Patient.* Form 471 DMH, 1/73.

New York State Department of Mental Hygiene: *Notice of Rights—Voluntary or Minor Voluntary Admission.* Form DMH 460 (4–78).

New York State Department of Mental Hygiene: *Notice of Status and Rights—Involuntary Admission.* Form DMH 461 (5–73).

New York State Department of Mental Hygiene. *Notice of Status and Rights—Emergency Admission.* Form DMH 474 (11–78).

New York State Department of Mental Hygiene: *Record of Emergency Admission.* Form DMH 474 (2–79).

New York State Department of Mental Hygiene: *Voluntary Request for Hospitalization.* Form DMH 472 (1–73).

Newhouse, P; Bridenbaugh, H: Pharmacologic characterization and lecten treatment of a patient with spontaneous oral-facial dyskinesia and dementia. *Am J Psychiatry,* 138:251–253, 1976.

Newton, RW: Physostigmine salicylate in the treatment of tricyclic antidepressant overdosage. *JAMA* 231:941–944, 1975.

Nierenberg, AA; Price, LH; Charney, DS, et al: After lithium augmentation: A retrospective follow-up of patients with antidepressant-refractory depression. *J Affective Disord,* 18:167–175, 1990.

Nies, A; Robinson, DS; Friedman, MJ; Green, R; Cooper, TB; Ravaris, CL; Ives, JO: Relationship between age and tricyclic antidepressant plasma levels. *Am J Psychiatry,* 134:790–793, 1977.

Niven, RG: Adolescent Drug Abuse. *Hospital and Community Psychiatry,* 37:596–607, 1986.

North, CS; Smith, EM; McCool, RE; Shea, JM: Short-term psychopathology in eyewitnesses to mass murder. *Hospital and Community Psychiatry,* 40:1293–1295, 1989.

North, CS; Clouse, RE; Spitznagel, EL; Alpers, DH: The relation of ulcerative colitis to psychiatric factors: A review of findings and methods. *Am J Psychiatry,* 147:974–981, 1990.

Noyes, R; Chaudry, DR; Domingo, DV: Pharmacologic treatment of phobic disorders. *J Clin Psychiatry,* 47:445–452, 1986.

Noyes, R; Clancy, J: Anxiety neurosis: A five-year follow-up. *J Nerv Ment Dis,* 162:200–205, 1976.

Noyes, R; Clancy, J; Crowe, R; Hoenk, PR; Slymen, DJ: The familial prevalence of anxiety neurosis. *Arch Gen Psychiatry,* 35:1057–1059, 1978.

Noyes, R; Clancy, J; Hoenk, PR; et al: The prognosis of anxiety neurosis. *Arch Gen Psychiatry,* 37:173–178, 1980.

Noyes, R; DuPont, RL; Pecknold, JC; Rifkin, A; et al: Alprazolam in panic disorder and agoraphobia: Results from a multicenter trial. *Arch Gen Psychiatry,* 45:423–428, 1988.

Nunes, EV; McGrath, PJ; Wager, S; et al: Lithium treatment for cocaine abusers with bipolar spectrum disorders. *Am J Psychiatry,* 147:655–657, 1990.

Nurnberg, HG: An overview of somatic treatment of psychosis during pregnancy and postpartum. *Gen Hosp Psychiatry,* 11:328–338, 1989.

Nurnberg, HG; Prudic, J; Fiori, M; Freedman, EP: Psychopathology complicating acquired immune deficiency syndrome (AIDS). *Am J Psychiatry,* 141:95–96, 1984.

Nutter, D; Brunswick, D: Relevancy of tricyclic antidepressant plasma levels. *Am J Psychiatry,* 138:526–527, 1981.

O'Brien, JP: Increase in suicide attempts by drug ingestion: The Boston experience, 1964–1974. *Arch Gen Psychiatry,* 34:1165–1169, 1977.

O'Connor v. Donaldson, 422 U.S. 563, 95 S. Ct. 2486 1975.

Odenheimer, GL: Acquired cognitive disorders of the elderly. *Geriatric Medicine, Medical Clinics of North America,* 73:1383–1411, 1989.

O'Dowd, MA; McKegney, FP: AIDS patients compared with others seen in psychiatric consultation. *Gen Hosp Psychiatry,* 12:50–55, 1990.

Ogata, SN; Silk, KR; Goodrich, S; Lohr, NE; et al: Childhood sexual and physical abuse in adult patients with borderline personality disorder. *Am J Psychiatry,* 147:1008–1013, 1990.

Ogden, M; Spector, MI; Hill, CA: Suicides and homicides among Indians. *Pub Health Rep,* 85:75–80, 1970.

Ogura, C; Nakazawa, K; Majima, K; et al: Lithium levels and exacerbations of bipolar illness. *Psychopharmacology,* 68:61–65, 1980.

O'Hara, MW: Social support, life events, and depression during pregnancy and the prepregnancy. *Arch Gen Psychiatry,* 43:569–573, 1986.

Okada, F: Depression after treatment with thiazide diuretics for hypertension. *Am J Psychiatry,* 142:1101–1102, 1985.

Okada, F; Ito, N; Tsukamoto, R: Two cases of transient partial amnesia in the course of transient global amnesia. *J Clin Psychiatry,* 48:449–450, 1987.

Okimato, JT, Barnes, RF; Veith, RC; et al: Screening for depression in geriatric medical patients. *Am J Psychiatry,* 139:799–802, 1982.

Okin v. Rogers, U.S. Ct. of Appeals 1st cir. (No. 77–1201). See also *"Okin v. Rogers." Mental Disability Law Reporter,* 2:43–50, 1977.

Okrasinski, H: Lithium acne. *Dermatologica,* 154:251–253, 1977.

Okuma, T; Yamushita, I; Takahaski, R; et al: A double-blind study of adjunctive carbamazepine versus placebo on excited states of schizophrenia and schizoaffective disorders. *Acta Psychiatric Scand,* 80:250–259, 1989.

Olin, GB; Olin, HS: Informed consent in voluntary mental hospital admissions. *Am J Psychiatry,* 132:938–941, 1975.

Orenstein, H; Peskind A; Raskind, MA: Thyroid disorders in female psychiatric patients with panic disorder or agoraphobia. *Am J Psychiatry,* 145:1428–1430, 1988.

Orenstein, H; Raskind, MA; Wylire, D; et al: Polysymptomatic complaints and Briquet's syndrome in polycystic ovary disease. *Am J Psychiatry,* 143:768–771, 1986.

Orr, SP; Clarbirn, JM; Altman, B: Psychometric profile of post-traumatic stress disorder, anxious, and healthy Vietnam veterans: Correlations with psychophysiologic responses. *Journal of Counseling and Clinical Psychology,* 58:1–7, 1990.

Osgood, NJ; Brant, BA: Suicidal behavior in long-term care facilities. *Suicide and Life-Threatening Behavior,* 20:123–137, 1990.

Ostroff, RB; Giller, E; Harkness, L; Mason, J: The norepinephrine-to-epinephrine ratio in patients with a history of suicide attempts. *Am J Psychiatry,* 142:224–227, 1985.

Ostrow, DG; Monjan, A; Joseph, J; VanRaden, M; et al: HIV-related symptoms and psychological functioning in a cohort of homosexual men. *Am J Psychiatry,* 146:737–742, 1989.

Othmer, E; DeSouza, C: A screening test for somatization disorder (hysteria). *Am J Psychiatry,* 142:1146–1149, 1985.

Ottman, R: Genetics of the partial epilepsies: A review. *Epilepsia,* 30:107–111, 1989.

Pablo, RY; Lamarre, CJ: Parasuicides in a general hospital psychiatric unit: Their demographic and clinical characteristics. *Gen Hosp Psychiatry,* 8:379–286, 1986.

Paffenbarger, RS; King, SH; Wing, AC: Chronic disease in former college students. IX. Characteristics in youth that predispose to suicide and accidental death in later life. *Am J Public Health,* 59:900–908, 1969.

Palmer, AB; Wohl, J: Voluntary admission forms: Does the patient know what he is signing? *Hospital and Community Psychiatry,* 23:38–40, 1972.

Parad, HJ; Caplan, G: A framework for studying families in crisis. In: *Crisis Intervention: Selected Readings.* New York, Family Service Association of America, 1965.

Parad, HJ: *Crisis Intervention: Selected Readings.* New York, Family Service Association of America, 1965.

Parham v. J. L., U.S.-47 LW, 4739, June 20, 1979.

Paris, J: Completed suicide in borderline personality disorder. *Psychiatric Annals,* 20:19–21, 1990.

Pariser, SF; Pinta, ER; Jones, BA: Mitral valve prolapse syndrome and anxiety neurosis/panic disorder. *Am J Psychiatry,* 135:246–247, 1978.

Parker, A: The meaning of attempted suicide to young parasuicides: A repertory grid study. *Br J Psychiatry,* 139:306–312, 1981.

Parker, G; Brown, L; Bignault, I: Coping behaviors as predictors of true course of clinical depression. *Arch Gen Psychiatry,* 43:561–565, 1986.

Parkes, CM: Risk factors in bereavement: Triplications for the prevention and treatment of pathologic grief. *Psychiatric Annals,* 20:308–313, 1990.

Parrish, H: Cause of death among college students: A study of 209 deaths at Yale University, 1920–1955. *Public Health Rep,* 71:1081–1085, 1956.

Parrish, HM: Epidemiology of suicide among college students. *Yale J Biol Med,* 29:585, 1957.

Parry, BL; Rosenthal, NE; Tamarkin, L; Wehr, TA: Treatment of patient with seasonal premenstrual syndrome. *Am J Psychiatry,* 144:762–766, 1987.

Pasamasnik, B; Scarpitti, F; Dinitry, S: *Schizophrenics in the Community.* New York, Appleton-Century-Crofts, 1967.

Pasnau, RO: Anxiety: The silent partner. *J Clin Psychiatry,* 50:3–45, 1989.

Pattison, EM; Kahan, J: The deliberate self-harm syndrome. *Am J Psychiatry,* 140:867–872, 1983.

Paul, SM: Anxiety and depression: A common neurobiological substrate? *J Clin Psychiatry,* 49:13–16, 1988.

Paulose, KP; Shaw, AA: Rapidly recurring seizures of psychogenic origin. *Am J Psychiatry,* 134:1145, 1977.

Paulson, GW: Steroid-sensitive dementia. *Am J Psychiatry,* 140:1031–1033, 1983.

Paykel, ES: Treatment of depression: The relevance of research for clinical practice. *Br J Psychiatry,* 155:754–763, 1989.

Pearlson, GD; Ross, CA; Lahr, WD; et al: Association between family history of affective disorder and the depressive syndrome of Alzheimer's disease. *Am J Psychiatry,* 147:452–456, 1990.

Peck, M; Schrut, A: Suicidal behavior among college students. *HSMHA Health Reports,* 86:149–156, 1971.

Pecknold, JC; Swinson, RP; Kuch, K; Lewis, CP: Alprazolam in panic disorder and agoraphobia: Results from a multicenter trial: III. Discontinuation effects. *Arch Gen Psychiatry,* 45:429–436, 1988.

Pederson, AM; Aruad, GA; Kindler, AR: Epidemiological differences between white and nonwhite suicide attempters. *Mental Health Digest,* 5:27–29, 1973.

Penick, EC; Powell, BJ; Siech, WA: Mental health problems and natural disaster tornado victims. *Journal of Community Psychology,* 4:64–67, 1976.

Penk, WE; Rabinowitz, R: Post-traumatic stress disorder (PTSD): Issues of utility, traumatogenicity, co-morbidity, teratogenicity vs. psychogenicity, ethnicity, "gendericity", and chronicity. *J Clin Psychology,* 45:688–690, 1989.

People v. Gorsehn, 51 Cal. 2d 716, 336 P. 2d 492, 1959.

People v. Wells, 33 Cal. 2d 330, 202 P. 2d 53, 1949.

Pepitone-Arreola-Rockwell, F; Rockwell, D; Core, N: Fifty-two medical student suicides. *Am J Psychiatry,* 138:198–201, 1981.

Perconte, ST; Goreczny, AJ: Failure to detect fabricated posttraumatic stress disorder with the use of the MMPI in a clinical population. *Am J Psychiatry,* 147:1057–1060, 1990.

Perelow, ED; Robins, C; Block, P; et al: Dysfunctional attitudes in depressed patients before and after clinical treatment and in normal control subjects. *Am J Psychiatry,* 147:439–444, 1990.

Perlmutter, RA; Jones, JE: Problem solving with families in psychiatric emergencies. *Psychiatric Quarterly,* 57:23–32, 1985.

Perris, C: Morbidity suppressive effect of lithium carbonate in cycloid psychosis. *Arch Gen Psychiatry,* 35:328–331, 1978.

Perry, SW; Jacobsen, P: Neuropsychiatric manifestations of AIDS-spectrum disorders. *Hospital and Community Psychiatry,* 37:135–142, 1986.

Perry, SW: Organic mental disorders caused by HIV: Update on early diagnosis and treatment. *Am J Psychiatry,* 147:695–710, 1990.

Perry, SW; Markowitz, J: Psychiatric interventions for AIDS-spectrum disorders. *Hospital and Comunity Psychiatry,* 37:101–106, 1986.

Perry, SW; Tross, S: Psychiatric problems of AIDS inpatients at the New York Hospital: Preliminary report. *Public Health Reports,* 99:200–204, 1984.

Perse, TL; Greist, JH; Jefferson, JW; Rosenfeld, R; et al: Fluvoxamine treatment of obsessive-compulsive disorder. *Am J Psychiatry,* 144:1543–1548, 1987.

Persild, H; Madsen, SN; Hansen, JEM: Irreversible myxedema after lithium carbonate. *Br Med J,* 1:1105–1109, 1978.

Pesslow, ED; Goldring, N; Fieve, RR; et al: The dexamethasone suppression test in depressed outpatients and normal control subjects. *Am J Psychiatry,* 140:245–247, 1983.

Peszke, MD: Is dangerousness an issue for physicians in emergency commitment? *Am J Psychiatry,* 132:825–828, 1975.

Peters, WD; Anderson, KD; Reid, PR; et al: Acute mental status changes caused by propranolol. *Johns Hopkins Med J,* 143:163–164, 1978.

Peterson, GA; Ballenger, JC; Cox, DP; Hucek A; et al: The dexamethasone suppression test in agoraphobia. *J Clin Psychopharmacol,* 5:100–102, 1985.

Peterson, LG; Peterson, M; O'Shanick, GJ; Swann, A: Self-inflicted gunshot wounds:Lethality of method versus intent. *Am J Psychiatry,* 142:228–231, 1985.

Peterson, MW: Imipramine treatment for hypersomnia. *Am J Psychiatry,* 136:984–985, 1979.

Petrie, WM; Maffucci, RJ Woosky, RL: Propranolol and depression. Am J Psychiatry, 139:92–94, 1982

Petty, LK; Asarnow, JR; Carlson, GA; Lesser, L: The dexamethasone suppression test in depressed, dysthymic, and nondepressed children. *Am J Psychiatry,* 142:631–633, 1985.

Pevnick, JS; Jasinski, DR; Haertzen, CA: Abrupt withdrawal from therapeutically administered diazepam. Report of a case. *Arch Gen Psychiatry,* 35:995–998, 1978.

Pfeffer, CR; Clinical perspectives in treatment of suicidal behavior among children and adolescents. *Psychiatric Annals,* 20:143–150, 1990.

Pfeffer, CR: Modabilities of treatment for suicidal children: An overview of the literature on current practice. *Am J Psychotherapy,* 38:364–371, 1984.

Pfeffer, CR: Suicidal fantasies in normal children. *J Nerv Ment Dis,* 173:78–83, 1985.

Pfeffer, CR: *The Suicidal Child.* New York, The Guilford Press, 1986.

Pfeffer, CR: Risk factors associated with youth suicide: A clinical perspective. *Psychiatric Annals,* 18:652–656, 1988.

Pfeffer, CR; Plutchik, R; Mirzruchi, MS; Lipkins, R: Suicidal behavior in child psychiatric inpatients and outpatients and in nonpatients. *Am J Psychiatry,* 143:733–738, 1986.

Pfefferbaum, B; Butler, PM; Mullins, D; Copeland, DR: Two cases of benzodiazepine toxicity in children. *J Clin Psychiatry,* 48:450–452, 1987.

Phillips, KA; Gunderson, JG; Hirshfeld, RMA; et al: A review of the depressive personality. *Am J Psychiatry,* 147:830–837, 1990.

Pillard, RC; Weinrich, JD: Evidence of familial nature of male homosexuality. *Arch Gen Psychiatry,* 43:808–812, 1986.

Pines, A; Maslach, C: Characteristics of staff burnout in mental health settings. *Hospital and Community Psychiatry,* 29:233–237, 1978.

Pitman, RK; Altman, B; Machlin, ML: Prevalence of posttraumatic stress disorder in wounded Vietnam Veterans. *Am J Psychiatry,* 146:667–669, 1989a.

Pitman, RK; Green, RC; Jenike, MA; Mesulam, MM: Clinical comparison of Tourette's disorder and obsessive–compulsive disorder. *Am J Psychiatry,* 144:1166–1171, 1987a.

Pitman, RK; Orr, SP; Forgue, OF; et al: Psychophysiologic assessment of post-traumatic stress disorder imagery in Vietnam combat veterans. *Arch Gen Psychiatry,* 44:970–975, 1987b.

Pitman, RK; Orr, SP; Stehetes, GS: Psychophysiological investigations of post-traumatic stress disorder imagery. *Psychopharmacology Bulletin,* 25:426–431, 1989b.

Pitman, RK; van der Kolk, BA; Orr, SP; Greenberg, MS: Naloxone-reversible analgesic response to combat-related stimuli in posttraumatic stress disorder: A pilot study. *Arch Gen Psychiatry,* 47:541–544, 1990.

Pitts, FN; Schuller, AB; Rich, CL; Pitts, AF: Suicide among U.S. women physicians, 1967–1972. *Am J Psychiatry,* 136:694–696, 1974.

Plante, ML: An analysis of "informed consent." *Fordham L Rev,* 36:639, 1968.

Platman, SR: A comparison of lithium carbonate and chlorpromazine in mania. *Am J Psychiatry,* 127:351–353, 1970.

Plaut, EA: A perspective on confidentiality. *Am J Psychiatry,* 131:1021–1024, 1974.

Plotkin, R: Limiting the therapeutic orgy: Mental patient's right to refuse treatment. *Northwestern University L Rev,* 72:461, 1977.

Plumb, M; Holland, J: Comparative studies of psychological function in patients with advanced cancer: Interviewers rated current and past psychological symptoms. *Psychosomatic Medicine,* 43:243–254, 1981.

Poland, RE; Rubin, RT; Lesser, IM; Lane, LA; et al: Neuroendocrine aspects of primary endogenous depression: II. Serum dexamethasone concentrations and hypothalamic-pituitary-adrenal cortical activity as determinants of the dexamethasone suppression test response. *Arch Gen Psychiatry,* 44:790–795, 1987.

Polchert, SE; Morse, RM: Pemoline abuse. *JAMA,* 254:946–947, 1985.

Pollit, J; Young, J: Anxiety state or masked depression? A study based on the action of monamine oxidase inhibitors. *Br J Psychiatry,* 119:143–149, 1971.

Pollock, DA; Rhodes, P; Boyle, CA, et al: Estimating the number of suicides among Vietnam veterans. *Am J Psychiatry,* 147:772–776, 1990.

Pope, HG; Hudson, JI; Jonas, JM; et al: Bulimia treated with imipramine: A placebo-controlled double-blind study. *Am J Psychiatry,* 140:554–558, 1983a.

Pope, HG; Jonas, JM; Hudson, JI: The validity of DSM-III borderline personality disorder: A phenomenologic family history, treatment response, and long-term follow-up study. *Arch Gen Psychiatry,* 40:23–30, 1983b.

Pope, HG; Ionescu-Pioggia, M; Aizley, HG; Varma, DK: Drug use and life style among college undergraduates in 1989: A comparison with 1969 and 1978. *Am J Psychiatry,* 147:998–1001, 1990.

Pope, HG; Katz, DL: Affective and psychotic symptoms associated with anabolic steroid use. *Am J Psychiatry,* 145:487–490, 1988.

Pope, HG; McElroy, SL; Satlin, A; Hudson, JI; et al: Head injury, bipolar disorder, and response to valproate. *Comprehensive Psychiatry,* 29:34–38, 1988.

Popkin, MK; Callies, AL: Psychiatric consultation to inpatients with "early-onset" type I diabetes mellitus in a university hospital. *Arch Gen Psychiatry,* 44:169–171, 1987.

Porkorny, AD: Prediction of suicide in psychotic patients: Report of a prospective study. *Arch Gen Psychiatry,* 40:249–257, 1983.

Porter, RA: Crisis intervention and social work models. *Community Mental Health Journal,* 2B:13, 1966.

Post, RM; Rubinow, DR; Uhde, TW; Roy-Byrne, PP; et al: Dysphoric mania: Clinical and biological correlates. *Arch Gen Psychiatry,* 46:353–358, 1989.

Post, RM: Sensitization and kindling perspectives for the course of affective illness: Toward a new treatment with the anticonvulsant carbamazepine. *Pharmacopsychiatry,* 23:3–17, 1990.

Potter, WZ; Murphy, DL; Wehr, TA; et al: Clorgyline: A new treatment for patients with refractory rapid-cycling disorder. *Arch Gen Psychiatry,* 39:505–510, 1982.

Powers, PS: Heart failure during treatment of anorexia nervosa. *Am J Psychiatry,* 139:1167–1170, 1982.

Prakash, R; Petrie, WM: Psychiatric changes associated with an excess of folic acid. *Am J Psychiatry,* 139:1192–1193, 1982.

Prasad, AJ; Kumar, N: Suicidal behavior in hospitalized schizophrenics. *Suicide and Life-Threatening Behavior,* 18:265–269, 1988.

Prasad, RB; Val, ER; Lahinezer, HW; et al: Associated diagnosis (comorbidity) in patients with borderline personality disorder. *Psychiatr J Univ Ottawa,* 15:22–27, 1990.

Prehn, RA: Medication refusal: Suggestions for intervention. *The Psychiatric Hospital,* 21:37–40, 1989.

Prentky, RA; Burgess, AW; Rolous, F; Lee, A; et al: The presumptive role of fantasy in serial sexual homicide. *Am J Psychiatry,* 146:887–891, 1989.

President's Commission for the Study of Ethical Problems in Medicine and Biochemical and Behavioral Research: *Making Health Care Decisions. A report on the Ethical and Legal Implications of Informed Consent in the Patient–Practitioner Relationship,* Vol 1. Washington, DC, Superintendent of Documents, October, 1982.

Prevnick, JS; Jasinski, DR; Haetzen, CA: Abrupt withdrawal from therapeutically administered diazepam. *Arch Gen Psychiatry,* 35:995–998, 1978.

Prezant, DW; Neimeyer, RA: Cognitive predictors of depression and suicide ideation. *Suicide and Life-Threatening Behavior,* 18:259–264, 1988.

Price, DM; Murphy, PA: Emotional depletion in critical care staff. *J Neurosurg Nurs,* 17:114–117, 1985.

Price, LH; Charney, DS; Delagado, PL; et al: Lithium and serotonin function: Implications for the serotonin hypothesis of depression. *Psychopharmacology,* 100:3–12, 1990.

Price, LH; Charney, DS; Heninger, GR: Efficacy of lithium-tranylcypromine treatment in refractory depression. *Am J Psychiatry,* 142:619–623, 1985.

Price, WA; DiMarzio, L: Premenstrual tension syndrome in rapid-cycling bipolar affective disorder. *J Clin Psychiatry,* 47:415–417, 1986.

Price, WA; Forejt, J: Neuropsychiatric aspects of AIDS: A case report. *Gen Hosp Psychiatry,* 8:7–10, 1986.

Price, WA; Heil, D: Estrogen-induced panic attacks. *Psychosomatics,* 29:433–435, 1988.

Price, WA; Zimmer, B; Conway,R; Szekely, B: Insulin-induced factitious hypoglycemic coma. *Gen Hosp Psychiatry,* 8:291–293, 1986.

Prien, RF; Point, P; Caffey, EM; et al: Comparison of lithium carbonate and chlorpromazine in the treatment of mania. *Arch Gen Psychiatry,* 26:136–153, 1972.

Privileged communication, *JAMA,* 297:257, 1966.

Privitera, MR; Springer, MO; Perlmutter, RA: To search or not to search: Is there a clinical profile of a patient harboring a weapon? *Gen Hosp Psychiatry,* 8:442–447, 1986.

Projects: Civil commitment of the mentally ill. *UCLA L Rev* 14:882, 1967.

Proudfoot, AT; Park, J: Changing patterns of drugs used for self-poisoning. *Br Med J,* 1:90–93, 1978.

Prouix, J: Sexual preference assessment of sexual aggressors. *Int J Law Psychiatry,* 12:275–280, 1989.

Prusoff, BA; Weissman, MM; Charney, J; et al: Speed of symptom reduction in depressed outpatients treated with amoxapine and amitriptyline. *Current Therapeutic Research,* 30:843, 1981.

Prusoff, BA; Williams, DH; Weissman, MM; et al: Treatment of secondary depression in schizophrenia: A double-blind, placebo-controlled trial of amitriptyline added to perphenazine. *Arch Gen Psychiatry* 36: 569–575, 1979.

Psychiatric News. Survey shows many community mental health centers lack emergency services. February 2, 1977.

Psychiatric News, New CMHC survey shows better emergency service. August 19, 1977.

Puig-Antich, J; Goetz, D; Davies, M; Kaplan T; et al: A controlled family history study of prepubertal major depressive disorder. *Arch Gen Psychiatry,* 46:406–418, 1989.

Putnam, FW; Guroff, JJ; Silberman, EK; Barban, L; et al: The clinical phenomenology of multiple personality disorder: Review of 100 recent cases. *J Clin Psychiatry,* 47:285–293, 1986.

Quitkin, F; Rifkin, A; Gochfeld, L; Klein, DF: Tardive dyskinesia: Are first signs reversible? *Am J Psychiatry,* 134:84–87, 1977.

Quitkin, F; Rifkin, A; Kane, J; et al: Long-acting oral vs. injectable antipsychotic drugs in schizophrenics. A one-year double-blind comparison in multiple-episode schizophrenics. *Arch Gen Psychiatry,* 35:889–892, 1978.

Quitkin, FM; Rifkin, A; Kaplan, J; et al: Phobic anxiety syndrome complicated by drug dependence and addiction: A treatable form of drug abuse. *Arch Gen Psychiatry,* 27:159–162, 172, 1972.

Rabiner, CJ; Wegner, JT; Kane, JM: Outcome study of first-episode psychosis: I. Relapse rates after 1 year. *Am J Psychiatry,* 143:1155–1158, 1986.

Rabkin, JG; Harrison, WM: Effect of imipramine on depression and immune status in sample of men with HIV infection. *Am J Psychiatry,* 147:495–497, 1990.

Rachlin, S; Fam, A; Milton, J: Civil liberties versus involuntary hospitalization. *Am J Psychiatry,* 132:189–192, 1975.

Racy, J; Ward-Racy, EA: Tinnitus in imipramine therapy. *Am J Psychiatry,* 137:854–855, 1980.

Rainey, JM: Disulfiram toxicity and carbon disulfide poisoning. *Am J Psychiatry,* 134:371–378, 1977.

Raj, A; Sheehan, DV: Medical evaluation of panic attacks. *J Clin Psychiatry,* 48:309–313, 1987.

Rampling, D: Aggression: A paradoxical response to tricyclic antidepressants. *Am J Psychiatry,* 135:117–118, 1978.

Rankel, HW; Rankel, LE: Carbamazepine in the treatment of catatonia. *Am J Psychiatry,* 145:361–362, 1988.

Rapaport, L: *The State of Crisis: Some Theoretical Consideration in Crisis Intervention: Selected Readings.* HJ Parad, ed. New York, Family Service Association of America, 1965.

Rapaport, R: Normal crisis, family structure and mental health. *Family Process,* 2:68, 1963.

Raphael, B: Preventive intervention with the recently bereaved. *Arch Gen Psychiatry,* 34:1450–1454, 1977.

Raphling, D; Lion, J: Patients with repeated admission to a psychiatric emergency service. *Community Ment Health J,* 6:313–318, 1970.

Rapoport, DJ; Covington, EC: Motor phenomena in benzodiazepine withdrawal. *Hospital and Community Psychiatry,* 40:1277–1279, 1989.

Rapoport, J: Serotonergic agents in obsessive-compulsive disorder: Fluvoxamine as an antiobsessional agent. *Psychopharmacology Bulletin,* 25:31–35, 1989.

Rapoport, JL; Berg, CJ; Ismond, DR; Zahn, TP; et al: Behavioral effects of caffeine in children. *Arch Gen Psychiatry,* 41:1073–1079, 1984.

Rapoport, JL; Buchsbaum, MS; Weingartner, H; et al: Dextroamphetamine: Its cognitive and behavioral effects in normal and hyperactive boys and normal men. *Arch Gen Psychiatry,* 37:933–943, 1980.

Rappolt, RT; Gay, GR; Farris, RD: Emergency management of acute phencyclidine intoxication. *JACEP,* 8:68–76, 1979.

Raskin, DE: Amphetamine use. *J Clin Psychopharmacol,* 3:262, 1983.

Rasking, MA; Risse, SC; Lampe, TH: Dementia and antipsychotic drugs. *J Clin Psychiatry,* 48:16–18, 1987.

Ratey, JJ; Morrill, R; Oxenkrug, G: Use of propranolol for provoked and unprovoked episodes of rage. *Am J Psychiatry,* 140:1356–1357, 1983.

Rathbone-McCuan, E; Voyles, B: Case detection of abused elderly parents. *Am J Psychiatry,* 139:189–192, 1982.

Rauch, PA; Stern, TA: Life-threatening injuries resulting from sleepwalking and night terrors. *Psychosomatics,* 27:62–64, 1986.

Rausch, JL; Pavlinac, DM; Newman, PE: Complete heart block following a single dose of trazodone. *Am J Psychiatry,* 141:1472–1473, 1984.

Ravaris, CL; Nies, A; Robinson, DS; et al: A multiple-dose, controlled study of phenelzine in depression-anxiety states. *Arch Gen Psychiatry,* 33:347–350, 1976.

Ravaris, CL; Robinson, DS; Ives, JO; et al: Phenelzine and amitriptyline in the treatment of depression: A comparison of present and past studies. *Arch Gen Psychiatry,* 37:1075–1080, 1980.

Raymond, ME; Slaby, AE; Lieb, J: Familial response to mental illness. *Soc Casework,* 56:492–498, 1975.

Raymond, ME; Slaby, AE; Lieb, J: Familial responses to mental illness. *Yale Psych Q,* 1(No. 2):4, 1977.

Raymond, ME; Slaby, AE; Lieb, J: Patterns of familial response to mental illness. In: *Inventory of Marriage and Family Literature,* MS Dahl, DHL Olson, eds. St. Paul, University of Minnesota Press, 1980.

Raymond, ME; Slaby, AE; Lieb, J: *The Healing Alliance,* New York, W. W. Norton Company, 1975.

Razani, J; White, KL; White, J; et al: The safety and efficacy of combined amitriptyline and tranylcypromine antidepressant treatment: A controlled trial. *Arch Gen Psychiatry,* 40:657–661, 1983.

Reasons sought for adolescent suicide increase. *The Washington Post,* Friday, June 4, 1976.

Reed, K; Smith, RC; Schoolar, JC; et al: Cardiovascular effects of nortriptyline in geriatric patients. *Am J Psychiatry,* 137:986–988, 1980.

Reed, SM; Wise, MIG; Timmerman, I: Choreoathetosis: A sign of lithium toxicity. *J Neuropsychiatry,* 1:57–66, 1989.

Reich, J; Tupin, JP; Abramowitz, SI: Psychiatric diagnosis of chronic pain patients. *Am J Psychiatry,* 140:1495–1498, 1983.

Reich, J; Yates, W: A pilot study of treatment of social phobia with alprazolam. *Am J Psychiatry,* 145:590–594, 1988.

Reich, P: Panic attacks and the risk of suicide. *N Engl J Med,* 321:1260–1261, 1989.

Reich, W: Soviet psychiatry on trial. *Commentary,* 40–48, January, 1978.

Reichard, CC; Elder, ST: The effects of caffeine on reaction time in hyperkinetic and normal children. *Am J Psychiatry,* 134:144–148, 1977.

Reiman, EM; Raichle, ME; Robins, E; Butler, FK; et al: The application of positron emission tomography to the study of panic disorder. *Am J Psychiatry,* 143:469–477, 1986.

Reisberg, B; Ferris, SH; Gershon, S: An overview of pharmacologic treatment of cognitive decline in the aged. *Am J Psychiatry,* 138:593–600, 1981.

Remick, RA; Wada, JA: Complex patrial and pseudoseizure disorders. *Am J Psychiatry,* 136:320–323, 1979.

Rennie v. Klein, 462 F. Supp. 1131 (1978).

Rennie v. Klein, 476 F. Supp. 1294 (D.N.J. 1979).

Resnik, HLP; Dizmang, LH: Observations on suicidal behavior among American Indians. *Am J Psychiatry,* 127:882–887, 1971.

Resnik, HLP: Erotized repetitive hangings, a form of self-destructive behavior. *Am J Psychiatry,* 127:882–887, 1971.

Resnik, HLP: *Suicidal Behavior: Diagnosis and Management.* Boston, Little, Brown and Co., 1968.

Resnik, HLP; Wittlin, BJ: Abortion and suicidal behaviors: Observations on the concept of "endangering the mental health of the mother". *Mental Hygiene,* 55:10–20, 1971.

Resnik, M; Burton, BT: Droperidol vs. haloperidol in the initial management of acutely agitated patients. *J Clin Psychiatry,* 45:298–299, 1984.

Reusch, J: Social factors in therapy. In: *Psychiatric Treatment,* Vol. 31, SB Wortis, H Herman, CC Hare, eds. Association for Nervous and Mental Diseases. Baltimore, Williams and Wilkins, 1953.

Reynolds, CF: Sleep disturbance in posttraumatic stress disorder: Pathogenetic or epiphenomenal? *Am J Psychiatry,* 146:695–696, 1989.

Reynolds, GP: Beyond the dopamine hypothesis: The neurochemical pathology of schizophrenia. *Br J Psychiatry,* 155:305–316, 1989.

Rich, CL: Self-induced vomiting: Psychiatric considerations. *JAMA,* 239:2688–2689, 1978.

Rich, CL; Fowler, RC; Young, D; Blenkush, M: San Diego suicide study: Comparison of gay to straight males. *Suicide and Life-Threatening Behavior,* 16:448–457, 1986a.

Rich, CL; Fowler, RC; Fogarty, LA; Young, D: San Diego suicide study: III.Relationships between diagnoses and stressors. *Arch Gen Psychiatry,* 45:589–592, 1988a.

Rich, CL; Ricketts, JE; Fowler, RC; Young, D: Some differences between men and women who commit suicide. *Am J Psychiatry,* 145:718–722, 1988b.

Rich, CL; Young, JG; Fowler, RC; Wagner, J; et al: Guns and suicide: Possible effects of some specific legislation. *Am J Psychiatry,* 147:342–346, 1990.

Rich, CL; Young, D; Fowler, RC: San Diego suicide study: I. Young vs. old subjects. *Arch Gen Psychiatry,* 43:577–582, 1986b.

Rickels, K; Case, WG; Werblowsky, J; et al: Amoxapine and imipramine in the treatment of depressed outpatients: A controlled study. *Am J Psychiatry,* 138:20–24, 1981.

Rickels, K; Canalosi, I; Greisman, P; et al: A controlled clinical trial of alprazolam for the treatment of anxiety. *Am J Psychiatry,* 140:82–85, 1983.

Rickels, K; Schweizer, E; Canalosi, I; Case WG; et al: Long-term treatment of anxiety and risk of withdrawal. *Arch Gen Psychiatry,* 45:444–450, 1988.

Rieger, W; Brady, JP; Weisberg, E: Hematologic changes in anorexia nervosa. *Am J Psychiatry,* 135:984–985, 1978.

Ries, RK; Boy-Byrne, PP; Ward, NG; Neppe, V; et al: Carbamazepine treatment for benzodiazepine withdrawal. *Am J Psychiatry,* 146:536–537, 1989.

Rifkin, A: Benzodiazepines for anxiety disorders: Are the concerns justified? *Postgrad Med,* 87:209–219, 1990.

Rifkin, A; Quitkin, F; Kane, J; et al: Are prophylactic antiparkinson drugs necessary? A continued study of procyclidine withdrawal. *Arch Gen Psychiatry,* 35:483–489, 1978.

Rifkin, A; Quitkin, F; Rabiner, CJ; et al: Fluphenazine decanoate, fluphenazine hydrochloride given orally, and placebo in remitted schizophrenics. I. Relapse rates after one year. *Arch Gen Psychiatry,* 34:43–47, 1977.

Rights of the mentally ill during incarceration: The developing law. (Note), *U Fla L Rev,* 25:494, 1973.

Rindell, JR; Wise, MG; Ursano, RJ: Three cases of AIDS-related psychiatric disorders. *Am J Psychiatry,* 143:777–778, 1986.

Ritvo, ER; Jorde, LB; Mason-Brothers, A; Freeman, BJ; et al: The UCLA-University of Utah epidemiologic survey of autism: Recurrence risk estimates and genetic counseling. *Am J Psychiatry,* 146:1032–1036, 1989.

Ritvo, ER; Freeman, BJ; Pingree, C; Mason-Brothers, A; et al: The UCLA-University of Utah epidemiologic survey of autism: Prevalence. *Am J Psychiatry,* 146:194–199, 1989.

Robbins, DR; Alessi, NE: Depressive symptoms and suicidal behavior in adolescents. *Am J Psychiatry,* 142:588–592, 1985.

Robbins, LN; Helzer, JE; Weissman, MM; Orvaschel, H; et al: Lifetime prevalence of specific psychiatric disorders in three sites. *Arch Gen Psychiatry,* 41:949–958, 1984.

Roberts, RE; Vernon, SW: Depression in the community. Prevalance and treatment. *Arch Gen Psychiatry,* 39:1407–1408, 1982.

Robertson, MM; Trimble, MR; Townsend, HRA: Phenomenology of depression in epilepsy. *Epilepsia,* 28:364–372, 1987.

Robins, E; Gentry, KA; Munoz, RA; Marten, S: A contrast of the three more common illnesses with the ten less common in a study and 18-month follow-up of 314 psychiatric emergency room patients. I. Characteristics of the sample and methods of study. *Arch Gen Psychiatry,* 34:259–264, 1977.

Robins, E; Gentry, KA; Munoz, RA; Marten, S: A contrast of the three more common illnesses with the ten less common in a study and 18-month follow-up of 314 psychiatric emergency room patients. II. Characteristics of patients with the three more common illnesses. *Arch Gen Psychiatry,* 34:269–281, 1977.

Robins, E; Gentry, KA; Munoz, RA; Marten, S: A contrast of the three more common illnesses with the ten less common in a study and 18 month follow-up of 314 psychiatric emergency room patients. III. Findings at follow-up. *Arch Gen Psychiatry,* 34:185–291, 1977.

Robins, LN; Kulbok, PA: Epidemiological studies in suicide. *Psychiatric Annals,* 18:619–627, 1988.

Robinson, DS; Nies, A; Ravaris, CL; et al: The monoamine oxidase inhibitor, phenelzine, in the treatment of depressive-anxious states. *Arch Gen Psychiatry,* 29:407–413, 1973.

Robinson, RG; Lipsey, JR; Rao, K; Price, TR: Two-year longitudinal study of poststroke mood disorders: Comparison of acute-onset with delayed onset depression. *Am J Psychiatry,* 143:1238–1244, 1986.

Robinson, RG; Starkstein, SE: Current research in affective disorders following stoke. *J Neuropsychiatry,* 2:1–13, 1990.

Robinson v. California, 370 U.S. 660 (1962).

Roca, RP: Bedside cognitive examination. *Psychosomatics,* 28:71–76, 1987.

Roehrich, H; Gold, MS: Diagnosis of substance abuse in an adolescent psychiatric population. *Int J Psychiatry Med,* 16:137–143, 1986–87

Roges v. Okin, 478 F. Supp. 1343 (1979).

Rogers, MP: Rheumatoid arthritis: Psychiatric aspects and use of psychotropics. *Psychosomatics,* 26:915–925, 1985.

Rome, HP: Personal reflections: Adolescent suicide. *Psychiatric Annals,* 20:118–119, 1990.

Roose, SP; Glassman AH; Walsh, BT; Woodring, S; et al: Depression, delusions, and suicide. *Am J Psychiatry,* 140:1159–1162, 1983.

Rose, DS: "Worse Than Death": Psychodynamics of rape victims and the need for psychotherapy. *Am J Psychiatry,* 143:817–824, 1986.

Rose, SP; Glassman, AH; Giardiner, EGV; et al: Cardiovascular effects of imipramine and bupropion in depressed patients with congestive heart failure. *J Clin Psychopharmacol,* 7:247–251, 1987.

Rosebush, P; Stewart, T: A prospective analysis of 24 episodes of neuroleptic malignant syndrome. *Am J Psychiatry,* 146:717–725, 1989.

Rosen, A: Case report: Symptomatic mania and phencyclidine abuse. *Am J Psychiatry,* 136:118–119, 1979.

Rosen, DH: Suicide survivors: A follow-up study of persons who survived jumping from the Golden Gate and San Francisco-Oakland Bay Bridges. *West J Med,* 122:289–294, 1975.

Rosen, PM; Walsh, BW: Patterns of contagion in self-mutilation epidemics. *Am J Psychiatry,* 146:656–658, 1989.

Rosenbaum, A; Hoge, SK: Head injury and marital aggression. *Am J Psychiatry,* 146:1048–1051, 1989.

Rosenbaum, AH; Schatzberg, AF; MacLaughlin, RA; Snyder, K; et al: The dexamethasone suppression test in normal control subjects: Comparison of two assays and effect of age. *Am J Psychiatry,* 141:1550–1555, 1984.

Rosenbaum, M: The role of depression in couples involved in murder-suicide and homicide. *Am J Psychiatry,* 147:1036–1039, 1990.

Rosenbaum, M: Crime and punishment - The suicide pact. *Arch Gen Psychiatry,* 40:979–982, 1983.

Rosenfeld, AA: Depression and psychotic regression following prolonged methylphenidate use and withdrawal: Case report. *Am J Psychiatry,* 136:226–228, 1979.

Rosenthal, J; Strauss, S; Minkoff, L; et al: Identifying lithium-response bipolar depressed patients using nuclear magnetic resonance. *Am J Psychiatry,* 143:779–780, 1986.

Rosenthal, LD; Merlotte, L; Young, DK; et al: Subjective and polysomnographic characteristics of patients diagnosed with narcolepsy. *Gen Hosp Psychiatry,* 12:191–197, 1990.

Rosenthal, MJ: Towards selective and improved performance of the mental status examination. *Acta Psychiatric Scand,* 80:207–215, 1989.

Rosenthal, NE; Carpenter, CJ; James SP; Parry, BL; et al: Seasonal affective disorder in children and adolescents. *Am J Psychiatry,* 143:356–358, 1986.

Rosenthal, NE; Sack, DA; Gillin, JC; Lewy, AJ; et al: Seasonal affective disorder: A description of the syndrome and preliminary findings with light therapy. *Arch Gen Psychiatry,* 41:72–80, 1984.

Rosenthal, NE; Wehr, TA: Seasonal affective disorders. *Psychiatric Annals,* 17:670–674, 1987.

Rosenthal, PA; Rosenthal S: Suicidal behavior by preschool children. *Am J Psychiatry,* 141:520–525, 1984.

Ross, CA; Heber, S; Anderson, G; et al: Differentiating multiple personality disorder and complex partial seizures. *Gen Hosp Psychiatry,* 11:54–58, 1989.

Ross, DR; Lewin, R; Gold, K; et al: The psychiatric uses of cold wet sheet packs. *Am J Psychiatry,* 145:242–245, 1988.

Ross, DR; Walker, JI; Peterson, J: Akathisia induced by amoxapine. *Am J Psychiatry,* 140:115–116, 1983.

Ross, HA: Commitment of the mentally ill: Problems of law and policy. *Michigan L Rev,* 57:945, 1959.

Ross, RJ; Ball, WA; Sullivan, KA; Caroff, SN: Sleep disturbance at the hallmark of posttraumatic stress disorder. *Am J Psychiatry,* 146:697–707, 1989.

Rossi, AM; Jacobs, M; Monteleone, M; Olsen, R; et al: Violent or fear-inducing behavior associated with hospital admission. *Hospital and Community Psychiatry,* 36:643–647, 1985.

Roth, LH; Meisel, A; Litz, CW: Tests of competency to consent to treatment. *Am J Psychiatry,* 134:279, 1977.

Roth, T; Zorick, F; Sicklesteel, J; et al: Effects of benzodiazepines on sleep and wakefulness. *Br J Pharm,* 11:318–355, 1981.

Rothberg, JM; Ursano, RJ; Holloway, HC: Suicide in the United States military. *Psychiatric Annals,* 17:545–548, 1987.

Rothschild, AJ: Mania after withdrawal of isocarboxazid. *J Clin Psychopharmacol,* 5:339–341, 1985.

Rothschild, AJ; Schatzberg, AF: Fluctuating postdexamethasone cortical levels in a patient with melancholia. *Am J Psychiatry,* 139:129–130, 1982.

Rounsaville, B; Lifton, N; Bieber, M: The natural history of a psychotherapy group for battered women. *Psychiatry,* 42:63–78, 1979.

Rounsaville, BJ; Kleber, HD: Untreated opiate addicts: How do they differ from those seeking treatment? *Arch Gen Psychiatry,* 42:1072–1077, 1985.

Rouse v. Cameron, 373 F. 2d 451 (1962).

Roy, A: Family history of suicide. *Arch Gen Psychiatry,* 40:971–974, 1983.

Roy, A: Rate of past loss in depression. *Arch Gen Psychiatry,* 38:301–302, 1981a.

Roy, A: Specificity of risk factors for depression. *Arch Gen Psychiatry,* 38:959–961, 1981b.

Roy, A: Adinoff, B; Roehrich, L; Lamparski, D; et al: Pathological gambling: A psychobiological study. *Arch Gen Psychiatry,* 45:369–373, 1988.

Roy, A; Pickar, D; DeJong, J; Karoum, F; et al: Suicidal behavior in depression: Relationship to noradrenergic function. *Biol Psychiatry,* 25:341–350, 1989.

Roy v. Hartogs, 173 (52) NYLJ (3–18–75) 17, Col. 7F (1975).

Roy-Byrne, PP; Dager, SR; Crowley, DS; Vitaliano, P; et al: Relapse and rebound following discontinuation of benzodiazepine treatment of panic attacks: Alprazolam versus diazepam. *Am J Psychiatry,* 146:860–865, 1989.

Roy-Byrne, PP; Geraci, Marilla; Uhde, TW: Life events and the onset of panic disorder. *Am J Psychiatry,* 143:1424–1427, 1986.

Roy-Byrne, PP; Post, RM; Hambrick, DD; Leverich, GS; et al: Suicide and course of illness in major affective disorder. *J Affective Disord,* 15:1–8, 1988.

Rubin, EH; Morris, JC; Storandt, M; Berg, L: Behavioral changes in patients with mild senile dementia of the Alzheimer's type. *Psychiatry Research,* 21:55–62, 1987.

Rubinow, DR; Roy-Byrne, P; Hoban, MC; Gold, PW; et al: Prospective assessment of menstrually related mood disorders. *Am J Psychiatry,* 141:684–686, 1984.

Rubinow, DR; Roy-Byrne, P: Premenstrual syndromes: Overview from a methodologic perspective. *Am J Psychiatry,* 141:163–172, 1984.

Rubinstein, N: Comparison of the level of possible post-traumatic stress disorder as measured by a questionnaire and a psychological survey between individuals who were victims of automobile accidents and individuals who admitted they were at fault for the accident. *Am J Psychiatry,* 147: 750–752, 1990.

Rudd, MD: The prevalence of suicidal ideation among college students. *Suicide and Life-Threatening Behavior,* 19:173–183, 1989.

Rudestam, KE; Imbroll, D: Societal reactions to a child's death by suicide. *J Consult Clin Psychol* 51(3):461–462, 1983.

Rudorfer, MV; Ross, RJ; Linnoila M; Sherer, MA; et al: Exaggerated orthostatic responsivity of plasma norepinephrine in depression. *Arch Gen Psychiatry,* 42:1186–1192, 1985.

Ruedrich, SL; Chu, CC; Wadle, CV: The amytal interview in the treatment of psychogenic amnesia. *Hospital and Community Psychiatry,* 36:1045–1046, 1985.

Rundell, JR; Wise, MG: Neurosyphilis: A psychiatric perspective. *Psychosomatics,* 26:287–295, 1985.

Ruskind, M; Peskind, E; Rivard, MF; et al: Dexamethasone suppression test and cortical circadian rhythm in primary degenerative dementia. *Am J Psychiatry,* 139:1468–1471, 1982.

Rynearson, EK: Psychological effecs of unnatural dying on bereavement. *Psychiatric Annals,* 16:272–275, 1986.

Rynearson, EK: Bereavement after homicide: A descriptive study. *Am J Psychiatry,* 141:1452–1454, 1984.

Sachs, MH; Selberstien, C; Weiler, P; et al: HIV-related risk factors in acute psychiatric inpatients. *Hospital and Community Psychiatry,* 41:445–451, 1990.

Sainsburg, P: *Suicide in London.* London, Chapman and Hall, 1955.

Sakinofsky, I; Roberts, RS: Why parasuicides repeat despite problem resolution. *Br J Psychiatry* 156:399–405, 1990.

Saks, BR; Frank, JB; Lowe, TL; Beman, W; et al: Depressed mood during pregnancy and the puerperium: Clinical recognition and implications for clinical practice. *Am J Psychiatry*, 142:728–731, 1985.

Salam, SA; Pillai, AK; Beresford, TP: Lorazepam for psychogenic catatonia. *Am J Psychiatry*, 144:1082–1083, 1987.

Salzman, C: Treatment of the elderly agitated patient. *J Clin Psychiatry*, 48:19–22, 1987.

Salzman, C: A primer on geriatric psychopharmacology. *Am J Psychiatry*, 139:67–74, 1982.

Salzman, C; Green, AI; Rodriguez-Villa, F; Jaskiw, GI: Benzodiazepines combined with neuroleptics for management of severe disruptive behavior. *Psychosomatics*, 27:17–22, 1986.

Salzman, C; Shader, RI; Greenblatt, DJ; et al: Long v. short half-life benzodiazepines in the elderly: Kinetics and clinical effects of diazepam and oxazepam. *Arch Gen Psychiatry*, 40:293–297, 1983.

Sanderson, WC; Beck, AT; Beck, J: Syndrome comorbidity in patients with major depression or dysthymia: Prevalence and temporal relationships. *Am J Psychiatry*, 147:1025–1028, 1990.

Sandman, CA; Barron, JL; Crinella, FM; Donnelly, FJ: Influence of naloxone on brain and behavior of a self-injurious woman. *Biol Psychiatry*, 22:899–906, 1987.

Sangiovanni, F; et al: Rapid control of psychotic excitement states with intramuscular haloperidol. *Am J Psychiatry*, 130:1155, 1973.

Sano, M; Stern,Y; Cole, L; et al: Depression in Parkinson's disease: A biochemical model. *J Neuropsychiatry*, 2:88–92, 1990.

Saravay, SM; Marke, J; Steinberg, MD; Rabiner, CJ: "Doom anxiety" and delirium in lidocaine toxicity. *Am J Psychiatry*, 144:159–163, 1987.

Sargant, W: The treatment of anxiety states and atypical depressions by the monoamine oxidase inhibitor drugs. *J Neuropsychiatry*, (Suppl) 1:96–103, 1962.

Sateia, MJ; Gustafson, DH; Johnsonn, SW: Quality assurance for psychiatric emergencies: An analysis of assessment and feedback methodologies. *Psychiatric Clin North Am*, 13(1):35–48, 1990.

Satel, SL; Gawin, FH: Seasonal cocaine abuse. *Am J Psychiatry*, 146:534–535, 1989.

Satterfield, JH; Cantwell, D; Schell, A; Blaschke, T: Growth of hyperactive children treated with methylphenidate. *Arch Gen Psychiatry*, 36:212–217, 1979.

Satterfield, JH; Hoppe, CM; Schll, AM: A prospective study of delinquency in 110 adolescent boys with attention deficit disorder and 88 normal adolescent boys. *Am J Psychiatry*, 139:795–798, 1982.

Satterfield, JH; Satterfield, BT; Cantwell, DP: Multimodality treatment: A two-year evaluation of 61 hyperactive boys. *Arch Gen Psychiatry*, 37:915–919,1980.

Scharf, MB; Khosla N; Brocker, N; Goff, P: Differential amnestic properties of short- and long-acting benzodiazepines. *J Clin Psychiatry*, 45:51–53, 1984.

Schatzberg, AF; Rothschild, AJ; Stake, JG; et al: The dexamethasone suppression test: Identification of subtypes of depression. *Am J Psychiatry*, 140:88–91, 1983.

Schatzberg, AF; Cole, JO: Benzodiazepines in depressive disorders. *Arch Gen Psychiatry*, 35:1359–1365, 1978.

Scheftner, WA; Young, MA; Endicott, J; Coryell, W; et al: Family history and five-year suicide risk. *Br J Psychiatry*, 153:805–809, 1988.

Schenk, L; Bear, D: Multiple personality and related dissociative phenomena in patients with temporal lobe epilepsy. *Am J Psychiatry*, 35:565–567, 1978.

Scher, M; Krieger, JN; Juergens, S: Trazadone and priapism. *Am J Psychiatry*, 140:1362–1363, 1983.

Schiffer, RB; Caine, ED; Bamford, KA; Levy, S: Depressive episodes in patients with multiple sclerosis. *Am J Psychiatry*, 140:1498–1500,1983.

Schiffer, RB; Wineman, M; Weitkamp, LR: Association between bipolar affective disorder and multiple sclerosis. *Am J Psychiatry*, 143:94–95, 1986.

Schlebusch, L; Wessels, WH: Hopelessness and low-intent in parasuicide. *Gen Hosp Psychiatry*, 10:209–213, 1988.

Schlesser, MA; Winokur, G; Sherman, BM: Hypothalamic-pituitary-adrenal axis activity in depressive illness: Its relationship to classification. *Arch Gen Psychiatry*, 37:737–743, 1980.

Schmideberg, M: The borderline patient. In: *American Handbook of Psychiatry*, S Arieto, ed. New York, Basic Books, 1959.

Schmidt, CW; Shaffer, JW; Zlotowitz, HI; et al: Suicide by vehicular crash. *Am J Psychiatry*, 134:175–178, 1977.

Schmidt, HS; Clak, RW; Hyman, PR: Protriptyline: An effective agent in the treatment of the narcolepsy-cataplexy syndrome and hypersomnia. *Am J Psychiatry,* 134:183–185, 1977.

Schneck, MK; Reisberg, B; Ferris, SH: An overview of current concepts of Alzheimer's disease. *Am J Psychiatry,* 139:165–173, 1982.

Schneider, SG; Farberow, NL; Kruks, GN: Suicidal behavior in adolescent and young adult gay men. *Suicide and Life-Threatening Behavior,* 19:381–384, 1989.

Schotte, DE; Stunkard, AJ: Bulimia vs bulimic behaviors on a college campus. *JAMA,* 258:1213–1215, 1987.

Schottenfeld, RS; Cullen, MR: Occupation-induced posttraumatic stress disorders. *Am J Psychiatry,* 142:198–202, 1985.

Schou, M; Juel-Nielsen, N; Stromgren, E; et al: The treatment of manic psychoses by the administration of lithium salts. *J Neurol Neurosurg Psychiat,* 126:1306–1310, 1970.

Schou, M; Weeke, A: Did manic-depressive patients who committed suicide receive prophylactic or continuation treatment at the time? *Br J Psychiatry,* 153:324–327, 1988.

Schuckit, MA: Alcoholic patients with secondary depression. *Am J Psychiatry,* 140:711–714, 1983a.

Schuckit, MA: Genetic and clinical implications of alcoholism and affective disorder. *Am J Psychiatry,* 143:140–147, 1986.

Schuckit, MA: The history of psychotic symptoms in alcoholics. *J Clin Psychiatry,* 43:53–57, 1982a.

Schuckit, MA: Prevalence of affective disorder in a sample of young men. *Am J Psychiatry,* 139:1431–1436, 1982b.

Schuckit, MA: Alcoholic men with no alcoholic first-degree relatives. *Am J Psychiatry,* 140:439–443, 1983b.

Schuckit, MA; Bernstein, LI: Sleep time and drinking history: a hypothesis. *Am J Psychiatry,* 138:528–530, 1981.

Schuckit, MA: *Drug and Alcohol Abuse: A Clinical Guide to Diagnosis and Treatment.* New York, Plenum Medical Book Co., 1979.

Schuckit, MA; Morrisey, ER: Drug abuse among alcoholic women. *Am J Psychiatry,* 136:607–611, 1979.

Schulberg, HC; Saul, M; McClelland, M; Ganguli, M; et al: Assessing depression in primary medical and psychiatric practices. *Arch Gen Psychiatry,* 42:1164–1170, 1985.

Schulsinger, F; Knop, J; Goodwin, DW; Teasdale, TW; et al: A prospective study of young men at high risk for alcoholism. *Arch Gen Psychiatry,* 43:755–760, 1986.

Schulz, SC; Pato, CN: Pharmacologic treatment of schizophrenia. *Psychiatric Annals,* 19:536–541, 1989.

Schwartz, A: Civil liability for causing suicide: A synthesis of law and psychiatry. *Vanderbilt L Rev,* 24:217, 1971.

Schwartz, D; Weiss, A; Miner, J: Community psychiatry and emergency service. *Am J Psychiatry,* 129:710–715, 1972.

Schwartz, GM; Gross-Braverman, B; Roth, B: Anxiety disorders and psychiatric referral in the general medical emergency room. *Gen Hosp Psychiatry,* 9:87–93, 1987.

Schwartz, HI; Legal and ethical issues in neuroleptic noncompliance. *Psychiatric Annals,* 16:588–595, 1986.

Schweizer, E; Case, WG; Rickels, K: Benzodiazepine dependence and withdrawal in elderly patients. *Am J Psychiatry,* 146:529–531, 1989.

Schweizer, E; Rickels, K: Failure of buspirone to manage benzodiazepine withdrawal. *Am J Psychiatry,* 143:1590–1592, 1986.

Schweizer, E; Winokur, A; Rickels, K: Insulin-induced hypoglycemia and panic attacks. *Am J Psychiatry,* 143:654–655, 1986.

Secunda, SK; Swann, A; Katz, MM; Koslow, SH; et al: Diagnosis and treatment of mixed mania. *Am J Psychiatry,* 144:96–98, 1987.

Segal, SP; Watson, MA; Goldfinger, SM; Averbuck, DS: Civil commitment in the psychiatric emergency room: II. Mental disorder indicators and three dangerousness criteria. *Arch Gen Psychiatry,* 45:753–758, 1988a.

Segal, SP; Watson, MA; Goldfinger, SM; Averbuck, DS: Civil commitment in the psychiatric emergency room: III. Disposition as a function of mental disorder and dangerousness indicators. *Arch Gen Psychiatry,* 45:759–763, 1988b.

Seiden, R: *Suicide Among Youth.* Washington, D.C. U.S. Government Printing Office, 1969.

Settle, EC; Settle, GP: A case of mania associated with fluoxetine. *Am J Psychiatry,* 141:280–281, 1984.

Setzler, CM; Ko, H; Royer, ME; et al: Bioavailability and pharmacokinetics or orally administered triazolam in normal subjects. *Clin Pharmacol Ther,* 21:111–112, 1977.

Shader, RI; et al: *Psychotic Drug Side-Effects,* Baltimore, Williams and Wilkins, 1970.

Shafi, M; Carrigan, S; Whittinghill, JR; Derrick, A: Psychological autopsy of completed suicide in children and adolescents. *Am J Psychiatry,* 142:1061–1064, 1985.

Shah, SA: Dangerousness and civil commitment of the mentally ill: Some public policy consideration. *Am J Psychiatry,* 132:501–505, 1975.

Shalman, R: An overview of folic acid deficiency and psychiatric illness. In: *Folic Acid in Neurology, Psychiatry, and Internal Medicine,* MI Botez, EH Reynold, eds. New York, Raven Press, 1979.

Shanok, SS; Malani, SC; Ninan, OP; et al: A comparison of delinquent and nondelinquent adolescent psychiatric inpatients. *Am J Psychiatry,* 140:582–585, 1983.

Shapiro, AK; Shapiro, E; Eisenkraft, GJ: Treatment of Gilles de la Tourette's syndrome with clonidine and neuroleptics. *Arch Gen Psychiatry,* 40:1235–1240, 1983.

Shapiro, WR: Remote effects of neoplasm on central nervous system: Encephalopathy. In: *Advances in Neurology,* Vol. 15, RA Thompson, JR Green, eds. New York, Raven Press, 1976.

Shaw, E: Lithium noncompliance. *Psychiatric Annals,* 16:583–587, 1986.

Shear, MK; Devereux, RB; Kramer-Fox, R; Mann, JJ; et al: Low prevalence of mitral valve prolapse in patients with panic disorder. *Am J Psychiatry,* 141:302–303, 1984.

Shear, MK; Kligfield, P; Harshfield, G; Devereux, RB; et al: Cardiac rate and rhythm in panic patients. *Am J Psychiatry,* 144:633–637, 1987.

Shear, MK; Sacks, MH: Digitalis delirium: Report of two cases. *Am J Psychiatry,* 135:1422–1423, 1978.

Sheard, MH: Clinical pharmacology of aggressive behavior. *Clin Neuropharmacol,* 11:483–492, 1988.

Shearer, SL; Peters, CP; Quaytman, MS; Wadman, BE: Intent and lethality of suicide attempts among female borderline inpatients. *Am J Psychiatry,* 145:1424–1427, 1988.

Sheehan, DV; Claycomb, JB; Surman, OS; Baer, L; et al: Panic attacks and the dexamethasone suppression test. *Am J Psychiatry,* 140:1063–1064, 1983.

Sheline, YI; Miller, MB: Catatonia relieved by oral diazepam in a patient with a pituitary microadenoma. *Psychosomatics,* 27:860–862, 1986.

Shenton, ME; Solovay, MR; Holzman, PS; Coleman, M; et al: Thought disorder in the relatives of psychotic patients. *Arch Gen Psychiatry,* 46:897–901, 1989.

Shephert, JT; Whiting, B: Beta-adrenergic blockage in the treatment of MAOI self-poisoning. *Lancet,* ii:1021, 1974.

Shiffman, S; Fischer, LB; Zetter-Segal, M; et al: Nicotine exposure among nondependent smokers. *Arch Gen Psychiatry,* 47:333–338, 1990.

Shimizu, T: Clinicopathologic studies on Behcet's disease in *Proceedings of an International Symposium.* Edited by Dilson, N; Konice, M; Ovul, C: Amsterdam, Excerpta Medica, 1979.

Shneidman, E; Faberow, N; Litman, R: *The Psychology of Suicide,* New York, Science House, 1970.

Shneidman, ES; Faberow, NL: The Los Angeles Suicide Prevention Center: A demonstration of public health feasibilities. *Am J Public Health,* 55:21–26, 1965.

Shneidman, ES; Mandelkom, P: *How to Prevent Suicide.* New York Public Affairs Pamphlet No. 407, 1967.

Shopsin, B; Gershon, S: Cogwheel rigidity related to lithium maintenance. *Am J Psychiatry,* 132:536–538, 1975.

Shopsin, B; Klein, H; Aaronson, M; et al: Clozapine, chlorpromazine, and placebo in newly hospitalized, acutely schizophrenic patients: A controlled double-blind comparison. *Arch Gen Psychiatry,* 36:657–664, 1979.

Shore, JH; Tatum, EL; Vollmer, WM: Psychiatric reactions to disaster: The Mount St. Helens experience. *Am J Psychiatry,* 143:590–595, 1986.

Showalter, CV; Thorton, WE: Clinical pharmacology of phencyclidine toxicity. *Am J Psychiatry,* 134:1134–1238, 1977.

Shubin, S: Burnout: The professional hazard you face in nursing. *Nursing,* 8:23–27, 1978.

Shuchter, SR; Zisook, S: Psychological reactions to the PSA crash. *Int J Psychiatry Med,* 14:293–301, 1984.

Shukla, S; Cook, BL; Hoff, AL; Aronson, TA: Failure to detect organic factors in mania. *J Affective Disord,* 15:17–20, 1988.

Sider, RC: Moral direction and misdirection for residents in the psychiatric emergency room. *Psychiatric Annals,* 16:405–407, 1986.

Siegel, K: AIDS: The social dimension. *Psychiatric Annals,* 16:168–172, 1986.

Siegel, RK: Cocaine hallucinations. *Am J Psychiatry,* 135:309–314, 1978.

Siever, LJ; Silverman, JM; Horvath, TB; et al: Increased morbid risk for schizophrenia-related disorders in relatives of schizotypal personality disordered patients. *Arch Gen Psychiatry,* 47:634–640, 1990.

Sigell, LT; Kapp, FT; Fusaro, EA; Nelson, ED; Falck, RS: Popping and snorting volatile nitrites: A current fact for getting high. *Am J Psychiatry,* 135:1216–1218, 1978.

Signer, SF; Benson, DF: Three cases of anorexia nervosa associated with temporal lobe epilepsy. *Am J Psychiatry,* 147:235–238, 1990.

Signer, SF: Capgras' Syndrome: The delusion of substitution. *J Clin Psychiatry,* 48:147–150, 1987.

Silber, E; Perry, SE; Block, DA: Patterns of parent-child interaction in a disaster. *Psychiatry,* 21:159–167, 1957.

Silberfarb, PM; Holland, JCB; Onbar, D; et al: Psychological response of patients receiving two drug regimens for lung cancer. *Am J Psychiatry,* 140:110–111, 1983.

Silberfarb, PM; Maurer, LH; Crouthamel, CS: Psychosocial aspects of neoplastic disease: I. Functional status of breast cancer patients during different treatment regimens. *Am J Psychiatry,* 137:450–455, 1980a.

Silberfarb, PM; Philibert, D; Levine, PM: Psychosocial aspects of neoplastic disease: II. Affective and cognitive effects of chemotherapy in cancer patients. *Am J Psychiatry,* 137:597–601, 1980b.

Silver, JM; Yudofsky, SC: Aggressive behavior in patients with neuropsychiatric disorders. *Psychiatric Annals,* 17:367–370, 1987.

Silverman, DC; Kalick, SM; Bowie, SI; Edbril, SD: Blitz rape and confidence rape: A typology applied to 1,000 consecutive cases. *Am J Psychiatry,* 145:1438–1441, 1988.

Simpson, GM; Pi, EH; Sramek, JJ: An update on tardive dyskinesia. *Hospital and Community Psychiatry,* 37:362–369, 1986.

Singer, MT; Ofshe, R: Thought reform programs and the production of psychiatric casualties. *Psychiatric Annals,* 20:188–193, 1990.

Singh, H: Treating a severely disturbed self-destructive adolescent with cold wet sheet packs. *Hospital and Community Psychiatry,* 37:287–288, 1986.

Siris, SG; Cooper, TB; Rifkin, AE; et al: Plasma imipramine concentrations in patients receiving concomitant fluphenazine decanoate. *Am J Psychiatry,* 139:104–106, 1982.

Siris, SG; vonKammen, DP; Docherty, JP: Use of antidepressant drugs in schizophrenia. *Arch Gen Psychiatry,* 35:1368–1377, 1978.

Sirois, F: Un symptome hysterique d: Astaxia abasia chez un jeune homme. *Psychiatr J Univ Ottawa,* 15:47–49, 1990.

Siskin, MI; Wynne, LC: Cult involvement as relational disorder. *Psychiatric Annals,* 20:199–203, 1990.

Skeen, WF: Acquired immunodeficiency syndrome and the emergency physician. *An Emerg Med,* 14:267–273, 1985.

Skodol, AE; Karasu, TB: Emergency psychiatry and the assaultive patient. *Am J Psychiatry,* 135;202–205, 1978.

Slaby, AE: Dementia. In: *Inpatient Psychiatry: Diagnosis and Treatment,* LI Sederer, ed. Baltimore, Williams and Wilkins, 139–156, 1983.

Slaby, AE: Dementia. In: *Neurologic, Neurogenic and Neuropsychiatric Disorders.* AJ Giannini, RL Gilliland, eds. Garden City, Medical Examination Publishing Company, 1982.

Slaby, AE: Diagnostic emergencies. In: *Baylor University Symposium on Emergency Psychiatry,* B Comstock, ed. Houston, Baylor University (1985).

Slaby, AE: Emergency psychiatry: An update. In: *The Psychiatric Knowledge and Skills Self-Assessment Program,* 5th ed. Washington, D.C., American Psychiatric Association, 1983.

Slaby, AE: Emergency psychiatry: An update. *Hospital and Community Psychiatry,* 32:687–698, October 1981.

Slaby, AE: Emergency psychiatry in the general hospital: Staffing, training and leadership issues. *Gen Hosp Psychiatry,* 3:306–309, 1981.

Slaby, AE: Evaluation and management of suicidal potential and attempts. In *Psychiatry in the Practice of Medicine,* H Leigh, ed. Addison Wesley & Company, Menlo Park, CA, 1981.

Slaby, AE: Medical disease presenting as a behavioral emergency. In: *Topics in Emergency Medicine.* Vol. 4, No. 4, RL Judd, MA Peszke, eds. Rockville, Maryland, Aspen Systems Corporation, January, 1983.

Slaby, AE: Pharmacotherapy. In: *The Psychotherapy Handbook,* R Herink, ed. New York, New American Library, 1980.

Slaby, AE: Prevention, early identification, and management of adolescent suicidal behavior. *R I Med J,* 69:463–470, 1986.

Slaby, AE: Psychiatric consequences of gynecologic surgery. In: *Clinical Problems, Injuries, and Complications of Gynecologic Surgery,* DH Nicols, ed. Baltimore, Williams and Wilkins, 1988.

Slaby, AE: Quality assurance and diagnostic psychiatry in the emergency setting. In: *Clinics of Emergency Medicine: Emergency Psychiatry,* W Dubin, ed. New York, Livingston-Churchill, 1983.

Slaby, AE: Research strategies in emergency psychiatry. *Psych Clin N Am,* 6:347–360, 1983.

Slaby, AE: The team approach to the treatment of the rape victim. *Connecticut Medicine,* 42:135–136, 1978.

Slaby, AE; Goldberg, RJ; Wallace, S: Interdisciplinary team approach to emergency psychiatric care. *Psychosomatics,* 24:(7) 627–637, 1983.

Slaby, AE; Lieb, J; Tancredi, JR: *Handbook of Psychiatric Emergencies,* 2nd ed. New York, Medical Examination Publishing Company, 1981.

Slaby, AE; Moreines, R: Emergency room evaluation and management of schizophrenia. In: *Handbook of Schizophrenia. Vol 4: Psychosocial Treatment of Schizophrenia,* 1990.

Slaby, AE; Perry, PL: Use and abuse of psychiatric emergency services. *Int J Psych Med,* 10:1–18, 1980.

Slaby, AE; Perry, PL: Use and abuse of psychiatric emergency services. Paper presented at the meetings of the American Psychiatric Association, Chicago, May, 1979.

Slaby, AE; Tancredi, LR: *Collusion for Conformity.* New York, Jason Aronson, 1975.

Slaby, AE; Wyatt, RJ: *Dementia in the Presenium,* Springfield, Illinois, Charles C. Thomas, 1974.

Slaby, AE: Emergency psychiatry: An update. *Hospital and Community Psychiatry,* 32:687–698, 1981.

Slater, E; Roth, M: *Mayer-Gross, Slater and Roth: Clinical Psychiatry,* 3rd ed. London, Bailiere, Tindall and Cassell, 1969.

Slater, E: The diagnosis of "hysteria." *Brit Med J,* 1395, 1965.

Slovenko, R (ed): *Sexual Behavior and the Law.* Springfield, Illinois, Charles C. Thomas, 1965.

Slovenko, R: *Psychiatry and Law.* Boston, Little, Brown and Co., 1973.

Slovenko, R: Psychotherapist-patient testimonial privilege: A Picture of misguided hope. *Catholic U L Rev,* 23:649–73, 1974.

Sluyter, GV: Stress and burnout among superintendents of public residential facilities. *Administration in Mental Health,* 12:174–183, 1985.

Smart, ADM: Megaloblastic madness. *Br Med J,* 2:1840–1845,1960.

Smith, EM; North, CS; McCool, RE; Shea, JM: Acute postdisaster psychiatric disorder: Identification of persons at risk. *Am J Psychiatry,* 147, 202–206, 1990.

Smith, GR; Braun, FW: Screening indexes in DSM-IIIR somatization disorder. *Gen Hosp Psychiatry,* 13:148–153, 1990.

Smith, K; Crawford, S: Suicidal behavior among "normal" high school students. *Suicide and Life-Threatening Behavior,* 16:313–325, 1986.

Smith, MC; Mitchell, J: Adolescent psychiatric disorders in the medical setting. *Psychiatric Annals,* 17:780–784, 1987.

Snider, WD; Simpson, DM; Nielsen, S; Gold, JWM; et al: Neurological complications of acquired immune deficiency syndrome: Analysis of 50 patients. *Ann Neurol,* 14:403–418, 1983.

Snole, L; et al: *Mental Health in the Metropolis.* New York, McGraw-Hill, 1962.

Snyder, S; Strain, JJ: Somatoform disorders in the general hospital inpatient setting. *Gen Hosp Psychiatry,* 11:288–293, 1989.

Snyder, S; Strain, JJ; Wolf, D: Differentiating major depression from adjustment disorder with depressed mood in the medical setting. *Gen Hosp Psychiatry,* 12:159–165, 1990.

Sohlberg, S; Norring, C; Holmgren, S; Rosmark, B: Impulsivity and long-term prognosis of psychiatric patients with anorexia nervosa/bulimia nervosa. *J Nerv Ment Dis,* 177:249–257, 1989.

Sokol, RS; Folks, DG; Herrick, RW; Freeman, AM: Psychiatric outcome in men and women after coronary bypass surgery. *Psychosomatics,* 28:11–16, 1987.

Soloff, PH; George A; Natham, S; Schulz, PM; et al: Progress in pharmacotherapy of borderline disorders. *Arch Gen Psychiatry,* 43:691–697, 1986a.

Soloff, PH; George, A; Nathan, RS; Schulz, PM; et al: Paradoxical effects of amitriptyline on borderline patients. *Am J Psychiatry,* 143:1603–1605, 1986b.

Soloff, PH; George, A; Nathan, RS: The dexamethasone suppression test in patients with borderline personality disorders. *Am J Psychiatry,* 139:1621–1623, 1982.

Soloff, PH; Millward, JW: Psychiatric disorders in the families of borderline patients. *Arch Gen Psychiatry,* 40:37–44, 1983.

Solomon, Z; Garb, R; Bleich, A; et al: Reactivation of combat-related posttraumatic stress disorder. *Am J Psychiatry,* 144:51–55, 1987a.

Solomon, JG; Solomon, S: Psychotic depression and bronchogenic carcinoma. 1 *Am J Psychiatry,* 135:859–860, 1978.

Solomon, K: Phenothiazine-induced bulbar palsy-like syndrome and sudden death. *Am J Psychiatry,* 134:308–311, 1977.

Solomon, Z; Weisenberg, M; Schwarzwald, J; Mikulincer, M: Posttraumatic stress disorder among front line soldiers with combat stress reaction: The 1982 Israeli experience. *Am J Psychiatry,* 144;448–454, 1987b.

Solursh, L: Combat Addiction: Post-traumatic stress disorder re-explored. *Psychiatr J Univ Ottawa,* 13:17–20, 1988.

Sorensen, B; Krogh-Sorensen, P; Larsen, NE; et al: The practical significance of nortriptyline plasma control: A prospective evaluation under routine conditions in endogenous depression. *Psychopharmacology,* 59:35–39, 1978.

Souder v. Brennan, 367 F Supp. 808 (D DC 1973).

Soulios, C; Firth, ST: Self-inflicted eye injury: Clinical and psychodynamic aspects. *Psychiatr J Univ Ottawa,* 11:238–242, 1986.

Sours, JA: Case reports of anorexia nervosa and caffeinism. *Am J Psychiatry,* 140:235–236, 1983.

Sours, JA; Vorhaus, LJ: Superior mesenteric artery syndrome in anorexia nervosa: A case report. *Am J Psychiatry,* 138:519–520, 1981.

Southwick, R: Hospital's responsibility. *Cleveland-Marshall L Rev,* 17:156, 1968.

Sparr, L; Pankratz, LD: Factitious posttraumatic stress disorder. *Am J Psychiatry,* 140:1016–1019, 1983.

Sparr, LF; Boehnlein, JK; Cooney, TG: The medical management of the paranoid patient. *Gen Hosp Psychiatry,* 8:49–55, 1986.

Specter, GA; Claiborn, WL: *Crisis Intervention.* New York, Behavioral Publications, 1973.

Spector, RG: Influence of folic acid on excitable tissues. *Nature (New Biol),* 240:247–249, 1972.

Spensley, J; Barter, JT; Werme, PH; Langsley, DG: Involuntary hospitalizatin: What for and how long? *Am J Psychiatry,* 131:219–223, 1974.

Spiegel, D; Hunt, T; Dondershine, HE: Dissociation and hypnotizability in posttraumatic stress disorder. *Am J Psychiatry,* 145:301–305, 1988.

Spielvogel, A; Wile, J: Treatment of the psychotic pregnant patient. *Psychosomatics,* 27:487–492, 1986.

Spier, SA; Tesar, GE; Rosenbaum, JF; Woods, SW: Treatment of panic disorder and agoraphobia with clonazepam. *J Clin Psychiatry,* 47:238–242, 1986.

Spiker, DG; Weiss, An; Chang, SS; et al: Tricyclic antidepressant overdose: Clinical presentation and plasma levels. *Clin Pharmacol Ther,* 18:539–546, 1975.

Spiker, DG, Weiss, JC; Dealy, RS; Griffin, SJ; et al: The pharmacological treatment of delusional depression. *Am J Psychiatry,* 142:430–436, 1985.

Spitzer, SP; Denzen, NK: *The Mental Patient: Studies in the Sociology of Deviance.* New York, McGraw Hill, 1968.

Spurlock, J: Adolescent suicide: Introduction. *Psychiatric Annals,* 20:120–121, 1990

Squire, LR: ECT and memory loss. *Am J Psychiatry,* 134:997–1001, 1977.

Squire, LR; Slater, PC; Miller, PC: Retrograde amnesia and bilateral electroconvulsive therapy. Long-term follow-up. *Arch Gen Psychiatry,* 38:89–95, 1981.

Sramek, JJ; Sayles, MA; Simpson, GM: Neuroleptic dosage for Asians: A failure to replicate. *Am J Psychiatry,* 143:535–536,1986.

Sramek, JJ; Baumgartner, WA; Tallow, JA; Ahrens, TN; et al: Hair analysis for detection of phencyclidine in newly admitted psychiatric patients. *Am J Psychiatry,* 142:950–953, 1985.

Stafford, MC; Weisheit, RA: Changing age patterns of U.S. male and female suicide rates, 1934–1983. *Suicide and Life-Threatening Behavior,* 18:149–163, 1988.

Stallines, L: Suicide mortality among Kentucky farmers, 1979–1985. *Suicide and Life-Threatening Behavior,* 20:156–163, 1990.

Stamm, WE; Handsfield, HH; Rompalo, AM; Ashley, RL; et al: The association between genital ulcer disease and acquisition of HIV infection in homosexual men. *JAMA,* 260:1429–1433, 1988.

Stangler, RS; Printz, AM: DSM-III: Psychiatric diagnosis in a university population. *Am J Psychiatry,* 137:937–940, 1980.

Stanley, M; Stanley, B: Reconceptualizing suicide: A biological approach. *Psychiatric Annals,* 18:646–651, 1988.

Stanton, A; Schwartz, M: *The Mental Hospital,* New York, Basic Books, 1954.

Starkman, MN; Schteingart, DE; Schork, MA: Correlation of bedside cognitive and neuropsychological tests in patients with Cushing's syndrome. *Psychosomatics,* 27:508–511, 1986.

State v. Thompson, Wright's Ohio Rep, 617, 1834.

Steer, RA; Beck, AT; Garrison, B; Lester, D: Eventual suicide in interrupted and uninterrupted attempter: A challenge to the cry-for-help hypothesis. *Suicide and Life-Threatening Behavior,* 18:119–128, 1988.

Stein, LI; Test, MA: Alternative to mental hospital treatment: I. Conceptual model, treatment program, and clinical evaluation. *Arch Gen Psychiatry,* 37:392–397, 1980.

Stein, MB: Panic disorder and medical illness. *Psychosomatics,* 27:833–840, 1986.

Stein, MB; Shea, CA; Uhde, TW: Social phobic symptoms in patients with panic disorder: Practical and theoretical implications. *Am J Psychiatry,* 146:235–238, 1989.

Stein, MB; Uhde, TW: Autoimmune thyroiditis and panic disorder. *Am J Psychiatry,* 146:259–260, 1989a.

Stein, MB; Uhde, TW: Depersonalization disorder: Effects of caffeine and response to pharmacotherapy. *Biol Psychiatry,* 26:315–320, 1989b.

Stein, MK; Rickels, K; Weise, CC: Maintenance therapy with amitriptyline: A controlled trial. *Am J Psychiatry,* 137:370–371, 1980.

Steingard, S; Frankel, FH: Dissociation and psychotic symptoms. *Am J Psychiatry,* 142:953–955, 1985.

Stern, TA; Purcell, JJ; Murray, GB: Complex partial seizures associated with Waldenstrom's macroglobulinemia. *Psychosomatics,* 26:890–892, 1985.

Sternberg, DE: Dual diagnosis: Addiction and affective disorders. *The Psychiatric Hospital,* 20:71–77, 1989.

Stevens, JR: Epilepsy, psychosis and schizophrenia. *Schizophrenia Research,* 1:79–89, 1988.

Stewart, DE; Addison, AM; Robinson, GE; Joffe, R; et al: Thyroid function in psychosis following childbirth. *Am J Psychiatry,* 145:1579–1581, 1988.

Stewart, MM: MAOI's and food-fact and fiction. *Adverse Drug Reaction Bull,* 58:200–203, 1976.

Stewart, RM; Brown, RIF: An outcome study of gamblers anonymous. *Br J Psychiatry,* 152:284–288,1988.

Stiffman, AR: Suicide attempts in runaway youths. *Suicide and Life-Threatening Behavior,* 19:147–159, 1989.

Stinson, DJ; Smith, WG; Amidjayo, I; Kaplan, JM: Systems of care and treatment outcomes for alcoholic patients. *Arch Gen Psychiatry,* 36:535–539, 1979.

Stockley, IH: Monoamine oxidase inhibitors: Interactions with sympathomimetic amines. *Pharmaceutical J,* 590–593, June, 1973.

Stone, AA: *Mental Health and Law: A System in Transition.* National Institute of Mental Health, DHEW Publication No. (ADM) 75–176, Washington, D.C. 1975.

Stone, A: (Comment on Peszke's: Is dangerousness an issue for physicians in emergency commitment?) *Am J Psychiatry,* 132:829–831, 1975.

Stone, A: The right to treatment and the medical establishment. *The Bulletin of the American Academy of Psychiatry and the Law,* 2:172, 1974.

Stoner v. Miller, 377 F. Supp. 177 (EDNY 1974).

Stotsky, BA: Relative efficacy of parenteral haloperidol and thiothixene for the emergency treatment of acutely excited and agitated patients. *Diseases of the Nervous System,* 38:967–973, 1977.

Stoudemire, A; Stork, M; Simel, D; et al: Neuro-ophthalmic systemic lupus erythematosus misdiagnosed as hysterical blindness. *Am J Psychiatry,* 139:1194–1196, 1982.

Stout, AL; Grady, TA; Steege, JF; Blazer, DG; et al: Premenstrual symptoms in black and white community samples. *Am J Psychiatry,* 143:1436–1439, 1986.

Streltzer, J; Hassell, H: Noncompliant hemodialysis patients: A biopsychosocial approach. *Gen Hosp Psychiatry,* 10:255–259, 1988.

Strober, M; Carlson, G: Bipolar illness in adolescents with major depression: Clinical, genetic, and psychopharmacologic predictors in a three to four-year prospective follow-up investigation. *Arch Gen Psychiatry,* 39:549–555, 1982.

Strober, M; Mirrell, W; Lampert, C; et al: Relapse following discontinuation of lithium maintenance therapy in adolescents with bipolar I illness: A naturalistic study. *Am J Psychiatry,* 147:457–461, 1990.

Sturner, WQ: Adolescent suicide fatalities. *R I Med J,* 69:471–474, 1986.

Sudak, HS; Ford, AB; Rushforth, NB: Adolescent suicide; An overview. *Am J Psychother,* 38(3):350–363, 1984.

Suicide: How to keep patients from killing themselves. Interviews with C. J. Frederick and H. Hendin. *Med World News,* pp. 86–95, July 1976.

Summers, WK; Reich, TC: Delirium after cataract surgery: review and two cases. *Am J Psychiatry,* 136:386–391, 1979.

Surman, OS: Psychiatric aspects of organ transplantation. *Am J Psychiatry,* 146:972–982, 1989.

Suspected rape. *ACOG Technical Bulletin.* No. 14, July, 1970.

Susser, E; Struening, EL; Conover, S: Psychiatric problems in homeless men. *Arch Gen Psychiatry,* 46:845–850, 1989.

Susser, M: *Community Psychiatry: Epidemiologic and Social Themes.* New York, Random House, 1968.

Suzuki v. Quisenberry, 411 F. Supp. 1113 (D. Hawaii, 1976).

Swartz, CM; Dunner, FJ: Dexamethasone suppression testing of alcoholics. *Arch Gen Psychiatry,* 39:1309–1312, 1982.

Swartz, M; Balzer, D; George, L; Landerman, R: Somatization disorder in a community population. *Am J Psychiatry,* 143:1403–1408, 1986.

Swartz, MS; McCraken, J: Emergency room management of conversion disordres. *Hospital and Community Psychiatry,* 37:828–832, 1986.

Swayze, VW; Yates, WR; Andreasen, NC; Alliger, RJ: CT Abnormalities in tardive dyskinesia. *Psychiatry Research,* 26:51–58, 1988.

Swedo, SE; Rappoport, JL; Cheslow, DL; Leonard, HL; et al: High prevalence of obsessive-compulsive symptoms in patients with Sydenham's chorea. *Am J Psychiatry,* 146:246–249, 1989.

Sweeney; Cowdry, RW; Gunderson, JG; Soloff, PH: Roundtable discussion. Psychopharmacology of borderline personality disorder: A Review. *J Clin Psychiatry,* 48:23–25, 1987.

Sweeny, S; Zamecnik, K: Predictors of self-mutilation in patients with schizophrenia. *Am J Psychiatry,* 138:1086–1089, 1981.

Swenson, JR; Erman, M; Labelle, J; Dimsdale, JE: Extrapyramidal reactions: Neuropsychiatric mimics in patients with AIDs. *Gen Hosp Psychiatry,* 11:248–253, 1989.

Swett, C; Cole, JO; Shapiro, S; Slone, D: Extrapyramidal side-effects in chlorpromazine recipients: Emergence according to benztropine prophylaxis. *Arch Gen Psychiatry,* 34:942–943, 1977.

Swett, D; Cole, JO; Hartz, SC; et al: Hypotension due to chlorpromazine. Relation to cigarette smoking, blood pressure and dosage. *Arch Gen Psychiatry,* 34:661–663, 1977.

Sylph, JA; Kedward, HB: Alternatives to the mental hospital: Use of residential facilities for long-term psychiatric care. *Arch Gen Psychiatry,* 34:909–912, 1977.

Szasz, TS: The communication of distress between child and parent. *Brit J Med Psychiatry,* 32:161, 1959.

Szymanski, HV: Prolonged depersonalization after marijuana use. *Am J Psychiatry,* 138:231–233, 1981.

Taffefson, GD: Hyperadrenergic hypomania consequent to the abrupt cessation of clonidine. *J Clin Psychopharmacol*, 1:93–95, 1981.

Takrani, LB: Cancer presenting as mental illness. *Psychiatr J Univ Ottawa*, 11:235–237, 1986.

Talley, JH: But what if a patient gets hooked? Fallacies about long-term use of benzodiazepines. *Postgrad Med*, 87:187–203, 1990.

Tamminga, CA; Crayton, JW; Chase, TW: Improvement in tardive dyskinesia after muscimol therapy. *Arch Gen Psychiatry*, 36:595–598, 1979.

Tamminga, CA; Smith, RC; Pandey, G; et al: A neuroendocrine study of supersensitivity in tardive dyskinesia. *Arch Gen Psychiatry*, 34:1199–1203, 1977.

Tancredi, LR: Emergency psychiatry and crisis intervention: Some legal and ethical issues. *Psychiatric Annals*, 12:799, 1982.

Tancredi, LR: Malpractice and tardive dyskinesia: A conceptual dilemma. *J Clin Psychopharmacol* 8(4) (Suppl):71–76, 1988.

Tancredi, LR; Slaby, AE: *Ethical Policy in Mental Health Care: Goal of Psychiatric Intervention.* New York, Neale Watson Academic Publications, 1977.

Tancredi, LR; Lieb, J; Slaby, AE: *Legal Issues in Psychiatric Care.* New York, Harper & Row Publishers, 1975.

Tancredi, LR; Slaby, AE: Ethical issues in mental health care. In: *Medical Ethics and the Law: Implications for Public Policy,* MD Hiller, ed. New York, Ballinger, 1981.

Tancredi, LR; Slaby, AE: Releasing the mentally ill: Justice or irresponsibility. *Connecticut Medicine,* 41:429–432, 1977.

Tancredi, LR; Slaby, AE: *Ethical Policy in Mental Health Care: The Goals of Psychiatric Intervention.* New York, Prodist, 1977.

Tancredi, LR; Woods, J: The social control of medical practice. In: *Economic Aspects of Health Care,* J McKinlay, ed. New York, Prodist, 1973.

Tangine, MD: Working with cult-affected families. *Psychiatric Annals*, 20:194–198, 1990.

Tanke, ED; Yesavage, JA: Characteristics of assaultive patients who do and do not provide visible cues of potential violence. *Am J Psychiatry*, 142:1409–1413, 1985.

Tarasoff v. Regents of the University of California, 529 P. 2d. 553 (1974).

Tarasoff v. Regents of the University of California, 551 P. 2d. 334 (1976). Wiley-Interscience, 1971.

Tardiff, K: A survey of psychiatrists in Boston and their work with violent patients. *Am J Psychiatry*, 131:1008, 1974.

Tardiff, K: Patterns and major determinants of homicide in the United States. *Hospital and Community Psychiatry*, 36:632–639, 1985.

Tardiff, K; Koenigsberg, HW: Assaultive behavior among psychiatric outpatients. *Am J Psychiatry*, 142:960–963, 1985.

Tardiff, K (ed): Seclusion and restraint. American Psychiatric Association Task Force Report No. 22, American Psychiatric Association, Washington, DC 1983.

Targum, SD: Capodanno, AE: The dexamethasone suppression test in adolescent psychotic inpatients. *Am J Psychiatry*, 140:589–591, 1983.

Tarter, RE; Hegedus, AM; VanThiel, DH; Schade, RR: Portal-systemic encephalopathy: Neuropsychiatric manifestations. *Int J Psychiatry Med*, 15:265–275, 1985–86.

Tasini, M: Complex partial seizures in a patient receiving trazodone. *J Clin Psychiatry*, 47:318–319, 1986.

Taylor, CB; Sheikh, J; Agras, WS; Roth, WT; et al: Ambulatory heart rate changes in patients with panic attacks. *Am J Psychiatry*, 143:478–482, 1986.

Taylor, MA; Abrams, R: Catatonia: Prevalence and importance in the manic phase of manic-depressive illness. *Arch Gen Psychiatry*, 34:1223–1225, 1977.

Taylor, WA; Gold, MS: Pharmacologic approaches to the treatment of cocaine dependence. *The Western Journal of Medicine*, 152:573–577, 1990.

Tefft, BM; Pederson, AM; Babigian, HM: Patterns of death among suicide attempters; a psychiatric population, and a general population. *Arch Gen Psychiatry*, 34:1155–1161, 1977.

Teicher, JD; Jacobs, J: The physician and the adolescent suicide attempter. *J School Health*, 36:406–415, 1966.

Teicher, JD; Jacobs, J: Adolescents who attempt suicide: Preliminary findings. *Am J Psychiatry*, 122:1248–1257, 1966.

Teicher, MH; Glod, C; Cole, J: Emergence of intense suicidal preoccupation during fluoxetine treatment. *Am J Psychiatry,* 147:207–210, 1990.

Tennant, FS: The clinical syndrome of marijuana dependence. *Psychiatric Annals,* 16:225–234, 1986.

Tesar, GE; Jenike, MA: Alprazolam as treatment for a case of obsessive–compulsive disorder. *Am J Psychiatry,* 141:689–690, 1984.

Tesar, GE; Murray, GB; Cassem, NH: Use of high-dose intravenous haloperidol in the treatment of agitated cardiac patients. *J Clin Psychopharmacol,* 5:344–347, 1985.

Test, MA; Stein, LI: Alternative to mental hospital treatment. III. Social cost. *Arch Gen Psychiatry,* 37:409–412, 1980.

Teusink, JP; Alexopoulous, GS; Shamoian, CA: Parkinsonian side effects induced by a monoamine oxidase inhibitor. *Am J Psychiatry,* 141:118–119, 1984.

Thackrey, M; Bobbitt, RG: Patient aggression against clinical and nonclinical staff in a VA medical center. *Hospital and Community Psyhiatry,* 41:195–197, 1990.

Thaker, GK; Nquzen, JA; Strauss, ME; et al: Clonazepam treatment on tardive dyskinesia: A practical GABA-mimetic strategy. *Am J Psychiatry,* 147:445–451, 1990.

Theodore, WH: Katz; D; Kufta, C; et al: Pathology of temporal lobe faci: Correlation with CT, MRI, and PET. *Neurology,* 40:797–803, 1990.

Theodore, WH: Pseudoseizures: Differential diagnosis. *J Neuropsychiatry,* 1:67–74, 1989.

Thienhaus, OJ; Hartford, JT: Depression in hyperprolactinemia. *Psychosomatics,* 27:663–664, 1986.

Thoa, NB: Wooten, GF; Axelrod, J; et al: Inhibition of release of dopamine-beta-hydroxylase and norepinephrine from sympathetic nerves by colchicine, vinblastine, or cytochalasin-B. *Proc Nat Acad Sci USA,* 69:520–522, 1972.

Thomas, CS; Weisman, GK: Emergency planning: The practical and theoretical backdrop to an emergency treatment unit. *Int J Soc Psychiatry,* 16:283, 1970.

Thomas, JM; Rubin, EH: Case report of a toxic reaction from a combination of tryptophan and phenelzine. *Am J Psychiatry,* 141:281–283, 1984.

Thompson, JW; Walker, RD: Adolescent suicide among American Indians and Alaska natives. *Psychiatric Annals,* 20:129–133, 1990.

Thomson, K; Shou, M: The treatment of lithium poisoning. In: *Lithium Research and Therapy,* FN Johnson, ed. New York, Academic Press, 1975.

Thornton, JE; Stahl, SM: Case report of tardive dyskinesia and Parkinsonism associated with amoxapine therapy. *Am J Psychiatry,* 141:704–705, 1984.

Ticknor, CB; Vogtsberger, KN: Development of psychosis during premature labor. *Hospital and Community Psychiatry,* 38:406–407, 1987.

Tiperman, A; Gilman, HE; Russakoff, LM: A case report of leukopenia associated with phenelzine. *Am J Psychiatry,* 141:806–807, 1984.

Tippin, J; Dunner, FJ: Biparietal infarctions in a patient with catatonia. *Am J Psychiatry,* 138:1386–1387, 1981.

Tishler, PV; Woodward, B; O'Connor, J; Holbrook, DA; et al: High prevalence of intermittent acute porphyria in a psychiatric patient population. *Am J Psychiatry,* 142:1430–1436, 1985.

Toenniessen, LM; Casey, DE; McFarland BH: Tardive dyskinesia in the aged: Duration of treatment relationships. *Arch Gen Psychiatry,* 42:278–284, 1985.

Tomlinson, BE; Blessed, G; Roth, M: Observations on the brains of demented old people. *J Neurol Sci,* 11:205–242, 1970.

Tonsic v. Wagner, 329 A. 2d 497(1974).

Treffert, DA: The Idiot Savant: A review of the syndrome. *Am J Psychiatry,* 145:563–572, 1988.

Trunquist, K; Frances, R; Rosenfeld, W; Mobarak, A: Pemoline in attention deficit disorder and alcoholism: A case study. *Am J Psychiatry,* 140:622–624, 1983.

Trzepacz, PT; Maue, FR; Coffman, G; Van Thiel, DH: Neuropsychiatric assessment of liver transplantation candidates: Delirium and other psychiatric disorders. *Int J Psychiatry Med,* 16:101–111, 1986–87.

Tsuang, MT: Suicide in schizophrenics, manics, depressives, and surgical controls: a comparison with general population suicide mortality. *Arch Gen Psychiatry,* 35:153–155, 1978.

Tsuang, MT; Boor, M; Fleming, JA: Psychiatric aspects of traffic accidents. *Am J Psychiatry,* 142:538–546, 1985.

Tsuang, MT; Woolson, RF: Excess mortality in schizophrenia and affective disorders. Do suicides and accidental deaths solely account for this excess? *Arch Gen Psychiatry,* 35:1181–1185, 1978.

Tune, LE; Strauss, ME; Leu, MF; et al: Serum levels of anticholinergic drugs and impaired recent memory in chronic schizophrenic patients. *Am J Psychiatry,* 139:1460–1462, 1982.

Turner, S; Daniels, L; Greer, S: Wernicke's encephalopathy in an 18 year-old woman. *Br J Psychiatry,* 154:261–262, 1989.

Turner, SM; Jacob, RG; Beidel, DC; Himmelhoch, J: Fluoxetine treatment of obsessive–compulsive disorder. *J Clin Psychopharmacol,* 5:207–212, 1985.

Tyrer, P; Candy, J; Kelly, D: Phenelzine in phobic anxiety: A controlled trial. *Psychol Med,* 3:120–124, 1973.

Uhl, V; Reus, VI; Fromm, JB: Psychiatric symptoms in Behcet's Syndrome. *Psychosomatics,* 26:547–549,1985.

Uhlenhuth, EH; DeWitt, H; Balter, MB; Johanson, CE; et al: Risks and benefits of long-term benzodiazepine use. *J Clin Psychopharmacol,* 8:161–167, 1988.

Ungerleider, J: The psychiatric emergency: Analysis of six months experience of a university hospital consultation service. *Arch Gen Psychiatry,* 3:593–601, 1960.

United States v. Brawner, 471 F. 2d 969 (1972).

United States v. George, 239 F. Supp. 752 (1964).

Urbaitis, JC: *Psychiatric Emergencies.* Norwalk, Appleton-Century-Crofts, 1983.

U.S.P.H.S.: Department of health education and welfare, NIMH: *Mental Health Statistics-Current Reports,* Series MHB-H-7, January, 1963.

Vaillant, GE; Milofsky, ES: Natural history of male alcoholism: IV Paths to recovery. *Arch Gen Psychiatry,* 39:127–133, 1982.

Valdes, M; Garcia, L; Treserra, J; dePablo, J; et al: Psychogenic pain and depressive disorders: An empirical study. *J Affecive Disord,* 16:21–25, 1989.

Valdiserri, EV; Carroll, KR; Hartl, AJ: A study of offenses committed by psychotic inmates in a county jail. *Hospital and Community Psychiatry,* 37:163–166, 1986.

Vandal, B; Vandel, S; Allers, G; et al: Interaction between amitriptyline and phenothiazines in man: Effect on plasma concentration of amitriptyline and its metabolite nortriptyline and the correlation with clinical response. *Psychopharmacotherapy,* (Berlin), 65:187–190, 1979.

Van Der Kolh, B; Greenberg, MS; Orr, SP; et al: Endogenous opioids, stress induced analgesia, and posttraumatic stress disorder. *Psychopharmacology Bulletin,* 125:417–421, 1989.

Van Dyke, C; Zilberg, N; McKinnon, JA: Posttraumatic stress disorder: A thirty-year delay in a World War II veteran. *Am J Psychiatry,* 142:1070–1073, 1985.

Van Kammen, DP; Peters, J; Yac, J; et al: Norepinephrine in acute exacerbations of chronic szhizophrenia. Negative symptoms resisted. *Arch Gen Psychiatry,* 47:161–168, 1990.

Van Patten, T; Marder, SR: Low-dose treatment strategies. *J Clin Psychiatry,* 47:12–16, 1986.

Van Patten, T; May, PRA: "A kinetic depression" in schizophrenia. *Arch Gen Psychiatry,* 35:1101–1107, 1978.

Van Patten, T; May, PRA: Marder, SR: Akathisia with haloperidol and thiothixene. *Arch Gen Psychiatry,* 41:1036–1039,1984.

van Praag, HM; Plutchik, R: Increased suicidality in depression: Group or subgroup characteristic? *Psychiatry Research,* 26:273–278,1988.

Van Scheyen, JD; Van Kammen, DP: Clomipramine-induced mania in unipolar depression. *Arch Gen Psychiatry,* 36:560–565, 1979.

Van Sweden, B; Mellerio, F: Toxic Ictal Delirium. *Biol Psychiatry,* 25:449–458, 1989.

Van Sweden, B; Peteghem, V: Psychopathology in baraneoplastic encephalopathy: An electroclinical observation. *J Clin Psychiatry,* 47:267–268, 1986.

VanValkenburg, C; Winokur, G: Hypertension and paranoia. Am J Psychiatry, 141:999–1000, 1984.

Varley, CK: Schizophreniform psychoses in mentally retarded adolescent girls following sexual assault. *Am J Psychiatry,* 141:593–595, 1984.

Varney, NR; Alexander, B: MacIndoe, JH: Reversible steroid dementia in patients without steroid psychosis. *Am J Psychiatry*, 141:369–372, 1984.

Vasavan Nair, NP; Suranyi-Cadotte, B; Schwartz, G; Thavundayil, JX; et al: A clinical trial comparing intramuscular haloperidol decanoate and oral haloperidol in chronic schizophrenic patients: Efficacy, safety, and dosage equivalence. *J Clin Psychopharmacol*, 6:30–37, 1986.

Vazquez-Barquero, JL; Acero, JAP; Ochoteco, A; Manrique, JFD: Mental illness and ischemic heart disease: Analysis of psychiatric morbidity. *Gen Hosp Psychiatry*, 7:15–20, 1985.

Verebey, K; Gold, MS; Mule, SJ: Laboratory testing in the diagnosis of marijuana intoxication and withdrawal. *Psychiatric Annals*, 16:234–241, 1986.

Vieweg, V; Glick, JL; Herring, S; Kerler, R; et al: Absence of carbamazepine-induced hyponatremia among patients also given lithium. *Am J Psychiatry*, 144:943–947, 1987.

Vincent, J; Varley, CK; Leger, P: Effects of methylphenidate in early adolescent growth. *Am J Psychiatry*, 147:501–502, 1990.

Virkkunen, M; DeJong, J; Bartko, J; Linnoila, M: Psychobiological concomitants of history of suicide attempts among violent offenders and impulsive fire setters. *Arch Gen Psychiatry*, 46:604–606, 1989a.

Virkkunen, M; DeJong, J; Bartko, J; Goodwin, FK; et al: Relationship of psychobiological variables to recidivism in violent offenders and impulsive fire setters: A Follow-up Study. *Arch Gen Psychiatry*, 46:600–603, 1989b.

Viswanathan, R; Kachur, EK: Development of agoraphobia after surviving cancer. *Gen Hosp Psychiatry*, 8:127–132, 1986.

Voineskos, G: New chronic patients in the emergency service. *Psychiatr J Univ Ottawa*, 10:95–100, 1983.

Volberg, RA; Steadman, HJ: Prevalence estimates of pathological gambling in New Jersey and Maryland. *Am J Psychiatry*, 146:1618–1619, 1989.

Volpe, R: Autoimmune thyroid disease. *Hospital Practice*, 141–158, Jan 1984.

Wade, DT; Legh-Smith, J; Hewer, RA: Depressed mood after stroke: A community study of its frequency. *Br J Psychiatry*, 151:200–205, 1987.

Wain, HJ: Pain control with hypnosis in consultation and liaison psychiatry. *Psychiatric Annals*, 16:106–109, 1986.

Wain, HJ; Amen, DG: Emergency room use of hypnosis. *Gen Hosp Psychiatry*, 8:19–22, 1986.

Wald, D; Lerner, J: Lithium in the treatment of periodic catatonia: A case report. *Am J Psychiatry*, 135:751–752, 1978.

Walker, JI: *Psychiatric Emergencies: Intervention and Resolution*. Philadelphia, J. B. Lippincott, 1983.

Walker, WR; Parsons, LB; Skelton, WD: Brief hospitalization on a crisis service: A study of patient and treatment variables. *Am J Psychiatry*, 130:896, 1973.

Wallace, SR; Goldberg, RJ; Slaby, AE: *Clinical Social Work in Health Care; New Biopsychosocial Approaches*. New York, Praeger Press, 1983.

Walsh, BT; Stewart, JW; Wright, L; et al: Treatment of bulimia with monoamine oxidase inhibitors. *Am J Psychiatry*, 36:555–559, 1979.

Walsh, BT; Roose, SP; Katz, JL; Dyrenfurth, I; et al: Hypothalamic-pituitary-adrenal-cortical activity in anorexia nervosa and bulimia. *Psychoneuroendocrinology*, 12:131–140, 1987.

Walsh, TL; Lavenstein, B; Licamele, WL; Bronheim, S; et al: Calcium antagonists in the treatment of Tourette's Disorder. *Am J Psychiatry*, 143:1467–1468, 1986.

Wamboldt, FS; Jefferson, JW; Wamboldt, MZ: Digitalis intoxication misdiagnosed as depression by primary care physicians. *Am J Psychiatry*, 143:219–221, 1986.

Wardle, J: Behavior therapy and benzodiazepines: Allies or antagonists? *Br J Psychiatry*, 156:163–168, 1990.

Watt, JAG: The relationship of paranoid states to schizophrenia. *Am J Psychiatry*, 142:1456–1458, 1985.

Watt, JAG: Hearing and premorbid personality in paranoid states. *Am J Psychiatry*, 142:1453–1455, 1985.

Way, BB; Banks, SM: Use of seclusion and restraint in public psychiatric hospitals: Patient characteristics and facility effects. *Hospital and Community Psychiatry*, 41:75–81, 1990.

Wasserman, D; Cullberg, J: Early separation and suicidal behavior in the parental homes of 40 consecutive suicide attempters. *Acta Psychiatr Scand*, 79:296–302, 1989.

Webster, A; Mawer, GE: Seizure frequency and major life events in epilepsy. *Epilepsia*, 30:162–167, 1989.

Wegner, JT; Catalano, F; Gibralter, J; Kane, JM: Schizophrenics with tardive dyskinesia: Neuropsychological deficit and family psychopathology. *Arch Gen Psychiatry,* 42:860–865, 1985.

Wehr, TA; Jocobsen, FM; Sack, DA; Arendt, J; et al: Phototherapy of seasonal affective disorder. *Arch Gen Psychiatry,* 43:870–875, 1986.

Wehr, TA; Rosenthal, NE: Seasonality and affective illenss. *Am J Psychiatry,* 146:829–839, 1989.

Wehr, TA; Sack DA; Rosenthal, NE: Sleep reduction as a final common pathway in the genesis of mania. *Am J Psychiatry,* 144:201–204, 1987a.

Wehr, TA; Sack, DA; Rosenthal, NE: Seasonal affective disorder with summer depression and winter hypomania. *Am J Psychiatry,* 144:1602–1603, 1987b.

Wehr, TA; Sack, DA; Rosenthal, NE; Cowdry, RW: Rapid cycling affective disorder: Contributing factors and treatment responses in 51 patients. *Am J Psychiatry,* 145:179–184, 1988.

Weiden, P; Bruun, R: Worsening of Tourette's Disorder due to neuroleptic-induced akathisia. *Am J Psychiatry,* 144:504–505, 1987.

Weiden, P; Harrigan, M: A clinical guide for diagnosing and managing patients with drug-induced dysphagia. *Hospital and Community Psychiatry,* 37:396–398, 1986.

Weiden, P; Roy, A: General vs specific risk factors for suicide in schizophrenia. Hillside Hospital, Long Island Jewish Medical Center, 1990.

Weiden, PJ; Mann, JJ; Haas, G; Mattson, M; et al: Clinical nonrecognition of neuroleptic-induced movement disorders: A cautionary study. *Am J Psychiatry,* 144:1148–1153, 1987.

Weiden, PJ; Shaw, E; Mann, JJ: Causes of neuroleptic noncompliance. *Psychiatric Annals,* 16:571–575, 1987.

Weilburg, JB; Bear, DM; Sachs, G: Three patients with concomitant panic attacks and seizure disorder: Possible clues to the neurology of anxiety. *Am J Psychiatry,* 144:1053–1056, 1987.

Weinberger, DR; Delisi, LE; Perman, GP; et al: Computed tomography in schizophreniform disorder and other acute psychiatric disorders. *Arch Gen Psychiatry,* 39:778–783, 1982.

Weiner, MF: Haloperidol, hyperthyroidism, and sudden death. *Am J Psychiatry,* 136:717–718, 1979.

Weiner, RD; Whanger, AD; Erwin, W; et al: Prolonged confusional state and EEG seizure activity following concurrent ECT and lithium use. *Am J Psychiatry,* 137:1452–1453, 1980.

Weingartner, H; Cohen, RM; Murphey, DC; et al: Cognitive processes in depression. *Arch Gen Psychiatry,* 38:42–47, 1981.

Weinstock, H: Phobias and their vicissitudes. *J Am Psychoanal Assoc,* 7:187–188, 1959.

Weintraub, MI: Regional pain is usually hysterial. *Arch Neurol,* 45:914–915, 1986.

Weisbrod, BA; Test, MA; Stein, LI: Alternative to mental hospital treatment. II. Economic benefit-cost analysis. *Arch Gen Psychiatry,* 37:400–405, 1980.

Weise, CC; Stein, MK; Pereira-Ogan, J; et al: Amitriptyline once daily vs. three times daily in depressed outpatients. *Arch Gen Psychiatry,* 37:555–560, 1980.

Weisman, G: Crisis houses and lodges: Residential treatment of acutely disturbed chronic patients. *Psychiatric Annals,* 15:642–647, 1985.

Weisman, G; Feirstein, A; Thomas, C: Three-day hospitalization - a model for intervention. *Arch Gen Psychiatry,* 21:620, 1969.

Weisman, M; Fox, K; Klerman, GL: Hostility and depression associated with suicide attempts. *Am J Psychiatry,* 130:450–455, 1973.

Weisman, MM: The epidemiology of suicide attempts, 1960 to 1971. *Arch Gen Psychiatry,* 30:737–746, 1974.

Weiss, G; Hectman, L; Perlman, T; Hopkins, J; Wener, A: Hyperactives as young adults: A controlled perspective ten-year follow-up of 75 children. *Arch Gen Psychiatry,* 36:675–681, 1979.

Weiss, NS: Recent trends in violent deaths among young adults in the United States. *Am J Epidemiol,* 103:416–422, 1976.

Weiss, RD; Goldenheim, PD; Mirin, SM; et al: Pulmonary dysfunction in cocaine smokers. *Am J Psychiatry,* 138:1110–1112, 1981.

Weiss, RD; Mirin, SM: The dual diagnosis alcoholic evaluation and treatment. *Psychiatric Annals,* 19:261–265, 1989.

Weissman, MM; Kidd, KK; Prusoff, BA: Variability in rates of affective disorders in relatives of depressed and normal probands. *Arch Gen Psychiatry,* 39:1397–1403, 1982.

Weissman, MM; Klerman, GL; Markowitz, S; et al: Suicidal ideation and suicide attempts in panic disorder and attacks. *N Engl J Med,* 321:1209–1214, 1989.

Weissman, MM; Klerman, GL; Prusoff, BA; et al: Depressed outpatients: Results one year after treatment with drugs and/or interpersonal psychotherapy. *Arch Gen Psychiatry,* 38:51–55, 1981a.

Weissman, MM; Merikangas, KR: The epidemiology of anxiety and panic disorders: An update. *J Clin Psychiatry,* 47:11–17, 1986.

Weissman, MM; Myers, JK; Thompson, WD: Depression and its treatment in a U.S. urban community—1975–1975. *Arch Gen Psychiatry,* 38:417–521, 1981b.

Weissman, MM; Prusoff, BA; Dimascio, A; et al: The efficacy of drugs and psychotherapy in the treatment of acute depressive episodes. *Am J Psychiatry,* 136:555–558, 1979.

Weissman, MM; Slaby, AE: Oral contraceptives and psychiatric disturbance: Evidence from research. *Br J Psychiatry,* 132:346, 1973.

Weller, RA; McKnelly, WV: Case report of withdrawal dyskinesia associated with amoxapine. *Am J Psychiatry,* 140:1515–1516, 1983.

Weller, RA; Welley, EB: Anorexia nervosa in a patient with an infiltrating tumor of the hypothalamus. *Am J Psychiatry,* 139:824–825, 1982.

Wells, CE: Diagnostic evaluation and treatment in dementia. In: *Dementia,* 2nd ed. CE Wells, ed. Philadelphia, F.A. Davis, 1977.

Wells, KB; Goldring, JM; Burnam, MA: Psychiatric disorder in a sample of the general population with and without chronic medical conditions. *Am J Psychiatry,* 145:976–981, 1988.

Wells, KB; Goldring, JM; Burnam, MA: Affective, substance use, and anxiety disorders in persons with arthritis, diabetes, heart disease, high blood pressure, or chronic lung conditions. *Gen Hosp Psychiatry,* 11:320–327, 1989.

Welner, A; Morten, S; Nochnick, E; et al: Psychiatric disorders among professional women. *Arch Gen Psychiatry,* 35:169–173, 1979.

Wender, PH; Reimherr, FW: Bupropion treatment of attention-deficit hyperactivity disorder in adults. *Am J Psychiatry,* 147:1018–1020, 1990.

Wender, PH; Reimherr, FW; Wood, D; Ward, M: A controlled study of methylphenidate in the treatment of attention deficit disorder, residual type, in adults. *Am J Psychiatry,* 142:547–552, 1985.

Wender, PH; Reimherr, FW; Wood, DR: Attention deficit disorder (minimal brain dysfunction) in adults. *Arch Gen Psychiatry,* 38:449–456, 1981.

Westermeyer, J; Peake, E: A ten-year follow-up of alcoholic native Americans in Minnesota. *Am J Psychiatry,* 140:189–194, 1983.

White, JH; O'Shanick, G: Juvenile manic-depressive illness. *Am J Psychiatry,* 134:1035–1036, 1977.

White, PD; Lewis, SW: Delusional depression after infectious mononucleosis. *Br Med J,* 295:97–98, 1987.

WHO Mental Health Collaborating Centers: Pharmacotherapy of depressive disorders. *J Affective Disord,* 17:197–198, 1989.

Widiger, TA; Rogers, JH: Prevalence and comorbidity of personality disorders. *Psychiatric Annals,* 19:132–136, 1989.

Wiesert, KN; Hendrie, HC: Secondary mania? A case report. *Am J Psychiatry,* 134:929–930, 1977.

Wilcox, JA; Nasrallah, HA: Childhood head trauma and psychosis. *Psychiatry Research,* 21:303–306, 1987.

Wilder, JF; Levin, G; Zwerling, I: A two-year follow-up evaluation of acute psychotic patients treated in a day hospital. *Am J Psychiatry,* 122:1095, 1966.

Wilder, JF; Plutchnik, R; Center, HR: Compliance with psychiatric emergency room referrals. *Arch Gen Psychiatry,* 34:930–933, 1977.

Wilkinson, CB: Introduction: The psychological consequences of disasters. *Psychiatric Annals,* 15:135–139, 1985.

Wilkinson, CB; Vera, E: The management and treatment of disaster victims. *Psychiatric Annals,* 15:174–184, 1985.

Willi, J; Grossmann, S: Epidemiology of anorexia nervosa in a defined region of Switzerland. *Am J Psychiatry,* 140:564–567, 1983.

Wilson, WH; Jefferson, JW: Thyroid disease, behavior, and psychopharmacology. *Psychosomatics,* 26:481–492, 1985.

Winberg, BG; Goldstein, S; Gepes, LE; Perel, JM: Imipramine and electrocardiographic abnormalities in hyperactive children. *Am J Psychiatry,* 132:542–545, 1975.

Wing, JK: Institutionalism in mental hospitals. In: *Mental Illness and Social Process,* T Scheff, ed. New York, Harper and Row, 1967.

Winkel, MF: Juvenile rheumatoid arthritis - parent support group: Do parents perceive a need? *Pediatric Nursing,* 14:131–132, 1988.

Winkelstein, W; Lyman, DM; Padian, N; Grant, R; et al: Sexual practices and risk of infection by the human immunodeficiency virus. *JAMA,* 257:321–325, 1987.

Winokur, A; March, V; Mendels, J: Primary affective disorder in relatives of patients with anorexia nervosa. *Am J Psychiatry,* 137:695–698, 1980a.

Winokur, A; Rickels, K; Greenblatt, DJ; et al: Withdrawal reaction from long-term, low-dosage administration of diazepam: A double-blind, placebo-controlled case study. *Arch Gen Psychiatry,* 37:101–105, 1980b.

Winokur, G: Unipolar depression: Is it divisible into autonomous subtypes? *Arch Gen Psychiatry,* 36:47–52, 1979.

Winters v. Miller, 466 F. 2d 65 (1971).

Winslow, RS; Stillner, V; Coons, DJ; Robinson, MW: Prevention of acute dystonic reactions in patients beginning high-potency neuroleptics. *Am J Psychiatry,* 143:706–710, 1986.

Winston, A; Pinsker, H; McCullough, L: A review of supportive psychotherapy. *Hospital and Community Psychiatry,* 37:1105–1114, 1986.

Wis. Stat. Ann. Secs. 51.001 and 51.75 art. II(f) (Supp. 1973).

Wittchen, HU; Burke, JD; Semler, G; Pfister, H; et al: Recall and dating of psychiatric symptoms. *Arch Gen Psychiatry,* 46:437–443, 1989.

Wittenborn, JR; Buhler, R: Somatic discomforts among depressed women. *Arch Gen Psychiatry,* 36:465–471, 1979.

Wofgang, ME: Suicide by means of victim-precipitated homicide. *J Clin Exp Psychopathol,* 20:335–349, 1959.

Wolcott, DL; Fawzy, FI; Pasnau, RO: Acquired immune deficiency syndrome (AIDS) and consultation-liaison psychiatry. *Gen Hosp Psychiatry,* 7:280–292, 1985.

Wolf, B; Grohmann, R; Biber, D; Brenner, PM; et al: Benzodiazepine abuse and dependence in psychiatric inpatients. *Pharmacopsychiatry,* 22:54–60, 1989.

Wolf, ME; Alavi, A; Mosnaim, AD: Posttraumatic stress disorder in Vietnam veterans clinical and EEG findings: Possible therapeutic effects of carbamazepine. *Biol Psychiatry,* 23:642–644, 1988.

Wolk-Wasserman, D: Contacts of suicidal neurotic and prepsychotic/psychotic patients and their significant others with public care institutions before the suicide attempt. *Acta Psychiatr Scand,* 75:358–372, 1987.

Wong, T; Tiessen, E; Math, B: Seizure in gradual clonazepam withdrawal. *Psychiatr J Univ Ottawa,* Vol 14, No. 3, 1989.

Woo, E; Greenblatt, DJ: Massive benzodiazepine requirements during acute alcohol withdrawal. *Am J Psychiatry,* 136:821–823, 1979.

Wood, D; Wender, PH; Reimherr, FW: The prevalence of attention deficit disorder, residual type, or minimal brain dysfunction in a population of male alcoholic patients. *Am J Psychiatry,* 140:95–98, 1983.

Wood, F; Novack, TA; Long, CJ: Post-concussion symptoms: Cognitive, emotional, and environmental aspects. *Int J Psychiatry Med,* 14:277–283, 1984.

Woodrow, KM: Gilles de la Tourette's Disease - A review. *Am J Psychiatry,* 131:1000, 1974.

Woods, JH; Katz, JL; Winger, G: Use and abuse of benzodiazepines: Issues relevant to prescribing. *JAMA,* 260:3476–3480, 1988.

Woods, SW: Catatonia in a patient with subdural hematomas. *Am J Psychiatry,* 137:983–984, 1980.

Woolfolk, RL; Grady, DA: Combat-related posttraumatic stress disorder: Patterns of symptomatology in help-seeking Vietnam veterans. *J Nerv Ment Disease,* 176:107–111, 1988.

Wyatt v. Stickney, 344 F. Supp. 373, 344 F. Supp. 387 1972.

Yacoub, O; Morrow, DH: Malignant hyperthermia and ECT. *Am J Psychiatry,* 143:1027–1029, 1986.

Yager, J; Kurtzman, F; Landsverk, J; Wiesmeier, E: Behavior and attitudes related to eating disorders in homosexual male college students. *Am J Psychiatry,* 145:495–497, 1988.

Yalles, SF: Suicide: A public health problem. In: *Suicidal Behaviors*. HLP Resnick, ed. Boston, Little, Brown and Co., 1968.

Yandow, V: Alcoholism in women. *Psychiatric Annals,* 19:243–247, 1989.

Yates, A; Musty, T: Preschool children's erroneous allegations of sexual molestation. *Am J Psychiatry,* 145:989–992, 1988.

Yedder (In re), Northampton Co., Orphans Court, Penna (1972) No. 1973–433 (June 6, 1973: Unreported opinion, Judge Alfred T. Williams, Jr.)

Yesavage, JA: Bipolar illness: Correlates of dangerous inpatient behavior. *Brit J Psychiatry,* 143:554–557, 1983.

Yesavage, JA: Correlates of dangerous behavior by schizophrenics in hospital. *J Psychiatr Res* 18(3):225–231, 1984.

Yesavage, JA: Dangerous behavior by Vietnam veterans with schizophrenia. *Am J Psychiatry,* 140:1180–1182, 1983.

Yesavage, JA: Differential effects of Vietnam combat experience vs. criminality on dangerous behavior by Vietnam veterans with schizophrenia. *J Nerv Ment Dis,* 171:382–384, 1983.

Yesavage, JA: Inpatient violence and the schizophrenic patient. A study of Brief Psychiatric Rating Scale scores and inpatient behavior. *Acta Psychiat Scand,* 67:353–357, 1983.

Yesavage, JA; Tanke, ED; Sheikh, JI: Tardive dyskinesia and steady-state serum levels of thiothixene. *Arch Gen Psychiatry,* 44:913–915, 1987.

Yesavage, JA; Tinklenberg, JR; Hollister, LE; Berger, PA: Vasodilators in senile dementias: A review of the literature. *Arch Gen Psychiatry,* 36:220–223, 1979.

Young, J; Williams, CL: When do mutual-help groups help? A typology of members. *Hospital and Community Psychiatry,* 39:1178–1182, 1988.

Young, LD; Feinsilver, DL: Male genital self-mutilation: Combined surgical and psychiatric care. *Psychosomatics,* 22:513–517, 1986.

Young, RC: Pharmacological treatment of depression. *Psychiatric Annals,* 20:102–107, 1990.

Young, RC; Alexopoulos, GS; Shamoian, CA; Dhar, AK; et al: Heart failure associated with high plasma 10 hydroxynortriptyline levels. *Am J Psychiatry,* 141:432–433, 1984.

Yu-Chin, R; Arcuni, OJ: Short-term hospitalization for suicidal patients within a crisis intervention service. *Gen Hosp Psychiatry,* 12:153–158, 1990.

Yudofsky, SC; Rosenthal, NE: ECT in a depressed patient with adult onset diabetes mellitus. *Am J Psychiatry,* 137:100–101, 1980.

Yudofsky, SC; Stevens, L; Silver, J; Barsa, J; et al: Propranolol in the treatment of rage and violent behavior associated with Korsakoff's psychosis. *Am J Psychiatry,* 141:114–115, 1984.

Zeanah, CH: Atypical panic attacks and lack of resolution of mourning. *Gen Hosp Psychiatry,* 10:373–377, 1988.

Zilber, N; Schufman, N; Lerner, Y: Mortality among psychiatric patients - the groups at risk. *Acta Psychiatr Scand,* 79:248–256, 1989.

Zimmerman, M; Coryell, W; Pfohl, B; Stangl, D: The reliability of the family history method for psychiatric diagnoses. *Arch Gen Psychiatry,* 45:320–322, 1988a.

Zimmerman, M; Pfohl, B; Coryell, W; Stangl, D; et al: Diagnosing personality disorder in depressed patients. *Arch Gen Psychiatry,* 45:733–737, 1988b.

Zimmerman, SL: The connection between macro and micro levels: States spending for hospitals and their suicide rates. *Suicide and Life-Threatening Behavior,* 20:16–30, 1990.

Zisook, S; Braff, DL; Click, MA: Monoamine oxidase inhibitors in the treatment of atypical depression. *J Clin Psychopharmacol,* 5:131–137, 1985.

Zitrin, CM; Klein, DF; Woerner, MG: Treatment of agoraphobia with group exposure in vivo and imipramine. *Arch Gen Psychiatry,* 37:63–72, 1980.

Zitrin, CM; Klein, DF; Woerner, MG: Behavior therapy, supportive psychotherapy, imipramine, and phobias. *Arch Gen Psychiatry,* 35:307–316, 1978.

Ziv, A; Israeli, R: Effects of bombardment on the manifest anxiety level of children living in Kibbutzim. *J Consult Clin Psychol,* 40:287–291, 1973.

Zohar, J; Shemesh, Z; Belmaker, RH: Utility of neuroleptic blood levels in the treatment of acute psychosis. *J Clin Psychiatry,* 47:600–603, 1986.

Zonana, H; Heinsz, JE; Levine, M: Psychiatric emergency services a decade later. *Psychiat in Med,* 4:273, 1973.

Zubenko, GS: Progression of illness in the differential diagnosis of primary dementia. *Am J Psychiatry,* 147:435–438, 1990.

Zubenko, GS; George, AW; Soloff, PH; Schulz, P: Sexual practices among patients with borderline personality disorder. *Am J Psychiatry,* 144:748–752, 1987.

Zusman, J; Shaffer, S: Emergency psychiatry hospitalization via court order: A critique. *Am J Psychiatry,* 130:1323–1326, 1974.

Zweben, JE: Recovery oriented psychotherapy: Facilitating the use of 12-step programs. *J Psychoactive Drugs,* 19:243–251, 1987.

Index